A Transdiagnostic Approach to Obsessions, Compulsions and Related Phenomena

"Top researchers from across the world have contributed to making *A Transdiagnostic Approach to Obsessions, Compulsions and Related Phenomena* the most comprehensive text published on this topic. The book, which is backed by the latest academic literature, provides a wide-ranging approach to treatment that incorporates psychopathologic, neurobiological, clinical and therapeutic elements.

Obsessive-compulsive disorder and associated mental illnesses can be difficult to diagnose. The book provides immense value in providing clinicians and researchers alike with the nuances necessary to identify and help patients to the best extent possible. It will undoubtedly be an indispensable reference document for professionals in this field for years to come."

Antonio E. Nardi, MD, PhD, Full Professor of Psychiatry, Federal University of Rio de Janeiro, Brazil

"Professors Fontenelle and Yücel compile an impressive comprehensive and authoritative source on the underpinnings and correlates of OCD and its related disorders. They advance cutting-edge reviews valuable to both clinicians and researchers. This volume represents a current and definitive reference work for these conditions. Uniquely, it also examines cross-diagnostic perspectives involving various contemporary nosologic systems (DSM-5, ICD-10, 11, RDoC, etc.) with respect to classification, treatment and prevention. Additionally, future investigative directions are presented for the multifaceted aspects of these disorders."

Edward C. Lauterbach, MD, FANPA, DFAPA, Professor Emeritus of Psychiatry and Neurology, Former Chief, Division of Adult and Geriatric Psychiatry, Founding Director Emeritus, Center for Translational Studies in Neurodegenerative Disease, Mercer University School of Medicine, USA

"This seminal volume covers virtually all aspects of obsessive-compulsive and related disorders from an innovative transdiagnostic perspective. Much more work is needed to advance this emerging field. But given the expertise of the more than sixty authors from across the globe, I am confident that this volume will become an invaluable resource for years to come both for practitioners as well as for researchers across a broad range of disciplines."

James F. Leckman, MD, PhD, Neison Harris Professor of Child Psychiatry, Psychology and Pediatrics, Yale University, USA

"A must-read reference to translational approaches to compulsive and obsessive phenomena in neuropsychiatry; Professors Fontenelle and Yücel represent the best clinician-scientists of our generation and assembled an all-star team to accomplish this challenging goal."

Jorge Moll, MD, PhD, Founder and Chairman of the Board of the D'Or Institute for Research and Education, Brazil

A Transdiagnostic Approach to Obsessions, Compulsions and Related Phenomena

Edited by

Leonardo F. Fontenelle

Federal University of Rio de Janeiro, Brazil

D'Or Institute for Research and Education, Brazil

Monash University, Australia

Murat Yücel

Monash University, Australia

CAMBRIDGE
UNIVERSITY PRESS

CAMBRIDGE
UNIVERSITY PRESS

University Printing House, Cambridge CB2 8BS, United Kingdom

One Liberty Plaza, 20th Floor, New York, NY 10006, USA

477 Williamstown Road, Port Melbourne, VIC 3207, Australia

314–321, 3rd Floor, Plot 3, Splendor Forum, Jasola District Centre, New Delhi – 110025, India

79 Anson Road, #06-04/06, Singapore 079906

Cambridge University Press is part of the University of Cambridge.

It furthers the University's mission by disseminating knowledge in the pursuit of education, learning, and research at the highest international levels of excellence.

www.cambridge.org
Information on this title: www.cambridge.org/9781107195776
DOI: 10.1017/9781108164313

First published 2019

Printed and bound in Great Britain by Clays Ltd, Elcograf S.p.A.

A catalogue record for this publication is available from the British Library.

Library of Congress Cataloging-in-Publication Data
Names: Fontenelle, Leonardo F., editor. | Yücel, Murat, editor.
Title: A transdiagnostic approach to obsessions, compulsions and related phenomena / edited by Leonardo F. Fontenelle, Murat Yücel.
Description: Cambridge, United Kingdom; New York, NY: Cambridge University Press, 2019. | Includes bibliographical references and index.
Identifiers: LCCN 2018029909 | ISBN 9781107195776 (hardback)
Subjects: | MESH: Obsessive-Compulsive Disorder | Compulsive Behavior – diagnosis | Compulsive Behavior – complications | Obsessive Behavior – diagnosis | Obsessive Behavior – complications
Classification: LCC RC533 | NLM WM 176 | DDC 616.85/227–dc23
LC record available at https://lccn.loc.gov/2018029909

ISBN 978-1-107-19577-6 Hardback

This book is dedicated to Isabela, Amanda, Olivia, Guiomar and Edson.
– Leonardo

I dedicate this book to Claudia, Melike, Eren, Leyla, Mikail and Semiha.
– Murat

Contents

List of Contributors *page* ix
Foreword xiii
Acknowledgments xvii

Section 1 – Theoretical Foundations of Obsessive-Compulsive and Related Disorders

1 **A Transdiagnostic Approach to Obsessions, Compulsions and Related Phenomena** 1
Leonardo F. Fontenelle and Murat Yücel

2 **The Philosophy of Compulsive Disorders: Compulsivity and Free Will** 14
Judy Luigjes and Damiaan Denys

3 **Family and Twin Studies of Obsessive-Compulsive and Related Disorders** 19
Danielle C. Cath, Nuno R. Zilhão, Dirk J. A. Smit and Dorret I. Boomsma

4 **The Molecular Genetics of Obsessive-Compulsive and Related Disorders** 29
Fabiana Barzotti Kohlrausch

5 **The Role of Environmental Factors in the Pathogenesis of Obsessive-Compulsive and Related Disorders** 39
Catarina Raposo-Lima and Pedro Morgado

6 **Immunology of Obsessive-Compulsive and Related Disorders** 51
Antonio L. Teixeira, Natalia P. Rocha and Andrea H. Marques

7 **Neurocognitive Basis of Compulsivity** 61
Martijn Figee, Judy Luigjes, Anneke Goudriaan, Ingo Willuhn and Damiaan Denys

8 **Structural Brain Imaging of Obsessive-Compulsive and Related Disorders** 74
Carles Soriano-Mas and Ben J. Harrison

9 **Functional Magnetic Resonance Imaging Studies of Obsessive-Compulsive and Related Disorders** 85
Jaewook Han and Jun Soo Kwon

Section 2 – Practical Aspects of Obsessive-Compulsive Disorder

10 **Epidemiology of Obsessive-Compulsive Disorder** 113
Roselind Lieb, Patrizia D. Hofer and Karina Wahl

11 **Symptoms, Diagnosis and Specifiers of Obsessive-Compulsive Disorder** 128
Leonardo F. Fontenelle

12 **The Natural History of Obsessive-Compulsive Disorder across the Lifespan** 144
Eesha Sharma and Y. C. Janardhan Reddy

13 **Sub-Diagnostic Obsessive-Compulsive Symptoms** 162
Albina R. Torres and Leonardo F. Fontenelle

14 **Assessment Instruments for Obsessive-Compulsive Disorder** 172
Andrew G. Guzick, Adam M. Reid and Eric A. Storch

15 **Pharmacological Treatments for Obsessive-Compulsive and Related Disorders: A Transdiagnostic Perspective** 183
Ricky A. Sachdev, Risha Ruparelia, Jemma E. Reid, Davis Mpavenda, Eduardo Cinosi and Naomi A. Fineberg

16 **Psychological Treatment of Obsessive-Compulsive Disorder: Efficacy, Mechanisms and Transdiagnostic Implications** 207
Jennifer L. Buchholz, Lillian Reuman, Shannon M. Blakey and Jonathan S. Abramowitz

17 **Innovative Cognitive Behavioral Treatments for Obsessive-Compulsive Disorder** 217
Kieron P. O'Connor, Catherine Ouellet-Courtois and Frederick Aardema

18 **Drug Augmentation Strategies for Treatment-Resistant Obsessive-Compulsive and Related Disorders** 229
Roseli Gedanke Shavitt and Juliana Belo Diniz

19 **Integrating Cognitive Behavioral Therapy and Medications for the Treatment of Obsessive-Compulsive Disorder** 242
Yael R. Stovezky, Marina Gershkovich, Reilly Kayser and H. Blair Simpson

20 **Deep Brain Stimulation, Transcranial Magnetic Stimulation and Transcranial Direct Current Stimulation for Obsessive-Compulsive Disorder** 255
Rebecca A. Segrave, Joshua J. Hendrikse and Linden Parkes

21 **Neurosurgery for Obsessive-Compulsive Disorder: Indications and Procedures** 279
Antonio Carlos Lopes

22 **Alternative Treatments for Obsessive-Compulsive Disorder: Nutraceuticals and Lifestyle Interventions** 292
Jerome Sarris and Georgina Oliver

Section 3 – Practical Aspects of Other Obsessive-Compulsive Related Disorders

23 **Transdiagnostic and Unique Clinical and Treatment Factors of Dysmorphophobia: Body Dysmorphic Disorder and Olfactory Reference Disorder** 307
Francesca Beilharz and Susan L. Rossell

24 **Hypochondriasis** 320
Vladan Starcevic

25 **Hoarding Disorder** 331
Lorena Fernández de la Cruz and David Mataix-Cols

26 **Transdiagnostic Factors in Obsessive-Compulsive Personality Disorder** 345
Michael G. Wheaton and Anthony Pinto

27 **Tourette's and Other Tic Disorders** 357
Andrea E. Cavanna

28 **Body-Focused Repetitive Behaviors** 367
Jon E. Grant and Samuel R. Chamberlain

29 **Stereotypic Movement Disorder** 376
Dan J. Stein

30 **The Clinical Neuropsychiatry of "Organic" Obsessive-Compulsive Disorder** 383
Leonardo F. Fontenelle

31 **Behavioral Addictions** 401
Samuel R. Chamberlain and Jon E. Grant

32 **Other Obsessive-Compulsive Related Disorders** 413
Ygor Arzeno Ferrão

Index 425

Contributors

Jonathan S. Abramowitz
University of North Carolina, Chapel Hill, NC, USA

Frederick Aardema
University Institute of Mental Health at Montreal, Montreal, Canada

Francesca Beilharz
Centre for Mental Health, Swinburne University of Technology, Melbourne, Australia

Shannon M. Blakey
University of North Carolina, Chapel Hill, NC, USA

Dorret I. Boomsma
Department of Biological Psychology, Vrije University, Amsterdam, the Netherlands

Jennifer L. Buchholz
University of North Carolina, Chapel Hill, NC, USA

Danielle C. Cath
Department of Psychiatry, Groningen University and University Medical Center Groningen, Groningen, the Netherlands

Andrea E. Cavanna
Department of Neuropsychiatry, BSMHFT and University of Birmingham, School of Life and Health Sciences, Aston Brain Centre, Aston University, Birmingham, UK
Sobell Department of Motor Neuroscience and Movement Disorders, Institute of Neurology and University College London, London, UK

Samuel R. Chamberlain
Department of Psychiatry, University of Cambridge, Cambridge, UK
Cambridge and Peterborough NHS Foundation Trust, Cambridge, UK

Eduardo Cinosi
Hertfordshire Partnership University NHS Foundation Trust, Highly Specialized OCD and Related Disorders Service, Welwyn Garden City, UK

Lorena Fernández de la Cruz
Department of Clinical Neuroscience, Karolinska Institute, Stockholm, Sweden

Damiaan Denys
Department of Psychiatry, Amsterdam University Medical Center, University of Amsterdam, the Netherlands
Netherlands Institute for Neuroscience, and Institute of the Royal Netherlands Academy of Arts and Sciences, Amsterdam, the Netherlands

Juliana Belo Diniz
Department and Institute of Psychiatry, University of Sao Paulo Medical School, Sao Paulo, Brazil

Ygor Arzeno Ferrão
Federal University of Health Sciences of Porto Alegre, Porto Alegre, Rio Grande do Sul, Brazil

Martijn Figee
Department of Psychiatry, Amsterdam University Medical Center, University of Amsterdam, the Netherlands
Department of Psychiatry, Icahn School of Medicine at Mount Sinai, NY, USA

Naomi A. Fineberg
Hertfordshire Partnership University NHS Foundation Trust, Highly Specialized OCD and Related Disorders Service, Welwyn Garden City, UK
Department of Postgraduate Medicine, University of Hertfordshire, Hatfield, UK
University of Cambridge, School of Clinical Medicine, Cambridge, UK

Leonardo F. Fontenelle
Obsessive, Compulsive, and Anxiety Spectrum Research Program, Institute of Psychiatry, Federal University of Rio de Janeiro, Brazil
D'Or Institute for Research and Education, Rio de Janeiro, Brazil
Turner Institute for Brain and Mental Health, School of Psychological Sciences, Monash University, Melbourne, Australia

Marina Gershkovich
Columbia University Medical Center at New York State Psychiatric Institute, New York, NY, USA

Anneke Goudriaan
Department of Psychiatry, University Medical Center, University of Amsterdam, the Netherlands

Jon E. Grant
Department of Psychiatry and Behavioral Neuroscience, University of Chicago, Chicago, IL, USA

Andrew G. Guzick
University of Florida Departments of Psychiatry and Clinical and Health Psychology, Gainesville, FL, USA

Jaewook Han
Department of Psychiatry, Seoul National University College of Medicine, Department of Neuropsychiatry, Seoul National University Hospital, Seoul, Republic of Korea

Ben J. Harrison
Melbourne Neuropsychiatry Centre, Department of Psychiatry, University of Melbourne, Melbourne, Australia

Joshua J. Hendrikse
Turner Institute for Brain and Mental Health, School of Psychological Sciences, Monash University, Melbourne, Australia

Patrizia D. Hofer
University of Basel, Department of Psychology, Division of Clinical Psychology and Epidemiology, Basel, Switzerland

Reilly Kayser
Columbia University Medical Center at New York State Psychiatric Institute, New York, NY, USA

Fabiana Barzotti Kohlrausch
Departament of General Biology, Institute of Biology, Federal Fluminense University, Niterói, Rio de Janeiro, Brazil

Jun Soo Kwon
Department of Psychiatry, Seoul National University College of Medicine, Department of Brain and Cognitive Sciences, Seoul National University College of Natural Science, Seoul, Republic of Korea

Roselind Lieb
University of Basel, Department of Psychology, Division of Clinical Psychology and Epidemiology, Basel, Switzerland

Antonio Carlos Lopes
Department and Institute of Psychiatry, University of Sao Paulo Medical School, Sao Paulo, Brazil

Judy Luigjes
Department of Psychiatry, Amsterdam University Medical Center, University of Amsterdam, the Netherlands

Andrea H. Marques
National Institute of Mental Health, Bethesda, MD, USA

David Mataix-Cols
Department of Clinical Neuroscience, Karolinska Institute, Stockholm, Sweden

Pedro Morgado
Life and Health Sciences Research Institute (ICVS), School of Medicine, University of Minho, ICVS-3Bs PT Government Associate Laboratory, Braga, Portugal

Davis Mpavenda
Hertfordshire Partnership University NHS Foundation Trust, Highly Specialized OCD and Related Disorders Service, Welwyn Garden City, UK

Kieron P. O'Connor
University Institute of Mental Health at Montreal, Montreal, Canada

Georgina Oliver
Department of Psychiatry, The Melbourne Clinic, University of Melbourne, Melbourne, Australia

Catherine Ouellet-Courtois
University Institute of Mental Health at Montreal, Montreal, Canada

Linden Parkes
Turner Institute for Brain and Mental Health, School of Psychological Sciences, Monash University, Melbourne, Australia

Anthony Pinto
Department of Psychiatry, Hofstra Northwell School of Medicine, Ambulatory Psychiatry Center, Zucker Hillside Hospital Hempstead, NY, USA

Catarina Raposo-Lima
Life and Health Sciences Research Institute (ICVS), School of Medicine, University of Minho, ICVS-3Bs PT Government Associate Laboratory, Braga, Portugal

Y. C. Janardhan Reddy
Obsessive-Compulsive Disorder (OCD) Clinic, Department of Psychiatry, National Institute of Mental Health and Neurosciences (NIMHANS), Bangalore, India

Adam M. Reid
Harvard Medical School, McLean Hospital, Department of Psychology Boston, MA, USA

Jemma E. Reid
Hertfordshire Partnership University NHS Foundation Trust, Highly Specialized OCD and Related Disorders Service, Welwyn Garden City, UK

Lillian Reuman
University of North Carolina, Chapel Hill, NC, USA

Natalia P. Rocha
Neuropsychiatry Program, Department of Psychiatry and Behavioral Sciences, University of Texas Health Science Center, Houston, TX, USA

Susan L. Rossell
Centre for Mental Health, Swinburne University of Technology, Monash Alfred Psychiatry Research Centre, Alfred Hospital and Monash University Central Clinical School, Department of Psychiatry, St Vincent's Hospital, Melbourne, Australia

Risha Ruparelia
Hertfordshire Partnership University NHS Foundation Trust, Highly Specialized OCD and Related Disorders Service, Welwyn Garden City, UK

Ricky A. Sachdev
Hertfordshire Partnership University NHS Foundation Trust, Highly Specialized OCD and Related Disorders Service, Welwyn Garden City, UK

Jerome Sarris
NICM Health Research Institute, Western Sydney University, Department of Psychiatry, The Melbourne Clinic, University of Melbourne, Melbourne, Australia

Rebecca A. Segrave
Turner Institute for Brain and Mental Health, School of Psychological Sciences, Monash University, Melbourne, Australia

Eesha Sharma
Department of Child and Adolescent Psychiatry, National Institute of Mental Health and Neurosciences (NIMHANS), Bangalore, India

Roseli Gedanke Shavitt
Department and Institute of Psychiatry, University of Sao Paulo Medical School, Sao Paulo, Brazil

H. Blair Simpson
Columbia University Medical Center at New York State Psychiatric Institute, New York, NY, USA

Dirk J. A. Smit
Amsterdam Medical Center, Department of Psychiatry, Amsterdam, the Netherlands

Carles Soriano-Mas
Department of Psychiatry, Bellvitge Biomedical Research Institute-IDIBELL, Mental Health Networking Biomedical Research Centre (CIBERSAM), Department of Psychobiology and Methodology of Health Sciences, Autonomous University of Barcelona, Barcelona, Spain

Vladan Starcevic
Faculty of Medicine and Health, Sydney Medical School, Nepean Clinical School, University of Sydney, Sydney, Australia

Dan J. Stein
Department of Psychiatry and MRC Unit on Risk & Resilience in Mental Disorders, University of Cape Town, Cape Town, South Africa

Eric A. Storch
Menninger Department of Psychiatry and Behavioral Sciences, Baylor College of Medicine, Houston, TX, USA

Yael R. Stovezky
Columbia University Medical Center at New York State Psychiatric Institute, New York, NY, USA

Antonio L. Teixeira
Neuropsychiatry Program, Department of Psychiatry and Behavioral Sciences, University of Texas Health Science Center, Houston, TX, USA

Albina R. Torres
Botucatu Medical School, São Paulo State University, São Paulo, Brazil

Karina Wahl
University of Basel, Department of Psychology, Division of Clinical Psychology and Epidemiology, Basel, Switzerland

Michael G. Wheaton
Department of Psychology, Barnard College, Columbia University, New York, NY, USA

Ingo Willuhn
Netherlands Institute for Neuroscience, an institute of the Royal Netherlands Academy of Arts and Sciences, Amsterdam, the Netherlands

Murat Yücel
Turner Institute for Brain and Mental Health, School of Psychological Sciences, Monash University, Melbourne, Australia

Nuno R. Zilhão
Department of Biological Psychology, Vrije Universiteit, Amsterdam, the Netherlands

Foreword

Clinicians who search for evidence-based findings to treat patients with mental disorders have struggled with the fact that, for a substantial number of patients, the current treatments offer only partial symptom relief, rather than a cure. A few patients will be totally incapacitated by their disease, and mental disorders therefore constitute one of the leading causes of disability. Research experts the world over have been trying to understand why the considerable money and effort invested in high-quality research have yet to translate into treatments that are more effective for those most severely affected by some of these conditions. The inscrutable nature of psychiatric disorders is frequently cited as the main reason for these disappointing results. In fact, after decades of research, we still do not have consistent biomarkers or objective measures to identify specific pathophysiological processes or the mechanisms of response to any pharmacological intervention in psychiatry (Chapter 15). In other words, there is a lack of specific, robust associations between how we define a given psychopathology and its underlying neurobiological processes [1,2,3].

Our inability to identify associations between psychiatric disorders and the mechanisms involved in their pathogenesis is also attributable to the current operational categorical approach to diagnosis, which fails to address the dimensional nature of many disorders and establishes boundaries between diagnostic categories that are often arbitrary and require substantial subjective judgment. In addition, there is a high rate of symptom overlap, which results in patients being diagnosed with multiple disorders simultaneously. Furthermore, the available diagnostic categories can be relatively unhelpful in distinguishing severity and subclinical cases are rarely addressed appropriately [4]. Moreover, data from recent large-scale, genome-wide association studies indicate that there is a marked overlap in liability across five major psychiatric disorders. Symptom domains that are known to be important in multiple disorders, such as executive function, are simply not captured by the current nosology [5]. Given that our nosology has been based on psychopathology since the nineteenth century, we have begun to seek alternative theoretical constructs to determine whether the use of the powerful twenty-first-century research tools translate into benefits for psychiatric patients [4].

One strategy is to completely revise the ways in which we define mental disorders and classify psychopathology. Initiatives in that vein include the Research Domain Criteria (RDoC) framework, sponsored by the United States National Institute of Mental Health [6], and the European Union Roadmap for Mental Health Research in Europe [7], to promote the development of better treatments. Therefore, rather than trying to understand the underlying biology of arbitrarily defined psychiatric disorders and proposing treatments focusing on syndromes, the RDoC initiative is developing a research classification system for psychopathological disorders based on the dimensions of neurobiology and observable behavior, using what is presently known about the molecular, cellular, circuit, physiological and cognitive bases of biologically valid brain systems to devise treatments that are more personalized and precise (Chapters 15, 20 and 21).

With the abovementioned issues in mind, Fontenelle and Yücel, in the company of the most erudite researchers in the area, invite the reader on a journey to reflect on these highly relevant topics in the interface between neuroscience and psychiatry. Using obsessive-compulsive and related disorders (OCRDs) as the motivating factor or as background, the book offers the reader a glimpse of the future of psychiatric diagnosis after the emergence of the RDoC and in the context of the recently issued *Diagnostic and Statistical Manual of Mental Disorders*, fifth edition (DSM-5) and the soon-to-be-issued 11th Revision of the International Classification of Diseases (ICD-11). In the DSM-5, obsessive-compulsive disorder (OCD) was moved from the anxiety disorders category to the newly created OCRD category (Chapter 11). The OCRDs include body dysmorphic disorder (BDD), hoarding disorder, hair-pulling disorder (also known as trichotillomania) and skin-picking disorder (also known as excoriation disorder).

This accessible book circumscribes the debate over a transdiagnostic approach to OCRDs, putting into perspective the available data on the putative overlaps in the presenting symptoms (i.e. repetitive thoughts and behavior), as well as etiologically relevant factors (e.g. risk factors, genes, neurotransmitter abnormalities and brain circuitry), reflecting on the question of whether identifying the dimensions of the observable symptoms that individuals with OCRDs do and do not have in common could provide the means for capturing this heterogeneity and lead to the development of individualized treatment plans (Chapter 15–22). Throughout this carefully curated collection of basic and clinical knowledge, psychiatrists, psychologists, behavioral neurologists and cognitive neuroscientists push nearly all the boundaries in the field. In the basic section, after learning the principles of the RDoC initiative and how they translate to a transdiagnostic approach (Chapter 1), the reader will be presented with knowledge on how OCRDs are influenced by philosophy (Chapter 2), family (Chapter 3), molecular genetics (Chapter 4), environmental factors (Chapter 5) and neuroimmunology (Chapter 6), as well as with the results of neuropsychology (Chapter 7) and the various neuroimaging approaches (Chapters 8 and 9). In the clinical section, the reader can learn about the history and nuances of the classification system that is currently used most widely in the field of psychiatry – the DSM system – from its inauguration to its most recent incarnation, as well as about the ICD system, including what can be expected in the ICD-11 (Chapter 11). Again, using OCD as a jumping-off point, and then extending to the other OCRDs, the book offers the most recent findings regarding the epidemiology (Chapter 10), natural history (Chapter 12) and subclinical forms of psychiatric disorders (Chapter 13). After the ways of assessing such disorders have been discussed (Chapter 14), several chapters deal with the current dilemmas involving the treatment of these conditions, such as the first-line pharmacological (Chapter 15) and psychological treatments (Chapters 16 and 17); combining psychological and pharmacological treatments (Chapter 19); treatment for resistant and refractory cases (Chapter 18); the use of neurostimulation techniques (Chapter 20) and neurosurgery (Chapter 21) and alternative treatments, including nutraceuticals, lifestyle interventions and other therapeutic strategies (Chapter 22).

In several chapters, OCD is taken as the example (because it is the disorder for which empirical data are more widely available) and comparisons are then drawn with the emerging data related to other OCRDs. However, the book goes beyond that, as subsequent chapters discuss in detail every disorder that is, in some way, on the same continuum with OCD (beyond the DSM), such as BDD; olfactory reference disorder (Chapter 23); hypochondriasis (Chapter 24); hoarding disorder (Chapter 25); obsessive-compulsive personality disorders (Chapter 26); Tourette's disorder and tic disorders (Chapter 27); body-focused repetitive disorders (Chapter 28); stereotyped movement disorders (Chapter 29); behavioral addictions (Chapter 31); BDD with actual flaws, BDD-like disorder without repetitive behavior, obsessional jealousy, shubo-kyofu (fear of a deformed face/body) and koro (fear that the penis – or labia, nipples or breasts in women – is shrinking or retracting and will disappear into the abdomen) (Chapter 32) and neurologic disorders (Chapter 30). Thus, the commonalities and differences in comparison with other OCRDs are discussed, the focus being on how a transdiagnostic approach could make sense for disorders that share phenomenological and neurobiological features. Likewise, there is a clear focus on translating the new knowledge into treatments, or rather, how we can put this new approach into practice when dealing with our patients.

For any professional in the field of mental health, clinical practices will certainly change with the advent of the new knowledge generated by the RDoC framework. However, certain questions remain. For example, will this approach make it possible to understand the nature of mental disorders and to discover novel treatments that are more effective? Undoubtedly, the RDoC initiative and its strategy to reveal neurobiological substrates constitute a heuristic approach but perhaps go too far by ignoring symptom-based approaches entirely. Decades of research have generated a nosology based on symptoms that allow us to establish specific treatments and prognoses. Because of the fragmentation of these concepts in different domains, there is no guarantee that treating each domain will translate to reduced suffering in the patient as a whole, nor that we will have more reliable ways of establishing the prognosis. As clinicians, our main focus is to relieve the suffering of our patients, which reflects their symptoms as they experience them [3]. As Fontenelle and Yücel mention in Chapter 1, only future therapeutic studies will be able to clarify whether concentrating on RDoC systems of classifying dysfunction is more beneficial than is using the current symptom-based approaches. Perhaps, rather than being applied exclusively, the DSM and RDoC approaches should be used in conjunction.

At the end of this journey, the reader will have a new perspective and be capable of deeper critical thinking about a subject that is central to our field. Some, like me, will then start revisiting certain chapters to get a better grasp on relevant information.

Euripedes C. Miguel

References

1. Hyman SE. Can neuroscience be integrated into the DSM-V? *Nat Rev Neurosci.* 2007;8:725–732.
2. Sanislow CA, Pine DS, Quinn KJ, Kozak MJ, Garvey MA, Heinssen RK, Wang PS, Cuthbert BN. Developing constructs for psychopathology research: research domain criteria. *J Abnorm Psychol.* 2010;119:631–639.
3. Gillan CM, Fineberg NA, Robbins TW. A trans-diagnostic perspective on obsessive-compulsive disorder. *Psychol Med.* 2017;47(9):1528–1548.
4. Craddock N, Owen MJ. Rethinking psychosis: the disadvantages of a dichotomous classification now outweigh the advantages. *World Psychiatry.* 2007;6(2):84–91.
5. McCoy TH, Castro VH, Rosenfield HR, Cagan A, Kohane IS, Perlis RH. A clinical perspective on the relevance of research domain criteria in electronic health records. *Am J Psychiatry.* 2015;172:316–320.
6. Insel T, Cuthbert B, Garvey M, Heinssen R, Pine DS, Quinn K, Sanislow C, Wang P. Research domain criteria (RDoC): toward a new classification framework for research on mental disorders. *Am J Psychiatry.* 2010;167:748–751.
7. Haro JM, Ayuso-Mateos JL, Bitter I, Demotes-Mainard J, Leboyer M, Lewis SW, et al. ROAMER: roadmap for mental health research in Europe. *Int J Methods Psychiatr Res.* 2014;23(S1):1–14.

Acknowledgments

In June 2015, the trustees of the David Winston Turner Endowment Fund made a generous philanthropic commitment to the Monash Institute of Cognitive and Clinical Neurosciences, enabling world-leading research into compulsive behaviors, with a particular emphasis on obsessive-compulsive disorder and addiction. We would like to thank the trustees of the fund for supporting our work, including the production of this book.

Leonardo would like to thank students and colleagues from the Anxiety, Obsessive, and Compulsive Research Program, Federal University of Rio de Janeiro; the D'Or Institute for Research and Education; the Brain and Mental Health Research Hub, Monash University and the Brazilian OCD Research Consortium. He is particularly indebted to Professor Euripedes C. Miguel, Professor Marcio Versiani (in memoriam), Dr. Jorge Moll Neto, Professor Kim Cornish and all the patients he was able to talk to in the past 20 years.

Murat would like to thank colleagues and trainees from the Brain and Mental Health Research Hub and Monash Institute of Cognitive and Clinical Neurosciences, Monash University. He is particularly indebted to Professor Kim Cornish, Professor Christos Pantelis, Assistant Professor Ben Harrison, Assistant Professor Alex Fornito and Dr. Rebecca Segrave.

Chapter 1

A Transdiagnostic Approach to Obsessions, Compulsions and Related Phenomena

Leonardo F. Fontenelle and Murat Yücel

Introduction

Obsessive-compulsive disorder (OCD) characteristic symptoms include obsessions (persistent and unwanted thoughts, images or urges) and compulsions (repetitive behaviors that are performed in response to obsessions or according to rigid rules). OCD is both frequent and disabling; it affects up to 3% of the general population and leads to decreased productivity and substantial decreases in quality of life. However, the impact of OCD's constituent symptoms (obsessions, compulsions and related phenomena) may be greater than the one associated with the disorder per se. For instance, obsessions and compulsions are frequently found in sub-threshold yet impactful forms. They also occur in conditions officially classified by the *Diagnostic and Statistical Manual of Mental Disorders*, 5th edition (DSM-5) [1] and the 11th Revision of the International Classification of Diseases (ICD-11) [2] as obsessive-compulsive and related disorders (OCRDs).

The fact that obsessive thoughts and compulsive behaviors may occur across a number of neuropsychiatric conditions has been well known since Kraepelin (for a list of conditions presenting OCD symptoms, see Table 1.1). However, it is only after the end of a strongly hierarchical approach to psychiatric diagnosis that clinicians have been able to officially diagnose OCD in the presence of conditions such as schizophrenia, major depressive disorder or Tourette's disorder. The recognition that neuropsychiatric disorders could be comorbid with one another has been a major advance in the field. It prompted clinicians not only to identify but also to treat comorbid OCD, thus leading to better outcomes. However, this is not exactly the transdiagnostic approach we deal with in this chapter.

Obsessions and compulsions are clinical constructs. Until now, they have proven to be reliable and useful. They are reliable for being consistent over time and between different clinicians, and useful for

Table 1.1 A few examples of neurologic, medical and psychiatric disorders that may give rise to obsessions and compulsions.

Predominant site of dysfunction	Disorder
Basal ganglia	Tourette's disorder
	Sydenham chorea (rheumatic fever)
	Huntington disease
	Neuroacanthocytosis
	Progressive supranuclear palsy
	Idiopathic striatal calcification (Fahr syndrome)
	Parkinson's disease
	Carbon monoxide poisoning
	Wasp venom
Frontal, anterior cingulate and temporal lobe	Stroke
	Brain contusions
	Degeneration (Pick's disease)
	Epilepsy
Generalized brain dysfunction	Diffusive axonal injury
	Gliomatosis cerebri
	Epilepsy
Psychiatric illness	Schizophrenia
	Depression (unipolar or bipolar)
	Anxiety disorders
	Trauma-related disorders (e.g. post-traumatic stress disorder)

being remediated by a series of strategies that, despite not being effective in some cases, can alleviate symptoms in many. However, rather than existing as "natural kinds," obsessions and compulsions may be the final products of multiple interrelating dysfunctional cognitive affective processes and corresponding neurobiological systems. Failure to recognize these complex interactions may explain lack of therapeutic response shown by many patients (e.g., only 40–60% of patients with OCD respond to an initial serotonin reuptake inhibitor trial) [3]. The acknowledgment of these and other limitations associated with a purely clinical approach have prompted the launch of Research Domain Criteria (RDoC) by the National Institute of Mental Health.

The RDoC, officially launched in 2010 [4], is an experimental classification system consisting of basic behavioral/cognitive functions and their corresponding biological correlates (e.g., genes, molecules, cells, brain circuits) [5]. The RDoC aim is to redefine the boundaries of DSM/ICD mental disorders on the basis of what is currently known about dysfunctional neurodomains, namely negative valence (responsible for responses to aversive situations), positive valence (which coordinates responses to positive motivational situations), cognitive processes, systems for social processes and arousal/regulatory systems [5]. Although it is not the official objective of the RDoC to compete with existing diagnostic systems (but rather to influence future ones), it is obviously critical to reflect upon strategies to narrow the gap between DSM/ICD OCRDs and the RDoC constructs [6].

Accordingly, a number of approaches have been proposed [6], including, for instance: (i) the adoption of more dimensional, biologically valid assessments in clinical practice (such as the recently proposed DSM-5 cross-cutting symptom measures); (ii) the study of experiential intermediate phenotypes that could, at least theoretically, be more comfortably accommodated by the RDoC or even (iii) the adoption of RDoC-based terminology in the clinic [6]. For instance, Yager and Feinstein [7] have provided a number of RDoC-friendly clinical questions that could elicit valuable biological information by translating high-order domains and constructs headings into clinically based language. They propose this assessment to be a part of mental status assessment akin to the review of systems, after the history of present illness.

However, it is also possible to dissect and "pareidolically" redesign complex and heterogeneous clinical phenomena like obsessions and compulsions into phenomena that can be more biologically valid. This may prove to be particularly relevant, as the current conceptualization of psychiatric signs and symptoms has remained basically the same for more than 100 years and has proved to be relatively far from the level of neuroscientific inquiry needed for the development of new treatments [6]. Thus, in this chapter, we have endeavored to break down the distinguishing features of obsessions and compulsions into RDoC-friendly ingredients that are shared by the cognitive and behavioral symptoms of other diagnoses. By doing this, we discuss potential targets for future treatment developments that could be more personalized and also offer clinicians an opportunity to think about differential diagnosis of symptoms that share features with obsessions and compulsions.

Abnormal Sense of Agency and Control

The RDoC has defined agency as the ability to recognize one's self as the agent of one's actions and thoughts, including the recognition of one's own body or body parts. Normally, human beings have both the sense of agency and ownership of their own thinking and behaviors. However, this sense of personal possession is never in the foreground of consciousness [8]. While the so-called first-rank symptoms (such as thought insertion, withdrawal and broadcasting) indicate that these abilities have been lost in schizophrenia, patients with OCD retain their capacity to recognize their symptoms as their own (despite their perception of lack of control). Similarly, individuals showing other psychopathological phenomena also present the feeling of being unable to control their symptoms, particularly generalized anxiety disorder (GAD) preoccupations or post-traumatic stress disorder (PTSD) flashbulb memories.

There is also a possibility that obsessions and first-rank symptoms share an underlying neuropsychological dysfunction that may be truly transdiagnostic. According to the "comparator model" of agency attribution, self-world distinction is based on a constant comparison between internal predictions ("efferent copies") and external information. Experimental findings in both schizophrenia [9] and OCD [10] samples have been interpreted as indicating a dysfunction of this "comparator." However, for some unknown reason, while patients with schizophrenia tend to rely more on external action signals (for example, visual feedback) than on internal cues (e.g., proprioception) when perceiving their own actions and inferring agency [11], patients with OCD tend to over-monitor their actions to secure goal attainment [10]. This difference could also explain why patients with schizophrenia self-attribute external sensory events to their own actions [11].

Self-Knowledge

The RDoC has defined self-knowledge as the ability to make judgments about one's current cognitive or emotional internal states, traits and/or abilities [12]. Self-knowledge can be described as a product of reflective consciousness [13,14]. Clinically, increased reflective consciousness (hyperreflexivity) can be seen in conditions as diverse as insomnia, OCD, hypochondria (health anxiety disorder), body dysmorphic disorder (BDD), depression and even schizophrenia [15]. However, in contrast to the former psychopathologies, increased reflective consciousness in schizophrenia is perceived more as an *ineffective* attempt to explain to one-self primary delusional experiences (e.g., loss of "familiarity with the world and with other people"), rather than as part of the primary pathological event itself [15]. For instance, while in OCD hyperreflexivity is generally associated with increased insight toward one's symptom (thus leading to increased ego-dystonicity), in schizophrenia the familiarity of things cannot be reproduced, and the personal environment seems increasingly alienated [15].

Despite being described as the prototypical mental disorder associated with hyperreflexivity, OCD may also be paradoxically characterized by poorer self-knowledge. For instance, a sizable proportion of OCD cases display decreased insight toward their symptoms (ego-syntonicity), thus leading the DSM-5 to allow the diagnosis of OCD with good or fair, poor, or absent insight/delusional beliefs.[1] Notably, the object of insight or awareness in OCD can be extremely variable, including the symptoms (obsessive thoughts or compulsive rituals), the resulting impairments or even the official medical diagnosis [16,17]. Alexithymia (i.e., the inability to "read" one's own emotional state) is a concept closely related to insight that has also been described in several OCD cases [18]. Using an RDoC framework, it would be interesting to investigate the activity of fronto-insular and anterior cingulate cortex (location of the so-called von Economo neurons [19]) in response to relevant stimuli both within patients with OCD with different levels of insight and across disorders exhibiting different profiles of self-knowledge.

Effort Valuation

The RDoC defines effort either as a "process by which the costs of obtaining an outcome are computed" or "the tendency to overcome response costs to obtain a reinforcer" [12]. Patients with OCD tend to resist unacceptable obsessive thoughts and to perform compulsive behaviors (or mental rituals) whose ultimate aim (reinforcer) is to decrease anxiety and fear. Thus, while avolitional patients tend to over-value effort, OCD can be conceptualized as under-valuing effort to obtain an outcome. The so-called myth of Sisyphus, who was punished for eternity to push a rock up a mountain, has been cited as a way of illustrating the endless efforts of patients with OCD [20]. In fact, most clinicians have seen patients with OCD who become absolutely exhausted fighting against time-consuming and sometimes very complex compulsions. Other OCRDs (e.g., BDD) patients pursue their objectives (e.g., cosmetic surgeries) with extreme tenacity. However, the diagnostic significance of resistance toward obsessive thoughts has been debated. Although the experience of internal struggle has been consistently reported as a distinguishing feature of OCD symptoms, increased severity has been associated with decreased resistance toward them [21]. Accordingly, the resistance item has been dropped from more recent assessment instruments [22,23].

Although there might be some sort of conceptual overlap between insight and effort valuation (i.e., one could argue that greater insight leads to greater efforts toward the suppression of compulsions), clinicians have seen many patients who do not resist their symptoms despite being fully aware of their absurdity. It is unfortunate that, to the best of our knowledge, no study has investigated the biological underpinnings of effort valuation in OCD, so only approximations are possible at this time. For instance, the most recent version of the famous Baxter's brain model of OCD [24], suggesting that direct corticosubcortical circuits are relatively hyperactive in relation to indirect corticosubcortical circuits, could provide a framework

[1] According to some authors, absent insight OCD cannot be described as delusional, as delusions are pre-reflexive, rather than a reflexive phenomenon [14].

for evaluating effort/resistance in OCD. According to Baxter [24], decreased resistance toward symptoms would be related to a reduced activity within indirect pathways, which would be further aggravated by comorbid depression. Thus, for Baxter et al. [24], Pierre Janet's name for OCD (psychasthenia) would actually be quite appropriate. Future work on effort valuation in OCD could benefit from including appropriate tasks (e.g., the effort–expenditure for rewards task) that could also incorporate OCD-related rewards.

Cognitive Control

Cognitive control refers to a system that modulates other cognitive and emotional systems in the service of goal-directed behavior [12]. Cognitive control is critical when prepotent modes of responding are not adequate to meet the demands of novel contexts and appropriate responses need to be selected among conflicting alternatives [12]. The RDoC matrix includes three different ways of conceptualizing cognitive control, namely: (i) goal selection, updating, representation and maintenance; (ii) response selection, and inhibition/suppression and (iii) performance monitoring [12]. Cognitive control (particularly performance monitoring) has been assessed on neurophysiological (event-related potentials N2 and N450), neuropsychological (Flanker, Simon and Stroop tasks) and neuroanatomical (anterior cingulate cortex/pre-supplementary motor area insula) levels. Error- (ERN) and correct-related negativities (CRN) are event-related potentials that peak on frontocentral electrodes just after erroneous or correct responses take place in response–conflict tasks, respectively [25].

It has been suggested that *doubt*, a well-known component of OCD since the late nineteenth century descriptions of *folie du doute*, is the most visible clinical manifestation of this enhanced error-monitoring phenotype [26]. In fact, early cybernetic models of OCD have suggested that doubt and incompleteness can be ascribed to the persistence of conflicting (high error) signals or mismatches that cannot be reduced to zero through behavioral output (compulsions) [26]. According to these models, compulsive behavior is repetitive because behavioral programs are executed over and over again as an unsuccessful attempt to reduce such error signals [26]. An increase in the amplitudes of ERN has been consistently reported in OCD [27], and other anxiety-related disorders, including GAD [28], separation anxiety disorder [29], social anxiety disorder [30] and illness anxiety disorder [25]. However, it is notable that increased CRN amplitudes have been restricted to OCD [25] and social anxiety disorder [30]. The latter finding has been interpreted as evidence of a more proactive, error-avoidant response style, particularly among OCD patients [25].

Perception

To the RDoC, perception refers to the process that performs computations on sensory data to: (i) construct and transform representations of the external environment; (ii) acquire information from, and make predictions about, the external world and (iii) guide action [12]. Although a critical aspect of the form of obsessive-compulsive symptoms (OCS) (i.e., "recurrent and persistent thoughts, urges, or *images*") [31], and BDD symptoms (i.e., a "preoccupation with one or more *perceived* defects or flaws") [1], only recently has greater attention been paid to the perceptive aspects of OCRDs. For instance, early studies suggest recurrent images to occur in only 17–26% of OCD samples [31,32], although more modern surveys, using standardized assessments, have shown them to be present in up to 81% of patients with OCD [33], 96% of those with BDD [34] and 78% of those with health anxiety disorder [35]. However, intrusive images do not seem to differ between patients with OCD and anxious controls in terms of frequency rates and number, although images in the first group have more frequently a repetitive nature, "a field perspective" (i.e., from one's own vantage point), "unacceptable ideas of harm" and a "dangerous self" meanings [36].

A concept related to OCD images (i.e., "sensory-laden obsessive thoughts") [37,38], has been associated with poorer insight [37], greater loudness of normal thoughts [37] and small to moderate positive correlations with severity of OCD (particularly the obsessions subscale of the Obsessive-Compulsive Inventory-Revised), suspiciousness (Paranoia Checklist) and depression (Patient Health Questionnaire) [38]. Recurrent images have also been related to exposure to previous adverse events, independently of diagnoses [33,34,35]. Thus, it is not surprising that successful attempts have been made to treat OCD [39] and BDD [40,41] images through re-scripting of memories (although randomized controlled trials are still lacking). These symptoms should be differentiated from the so-called "sensory phenomena", which are described as uncomfortable, distressing and subjective experiences that precede, accompany or follow and are usually relieved by repetitive behaviors such as tics (in up to 90% of cases) [42] or OCD compulsions (in 65% of cases) [43].[2] In a study with 1001 patients with OCD, "sensory phenomena" has been associated with higher frequency and greater severity of the symmetry/ordering and contamination/washing symptom dimensions; comorbid Tourette's disorder and a family history of tic disorders [43].

Aside from being a key ingredient of DSM and ICD criteria for many OCRD symptoms, disturbed perception is also described as an underlying neuropsychological deficit in this same population. For instance, although patients with OCD seem to perform poorly in tests tapping many different cognitive domains, the largest effect sizes are found for visual (non-verbal) memory [44]. However, these deficits seem to result from deficient executive function-related organizational impairments [44], which may be related to an underlying orbitofrontal cortex dysfunction [45]. In other words, the inability of patients with OCD to recall visual information is related to their tendency to focus on minutiae instead of breaking down "the big picture" into simpler components that are easier to remember. Similar deficits have been described in BDD [46] and anorexia nervosa [47] samples. Based on this model, cognitive training, whereby patients learn to appreciate the *gestalt* of any given context, has been proposed as a treatment of OCD [48] and may be potentially helpful in other OCRDs with similar cognitive deficits. Despite the heuristic value of the non-verbal memory model of OCD, it is difficult to reconcile it with OCD symptoms that are primarily verbal or auditory (e.g., obsessive thoughts).

Reward Valuation, Expectancy and Responsiveness

The RDoC has broken down reward-related constructs into three to four subconstructs, namely: (i) the "processes by which the probability and benefits of a prospective outcome are computed and calibrated by reference to external information, social context and/or prior experience" (*reward valuation*) [12]; (ii) "a state triggered by exposure to internal or external stimuli, experiences or contexts that predict the possibility of reward (*reward expectation*) [12] and (iii) the "Mechanisms/processes associated with hedonic responses as reflected in subjective experiences, behavioral responses and/or engagement of the neural systems to a positive reinforce and culmination of reward seeking" (*initial responsiveness to reward attainment*) [12]. Although obsessive thoughts and compulsive rituals have been traditionally ascribed to fears of harm and feelings of incompleteness interest in the role of reward in OCD is not new [49]. For instance, commenting on the gratification obtained by patients with OCD when performing their rituals, Sandor Rado argued that "no man can stay alive without satisfying, one way or another, the organism minimal hedonic requirements, and so the patient is forced to find solace and high moral gratification in the fact that he is a fine man" [50]. However, a renewed interest in a protagonism of reward (particularly reward expectation) as a motivator for OCD behaviors has been noted in the last few years, not only in terms of symptom expression but also in relation to the role of the reward system in the pathophysiology of OCD [51]. For instance, in a preliminary report, we found that most patients with OCD from a relatively small sample (n = 22) reported an increase of positive affect, as measured by the Positive and Negative Affective Schedule in anticipation of the performance of their compulsive behaviors [52]. This finding was expanded and fleshed out in a subsequent study of reward mechanisms in patients with OCD, this time using a clinician-administered interview and a significantly larger and more well-characterized sample (n = 73). In the latter study, we found that almost half (49%) of our patients with OCD (particularly washers) endorsed that they *anticipated* obtaining a reward (i.e., positive affect) from the enactment of their dominant compulsive behavior. Also, washers stood out among other OCD subtypes in that their positive affects during and after compulsive behaviors were highly (and positively) correlated with duration of illness [51].

An earlier functional magnetic resonance imaging (fMRI) study found hypoactivation in the nucleus accumbens [53] during reward *anticipation*

[2] In OCD, sensory phenomena included "just-right" perceptions triggered by tactile, visual, or auditory input (51.8%), tactile and musculoskeletal sensations (37.1%), "just right" perceptions triggered by internal feelings of incompleteness (17.6%), "energy release" sensations (14.4%) and an "urge only" phenomenon (24.0%) [43].

in patients with OCD (particularly the washing subtype) compared with healthy controls [54]. However, another investigation did not find ventral striatal activation during reward anticipation in patients with OCD compared with controls, but increased ventral striatal activation in a loss avoidance contrast that correlated significantly and positively with severity of compulsions [55]. In another fMRI study, the performance of OCD and healthy controls on a monetary reward-based spatial learning task did not differ but, unlike controls, patients with OCD did not display activation in the left ventral putamen and amygdala during reward anticipation and in the left hippocampus, amygdala and ventral putamen during unexpected reward attainments [56]. Further, participants with OCD who had the most severe doubt/checking symptoms showed less activation in both the left hippocampus and ventral putamen during the attainment of unexpected rewards. Finally, a sham controlled study showed deep brain stimulation of the nucleus accumbens to effectively treat refractory OCD [57]. Taken together, these findings suggest that the reward system may be involved in the normal relief that results from performing an OCD behavior, thereby contributing to difficulty controlling the urge to repeat it.

Sustained Threat

Broadly speaking, all RDoC sub-constructs related to threat may be involved in OCD, including acute threat or "fear" ("activation of the brain's defensive motivational system to promote behaviors that protect the organism from perceived danger") [12], potential threat or "anxiety" ("activation of a brain system in which harm may potentially occur but is distant, ambiguous or low/uncertain in probability") [12] and sustained threat ("an aversive emotional state caused by prolonged … exposure to internal and/or external condition(s), state(s), or stimuli that are adaptive to escape or avoid") [12]. For instance, acute exposure to stimuli that patients with OCD are afraid of (e.g., dirtiness) may result in panic attacks (acute threat), intolerance to uncertainty (potential threat) has been proposed to be an underlying vulnerability factor for OCD and the cognitive and emotional changes caused by threatening stimuli tend to persist in people with OCD even after the stimuli have been completely removed (sustained threat). Nevertheless, and despite of all these considerations, it has been suggested that sustained threat seems to exemplify more clearly the recalcitrant and repetitive experiences that are core to OCD (i.e., thoughts that increase and behaviors that decrease threat).

Accordingly, structures involved in the pathophysiology of OCD [58] seem to significantly overlap with the ones reported to mediate sustained threat, including the ventral striatum, the cingulate and the amygdala [12]. In addition, animal studies (as reviewed by Avery et al. [59]) suggest that another structure, i.e., the *bed nucleus of stria terminalis*, is key to both sustained threat monitoring and to the withdrawal and relapse stages of addiction. Therefore, though more research on this topic seems advisable, sustained threat may be an interesting cross-diagnostic endophenotype linking OCRDs compulsive behaviors to behaviors in substance-related and addictive disorders (SRAD). On a behavioral level [12], sustained threat seems to express itself as attentional bias to threat [60], avoidance [61], conflict detection [62],[3] and perseverative behavior [63], all constructs previously reported in OCD. Unfortunately, the RDoC does not include any self-report of sustained threat. It is also unfortunate that other potential tools (i.e., the Sensitivity to Punishment and Sensitivity to Reward Questionnaire) [64] are not psychometrically sound or do not seem to reflect the core psychopathology related to sustained threat [65].

Habit

Healthy decision making is thought to arise from a flexible balance between model-based (goal-directed) and model-free (habitual) reinforcement learning [66]. This distinction has been based on outcome devaluation studies, which investigate habits formation via persistence compared with disappearance of learned behaviors according to motivational changes [67]. The RDoC has defined habits as "Sequential, repetitive, motor, or cognitive behaviors elicited by external or internal triggers that, once initiated, can go to completion without constant conscious oversight" [12]. While habit can be adaptive for freeing up cognitive resources, it can also become resistant to changes and result in problematic behaviors. It is beyond the scope

[3] The RDoC suggest the neurophysiological underpinning of conflict detection to be ERN, already addressed in this chapter under cognitive control.

of this chapter to examine in a detailed fashion the science showing increased habit formation in OCRDs and SRAD (which is discussed more in depth in other chapters of this book, e.g., Chapter 8). However, since a propensity toward increased habit formation cuts across different compulsive disorders [66], we thought it would be appropriate to address here some issues related to the psychobiology of habits that could help illuminate compulsivity as a whole.

For instance, substance addictions have been conceptualized as strong stimulus–response drug-seeking habits that are driven by positive reinforcement [68]. The same might hold true for other behavioral addictions, such as gambling disorder [69]. However, at a first glance, it might not seem easy to reconcile OCD with the habit-formation model, as OCD behaviors are traditionally seen as driven by negative, rather than positive, reinforcement. Yet, patients with OCD have also developed greater ("avoidance") habits than controls in a shock avoidance task designed to induce habits through overtraining [70]. Also, in a sample of 73 patients with OCD, we have found that their Self-Report Habit Index (SRHI) scores correlated positively with indexes of OCD severity (Obsessive-Compulsive Inventory short version total scores and the Yale–Brown Obsessive Compulsive Scale compulsions sub-scores), even after redundant SRHI items were excluded [51]. In the latter study, there was also correlation between duration of illness and severity of checking symptoms and not severity of other symptoms [51]. A relationship between habits and checking has been highlighted in at least one study with non-clinical controls and deserves further investigation [71].

The habit system may also be involved in another feature deemed relevant for the differential diagnosis of OCRDs and SRAD, namely, the increased behavioral complexity associated with most OCRD rituals, including washing, checking and ordering behaviors. Although the traditional neurobehavioral examination has emphasized the assessment of the inability to perform complex motor sequences (i.e., ideational apraxia) in cognitive disorders, it has apparently neglected the possibility that complex OCD rituals represents a mirror phenomenon; that is, an excessive execution of a sequence or complex motor acts (i.e., behavioral routines that are encapsulated in "chunks" limited by action boundary, beginning-and-end, signals from the striatum and the prefrontal cortex) [72]. Smith and Graybiel [68] speculated that these behaviors could results from chunking-related activity in the dorsolateral striatum or infralimbic cortex, loss of error-corrective signaling in the dorsolateral striatum or inflexibility in the infralimbic-related habit-promoting process.

A Synthesis of the Transdiagnostic Approach to Obsessions and Compulsions

We believe that an in-depth discussion on the transdiagnostic aspects of obsessions and compulsions (rather than one that focuses on full-blown DSM-5 OCD) poses significant challenges. For instance, we acknowledge that, as advocated by the RDoC matrix, clinical and subthreshold forms of psychopathology are likely to share the same underlying neurobiology (for a review see Chapter 15). However, clinicians still specify what is classifiable or diagnosable and what does not need any specific therapeutic intervention. Although diagnostic constructs can be dimensional, and obsessionality and compulsivity are clear examples of these sorts of symptoms/traits, the decision of treating or not treating a patient remains a categorical one. Thus, a dimensional approach poses practical and ethical questions, such as where the lines should be drawn and the associated risks of over- or undertreatment. This dilemma has been faced by previous psychiatric classificatory schemes and should not be ignored.

Yet, if one wants to discuss the implications of the transdiagnostic aspects of obsessions and compulsions, one should operationalize the concepts of obsessionality and compulsivity. In lay terms, obsessionality could be simply described as the tendency to think excessively, while compulsivity could be defined as propensity toward exhibiting behavioral excesses. However, these "common sense" definitions do not seem to have much clinical utility, as they encompass several unrelated cognitive (e.g., depressive rumination) and behavioral (e.g., psychomotor agitation) symptoms. Also, they cannot guide treatment, as there is no therapeutic approach that is able to remediate all abnormally persistent cognitions and excessive behaviors indiscriminately. However, if, as we propose, obsessionality and compulsivity are construed as traits that partially overlap with what has been technically known as obsessions and compulsions, we believe that a few advances can be made, at least if the critical components of the later constructs are identified and described. Thus, there may be different types and definitions of obsessionality and compulsivity. This was our approach in this chapter, where we refer to different RDoC dimensions. Symptoms that could be subsumed under obsessionality and compulsivity are listed in Tables 1.2 and 1.3, respectively.

Deconstructing obsessions and compulsions into their key components has theoretical (pathophysiological) and practical (diagnostic and therapeutic) implications. First, DSM-5 OCD may have different neurobiological systems implicated in its pathophysiology depending on whether a specific set of symptoms (e.g., obsessions, compulsions or both) predominates. For instance, obsessive images may be more trauma related [36], whereas compulsive behaviors may be more neurodevelopmentally based [73]. Notably, this approach might have implications for other conditions that share features with OCD; for example, OCD obsessive images and PTSD intrusive images may both result from dysfunction in similar brain circuits (Table 1.2) [74]. Second, a transdiagnostic approach to obsessions and compulsions may also have diagnostic consequences, as the differential diagnosis of OCD may be more precisely performed if cognitions (e.g., thought alienation) or behaviors (e.g., stereotypies) that characterize other disorders (e.g., schizophrenia) are disentangled from obsessional thoughts or compulsive rituals that are core to OCD.

Most critically, however, a transdiagnostic approach to obsessions and compulsions could help to illuminate the neurobiology of different psychiatric disorders, thus leading to better treatments, in line with RDoC guidelines. For instance, patients with OCD recognize obsessions, along with several other cognitive symptoms that share the feature of being persistent and distressing, as their own experience, and not as someone else's as in thought alienation. Thus, it makes sense to contrast OCD with schizophrenia samples to clarify the biology that underlies abnormal agency. Similarly, compared with delusions, which are prereflexive phenomena ("delusional patients express conviction and certainty about certain statements rather than admit that these statements may be subject to discussion and inquiry" [75]), obsessions involve an intense internal dialog, thus suggesting that patients with OCD can be contrasted with psychotic patients to illuminate the biology of insight and self-knowledge. Further, like many obsessions, the preoccupations of GAD include doubt, elements that are lacking in auditory hallucinations and paraphilic fantasies and could be studied under the construct of cognitive control and sustained threat.

All behaviors listed in Table 1.3 can be executed with a certain degree of automaticity, but compulsive, avoidant and addictive behaviors are the only ones more clearly performed to decrease fear and distress. Thus, it seems reasonable to contrast patients with the latter conditions to samples with other automatic behaviors to clarify the biological basis of sustained threat and to develop anti-fear treatments. It is also interesting that behaviors associated with the so-called sensory phenomena, such as OCD compulsions, Tourette's tics and trichotillomania grooming behaviors have been shown to be genetically linked [76]. Further, it has been demonstrated that impulsivity is a risk factor for addiction, and both may be related to poor cognitive control and lack of foresight. Finally, while addictive, grooming and *punding* behaviors are all well known to be associated with reward valuation expectancy and responsiveness, it has been increasingly recognized that OCD compulsions and anxiety disorder avoidance can also be associated with reward processing abnormalities. Thus, it seems sensible to test approaches targeting anticipatory (dopaminergic) and/or consummatory (opioidergic) transmission in the latter conditions.

We must acknowledge that, instead of resulting from the combination of multiple dysfunctional neurobiological systems, OCD may be ascribed to a still unrecognized and broad obsessionality and/or compulsivity RDoC construct/sub-construct. However, there is yet no full consensus on how these concepts should be understood; that is, as symptom phenomena, as personality traits or as neuropsychological constructs [77]. Although the RDoC approach is particularly interested in addressing the abnormal biology underlying symptoms (rather than on obsessions or compulsions per se), it is conceptually difficult to disentangle obsessionality and compulsivity from the concept with which it is intrinsically intermingled (i.e., a symptom complex). In other words, searching for the biology of obsessionality and compulsivity and not for obsessions and compulsions could be a mere semantic exercise that does not capture the underlying biology of OCRDs. However, only future therapeutic studies will be able to clarify whether concentrating on dysfunctional RDoC systems underlying obsessionality and compulsivity will prove more beneficial to

Table 1.2 Overview of persistent and distressing cognitive symptoms sharing a few features with obsessions.

RDoC systems	Symptom feature	Thought alienation	Delusions and overvalued ideas	Preoccupations	Ruminations	Obsessive thoughts	Obsessive images	Fantasies	Flashbulb memories	Hallucinations
Agency	Symptom associated with ***possession*** or ownership	---	++++	++++	++++	++++	++++	++++	++++	---
Self-knowledge	Product of increased ***reflective*** consciousness	---	---	++++	++++	+–++	++	++++	++	---
	Increased ***insight*** toward symptom	---	---	++	++	+++	+++	++++	+++	---
Effort valuation	Increased ***resistance*** toward symptom	---	---	+	+	++	++	---	---	---
Cognitive control	Increased doubt and anxious apprehension	---	---	++++	+	+++	+++	---	---	---
Perception	Increased ***perceptual*** symptom component	---	+	---	---	+	++++	++++	++++	++++
Reward valuation, expectancy and responsiveness	***Reward*** in anticipation/ during symptom	---	---	---	---	+	+	++++	---	---
Sustained threat	Increased fear or distress resulting from symptom	---	---	++++	++	+++	+++	---	++++	+++
Examples		Schizophrenia	Schizophrenia, delusional disorder, BDD; hypochondria	GAD, other anxiety disorders	Major depressive disorder	OCD	OCD	Paraphilia, paraphilia-related disorders	PTSD	Schizophrenia

Legend: ++++: Always or almost always present; +++: Present in majority of cases; ++: May be present or absent; +: Present in a minority of cases: ---: Absent.
BDD, body dysmorphic disorder; GAD, generalized anxiety disorder; OCD, obsessive-compulsive disorder; PTSD, post-traumatic stress disorder; RDoC, Research Domain Criteria.

Table 1.3 Overview of repetitive behaviors sharing a few features with compulsions.

RDoC systems	Symptom features	Stereotypies and mannerisms	Simple tics	Grooming behaviors	Addictive behaviors	Punding behaviors	Impulsive behaviors	Complex tics	Compulsive behaviors	Avoidant behaviors
Sustained threat	Performance decreases *fear/distress*	---	---	---	++	---	---	---	+++	++++
Perception	Associated with *sensory phenomena*	---	++++	+	---	---	---	++++	++	---
Perception monitoring and perception and understanding of Self	*Increased awareness* into behavior	---	++	+	---	---	---	++	+++	+++
Cognitive control	Performance is devoid of *foresight*	---	+	+++	+++	+	++++	+	+	+
Reward valuation, expectancy and responsiveness	Performance increases *reward*	---	---	+++	++++	++	+++	---	+	+
Habit system	Performance is (or can be) automatic	++++	++	+++	++++	+++	+++	++	++	++
	Increased behavioral complexity	---	---	---	++	++	+	+++	+++	---
Examples		Schizophrenia, autism spectrum disorders, mental restriction	Tic disorders (Tourette's disorder)	Trichotillomania (hair pulling disorder), excoriation (skin picking) disorder	Substance and behavioral addictions (pathological gambling)	Dopaminergic therapy	Kleptomania and pyromania	Tic disorders (Tourette's disorder)	OCD, BDD	Anxiety disorders; social phobia; hoarding disorder

Legend: ++++: Always or almost always present; +++: Present in majority of cases; ++: May be present or absent; +: Present in a minority of cases: ---: Absent.
BDD, body dysmorphic disorder; OCD, obsessive-compulsive disorder.

patients than concentrating on obsessions and compulsions per se.

References

1. American Psychiatric Association. *Diagnostic and Statistical Manual of Mental Disorders,* 5th ed. Washington, DC: APA; 2013.
2. World Health Organization. International Classification of Diseases, 11th Revision. Geneva: WHO; 2018.
3. Arumugham SS, Reddy JY. Augmentation strategies in obsessive-compulsive disorder. *Expert Rev Neurother.* 2013;13(2):187–202.
4. Insel T, Cuthbert B, Garvey M, et al. Research domain criteria (RDoC): toward a new classification framework for research on mental disorders. *Am J Psychiatry.* 2010;167(7):748–751.
5. Cuthbert BN. Research Domain Criteria: toward future psychiatric nosologies. *Dialogues Clin Neurosci.* 2015;17(1):89–97.
6. Maj M. Narrowing the gap between ICD/DSM and RDoC constructs: possible steps and caveats. *World Psychiatry.* 2016;15(3):193–194.
7. Yager J, Feinstein RE. Potential applications of the National Institute of Mental Health's Research Domain Criteria (RDoC) to clinical psychiatric practice: how RDoC might be used in assessment, diagnostic processes, case formulation, treatment planning, and clinical notes. *J Clin Psychiatry.* 2017;78(4):423–432.
8. Fish F. *Clinical Psychopathology: Signs and Symptoms in Psychiatry,* 2nd ed. Hamilton M, ed. Bristol: John Wright; 1985.
9. Synofzik M, Voss M. Disturbances of the sense of agency in schizophrenia. In: Balconi M, ed. *Neuropsychology of the Sense of Agency.* Milan: Springer; 2010:145–155.
10. Belayachi S, Van der Linden M. Looking for outcomes: the experience of control and sense of agency in obsessive-compulsive behaviors. In: Balconi M, ed. *Neuropsychology of the Sense of Agency.* Milan: Springer; 2010:157–171.
11. Balconi M. Disruption of the sense of agency: from perception to self-knowledge. In: Balconi M, ed. *Neuropsychology of the Sense of Agency: From Consciousness to Action.* Milan: Springer; 2010:125–143.
12. National Institute of Mental Health. Research Domain Criteria (RDoC). 2017; www.nimh.nih.gov/research-priorities/rdoc/index.shtml (accessed January 26, 2017).
13. Störring GE. Transtornos de la conciencia. In: Reichardt M, ed. *Psiquiatria general y especial.* Madrid: Editorial Gredos; 1958:72–82.
14. Denys D. Obsessionality and compulsivity: a phenomenology of obsessive-compulsive disorder. *Philos Ethics Humanit Med.* 2011;6:3.
15. Fuchs T. The psychopathology of hyperreflexivity. *J Speculative Philosophy.* 2010;24(3):239–255.
16. Markova IS, Jaafari N, Berrios GE. Insight and obsessive-compulsive disorder: a conceptual analysis. *Psychopathology.* 2009;42(5):277–282.
17. Fontenelle JM, Harrison BJ, Santana L, Conceicao do Rosario M, Versiani M, Fontenelle LF. Correlates of insight into different symptom dimensions in obsessive-compulsive disorder. *Ann Clin Psychiatry.* 2013;25(1):11–16.
18. Robinson LJ, Freeston MH. Emotion and internal experience in obsessive compulsive disorder: reviewing the role of alexithymia, anxiety sensitivity and distress tolerance. *Clin Psychol Rev.* 2014;34(3):256–271.
19. Allman JM, Tetreault NA, Hakeem AY, et al. The von Economo neurons in the frontoinsular and anterior cingulate cortex. *Ann N Y Acad Sci.* 2011;1225:59–71.
20. Simon EM. *The Myth of Sisyphus: Renaissance Theories of Human Perfectibility.* Cranbury, NJ: Fairleigh Dickinson University Press; 2007.
21. Woody SR, Steketee G, Chambless DL. Reliability and validity of the Yale–Brown Obsessive-Compulsive Scale. *Behav Res Ther.* 1995;33(5):597–605.
22. Rosario-Campos MC, Miguel EC, Quatrano S, et al. The Dimensional Yale-Brown Obsessive-Compulsive Scale (DY-BOCS): an instrument for assessing obsessive-compulsive symptom dimensions. *Mol Psychiatry.* 2006;11(5):495–504.
23. Abramowitz JS, Deacon BJ, Olatunji BO, et al. Assessment of obsessive-compulsive symptom dimensions: development and evaluation of the Dimensional Obsessive-Compulsive Scale. *Psychol Assess.* 2010;22(1):180–198.
24. Baxter Jr. LR, Ackermann RF, Swerdlow NR, et al. Specific brain system mediation of obsessive-compulsive disorder responsive to either medication or behavior therapy. In: Goodman WK, Rudorfer MV, Maser JD, eds. *Obsessive-Compulsive Disorder: Contemporary Issues in Treatment.* Mahwah, NJ: Lawrence Erlbaum Associates; 2000:573–609.
25. Riesel A, Goldhahn S, Kathmann N. Hyperactive performance monitoring as a transdiagnostic marker: results from health anxiety in comparison to obsessive-compulsive disorder. *Neuropsychologia.* 2017;96:1–8.

26. Pitman RK. A cybernetic model of obsessive-compulsive psychopathology. *Compr Psychiatry.* 1987;28(4):334–343.

27. Endrass T, Ullsperger M. Specificity of performance monitoring changes in obsessive-compulsive disorder. *Neurosci Biobehav Rev.* 2014;46(Pt 1):124–138.

28. Weinberg A, Kotov R, Proudfit GH. Neural indicators of error processing in generalized anxiety disorder, obsessive-compulsive disorder, and major depressive disorder. *J Abnorm Psychol.* 2015;124(1):172–185.

29. Carrasco M, Hong C, Nienhuis JK, et al. Increased error-related brain activity in youth with obsessive-compulsive disorder and other anxiety disorders. *Neurosci Lett.* 2013;541:214–218.

30. Endrass T, Riesel A, Kathmann N, Buhlmann U. Performance monitoring in obsessive-compulsive disorder and social anxiety disorder. *J Abnorm Psychol.* 2014;123(4):705–714.

31. Akhtar S, Wig NN, Varma VK, Pershad D, Verma SK. A phenomenological analysis of symptoms in obsessive-compulsive neurosis. *Br J Psychiatry.* 1975;127:342–348.

32. Shooka A, al-Haddad MK, Raees A. OCD in Bahrain: a phenomenological profile. *Int J Soc Psychiatry.* 1998;44(2):147–154.

33. Speckens AE, Hackmann A, Ehlers A, Cuthbert B. Imagery special issue: intrusive images and memories of earlier adverse events in patients with obsessive-compulsive disorder. *J Behav Ther Exp Psychiatry.* 2007;38(4):411–422.

34. Osman S, Cooper M, Hackmann A, Veale D. Spontaneously occurring images and early memories in people with body dysmorphic disorder. *Memory.* 2004;12(4):428–436.

35. Muse K, McManus F, Hackmann A, Williams M, Williams M. Intrusive imagery in severe health anxiety: prevalence, nature and links with memories and maintenance cycles. *Behav Res Ther.* 2010;48(8):792–798.

36. Lipton MG, Brewin CR, Linke S, Halperin J. Distinguishing features of intrusive images in obsessive-compulsive disorder. *J Anxiety Disord.* 2010;24(8):816–822.

37. Moritz S, Claussen M, Hauschildt M, Kellner M. Perceptual properties of obsessive thoughts are associated with low insight in obsessive-compulsive disorder. *J Nerv Ment Dis.* 2014;202(7):562–565.

38. Rohlinger J, Wulf F, Fieker M, Moritz S. Sensory properties of obsessive thoughts in OCD and the relationship to psychopathology. *Psychiatry Res.* 2015;230(2):592–596.

39. Veale D, Page N, Woodward E, Salkovskis P. Imagery rescripting for obsessive compulsive disorder: a single case experimental design in 12 cases. *J Behav Ther Exp Psychiatry.* 2015;49(Pt B):230–236.

40. Ritter V, Stangier U. Seeing in the mind's eye: imagery rescripting for patients with body dysmorphic disorder. A single case series. *J Behav Ther Exp Psychiatry.* 2016;50:187–195.

41. Willson R, Veale D, Freeston M. Imagery rescripting for body dysmorphic disorder: a multiple-baseline single-case experimental design. *Behav Ther.* 2016;47(2):248–261.

42. Houghton DC, Capriotti MR, Conelea CA, Woods DW. Sensory phenomena in Tourette syndrome: their role in symptom formation and treatment. *Curr Dev Disord Rep.* 2014;1(4):245–251.

43. Ferrao YA, Shavitt RG, Prado H, et al. Sensory phenomena associated with repetitive behaviors in obsessive-compulsive disorder: an exploratory study of 1001 patients. *Psychiatry Res.* 2012;197(3):253–258.

44. Abramovitch A, Abramowitz JS, Mittelman A. The neuropsychology of adult obsessive-compulsive disorder: a meta-analysis. *Clin Psychol Rev.* 2013;33(8):1163–1171.

45. Choi JS, Kang DH, Kim JJ, et al. Left anterior subregion of orbitofrontal cortex volume reduction and impaired organizational strategies in obsessive-compulsive disorder. *J Psychiatr Res.* 2004;38(2):193–199.

46. Deckersbach T, Savage CR, Phillips KA, et al. Characteristics of memory dysfunction in body dysmorphic disorder. *J Int Neuropsychol Soc.* 2000;6(6):673–681.

47. Sherman BJ, Savage CR, Eddy KT, et al. Strategic memory in adults with anorexia nervosa: are there similarities to obsessive-compulsive spectrum disorders? *Int J Eat Disord.* 2006;39(6):468–476.

48. Buhlmann U, Deckersbach T, Engelhard I, et al. Cognitive retraining for organizational impairment in obsessive-compulsive disorder. *Psychiatry Res.* 2006;144(2–3):109–116.

49. Bragdon LB, Coles ME. Examining heterogeneity of obsessive-compulsive disorder: evidence for subgroups based on motivations. *J Anxiety Disord.* 2017;45:64–71.

50. Rado S. So-called obsessive-compulsive neurosis. In: Arieti S, ed. *American Handbook of Psychiatry,* 2nd ed. Volume 3. New York, NY: Basic Books; 1974:195–208.

51. Ferreira GM, Yücel M, Dawson A, Lorenzetti V, Fontenelle LF. Investigating the role of anticipatory reward and habit strength in obsessive-compulsive disorder. *CNS Spectr.* 2017;22(3):295–304.

52. Fontenelle LF, Oostermeijer S, Ferreira GM, Lorenzetti V, Luigjes J, Yücel M. Anticipated reward in obsessive-compulsive disorder: are compulsions rewarding? *J Clin Psychiatry.* 2015;76(9):e1134–1135.

53. Berridge KC, Kringelbach ML. Pleasure systems in the brain. *Neuron.* 2015;86(3):646–664.

54. Figee M, Vink M, de Geus F, et al. Dysfunctional reward circuitry in obsessive-compulsive disorder. *Biol Psychiatry.* 2011;69(9):867–874.

55. Jung WH, Kang DH, Han JY, et al. Aberrant ventral striatal responses during incentive processing in unmedicated patients with obsessive-compulsive disorder. *Acta Psychiatr Scand.* 2011;123(5):376–386.

56. Marsh R, Tau GZ, Wang Z, et al. Reward-based spatial learning in unmedicated adults with obsessive-compulsive disorder. *Am J Psychiatry.* 2015;172(4):383–392.

57. Denys D, Mantione M, Figee M, et al. Deep brain stimulation of the nucleus accumbens for treatment-refractory obsessive-compulsive disorder. *Arch Gen Psychiatry.* 2010;67(10):1061–1068.

58. Frydman I, de Salles Andrade JB, Vigne P, Fontenelle LF. Can neuroimaging provide reliable biomarkers for obsessive-compulsive disorder? A narrative review. *Curr Psychiatry Rep.* 2016;18(10):90.

59. Avery SN, Clauss JA, Blackford JU. The human BNST: functional role in anxiety and addiction. *Neuropsychopharmacology.* 2016;41(1):126–141.

60. Bradley MC, Hanna D, Wilson P, Scott G, Quinn P, Dyer KF. Obsessive-compulsive symptoms and attentional bias: an eye-tracking methodology. *J Behav Ther Exp Psychiatry.* 2016;50:303–308.

61. Starcevic V, Berle D, Brakoulias V, et al. The nature and correlates of avoidance in obsessive-compulsive disorder. *Aust N Z J Psychiatry.* 2011;45(10): 871–879.

62. Ursu S, Stenger VA, Shear MK, Jones MR, Carter CS. Overactive action monitoring in obsessive-compulsive disorder: evidence from functional magnetic resonance imaging. *Psychol Sci.* 2003;14(4):347–353.

63. Stern ER, Taylor SF. Cognitive neuroscience of obsessive-compulsive disorder. *Psychiatr Clin North Am.* 2014;37(3):337–352.

64. Fullana MA, Mataix-Cols D, Caseras X, et al. High sensitivity to punishment and low impulsivity in obsessive-compulsive patients with hoarding symptoms. *Psychiatry Res.* 2004;129(1):21–27.

65. Watson D, Stanton K, Clark LA. Self-report indicators of negative valence constructs within the research domain criteria (RDoC): a critical review. *J Affect Disord.* 2017;216:58–69.

66. Voon V, Derbyshire K, Ruck C, et al. Disorders of compulsivity: a common bias towards learning habits. *Mol Psychiatry.* 2015;20(3):345–352.

67. Gillan CM, Otto AR, Phelps EA, Daw ND. Model-based learning protects against forming habits. *Cogn Affect Behav Neurosci.* 2015;15(3):523–536.

68. Smith KS, Graybiel AM. Habit formation. *Dialogues Clin Neurosci.* 2016;18(1):33–43.

69. Goudriaan AE, Yücel M, van Holst RJ. Getting a grip on problem gambling: what can neuroscience tell us? *Front Behav Neurosci.* 2014;8:141.

70. Gillan CM, Morein-Zamir S, Urcelay GP, et al. Enhanced avoidance habits in obsessive-compulsive disorder. *Biol Psychiatry.* 2014;75(8):631–638.

71. Snorrason I, Lee HJ, de Wit S, Woods DW. Are nonclinical obsessive-compulsive symptoms associated with bias toward habits? *Psychiatry Res.* 2016;241:221–223.

72. Burguiere E, Monteiro P, Mallet L, Feng G, Graybiel AM. Striatal circuits, habits, and implications for obsessive-compulsive disorder. *Curr Opin Neurobiol.* 2015;30:59–65.

73. Pauls DL, Abramovitch A, Rauch SL, Geller DA. Obsessive-compulsive disorder: an integrative genetic and neurobiological perspective. *Nat Rev Neurosci.* 2014;15(6):410–424.

74. Lipinski JF, Jr., Pope HG, Jr. Do “flashbacks” represent obsessional imagery? *Compr Psychiatry.* 1994;35(4):245–247.

75. Spitzer M. On defining delusions. *Compr Psychiatry.* 1990;31(5):377–397.

76. Ferrao YA, Miguel E, Stein DJ. Tourette’s syndrome, trichotillomania, and obsessive-compulsive disorder: how closely are they related? *Psychiatry Res.* 2009;170(1):32–42.

77. Chamberlain SR, Leppink EW, Redden SA, Grant JE. Are obsessive-compulsive symptoms impulsive, compulsive or both? *Compr Psychiatry.* 2016;68:111–118.

Chapter 2

The Philosophy of Compulsive Disorders: Compulsivity and Free Will

Judy Luigjes and Damiaan Denys

Defining Compulsivity

Compulsivity is a hot topic in psychiatry. Many disorders display compulsive behaviors such as addiction, eating disorders, paraphilic disorders and obsessive-compulsive and related disorders [1,2,3]. Since compulsive behaviors differ greatly between disorders, compulsivity may refer to drug or alcohol use as well as to gambling, to ritualistic behaviors and repetitive acts such as cleaning, counting or checking (i.e., compulsions), to restrictive eating behavior, as well as overeating. Despite the broad diversity in behavioral expression, we all, intuitively, have an impression of what the word compulsive stands for. In obsessive-compulsive disorder, the prototypical compulsive disorder, it is the perseverative nature of compulsions despite explicit awareness of their irrationality. In addiction, the word compulsive brings to mind the addict who keeps on using drugs while pleasure declines and despite realizing the destructive effects of the drugs. Despite our commonsense intuition, it is difficult to define when a particular behavior precisely is compulsive. First, there are no well-accepted, validated definitions of compulsivity. Second, there is a lack of neuropsychological tasks or questionnaires that assess compulsivity transdiagnostically across disorders [4]. Thus, though compulsivity is commonly used in recent literature and scientific symposia, its definition still is elusive.

To ensure consensus about the precise meaning of compulsivity, a well-accepted, validated definition is needed at a minimum to clarify two important questions. First, how do we demarcate compulsive behavior from other types of behavior? Second, what exactly is the commonality between the different types of compulsive behavior? With this aim in mind, we conducted a study exploring the definitions of compulsivity used in studies that investigated compulsivity over different disorders [5]. First, we found that 10 of 28 articles that focused on transdiagnostic compulsivity (in at least 3 or more disorders) did not even define compulsivity. Second, we noticed that studies conceptualized compulsivity in different ways. The most striking difference was the contrast between the phenomenological and the observational approach. The first approach focused on the subjective experience of the patient while the latter focused on how the behavior would be described from an objective, outside perspective. An example of a phenomenological definition is Denys [6], who aimed to find the essence of compulsivity by stripping away all the elements not present in all forms of compulsivity. He then defined compulsivity as the "inability to not perform an act, with a subjective feeling of loss of control vis-à-vis oneself". While Grant et al. [7], in an article about new treatment models for compulsivity, defined compulsivity observationally by "actions, which are persistently repeated despite adverse consequences". Other definitions use both observational and phenomenological elements.

These examples illustrate that compulsivity may be conceptualized from two perspectives: from a third person or objective perspective where compulsivity is perceived as a particular behavior with certain observational characteristics but also from a first-person subjective perspective where compulsivity is a particular mindset that is characterized by a certain experience. This aligns with reports of patients. Some of their suffering results from the consequences of the behavior and the loss of control this entails. But there is also a more direct suffering in the experience of having to do something that one does not want to do. This compulsivity is the experience of loss of control over one's own behavior, the inability to choose and steer one's actions freely, which gives rise to feelings of powerlessness and shame. Because the suffering in compulsivity is inherent to the experience, compulsivity differs from impulsivity where suffering is caused by the consequences of the behavior and not the experience of doing the behavior.

The common and wide use of compulsivity may give the wrong impression that we refer to one clear singular construct, and that we agree on its meaning. The difficulty in defining compulsivity might be related to the wide variety of behaviors to which it refers but also to the importance of both the third- and first-person perspective. The aim of this chapter is twofold: to explore the implications of understanding compulsivity from a third- and first-person perspective, and second to explore and better understand when behavior is experienced as compulsive. The observational third-person perspective puts emphasis on the dysfunctional nature of compulsivity, thereby contrasting it with functional behavior. The phenomenological first-person perspective stresses the subjective experience setting up a contrast between compulsive and free behavior.

Compulsivity as Dysfunctional Behavior

A commonly used observational definition is that compulsivity involves repetitive actions despite negative consequences, or being inappropriate to the situation [3,7,8,9]. This observational definition focuses on dysfunction: the behavior leads to negative consequences or makes little or no sense within the context. For instance, according to this definition one would display compulsive behavior if one loses one's job as a result of drug use. It is of note that the subjective experience of the drug user has no role in this definition. His behavior is described as compulsive, independent of whether or not he perceives his behavior as problematic, or experiences himself as having lost control. It is scientifically attractive to have a definition that allows one to tick-off observational characteristics and that is independent of subjective reports, which are changeable and less reliable. Moreover, the mere use of observational characteristics makes it possible to translate this definition to animal models. Yet the question remains whether the essence of compulsivity is sufficiently captured by such an observational approach. Since an observational definition requires an external agent to assess what is appropriate and functional, this assessment may differ from the patient's own view, and is additionally dependent on cultural norms, since what is judged to be functional behavior may differ across cultures.

Compulsivity as Lack of Experienced Freedom

The phenomenological definition of compulsivity aims to capture the subjective experience of the patient, which is possibly its most puzzling aspect. Patients feel that they have to perform actions that they do not want to perform. Experiencing the inability to stop their own behavior, and the resulting lack of control, significantly adds to the suffering of patients. It evokes shame, self-doubt and frustration. It is the reflection upon one's own inability to adapt one's behavior and the resulting lack of control that brings about the heavy burden of compulsive behavior. However, it is hard to make generalizations about under what conditions people experience their behavior as free or compulsive. The phenomenological definition requires reflections on philosophical themes of free will, autonomy and identity. For example, the drug user from the above example may be dysfunctional but may not feel compulsive. Perhaps he wants to use drugs and cares little about the job he has lost. As humans, we have the capacity to relate to our behavior and distinguish between behavior (and its motive) resulting from our will and behavior over which we feel little or no control. Therefore, from a phenomenological viewpoint, the same behavior, context and consequences may go together with different levels of compulsivity. For instance, an extensive ritual around bedtime to check the locks multiple times may for one person feel free and for the other compulsive. Whether one experiences behavior as free or compulsive may relate to the degree it serves one's overall cares and concerns (goals and values), but also to a broader question of when behaviors are viewed as one's own.

We conclude that there are differences in what is judged to be compulsive from a first- and third-person perspective. It is possible that behavior is seen from a third-person perspective as compulsive without the person experiencing compulsivity; the behavior may even be experienced as goal driven. Thus, merely using the third-person perspective could result in a definition of compulsivity that describes behavior with similar observational characteristics but with underlying motivational states that differ significantly. A related question is whether the severity of compulsivity is dependent on the behavior's dysfunction or on the compulsivity experienced by the patient or a combination of the two. We propose that, for a complete understanding of the compulsive patient's suffering, we need to include the phenomenological perspective.

Practical Identity

When do we experience behavior as compulsive? How can one feel internally forced to perform a certain behavior? Every agent, including non-human animals, can be seen as the cause of their actions. Yet, to determine those actions as free or compulsive, or to make any hierarchical order in terms of freedom, we need the capacity to relate to or on our behavior and its motives. Without this awareness there would not be any question about freedom or compulsivity; one would just act on whatever inclination is strongest. The capacity to determine ourselves to be the cause of our acts is what Christine Korsgaard calls *human* agency [10]. For this, we need a reflective awareness of our mental states, or, in other words, self-consciousness. Only when we are aware that we are inclined to act a certain way, do we have the choice to act upon it or not. To experience actions as free we need to feel they *come from us* in a different sense than to simply say we performed them. They have to match with who we think we are, or in other words, to come from an identity that we constitute ourselves. Korsgaard argues that we continually constitute ourselves in practical identities: an idea of yourself "under which you find your life to be worth living and your actions to be worth undertaking" [10,11]. This identity can include different roles, like that of a father or professional, relationships, members of certain groups, vocations and so on. We check whether our behavior is consistent with this identity, and this identity is constantly shaped by endorsing and rejecting potential motives when we act. Thus, not only does our practical identity shape our behavior but our behavior also shapes our identity. Therefore, a practical identity is not a static construct but is a continuing, interactional process that gives us a sense of unity. This sense of unity is necessary to perceive our acts as arising from *a self*, a whole that constitutes a person. We experience compulsivity when we feel we have to perform an act that is incompatible with this identity. So, while the compulsive patient is fully aware that she is performing the act, it does not feel as if it is her choice. Our self-consciousness makes it possible to perceive our actions as resulting from ourselves (as agents) but also from forces that work on or in us.

Conflicting Motives

Under what circumstances do we perform acts incompatible with our practical identities? An important reason for us to become aware of and relate to our behavior is when we experience conflicting motives. This is something we also observe in patients. An addicted patient can have a strong desire to use drugs, but at the same time can realize that his drug abuse impedes other goals. A patient with anorexia may wish to eat lasagna, yet, at the same time be determined not to gain another ounce. But conflicting motivations are not necessarily a thread for our sense of unity. For instance, I can endorse both the motives of caring for my weight and desiring chocolate, and thereby endorse the inner conflict that I experience when I encounter chocolate cake as my own. It becomes a problem when I go on a diet and value my weight over my desire for chocolate, yet keep eating the chocolate cake. In this situation, it is more likely that I will experience loss of control, since I feel unable to choose an option that fits with my overall preferences. Yet, if I am still able to match my desire for chocolate with my practical identity I may still preserve a sense of freedom. For instance, if I acknowledge that my desire for chocolate may regularly outweigh my goal of losing weight, the experience of compulsivity will be less pronounced than when I strongly identify with the goal of losing weight while rejecting the desire for the cake. In the latter case, I might find my strong urge to eat chocolate cake abhorrent, and this urge more likely feels intrusive and threatening to my freedom. Therefore, the degree of compulsivity (or freedom) seems to be related to the degree to which behavior aligns with our practical identities: the concept of ourselves that captures what we care for in life [12]. In its broadest sense, the experience of compulsivity depends on the degree to which we can *own* our behavior. The more we view our (motives for) behaviors as an intelligible part of ourselves the less likely they compromise our freedom and control.

How people construct personal identities can vary greatly. These differences may have their own problems. Some people may be inflexible by having narrowly defined identities and easily reject behavior as incompatible with who they are. Others may be overly flexible by taking any inclination as a good motive to act and thereby constructing their identities to match any (inconsistent) behavior. Therefore, people may differ in how they grapple with conflicting motives. We will clarify this distinction by discussing two polar opposites on this spectrum. Patients who are very flexible in constructing their identities will be less inclined to experience their behavior as compulsive. At the same time it may also make them less likely to change dysfunctional behavior, and they may experience less unity in what they care for. For instance the addicted individual that one day wants to quit her drug use to build up a professional and family life while the next day embraces her life as drug user, might find it difficult to change her drug use. Pointing out these inconsistencies and stimulating patients to more narrowly construct these identities is used as a strategy by motivational therapy to treat addictive disorders. On the other side are the patients with a strong tendency to reject motives that do not perfectly align with their identities. This may induce feelings of shame, control loss and increase suffering, which could also hamper behavioral change. An extreme example is a patient with severe contamination fear and cleaning compulsions, who experienced a decrease of more than 16 hours of compulsive behavior daily following successful deep brain stimulation. After treatment, she spent no more than 15 minutes on cleaning. However, she insisted that she still continued to experience compulsions and rituals and requested additional treatment. It appeared that she experienced her regular daily activities of house cleaning, organizing and checking as compulsive since she did not identify with the motives of performing these behaviors. Therefore, even with these functional behaviors she felt as if she "had to" do them instead of wanting to do them. Mindfulness tries to increase (nonjudgmental) awareness of one's motives that can help to incorporate them into one's identity. Therefore, next to the traditional approach of focussing on decreasing dysfunctional behavior, an additional possible approach in changing one's experienced compulsivity might be changing one's relation to the behavior.

Why Are These Different Viewpoints on Compulsivity Important?

In recent years, the interest in compulsive behavior increased since it transcends traditional psychiatric diagnostic categories. Therefore it fits within the strategic plan of the US National Institute of Mental Health, which aims to establish a new classification of psychiatry for research purposes based on dimensions of observable behavior and neurobiological measures instead of diagnostic categories [13]. The driving idea is that the difficulties of finding neurological and cognitive differences between current diagnostic categories of psychiatry can be explained by the heterogeneity of symptoms within groups and overlap between the groups. A more successful approach is expected from studying behavioral and symptom dimensions that cross diagnostic boundaries because these may map more closely to neurological and cognitive findings.

However, investigating compulsive behavior and its neural correlates will directly be affected by how it is defined. The definition of compulsive behavior as repetitive action despite negative consequences or inappropriateness would include a large variability in the motives that underlie the behavior or the experience that accompanies it. This may be a sensible approach for studying why certain individuals are generally prone to continue to perform dysfunctional repetitive actions. However, it may fail to explain why people persist in behavior they do not want to perform. For this question, we need (to include) a phenomenological description of compulsivity, for which we need a better understanding of when behavior is experienced as compulsive. We proposed that behavior is experienced as compulsive when the individual perseverates while it is incompatible with their identity. Yet, we need qualitative research to confirm these hypotheses and to further explore the experience of compulsivity.

Acknowledgments

We would like to thank Julian Kiverstein, whose comments greatly improved the chapter. JL was financed by the Amsterdam Brain and Cognition Talent Fund.

References

1. Robbins TW, Gillan CM, Smith DG, de Wit S, Ersche KD. Neurocognitive endophenotypes of impulsivity and compulsivity: towards dimensional psychiatry. *Trends Cogn Sci.* 2010;16:81–91.
2. Skodol AE, Oldham JD. Phenomenology, differential diagnosis, and comorbidity of the impulsive-compulsive spectrum of disorders. In: Hollander E, Cohen LJ, eds. *Impulsivity and Compulsivity.* Washington, DC: American Psychiatric Association Publishing; 1996:1–36.
3. Fineberg NA, Chamberlain SR, Goudriaan AE, et al. New developments in human neurocognition: clinical, genetic, and brain imaging correlates of impulsivity and compulsivity. *CNS Spectr.* 2014;19:69–89.

4. Yücel M, Fontenelle LF. Compulsivity as an endophenotype: the search for a hazy moving target. *Addiction.* 2012;107:1735–1736.
5. Luigjes J, Lorenzetti V, De Haan S, et al. Defining compulsive behavior. Unpublished.
6. Denys D. Compulsivity and free will. *CNS Spectr.* 2014;19(1):8–9.
7. Grant JE, Fineberg N, van Ameringen M, et al. New treatment models for compulsive disorders. *Eur Neuropsychopharmacol.* 2016;26(5): 877–884.
8. Fineberg NA, Potenza MN, Chamberlain SR, et al. Probing compulsive and impulsive behaviors, from animal models to endophenotypes: a narrative review. *Neuropsychopharmacology.* 2010;35:591–604.
9. Dalley JW, Everitt BJ, Robbins TW. Impulsivity, compulsivity, and top-down cognitive control. *Neuron.* 2011;69:680–694.
10. Korsgaard CM. *Self-Constitution : Agency, Identity, and Integrity.* Oxford University Press; 2009.
11. Korsgaard CM. *The Sources of Normativity.* Cambridge University Press; 1996:100–102.
12. Slors MVP. *You Would Have Thought so! Brain, Consciousness and Free Will in Philosophical Perspective.* Amsterdam: Boom; 2012.
13. National Institute of Mental Health. The National Institute of Mental Health Strategic Plan, 2008. Available from: www.nimh.nih.gov/about/strategic-planning-reports/index.shtml#strategic-objective4 (accessed June 30, 2018).

Chapter 3

Family and Twin Studies of Obsessive-Compulsive and Related Disorders

Danielle C. Cath, Nuno R. Zilhão, Dirk J. A. Smit and Dorret I. Boomsma

Introduction

The current definition of obsessive-compulsive disorder (OCD) was introduced in the 1980s in the *Diagnostic and Statistical Manual of Mental Disorders*, third edition (DSM-III) [1]. Until then, OCD was commonly referred to as "obsessive compulsive neurosis", or "psychasthenia". According to the fourth edition, DSM-IV) [2], OCD was classified as an anxiety disorder, characterized by persistent, repetitive and intrusive thoughts/images (obsessions) that cause anxiety and or tension and are in over 80% of cases followed by anxiety/tension reducing actions and ritualized behaviors (compulsions). Relief from carrying out compulsions is usually brief and the repetitive behavior by and in itself fuels subsequent repetitive behavior [3], with the person getting caught in a cycle of fear, doubt, worry and distress, leading to high levels of social impairment. Whereas in DSM-IV OCD was classified among the anxiety disorders, the new edition (DSM-5) [4] includes OCD in its own category (OCD and related disorders) alongside hoarding disorder, excoriating disorder, body dysmorphic disorder and trichotillomania, assuming commonalities with respect to underlying genetic and environmental factors contributing to occurrence and maintenance of the disease. What are the most important comorbidities of OCD? OCD is mostly accompanied by concurrent major depression (31%), anxiety disorders (25%), hoarding disorder (18–19%) and between 12% and 20% of patients have comorbid Tourette's disorder or tics [5,6,7,8,9,10,11]. An important next question is to find out to what extent those comorbid disorders actually share underlying genetic or environmental risk factors, or are genetically distinct. One of the most powerful tools to study this question entails family and twin studies. Family studies are particularly relevant to investigate whether a specific (comorbid) trait B runs in families with trait A more frequently than expected by chance. When that occurs, it is likely that trait B shares some genetic risk with trait A, although an increased co-occurrence as a result of common underlying family environmental factors cannot be ruled out. An advantage of family-based clinical studies is that families are selected through probands with the disorder, who are likely to carry increased genetic load for a trait. On the other hand, the epidemiological twin model in which correlations within and between monozygotic (MZ) and dizygotic (DZ) twins for multiple traits are compared using model fitting approaches (structural equation modeling) has the advantage that 100% of the phenotypic variation of a (comorbid) trait is being explained by the combination of additive genetic effects, by common (family) environment and by unique environmental effects. Thus, epidemiological twin studies can disentangle genetic from family environment effects. They give a "helicopter" view of the contribution of these three underlying effects [12], providing a valuable first directional step to estimate the presence and proportion of shared genetic and environmental influences on a trait, often expressed in genetic and environmental correlations. However, they are unable to provide information on *which* genetic or environmental effects might be operant, since no molecular ("wet") genetics are involved.

Here, we provide an overview of the family and genetic epidemiological twin family studies of OCD and its comorbidities. Those comorbid disorders that have been most extensively studied are: tics, hoarding disorder and attention deficit and hyperactivity disorder (ADHD). Based on the high comorbidity rates with anxiety and depression, one would assume that family and twin studies would have been directed toward the comorbidities with these disorders. However, this is not the case, for several reasons. Historically, research has focused on the relationship between OCD and tics [13,14,15]. Specific explorations of comorbidities between OCD, Tourette's disorder, ADHD and hoarding disorder have been the result of the notion that these disorders share commonalities with respect to dysfunctional corticostriatothalamocortical circuitry [16,17]. Finally, during the recent debates regarding the development of the DSM-5 classification system, several field trials explored a more logical placement of OCD among OCD spectrum disorders, away from the anxiety disorders, which led to new insights on the relationship between OCD and hoarding disorder [18,19]. This chapter particularly focuses on the relationship between OCD and these disorders, including new insights on magnitude of genetic influences on the stability of OCD in time.

Recent Research Findings

Family and Twin Studies of OCD: Genetic Architecture

Applications of genetic structural equation modeling [20] have advanced the field of psychiatric genetic research. Both family-based and epidemiological twin studies have sought to estimate the contribution of genetic and environmental influences to variation in the phenotype, often specified as the heritability of the liability to develop the disease. Collaborative psychiatric genetic research further contributed to the insight into the genetic basis of OCD, as well as the shared underlying etiology with some of its comorbidities [21,22,23,24]. This rapidly growing field now aims at finding the genetic DNA variants that help to identify pathways of disease development.

Family studies investigate clustering of a trait within families (i.e., in biological and possibly non-biological relatives), and provide a first insight into the possible contribution of genetic factors to the etiology of complex disorders. However, increased familial aggregation is in itself not sufficient to prove a genetic origin of a disorder, because phenotypic resemblance between family members may also be due to family members sharing a common environment. Only in those instances where non-biological family members are included into the design (e.g., adopted children), the influence of shared genes and shared environment can be distinguished. Currently, studies that include adopted family members are not available for OCD spectrum disorders.

The first family studies reported in OCD were based solely on family *history* data without directly interviewing the relatives of patients themselves. Although these studies tend to underestimate the real disease rate within families, they have generated consistent conclusions on the familiarity of OCD. Subsequently, various family study reports have appeared in the literature, both in adults and in children or adolescents, using *direct* interviews with at least one family member, in some instances combined with family history data [15,25,26]. Overall, the results showed an up to ten-fold increased rate of OCD in first-degree relatives of children/adolescents with OCD and a two-fold increase in relatives of adults with OCD. Thus, prevalence rates in first-degree family members of a child with OCD was 22.5% (vs. 2.6% in matched controls) [27], and in adult probands with OCD, frequencies of OCD in their first-degree relatives were 10–11.7% compared with 1.9–2.7% in control relatives, which is comparable to estimates in the general population [15,25]. Interestingly, within families of affected male probands, male relatives tend to report more tic symptoms, while female relatives more often present obsessive-compulsive behavior [15].

Twin studies can distinguish genetic and shared environmental factors by modeling the differences in correlations between MZ and DZ twins [28]. MZ twins are genetically identical, while DZ twins share on average 50% of their segregating genes, which is similar to the resemblance of any non-twin siblings. If MZ twins resemble each other more than DZ twins, this is indicative for the importance of genetic influences on the trait under consideration. Twin studies of OCD go back to 1929, with the first report on obsessive-compulsive symptoms (OCS) of twins by Lange. In the following 40 years, a number of clinical twin studies were published in OCD (for a historical overview, see van Grootheest et al. [29]). Two of the largest clinical twin studies in the period of the DSM-III diagnostic system [31] reported concordance rates for OCD of 45% in MZ pairs and 15% in DZ pairs [30], and of 33% in MZ pairs and 7% in DZ pairs [31], respectively, indicating a genetic background for OCD.

Other twin studies on the heritability of OCD focused on OCS rather than OCD [32,33,34]. By using continuous data from self-report questionnaires of a variety of OCS, and population-based epidemiological samples, as opposed to clinically based samples, larger samples could be recruited. Figure 3.1 summarizes the heritability estimates obtained from twin studies in OCD and OCS.

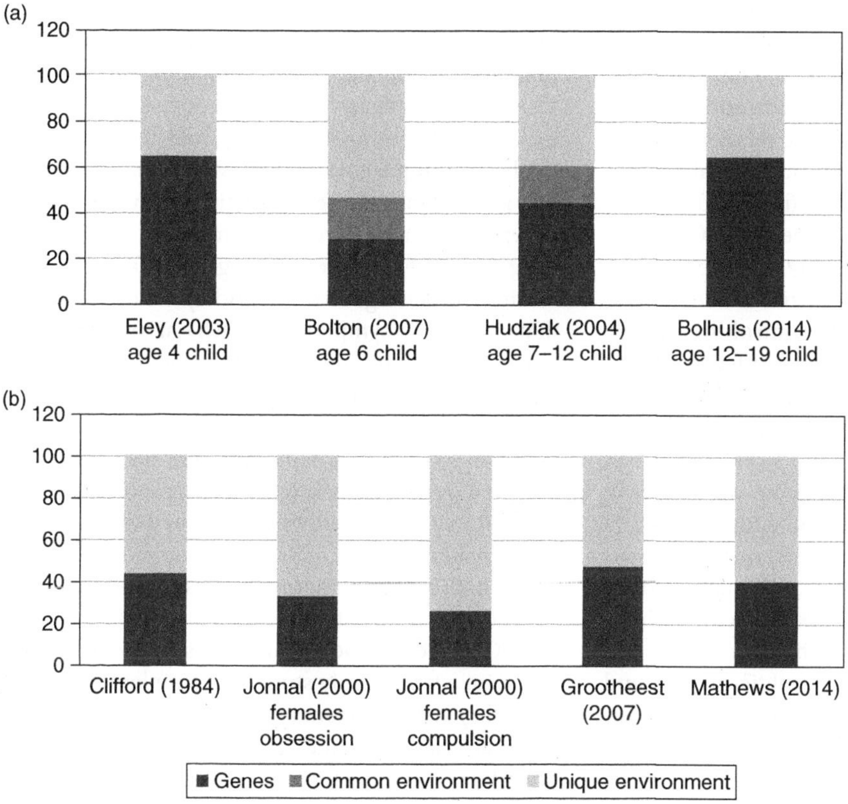

Figure 3.1 Heritabilities of obsessive-compulsive disorder: (a) Twin studies in children. (b) Twin studies in adults.

Clifford and colleagues conducted the first relatively large study of OCS in an epidemiological sample of 419 twin pairs [35]. Using genetic structural equation modeling, the study obtained heritability estimates for obsessional traits (44%) and OCS (47%). Subsequent studies, using larger epidemiological sample sets, provided heritability estimates ranging between 26% and 65%, depending on ages and sex of the sample population [32,33,34,36,37]. Generally, in children, the genetic contribution to variation in the obsessive-compulsive phenotype was estimated to be between 45% and 65%; in adults, these proportions were considerably lower, estimated to be between 27% and 47%, suggesting that environmental contributions to the obsessive-compulsive phenotype increase with age. No qualitative sex differences were detected; that is, there were no indications that boys/men differ from girls/women with respect to the underlying genes themselves. One study found quantitative sex differences, with higher heritabilities in women (50%) than in men (39%) [34].

In recent years, three studies have added a longitudinal perspective to the twin design in cohorts of children, adolescents and adults [38,39,40]. Stability, as expressed by longitudinal phenotypic correlations, was between 0.50 and 0.63, with substantial genetic contributions to symptom persistence (34–56%), indicating that stability of OCS over time has a substantial genetic component. In children, stability of OCS was estimated at between 35% and 51% for boys and between 28% and 34% for girls [34]. Interestingly, a modest effect of family environment was detected at 12 years of age in the van Grootheest et al. study [29].

Family and Twin Studies of Obsessive-Compulsive Disorders and their Comorbid Disorders

Comorbidities Between Obsessive-Compulsive Disorder, Anxiety and Depressive Disorders

Except for bipolar disorder, all types of anxiety and affective disorders seem to occur more frequently in patients with OCD than in healthy people, with rates of current major depressive disorder (MDD) found to be between 16% and 30%, and rates of anxiety disorders up to 20% [41,42,43], depending on age and sex of the sample population. Thus, the next question is to what extent these increased comorbidities reflect commonalities in underlying genetic relationships, or shared environmental risk factors. Hanna et al. studied lifetime MDD occurrence in 600 first- and second-degree family members of 35 children with OCD and 17 healthy comparison children, by interviewing the parents of these children [44]. Lifetime MDD prevalence was higher in cases than in control first-degree relatives (30.4% vs. 15.4%). Further, lifetime MDD prevalence was higher in first-degree relatives of case probands *with* MDD than in first-degree relatives of case probands *without* MDD (46.3% vs. 19.7%). In line with this, lifetime MDD prevalence was higher in second-degree relatives of case probands *with* MDD than in second-degree relatives of case probands *without* MDD (31.9% vs. 16.8%) or control second-degree relatives (31.9% vs. 15.4%). These findings point to a complex relationship between OCD and MDD, in which some common genetic background might play a role but in which the alternative possibility, that is, of MDD being secondary to OCD, is likely as well.

Nestadt et al. examined a large adult cohort of patients with OCD (n = 80) and 260 first-degree relatives (n = 343), comparing them with a healthy comparison group (n = 73) and their first-degree relatives (n = 300), using direct interviewing [41]. Generalized anxiety disorder (GAD), panic disorder, agoraphobia, separation anxiety disorder (SAD) and recurrent major depression were more common in the relatives of patients with OCD than in relatives in the control group. These disorders occurred more frequently if the relative was diagnosed with OCD. Only GAD and agoraphobia were more frequent in relatives of those with OCD *independent* of OCD in the proband, signifying that these two disorders are likely to share underlying genetic relationships with OCD and that these anxiety disorders are not a direct consequence of the person suffering from OCD.

To the best of our knowledge, only one genetic epidemiological twin study has been performed to date using structural equation modeling to study the underlying shared architecture between OCD and depressive disorders [38]. In this study, both cross-sectional and longitudinal relationships between obsessive-compulsive and depressive symptoms have been studied in a sample of 2651 adolescents (12–19 years) and 4920 adults. Interestingly, it was found that longitudinal associations between OCS at timepoint 1 and depressive symptoms at timepoint 2 in the adolescent group were driven by genetic factors contributing to these associations, and not by shared unique environmental factors. Likewise, in this group most of the correlations between OCS at timepoint 1 and depressive symptoms at timepoint 2 (up to 65%) were driven by genetic factors. These findings argue against the widely held hypothesis that depressive symptoms in OCD arise as a consequence of the burden of suffering from OCD; instead they are in favor of shared *genetic* factors that drive the relationship between obsessive-compulsive and depressive symptoms. Moreover, one 2018 study [45] has used polygenic risk score calculation to estimate to what extent the individual risk of MDD has predictive value toward OCS in the same individual. The polygenic risk score approach assesses to what extent the individual risk of these traits has predictive value for OCS. To do so, polygenic scores were constructed based on a twin family study [21] supplemented with summary statistics from available published genome-wide association studies on a variety of psychiatric disorders. The study focused on various traits that are epidemiologically related to OCS and investigated the ability of MDD scores to effectively predict OCS, considering genetic correlations between MDD scores and OCS. The polygenic scores for MDD ($P = 5.6 \times 10^{-5}$) were significant after correction for multiple testing ($\alpha = 0.006$). This result means that the genetic liability for MDD also results in increased OCS, and highlights the genetic overlap between these symptoms and MDD and OCS. Overall, polygenic scores including MDD explained 0.38–0.79% of the total variance of OCS.

Comorbidities Between Obsessive-Compulsive Disorder and Attention Deficit and Hyperactivity Disorder

Although prevalence rates of ADHD in OCD have been somewhat inconsistent [7,46,47,48], they are significantly increased, with reports between 36% and 57% for ADHD combined type, between 30% and 48% for the inattentive subtype of ADHD and lower prevalence rates (13%) for ADHD hyperactive subtype [49]. Moreover, one small-scale clinical study in young children (below age 3 years) with OCD indicated that rates of ADHD of up to 60% can be expected [50]. A next step is to study shared underlying liabilities between OCS and subtypes of ADHD.

Geller et al., using family study methodology, examined the relationship between OCD and ADHD in 1533 first-degree relatives of three groups of index children (between 6 and 17 years): those with ADHD and OCD, those with ADHD but no OCD and matched healthy controls [51]. They found the risk for ADHD to be similarly elevated in families of young people with ADHD with (18.9%) and without OCD (20.1%), and both groups had somewhat increased rates of ADHD compared with controls (4.6%), indicating a strong familial risk for ADHD. The risk for OCD was significantly elevated only among relatives of young people with ADHD and OCD (13.0%) compared with controls (0.5%), showing a strong familial risk for OCD. Relatives affected with ADHD had a significantly elevated risk for OCD in comparison with relatives unaffected by ADHD (7.4% vs. 1.3%), suggestive of co-segregation between these disorders.

The only large-scale genetic epidemiological twin study (n = 21,911 twins) has examined underlying shared genetic and environmental vulnerabilities between OCD and ADHD in the Swedish Twin Registry, looking at the underlying genetic and environmental contributions to OCS, ADHD and tics [47]. Model fitting suggested a latent liability factor underlying the three phenotypes, with modest correlations between the three phenotypes ranging between 0.24 and 0.45, and correlations being strongest between OCS and tics. Significantly less of the variance of ADHD symptom liability than of obsessive-compulsive or tic symptom liability was explained by this common factor, and the majority of the genetic variance between OCS, tics and ADHD was disorder specific rather than shared. Moreover, the largest proportion of variance in liability of tics, ADHD and OCS was attributed to specific non-shared environmental influences. To conclude, these phenotypes do not appear to be alternative expressions of the same underlying genetic liability. In line with this notion, in DSM-5, similar to previous editions of DSM, ADHD and OCD are placed in different disorder categories: ADHD in the neurodevelopmental section and OCD in the section for OCD spectrum disorders.

Comorbidities Between Obsessive-Compulsive Disorder and Tics

The best-studied comorbidities in OCD have been between OCD and tics, with various family and twin studies performed to date. Prevalence rates of tics/Tourette's disorder in OCD range between 28% and 49% of OCD/symptoms in Tourette's, and reversely, of 10% and 20% of tics in OCD [52,53,54], which is considerably increased relative to what one would expect by chance. The first family study on the relationship between OCD and tics, with individuals with Tourette's disorder as a starting point found similar rates of Tourette's, OCD and chronic multiple tics in relatives of Tourette's probands with OCD compared with relatives of Tourette's probands without OCD [13]. Further, they found elevated rates of OCD *without* Tourette's disorder or chronic multiple tics among first-degree relatives of probands with both Tourette's disorder and OCD and Tourette's without OCD, suggesting that, in families with Tourette's disorder, OCD may represent an alternative expression of the genetic factors responsible for Tourette's and/or chronic multiple tics. Since then, several family and twin studies have examined underlying commonalities in comorbid disease liability between OCD and tics in families of OCD probands [15,20,46,47,52,55,56].

Browne et al. investigated a very large population-based Danish sample and examined how OCD and tics cluster in families [56]. They found a mean sibling recurrence risk for Tourette's/chronic multiple tics across all birth years of 9.88% and for OCD of 4.01%. The sibling relative risk ratio for tics was considerably higher than for OCD (18.63 vs. 4.89), and also for parent–offspring relative risk ratios (61.02 for Tourette's/chronic multiple tics vs. 6.25 for OCD). Thus, the familial aggregation of Tourette's/chronic multiple tics is substantially higher than for OCD. The sibling and parent-offspring *cross-disorder* risks were elevated, ranging from 3.20 to 10.27.

Overall, clinical OCD family study results have shown an up to ten-fold increased rate of OCD in first-degree relatives of children/adolescents with OCD, and a two-fold increase in relatives of adults with OCD. Interestingly, within families of affected male OCD probands, male relatives tend to report more tic symptoms, especially in relatives of early onset cases, while female relatives more often present with typical OCS [15,52,55,56]. The overall picture emerging from these clinical studies is of OCD being characterized by highly familial early-onset subtypes that – especially in males – might be tic-related as well as -unrelated, and of fewer familial late-onset subtypes in which individual-specific environmental adversities play a more dominant role.

Twin studies on the relationship between OCS and tics [20,47,57,58,59] have been carried out both in children and adults. Bolton et al. investigated familial aggregation of OCS, tics and anxiety disorders in a community sample of 6-year-old twins using a two-phase design in which 4662 twin pairs were identified and 854 pairs were assessed in the second phase by maternal-informant diagnostic interview using DSM-IV criteria [58]. There were strong familial aggregations, both between OCS and tics, and between OCS and other anxiety disorders (80% and 97% respectively), suggesting – in line with the family study by Pauls et al. [15] – the presence of an early-onset genetically mediated form of OCD and tics, and also a familial early-onset anxiety-related form of OCD. A 2016 population-based twin family study with data from the Swedish Twin Registry (n = 20,821) has specifically addressed the proportion of shared genetic and environmental factors underlying the liability to chronic tics, ADHD and OCS [47]. A substantial correlation of 0.45 was found between tics and OCS. Two genetic epidemiological studies of OCS and tics have been carried out in adult twin families at the Dutch Twin Register, of which one study specifically addressed the relationship between tics and OCS [20]. In line with Pinto et al. [47], substantial genetic correlations of 0.37 were found between OCS and tics. Interestingly, tics were mostly influenced by unique environmental factors *un*shared with OCS.

From another line of research, single nucleotide polymorphism (SNP)-based results of genome-wide association studies (GWAS) have been used to identify commonly occurring SNP-based genetic variation and to estimate the heritability of a trait from all measured and imputed SNPs (referred to as SNP-based heritability) across the genome. This method – referred to as genome-wide complex trait analysis (GCTA) – calculates the genetic similarity between individuals based on the measured SNPs, and estimates how much similarity explains their phenotypic similarity. In the bivariate situation, a genetic correlation between traits can be estimated based on the SNP-based information. Results from GWAS of large clinical samples of patients with Tourette's disorder and OCD have been analyzed in this way, and a genetic correlation was found between OCD and Tourette's disorder of 0.41 [24]. Further, for this same group, Yu et al. sought to characterize common genetic variants that were shared among Tourette's disorder and OCD [60]. Although no specific variants were identified, the combined GWAS signals were significantly enriched for functional alleles, suggesting that Tourette's disorder and OCD share a substantial proportion of genetic risk variants [60]. Finally, a 2016 twin-family genetic epidemiological study from our group found, fully in line with these previous findings, substantial genetic correlations of 0.37 between OCS and tics [20].

A remark can be made in light of the fact that within the DSM-5 classification system, Tourette's disorder and OCD have been positioned in two separate categories of disorders; that is, in the neurodevelopmental disorder category (Tourette's) and in the OCD spectrum disorder category (OCD) respectively. Interestingly, Iervolino et al. have argued that a genetic correlation between two disorders under .50 argues in favor of the one disorder being a separate, but related entity as it is currently defined in DSM-5 [61]. With the consistently and repeatedly found significant genetic correlations between Tourette's disorder and OCD, albeit less than .50, this would mean that it would be logical to place both disorders as separate but related disorders within the same category in DSM-5; that is, to place Tourette's disorder within OCD spectrum disorders or OCD within neurodevelopmental disorders. However, other choices have been made.

Comorbidities Between Obsessive-Compulsive Disorder, Hoarding Disorder and Behavior

Between 18% and 42% of patients in clinical and epidemiological studies of OCD report hoarding behaviors, depending on phenotypic definition [62,63,64,65,66], and, conversely, OCD is reported in 12–20% of patients with hoarding disorder [11,67,68,69]. Two studies by Iervolino et al. in a sample consisting predominantly of female twins from the TwinsUK twin registry have specifically examined the genetic and environmental overlap between OCS and hoarding behavior (4459 female twins, mean age of 55.0 years) [61,70]. Forty-five percent of the genetic variance was shared between hoarding and OCS. A 2016 twin study from the Netherlands Twin Register assessed the unique and shared genetic contributions to hoarding behavior and OCS in a sample of 7567 twins (2270 males, 5297 females, mean age of 33.2 years) [20]. The authors found very similar genetic correlations of 0.44 compared with Iervolino et al. (0.45). Further, 42% of the variance in unique environmental factors was shared between OCS and hoarding, and 50.4% of the total *phenotypic* variance between OCS and hoarding was explained by genetic factors.

In DSM-5, hoarding disorder and OCD have been positioned – in contrast to DSM-IV – as separate although related disorders in the category of OCD spectrum disorders. One could argue, according to Iervolino et al., that a genetic correlation between OCD and hoarding disorder of less than .50 argues in favor of hoarding being a separate, but related entity, as it is currently defined in DSM-5. Our data on the relationship between hoarding disorder and OCS support this view.

Cross-Diagnostic Approaches and Their Implications for Classification and Diagnosis

Two studies have performed complex trivariate analyses to investigate shared variance underlying OCD, hoarding and tics [20] and underlying OCS, ADHD symptoms and tics [47]. For the results of the Pinto et al. study [47], see the paragraph above on OCD and ADHD. Zilhão et al. [20] estimated the degree of common and unique genetic factors contributing to the etiology of OCS, hoarding and tics, using data from adult participants in the Netherlands Twin Register. The sample comprised adult monozygotic ($n = 2460$) and dizygotic ($n = 2833$) twin pairs (mean age 33.61 years). A liability threshold model was fitted to the twin data using Mplus, analyzing heritability of phenotypes and of their comorbidity. Genetic correlations were 0.30 between hoarding disorder and OCD, 0.15 between hoarding and tics and 0.25 between OCD and tics. In sum, 31.5–43.0% of the total genetic variance was shared across hoarding, OCD and tics. This means that across these phenotypes, the contribution of genetic factors unique to each phenotype was substantially higher; 0.57 for OCS, 0.61 for hoarding and 0.68 for tics. Strikingly, estimates of the shared environmental factors between OCS–hoarding, hoarding–tics and OCS–tics revealed 0.42 of the environmental variance to be shared between OCS and hoarding, and only 0.04 (4%) between OCS–tics and hoarding–tics. Thus, tics were mostly influenced by specific environmental factors unshared with OCS and hoarding.

Conclusions and Future Directions

Heritability estimates of OCD and its comorbid disorders, based on genetic epidemiological population-based studies, range between .27 and .45, and although there are significant genetic correlations between OCD, tics, ADHD and hoarding, these correlations are variable, being highest between OCD and tics, and between OCD and hoarding, and lower between OCD and ADHD. Strikingly, genetic variance unique to each phenotype contributed more to genetic variance than the shared genetic variance. Our findings do not therefore fully support generalist genes hypotheses stating that, as a result of pleiotropy, the same genes underlie a broad range of developmental mental disorders. Although, based on the studies described above, there is a proportion of shared genetic variance across the studied disorders, the majority of genetic effects are trait specific. These findings have consequences for molecular studies; more genetic variance seems to be shared between OCD and tics and between OCD and hoarding, and thus it seems to make more sense to conduct common molecular genetic studies between these disorders than across, for instance, OCD and ADHD.

A first issue in the estimation of heritability that is only partly understood entails the discrepancies between the lower heritability estimates found in epidemiological twin studies and clinical OCD twin/family studies. Explanations might be a larger amount of measurement error in the epidemiological samples (as a result of retrospective self-report measures used in lifetime trait occurrence) than in clinical samples with the actual disorder. Generally, measurement error adds to inflated estimates of unique environmental influence, and lower heritability estimates. Alternatively, the discrepancy between clinical and epidemiological samples might reflect the fact that, in OCD family studies, it is highly likely that participants with persistent OCD are over-represented, in stemming from families associated with increased genetic load. By contrast, the epidemiological studies may be genetically more heterogeneous, or may represent a group in which environmental factors play a larger role.

A second issue concerns discrepancies between heritability estimates using either statistical estimates (structural equation modeling) compared with SNP-based methods. In general, estimates from SNP-based methods are lower than the genetic epidemiological methods described in this chapter. This is a result of the SNP-based method, which captures only similarities based on SNP resemblance across individuals with a particular trait.

To conclude, we have witnessed remarkable progress in our conceptualization of OCD and its comorbidities in the past few decades. It is now largely agreed that OCD is highly heterogeneous in its phenotypic expression, and mediated by large numbers of common SNPs of small effect, with only limited influences of Copy Number Variants and rare variants. Further, OCD, in contrast to previous assumptions [15,71], only partly shares genetic architecture or environmental risk factors with Tourette's disorder. We expect that OCD will reveal a similar scenario when studied in coherence with other psychiatric disorders such as schizophrenia. Within less than a decade after the first GWAS was published, more than 100 loci were identified in schizophrenia as a result of huge sample sizes (n = 37,000 cases and 113,000 controls) in collaborative GWAS meta-analytic efforts [72]. In the near future, increased sample sizes due to worldwide consortia might equally yield results with respect to gene pathways involved in both disorders.

Finally, the fast development of new genetic techniques to target other genetic variation than common SNPs, will generate new insightful results. These new genetic techniques move beyond variation in the DNA sequence, including among others copy number variations, *de novo* mutations or rare variants and micro-RNAs, methylation and RNA expression, supplemented by pathway and network approaches.

References

1. American Psychiatric Association. *Diagnostic and Statistical Manual of Mental Disorders.* 3rd rev. ed. Washington, DC: APA; 1987.
2. American Psychiatric Association. *Diagnostic and Statistical Manual of Mental Disorders.* 4th ed. Washington, DC: APA; 1994.
3. van den Hout M, Kindt M. Repeated checking causes memory distrust. *Behav Res Ther.* 2003;41:301–316.
4. American Psychiatric Association. *Diagnostic and Statistical Manual of Mental Disorders.* 5th ed. Washington, DC: APA; 2013.
5. Angst J, Gamma A, Endrass J, et al. Obsessive-compulsive severity spectrum in the community: prevalence, comorbidity, and course. *Eur Arch Psychiatry Clin Neurosci.* 2004;254:156–164.
6. Emmelkamp PMG, Bouman TK, Scholing MA. *Angst, fobieen en dwang.* Deventer: Van Loghum Slaterus; 1989.
7. Geller D, Petty C, Vivas F, et al. Further evidence for co-segregation between pediatric obsessive compulsive disorder and attention deficit hyperactivity disorder: a familial risk analysis. *Biol Psychiatry.* 2007, 61:316–321.
8. Langley AK, Lewin AB, Bergman RL, et al. Correlates of comorbid anxiety and externalizing disorders in childhood obsessive compulsive disorder. *Eur Child Adolesc Psychiatry.* 2010;19:637–645.
9. Pallanti S, Grassi G, Sarrecchia ED, et al. Obsessive-compulsive disorder comorbidity: clinical assessment and therapeutic implications. *Front Psychiatry.* 2011;2:70.
10. Storch EA, Larson MJ, Muroff J, et al. Predictors of functional impairment in pediatric obsessive-compulsive disorder. *J Anxiety Disord.* 2010;24:275–283.
11. Mathews CA, Delucchi K, Cath DC, et al. Partitioning the etiology of hoarding and obsessive-compulsive symptoms. *Psychol Med.* 2014;44:2867–2876.
12. Kendler KS. Psychiatric genetics: a methodologic critique. *Am J Psychiatry.* 2005;162:3–11.
13. Pauls DL, Towbin KE, Leckman JF, et al. Gilles de la Tourette's syndrome and obsessive-compulsive disorder. *Arch Gen Psychiatry.* 1986;43:1180–1182.
14. Pauls DL, Raymond CL, Stevenson JM, et al. A family study of Gilles de la Tourette syndrome. *Am J Hum Genetics.* 1991;48:154–163.
15. Pauls DL, Alsobrook JP, Goodman W, et al. A family study of obsessive-compulsive disorder. *Am J Psychiatry.* 1995;152:76–84.
16. Langen M, Kas MJ, Staal WG, et al. The neurobiology of repetitive behavior: of mice ... *Neurosci Biobehav Rev.* 2011;35:345–355.
17. Langen M, Durston S, Kas MJ, et al. The neurobiology of repetitive behavior: ... and men. *Neurosci Biobehav Rev.* 2011;35:356–365.
18. Pertusa A, Fullana MA, Singh S, et al. Compulsive hoarding: OCD symptom, distinct clinical syndrome, or both? *Am J Psychiatry.* 2008; 165:1289–1298.
19. Mataix-Cols D, Frost RO, Pertusa A, et al. Hoarding disorder: a new diagnosis for DSM-V? *Depress Anxiety.* 2010;27:556–572.
20. Zilhao NR, Smit DJ, Boomsma DI, et al. Cross-disorder genetic analysis of tic disorders, obsessive-compulsive, and hoarding symptoms. *Front Psychiatry.* 2016;7:120.
21. den Braber A, Zilhao NR, Fedko IO, et al. Obsessive-compulsive symptoms in a large population-based twin-family sample are predicted by clinically based polygenic scores and by genome-wide SNPs. *Transl Psychiatry.* 2016;6:e731.
22. Zilhao NR, Smit DJ, den Braber A, et al. Genetic and environmental contributions to stability in adult obsessive compulsive behavior. *Twin Res Hum Genet.* 2015;18:52–60.

23. Stewart SE, Yu D, Scharf JM, et al. Genome-wide association study of obsessive-compulsive disorder. *Mol Psychiatry.* 2013;18:788–798.
24. Davis LK, Yu D, Keenan CL, et al. Partitioning the heritability of Tourette syndrome and obsessive compulsive disorder reveals differences in genetic architecture. *PLoS Genet.* 2013;9:e1003864.
25. Nestadt G, Samuels J, Riddle MA, et al. A family study of obsessive-compulsive disorder. *Arch Gen Psychiatry.* 2000;57:358–363.
26. Reddy PS, Reddy YC, Srinath S. A family study of juvenile obsessive-compulsive disorder. *Can J Psychiatry.* 2001;46:346–351.
27. Hanna GL, Himle JA, Curtis GC, et al. A family study of obsessive-compulsive disorder with pediatric probands. *Am J Med Genet B Neuropsychiatr Genet.* 2005;134:13–19.
28. Boomsma DI, Busjahn A, Peltonen L. Classical twin studies and beyond. *Nat Rev Genet.* 2002;3:872–882.
29. van Grootheest DS, Cath DC, Beekman AT, et al. Twin studies on obsessive-compulsive disorder: a review. *Twin Res Hum Genet.* 2005;8:450–458.
30. Carey G, Gottesmann II. Twin and family studies of anxiety, phobic and obsessive disorders. In: Klein DF, Rabkin JG, eds. *Anxiety: New Research and Changing Concepts.* New York, NY: Raven Press; 1981:117–136.
31. Skre I, Onstad S, Torgersen S. A twin study of DSM-III-R anxiety disorders. *Acta Psychiatr Scand.* 1993;88:85–92.
32. Eley TC, Bolton D, O'Connor TG, et al. A twin study of anxiety-related behaviours in pre-school children. *J Child Psychol Psychiatry.* 2003;44:945–960.
33. Hudziak JJ, van Beijsterveldt CE, Althoff RR, et al. Genetic and environmental contributions to the Child Behavior Checklist Obsessive-Compulsive Scale: a cross-cultural twin study. *Arch Gen Psychiatry.* 2004;61:608–616.
34. van Grootheest DS, Bartels M, Cath DC, et al. Genetic and environmental contributions underlying stability in childhood obsessive-compulsive behavior. *Biol Psychiatry.* 2007;61:308–315.
35. Clifford CA, Murray RM, Fulker DW. Genetic and environmental influences on obsessional traits and symptoms. *Psychol Medicine.* 1984;14:791–800.
36. Jonnal AH, Gardner CO, Prescott CA, et al. Obsessive and compulsive symptoms in a general population sample of female twins. *Am J Med Genet.* 2000;96:791–796.
37. van Grootheest DS, Boomsma DI, Hettema JM, et al. Heritability of obsessive-compulsive symptom dimensions. *Am J Med Genet B Neuropsychiatr Genet.* 2008;147B:473–478.
38. Bolhuis K, McAdams TA, Monzani B, et al. Aetiological overlap between obsessive-compulsive and depressive symptoms: a longitudinal twin study in adolescents and adults. *Psychol Med.* 2014;44:1439–1449.
39. van Grootheest DS, Cath DC, Hottenga JJ, et al. Genetic factors underlie stability of obsessive-compulsive symptoms. *Twin Res Hum Genet.* 2009;12:411–419.
40. Zilhão NR, Smit DJ, den Braber A, et al. Genetic and environmental contributions to stability in adult obsessive compulsive behavior. *Twin Res Hum Genet.* 2015;18:52–60.
41. Nestadt G, Samuels J, Riddle MA, et al. The relationship between obsessive-compulsive disorder and anxiety and affective disorders: results from the Johns Hopkins OCD Family Study. *Psychol Med.* 2001;31:481–487.
42. Rickelt J, Viechtbauer W, Lieverse R, et al. The relation between depressive and obsessive-compulsive symptoms in obsessive-compulsive disorder: results from a large, naturalistic follow-up study. *J Affect Disord.* 2016;203:241–247.
43. Saraf G, Paul I, Viswanath B, et al. Bipolar disorder comorbidity in patients with a primary diagnosis of OCD. *Int J Psychiatry Clin Pract.* 2017;21:70–74.
44. Hanna GL, Himle JA, Hanna BS, et al. Major depressive disorder in a family study of obsessive-compulsive disorder with pediatric probands. *Depress Anxiety.* 2011;28:501–508.
45. Hirschtritt ME, Lee PC, Pauls DL, et al. Lifetime prevalence, age of risk, and genetic relationships of comorbid psychiatric disorders in Tourette syndrome. *JAMA Psychiatry.* 2015;72:325–333.
46. Pinto R, Monzani B, Leckman JF, et al. Understanding the covariation of tics, attention-deficit/hyperactivity, and obsessive-compulsive symptoms: a population-based adult twin study. *Am J Med Genet B Neuropsychiatr Genet.* 2016;171:938–947.
47. McKay D, Abramowitz JS, Calamari JE, et al. A critical evaluation of obsessive-compulsive disorder subtypes: symptoms versus mechanisms. *Clin Psychol Rev.* 2004;24:283–313.
48. Geller D, Biederman J, Griffin S, et al. Comorbidity of juvenile obsessive-compulsive disorder with disruptive behavior disorders: a review and a report. *J Am Acad Child Adolesc Psychiatry.* 1996;35:1637–1646.
49. Coskun M, Zoroglu S, Ozturk M. Phenomenology, psychiatric comorbidity and family history in referred preschool children with obsessive-compulsive disorder. *Child Adolesc Psychiatry Ment Health.* 2012;6:36.
50. Geller D, Petty C, Vivas F, et al. Examining the relationship between obsessive-compulsive disorder

and attention-deficit/hyperactivity disorder in children and adolescents: a familial risk analysis. *Biol Psychiatry.* 2007;61:316–321.

51. do Rosario-Campos MC, Leckman JF, Curi M, et al. A family study of early-onset obsessive-compulsive disorder. *Am J Med Genet B Neuropsychiatr Genet.* 2005;136:92–97.

52. Como PG, LaMarsh J, O'Brien KA. Obsessive-compulsive disorder in Tourette's syndrome. *Adv Neurol.* 2005;96:249–261.

53. Jaisoorya TS, Reddy YC, Srinath S, et al. Obsessive-compulsive disorder with and without tic disorder: a comparative study from India. *CNS Spectr.* 2008;13:705–711.

54. Grados M, Riddle MA, Bienvenue J, et al. The familial phenotype of obsessive-compulsive disorder in relation to tic disorders: the Hopkins OCD family study. *Biol Psychiatry.* 2001;50:559–565.

55. Browne HA, Hansen SN, Buxbaum JD, et al. Familial clustering of tic disorders and obsessive-compulsive disorder. *JAMA Psychiatry.* 2015;72:359–366.

56. Nestadt G, Lan T, Samuels J, et al. Complex segregation analysis provides compelling evidence for a major gene underlying obsessive-compulsive disorder and for heterogeneity by sex. *Am J Hum Genetics.* 2000;67:1611–1616.

57. Bolton D, Rijsdijk F, O'Connor TG, et al. Obsessive-compulsive disorder, tics and anxiety in 6-year-old twins. *Psych Med.* 2007;37:39–48.

58. Zilhao NR, Olthof MC, Smit DJ, et al. Heritability of tic disorders: a twin-family study. *Psychol Med.* 2017;47:1085–1096.

59. Yu D, Mathews CA, Scharf JM, et al. Cross-disorder genome-wide analyses suggest a complex genetic relationship between Tourette's syndrome and OCD. *Am J Psychiatry.* 2015;172:82–93.

60. Iervolino AC, Rijsdijk FV, Cherkas L, et al. A multivariate twin study of obsessive-compulsive symptom dimensions. *Arch Gen Psychiatry.* 2011;68:637–644.

61. Frost RO, Hartl TL. A CBT model of compulsive hoarding. *Behav Res Ther.* 1996;34:341–350.

62. Frost RO, Steketee G, Cohn L, et al. Personality traits in subclinical and non-obsessive-compulsive volunteers and their parents. *Behav Res Therapy.* 1994;32:47–56.

63. Lochner C, Kinnear CJ, Hemmings SM, et al. Hoarding in obsessive-compulsive disorder: clinical and genetic correlates. *J Clin Psychiatry.* 2005;66:1155–1160.

64. Rasmussen SA, Eisen JL. Epidemiology and clinical features of obsessive-compulsive disorders. *Psychiatr Clin North Am.* 1992;15(4):743–758.

65. Samuels J, Bienvenu III OJ, Riddle MA, et al. Hoarding in obsessive compulsive disorder: results from a case-control study. *Behav Res Ther.* 2002;40:517–528.

66. Frost RO, Steketee G, Tolin DF. Diagnosis and assessment of hoarding disorder. *Annu Rev Clin Psychol.* 2012;8:219–242.

67. Ivanov VZ, Mataix-Cols D, Serlachius E, et al. Prevalence, comorbidity and heritability of hoarding symptoms in adolescence: a population based twin study in 15-year-olds. *PLoS One.* 2013;8:e69140.

68. Cath DC, Nizar K, Boomsma DI, et al. Age-specific prevalence of hoarding and obsessive compulsive disorder: a population-based study. *Am J Geriatr Psychiatry.* 2017;25:245–255.

69. Iervolino AC, Perroud N, Fullana MA, et al. Prevalence and heritability of compulsive hoarding: a twin study. *Am J Psychiatry.* 2009;166:1156–1161.

70. Pauls DL, Leckman JF. The inheritance of Gilles de la Tourette syndrome and associated behaviors: evidence for an autosomal dominant transmission. *N Engl J Med.* 1986;315:993–997.

71. Ripke S, O'Dushlaine C, Chambert K, et al. Genome-wide association analysis identifies 13 new risk loci for schizophrenia. *Nat Genet.* 2013;45:1150–1159.

Chapter 4

The Molecular Genetics of Obsessive-Compulsive and Related Disorders

Fabiana Barzotti Kohlrausch

Introduction

As in all complex diseases, the genetic susceptibility for major psychiatric disorders, such as schizophrenia or bipolar disorders, is determined by multiple genes with a small to moderate effect impacting on the risk of developing these conditions, genotype–environment interactions and risk behaviors. Further, given its complexity and associated clinical heterogeneity, obsessive-compulsive disorder (OCD) may pose a greater challenge for researchers attempting to link genetics to dysfunctional brain circuits, as OCD may be associated with several distinct genetic abnormalities, multiple dysfunctional brain systems and a plethora of resulting phenotypes [1].

The same difficulty is faced by researchers studying other obsessive-compulsive related disorders (OCRDs), including body dysmorphic disorder (BDD), hoarding disorder, trichotillomania and skin-picking disorder, among others. Fortunately, twin and family studies have all demonstrated the importance of genetic factors in the expression of OCRDs [2,3]. However, what is currently known about the molecular basis of the broad category of OCRDs has been based mostly on studies performed with OCD samples (Figure 4.1). Animal models, linkage studies and family or case–control association studies have all suggested a role for specific genes in the pathophysiology of OCD, but less so in other OCRDs. Therefore, owing to the complexity of OCRDs, many gaps still exist in the knowledge of the genetic basis of these disorders.

Recent Research Findings

Molecular Studies

Molecular studies in multifactorial diseases aim to search for genomic regions or specific genetic variations involved in different human diseases. In this context, there are two main categories of studies: linkage studies and association studies. These studies have been carried out with OCD over at least two decades, and heterogeneous results have been observed.

Linkage Studies

Linkage studies (genome scans) aim to identify chromosomal regions likely to contain susceptibility loci for multifactorial disorders transmitted in families. This approach is an unbiased search of the entire genome, without previous knowledge about the role of specific genes in the disorder. Published genome scans have identified genomic regions associated with OCD phenotype including 1p [4,5], 1q [6], 2p14 [5], 3q [7], 5q13 [5], 6p25 [5], 6q [7], 7p [7], 9p24 [8,9], 10p13 [5], 11p15 [10], 15q [4,7], 16q24 [4], 17p12 [4] and 19p13 [11]. However, these findings have not been replicated, nor did any of these associations reach accepted levels of statistical significance. One study provided suggestive evidence for early-onset OCD linkage on chromosome 10p15 [12].

It is likely that the lack of replication of the genomic regions in all these studies results from different genetic models, variation of the recurrence risk in the families, clinical heterogeneity and ethnicity [13]. As these confounders may have interfered with the results, this information must be interpreted with caution. Concerning non-OCD OCRDs, only hoarding as a symptom has been evaluated in linkage studies, but only in families with OCD members. Samuels et al. [14] identified a region on chromosome 14 linked with compulsive hoarding behavior in families with OCD. Linkage studies are not ideal to detect small- or moderate-effect genes; to this end, the identification of candidate genes by association studies may generate more useful information to elucidate the genetic basis of OCRDs.

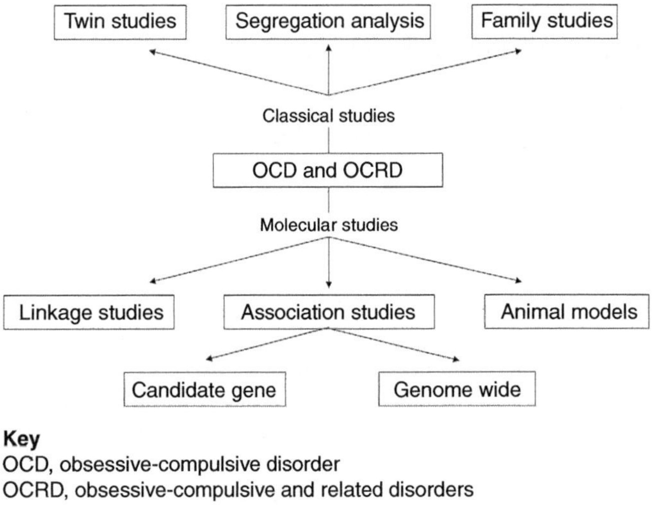

Figure 4.1 Flowchart for unraveling genetic basis of obsessive-compulsive and related dis orders.

Candidate Gene Studies

Candidate gene studies are the most commonly employed for assessing the association between a particular gene (or set of genes) and a psychiatric disorder. The main focus of these studies is the investigation of gene polymorphisms, genetic variations found in more than 1% of the general population. There are several types of polymorphisms, such as duplications, insertions or deletions of nucleotides (INDELS), repeated nucleotide patterns (variable number of tandem repeats and short tandem repeats), copy number variations and single nucleotide polymorphisms (SNPs). SNPs represent a difference in a single DNA nucleotide and are the most common of all polymorphisms in the human genome, occurring once every 300 base pairs on average.

Candidate gene studies in OCD have focused mainly on genes involved in the serotonergic, dopaminergic, glutamatergic and immune pathways, and in neurotrophic and neurodevelopmental processes [2,15]. The anti-obsessional efficacy of serotonin reuptake inhibitors (SRIs) suggests that serotonin might have a role in the pathophysiology of OCD [16]. One of the most promising candidates among the serotonergic genes in OCD is the serotonin transporter (solute carrier family 6 member 4, *SLC6A4*). The last comprehensive meta-analysis evaluating OCD and all previously published polymorphisms confirmed that OCD is associated with polymorphisms of *SLC6A4* (5-HTTLPR), 5-hydroxytryptamine receptor 2A gene (*HTR2A*) and catechol-*O*-methyltransferase (*COMT*; only in males) [17].

The belief that the dopaminergic system may be involved in the pathophysiology of OCD is based on therapeutic benefits of the addition of dopaminergic blockers to the therapeutic regimen of individuals who fail to show adequate responses to SRIs and on the exacerbation of OCD symptoms during use of amphetamine or cocaine [18], among other factors. Dopamine transporter gene (solute carrier family 6 member 3, *SLC6A3*), dopamine receptor genes *DRD2*, *DRD3* and *DRD4*, and genes involved in the catabolic pathways for dopamine (*COMT* and monoamine oxidase A, *MAOA*) were previously evaluated in OCD, but results have been only partially replicated and therefore none of them have been considered strong candidate genes for OCD [2,3].

Studies also suggest that abnormalities in glutamate homeostasis and neurotransmission may be implicated in the pathophysiology of OCD [19,20,21,22]. The glutamate is the main neurotransmitter in the corticostriatal-thalamocortical (CSTC) loops, a group of neurocircuits thought to be critical to the mediation of obsessive-compulsive symptoms. A widely replicated candidate gene, located in a region previously linked to OCD (9p24) [8,9] is the glutamate transporter gene or solute carrier family 1 member 1 (*SLC1A1*). This gene codes for the excitatory amino acid carrier EAAC1 and is highly expressed within the cerebral cortex, striatum and thalamus [23].

However, a 2013 meta-analysis was unable to find sufficient evidence supporting the role of *SLC1A1* in the pathophysiology of OCD [24]. Another glutamatergic gene, glutamate receptor, ionotropic, N-methyl-D-aspartate 2B (*GRIN2B*) is highly expressed in adult brain regions implicated in the pathogenesis of OCD [25] and therefore has been considered a candidate gene for OCD studies. Accordingly, a handful of studies found evidence of an association between OCD and *GRIN2B* [26,27,28,29]. Dysfunction of these proteins due to genetic variations might result in an imbalance between the direct and indirect pathways of the CSTC [30], which contributes to the expression of obsessive-compulsive symptoms.

Additional data suggest that polymorphisms related to gamma-aminobutyric acid, acetylcholine, neurotrophins, myelinization and immunological factors might be associated with OCD or distinct OCD sub-phenotypes [2]. However, many of these results are based on single studies and need further evaluation. Unfortunately, lack of replication, distinct phenotyping methods and small sample sizes negatively affect most candidate gene studies, making it difficult to draw accurate conclusions about the results. However, it is plausible that some of these gene polymorphisms may be specific to obsessive-compulsive symptoms rather than OCD as a whole.

Genome-Wide Association Studies

Genome-wide association studies (GWAS) represent a promising way to study complex disorders. These studies examine hundreds or thousands of SNPs at the same time across the genome, and have already identified strong candidate genes in OCD. The first GWAS performed to identify common variants associated with OCD was conducted by the International OCD Foundation Genetic Collaborative (IOCDF-GC) study. It comprised 1465 patients with OCD, 5557 ancestry-matched controls and 400 trios [31]. The strongest association was detected with SNPs in *DLGAP1*, and near to *BTBD3* and *FAIM2*.

In 2015, the OCD Collaborative Genetics Association Study (OCGAS) performed the second OCD GWAS [32], comprising 1406 patients, 1984 unrelated controls and 460 trios. This study identified a few candidate genes for OCD, such as a marker on chromosome 9, near PTPRD, which promotes the differentiation of glutamatergic synapses and interacts with SLITRK3. However, no SNP was associated with OCD at genome-wide significance level ($P \leq 5 \times 10^{-8}$) [33,34]. Interestingly, 12 signals showed the same associations in both IOCDF-GC and OCGAS analyses, suggesting that a subset of these variants might be truly involved in the susceptibility to OCD.

A more recent GWAS evaluated obsessive-compulsive symptom scores and found four genes (*MEF2BNB*, *RFXANK*, *MEF2BNB-MEF2B* and *MEF*) to be significantly associated with OCD [11]. Since these four genes are in the same chromosomal region, 19p13.11 was suggested to be the susceptibility locus for obsessive-compulsive symptoms. In this study, the authors did not replicate the previous findings reported by Stewart et al. [31] and Mattheisen et al. [32].Two 2016 studies described an exon-based GWAS of OCD samples. Costas et al. [35] evaluated 370 OCD cases and 443 controls from Spain, and concluded that *DNM3* may increase the risk of OCD. This study did not replicate the findings of the two previous GWAS.

Cappi et al. [36] evaluated 20 OCD sporadic trios and identified rare *de novo* single-nucleotide variants. The rate of these *de novo* variants (2.51×10^{-8} per base per generation) was significantly higher in patients with OCD than among unaffected people, using the same platform. By using a protein–protein interaction network analysis, Cappi et al. [36] were also able to find evidence suggesting that these single-nucleotide variants may lead to perturbations of integrated molecular networks implicated in both immunological and neurodevelopmental processes thought to be relevant for the pathophysiology of OCD.

A common characteristic of GWAS is the low power to detect significant association signals for small effect sizes due to limited sample sizes. Therefore, larger collaborative studies should be performed to maximize sample sizes and increase power to detect genome-wide significant associations in OCD and other neuropsychiatric disorders. Indeed, a GWAS with 35,000 cases of schizophrenia identified 108 independent associations in 97 genes [37], showing that increasing the sample size is the best alternative to detect the effect of small risk variants influencing the expression of complex psychiatric disorders.

Animal Models

The study of animal models (e.g., knockout or transgenic mice) for complex psychiatric disorders such as OCRDs is a very valuable tool. Despite intrinsic limitations, such as the inability to reproduce reliably some of the experiences lived by patients with OCD (such as the resistance to obsessions and the feeling of being forced to perform a compulsive behavior), animal models may allow more invasive monitoring of structural and molecular changes associated with

OCD, and an early assessment of the efficacy of novel medications that would be impossible to test in human beings for ethical reasons [38]. Genetic engineering in animals that exhibit both corticostriatal dysfunction and OCD-like behavior supports candidate gene studies in the pathogenesis of OCD [39].

Different animal models of OCD or obsessive-compulsive-like behaviors have been developed. Grooming was the main behavior evaluated in these animals, since excessive grooming may lead to self-injury in mice and to motorically focused OCRDs such as trichotillomania and onychophagia in humans [40,41]. The first mouse genetic model of self-injurious and excessive grooming, resulting in extensive hair loss and skin lesions, was created by the homozygous deletion of *Hoxb8* [42]. *Hoxb8* encodes a member of the Homeobox (Hox) transcription factors (Hoxb8), which has a developmental function in patterning of the anterior–posterior axis [43]. The symptoms can be rescued by bone marrow transplantation from wild-type mice, underlining the importance of this gene in OCD or OCD-like behaviors.

The *Sapap3* knockout mouse may be conceptualized as a model of obsessive-compulsive-spectrum behavior [44], for exhibiting similar behaviors to patients with OCD (such as perseverative grooming phenotype resulting in open skin wounds, and increased anxiety-like behavior) and also showing cortico-striatal glutamatergic transmission abnormalities [45]. These synaptic abnormalities concur with previous results showing that individuals with OCD appear to have dysfunction in this circuit [3,30,46]. Another study has also observed that, unlike corticostriatal synapses, thalamostriatal synaptic activity is not affected [47]. An optogenetic approach to block repetitive compulsive behavior in a mouse model of *Sapap3* deletion, through stimulation of the lateral orbitofrontal cortex in the striatum, resulted in the restoration of the behavioral response inhibition and of the defective downregulation of striatal projection neuron activity [48]. The excessive grooming in *Sapap3* knockout animals was alleviated by subchronic administration of fluoxetine [45].

The *Slitrk5* null mice displayed increased anxiety-like behaviors and elevated grooming resulting in skin lesions and facial hair loss [49]. These animals show dysfunctions in the CSTC circuit implicated in OCD, such as increased orbitofrontal cortex activity, decreased striatal volume and defective corticostriatal transmission. The molecular or cellular processes leading to the grooming phenotype in *Slitrk5* deficient mice remain unclear, but they might also be reversed by chronic treatment with fluoxetine.

Although mice lacking *SLC1A1* do not exhibit altered obsessive-compulsive-like behaviors [50], there are several studies implicating the human *SLC1A1* gene in at least some cases of OCD (as reviewed above).

Cross-Diagnostic Approaches and Their Implications for Classification and Diagnosis

Decades of research in epidemiological and molecular/clinical genetics, and the development of new techniques, have all improved our knowledge of the genetics of OCRDs. Given the current state of knowledge, most candidate genes are involved in brain development or functioning. From the perspective of inheritance, the risk of OCD is significantly higher among relatives of patients with early-onset OCD. In fact, results from a number of independent studies have demonstrated that childhood-onset OCD is more familial than adult onset, and probably more genetic variants are involved in early development of OCD. Additionally, different clusters of symptoms that comprise the OCD phenotype also appear to be heritable. Therefore, it is likely that different genes influence different components of OCD [2]. If genetic tests for OCD become available in the future, perhaps their application will be more effective in the evaluation of these sub-types of OCD rather than for OCD as a single phenotype. It is important to note that genetic counseling provides helpful family guidance and further clarification about biological and environmental factors involved in the development of OCRDs.

To date, the strongest candidate gene in OCD is *SLC1A1*, but the results of the different studies are still contradictory, possibly because of differences across studies and a lack of statistical power. The most recent meta-analysis reported significant associations between OCD and *SCL6A4* (HTTLPR), *HTR2A* and *COMT* (Val166Met; in males) [17]. However, it is important to note that most polymorphisms that have been associated with OCD have also been related to other disorders, such as schizophrenia, depression and bipolar disorder. Thus, it is important to investigate which factors will determine which subjects with these polymorphisms are going exhibit OCD or, alternatively, any other of these conditions.

From the genetic point of view, OCRDs are among the least studied neuropsychiatric disorders. In fact, the genetics of OCRDs could learn from other equally complex psychiatric disorders, such as schizophrenia and bipolar disorders. The International Schizophrenia Consortium, part of the Psychiatric Genomics Consortium, calculated that a composite genetic risk profile score derived from all independent nominally significant associated alleles ($P < 0.05$) captures about 7% of total liability for the disorder in people of European ancestry, and less than 7% in people of non-European ancestry [51]. From the perspective of effect sizes, individuals with higher genetic risk profiles had approximately 4–5 times higher risk of developing schizophrenia than average. Thus, the more variables found by large studies, the more combinations can be made, generating more complete predictions [52].

Despite all progress, success in elucidating the genetic basis of OCRDs will certainly depend on the recruitment of large, carefully and homogeneously phenotyped sets of families, cases and controls; use of advanced genome-wide techniques and methods for the analysis of data, and development of powerful statistical and bioinformatic tools to analyze these types of complex data. The fact that genetic variations are probably related to obsessive-compulsive symptoms rather than to full-blown OCD should also be considered relevant for the classification of OCD, as genetic tests will probably be unable to confirm or refute categorical diagnosis as it is currently conceived. Although age of onset of OCRDs and gender may be under different genetic influences within the larger phenotype of OCD [15], the lack of identification of major gene(s) linked to these variables precludes the application of genetics as a tool in the diagnosis and classification of OCD.

Clinical Implications of Cross-Diagnostic Approaches for Treatment and Prevention

The efficacy of approved drugs in OCD (such as SRIs) is well documented. However, up to 40% of patients do not respond properly to a first SRI trial, which might lead to persistent impairment or even treatment dropout [53,54,55,56]. Decisions about the best treatment to be employed still follow trial-and-error, an approach that submits patients with OCD to ineffective treatments, with a risk of suffering unpleasant or serious adverse effects. The effect of drug treatment depends on several individual factors, which influence the response to treatment in several ways. The observed heterogeneity in drug response results partly from physiological and environmental factors, such as age, gender, ethnicity, hepatic and renal function, diet, concomitant use of different medications, severity and type of illness, alcohol consumption and smoking [57]. However, in some cases, the heterogeneity of the response may not be fully explained by these factors, and genetic factors should be considered as an additional source of response variability.

Genetic variations in patients under pharmacological treatment can substantially influence efficacy and toxicity of drug therapies. Pharmacogenetic approaches provide a new methodology for uncovering the heterogeneity of responses to psychotropic medications, since genetic factors may modify the pharmacokinetic and pharmacodynamic effects of drugs. Pharmacokinetics is the dissemination of a drug in an organism, which depends on absorption, distribution, metabolism and excretion processes, which will ultimately lead to the final plasma concentration of the drug. On the other hand, pharmacodynamics refers to the impact of the drug on the body, which depends on the interaction of the drugs with receptors as well as on the cellular and physiological changes subsequent to this interaction.

Genetic factors influencing antidepressant responses have been well studied in major depressive disorder, but there are few studies searching for genetic predictors of antidepressant response on OCD, not to mention other OCRDs. Since SRI pathways involve the serotonergic system, the most frequently studied gene in OCD pharmacogenetics is the serotonin transporter (*SLC6A4*), particularly the functional promoter polymorphism, HTTLPR [58,59,60,61,62,63,64]. Indeed, the results observed are inconsistent, and the influence of HTTLPR on treatment response in OCD requires further study. Additional serotonergic genetic variants have been suggested to influence antidepressant response in OCD, such as *HTR1B* and *HTR2A* receptor genes [64,65,66]. In terms of polymorphisms involved in other neurotransmitter pathways, *SLC1A1*, *BDNF*, *COMT*, *MAOA*, *C9orf68*, *DLGAP2* and *SLITRK5*, have all been significantly associated with response to different SRIs, mostly in single studies [54,55].

In relation to pharmacokinetic genes, a case report described a relationship between a genetic polymorphism of the *CYP2D6* gene that resulted in impaired drug metabolism and a fluoxetine-related death in a child with attention-deficit hyperactivity disorder, OCD and Tourette's disorder [67]. Another case report described a CYP2D6 poor metabolizer patient with OCD who had high sertraline plasma levels and induction of an epileptic seizure under sertraline treatment [68]. Further association studies failed to detect significant associations between predicted (by polymorphisms) CYP2D6 metabolizer status and plasma levels or response to SRIs in OCD [69,70,71]. However, Brandl et al. [69] observed more failed medication trials in CYP2D6 non-extensive compared with extensive metabolizers, and Müller et al. [71] observed a lack of response and/or occurrence of adverse effects in most poor metabolizer and ultra-rapid metabolizer patients with OCD.

To date, the only GWAS performed in terms of OCD pharmacogenetics evaluated 524 responders and 290 non-responders to SRIs [56]. The top-ranked SNP was located in proximity to *DISP1*, and suggestive signals were found near to *PCDH10*, *GRIN2B* and *GPC6* genes. Enrichment analysis indicated the importance of genes involved in the glutamatergic and serotonergic neurotransmission pathways. As pharmacogenetic studies of antidepressant response in OCD are still scarce and limited by small sample sizes and infrequent assessments of drug plasma levels, most results were not replicated in homogeneous populations, and it may be premature to determine the validity of the previous individual associations of therapeutic response and genetic polymorphisms. However, the development of biomarker tests that can adequately predict the individual risk for SRI response in OCD may potentially improve the therapy in the future.

We must bear in mind that the screening of ethnically diverse populations for the identification of the human genetic variation is also an important bottleneck in pharmacogenetic studies of patients with OCD. For instance, since some polymorphisms are representative or restricted to a single group, the application of some pharmacogenetic data may be restricted to these very specific ethnic groups. Meanwhile, prospective studies are required to contribute to a better understanding of the molecular basis underlying the large interindividual variation in OCD drug treatment response. Genetic predictors can only be used in routine clinical practice after these studies are performed. Actually, pharmacogenetic knowledge and clinical practice have not advanced as rapidly as the corresponding technology, and few applications have been performed to date in disease management and drug development.

Future Directions

Specific genes causing OCRDs have not yet been reliably established. Clinical and etiologic heterogeneity of these conditions, as well as gene–gene and gene–environmental interactions, further complicate the search for genes involved in obsessive-compulsive symptoms. The GWAS findings in OCD have also been frustrating as no specific gene could exceed the minimum threshold for significant association.

All these limitations point to the need to reevaluate the roles of environmental factors in OCRDs and other psychiatric conditions [72]. Environmental factors that may impact the brain development/functions through epigenetic mechanisms and result in psychiatric disorders should be further investigated. To date, individual genetics alone do not respond to the development of these complex psychiatry phenotypes.

A wide variety of diseases, conditions and behaviors have been linked to epigenetic mechanisms, such as cancers, cognitive dysfunction, cardiovascular diseases and neurobehavioral disorders. The term "epigenetics" refers to any process that alters gene activity without changing the DNA sequence, leading to modifications potentially transmitted to daughter cells [73]. Epigenetic mechanisms include DNA methylation, histone modifications, RNA editing and non-coding microRNA (miRNA) interference [74].

Aberrant epigenetic markers in individuals with psychiatric disorders have been detected in gene-specific or whole-genome epigenetic analyses [72]. For example, patients with schizophrenia and/or bipolar disorder showed aberrant DNA methylation in several genes in brain or blood, such as *COMT*, *HTR2A*, *HTR1E*, *DTNBP1*, *NOS1*, *SLC6A4* and others [72,75,76,77,78], aberrant expression of several histone genes [79,80], and increased expression of several miRNAs in postmortem brains [81,82,83]. Unfortunately, the origins of these dysregulations remain to be identified for therapeutic or preventive applications.

In addition to the influence of epigenetics, abnormalities of splicing may also contribute to the etiology of psychiatric disorders. This is important, since the way in which exons are spliced together is a fundamental determinant of protein functions [84]. For example, the *DRD2* gene presents two most common isoforms, $D2_{short}$ and $D2_{long}$, both with essential functions in brain. Perhaps gene polymorphisms may disturb the production of these isoforms, impairing important dopaminergic pathways and contributing to the expression of psychiatric conditions. In fact, Zhang et al. [85] found that two polymorphisms (in intron 6 and 5) were associated with decreased expression of the $D2_{short}$ splice variant, through favored inclusion of exon 6. Additionally, besides disorder-specific alterations, studies have observed splicing abnormalities common to both schizophrenia and bipolar disorder [86].

In the field of OCD treatment, scientific advances are being made in the gene–response connection, and pharmacogenetics has become progressively popular. With the advancement of high-throughput technologies, new dimensions in the search for multiple genes and their expression affecting the response to medication will be generated. These data, when combined with environmental factors that show an impact on treatment response, could be used to construct algorithms for calculating dose adjustments of drugs commonly used in the treatment of OCRDs.

In conclusion, the interaction among epigenetic markers, genome variations and environmental factors makes the study of complex psychiatric diseases even more complex than we expected. However, the advancement of modern technologies such as next generation sequencing might help to combine genetic and epigenetic alterations related to OCRDs, encouraging diagnostic, preventive and therapeutic applications in the future.

References

1. Grunblatt E, Hauser TU, Walitza S. Imaging genetics in obsessive-compulsive disorder: linking genetic variations to alterations in neuroimaging. *Prog Neurobiol.* 2014;121:114–124.
2. Pauls DL, Abramovitch A, Rauch SL, et al. Obsessive-compulsive disorder: an integrative genetic and neurobiological perspective. *Nat Rev Neurosci.* 2014;15:410–424.
3. Browne HA, Gair SL, Scharf JM, et al. Genetics of obsessive-compulsive disorder and related disorders. *Psychiatr Clin North Am.* 2014;37:319–335.
4. Ross J, Badner J, Garrido H, et al. Genomewide linkage analysis in Costa Rican families implicates chromosome 15q14 as a candidate region for OCD. *Hum Genet.* 2011;130:795–805.
5. Mathews CA, Badner JA, Andresen JM, et al. Genome-wide linkage analysis of obsessive-compulsive disorder implicates chromosome 1p36. *Biol Psychiatry.* 2012;72:629–636.
6. Shugart YY, Samuels J, Willour VL, et al. Genomewide linkage scan for obsessive-compulsive disorder: evidence for susceptibility loci on chromosomes 3q, 7p, 1q, 15q, and 6q. *Mol Psychiatry.* 2006;11:763–770.
7. Nestadt G, Samuels J, Riddle M, et al. A family study of obsessive-compulsive disorder. *Arch Gen Psychiatry.* 2000;57:358–363.
8. Hanna GL, Veenstra-VanderWeele J, Cox NJ, et al. Genome-wide linkage analysis of families with obsessive-compulsive disorder ascertained through pediatric probands. *Am J Med Genet.* 2002;114:541–552.
9. Willour VL, Yao Shugart Y, Samuels J, et al. Replication study supports evidence for linkage to 9p24 in obsessive-compulsive disorder. *Am J Hum Genet.* 2004;75:508–513.
10. Wang Y, Samuels JF, Chang YC, et al. Gender differences in genetic linkage and association on 11p15 in obsessive-compulsive disorder families. *Am J Med Genet B Neuropsychiatr Genet.* 2009;150B:33–40.
11. den Braber A, Zilhao NR, Fedko IO, et al. Obsessive-compulsive symptoms in a large population-based twin-family sample are predicted by clinically based polygenic scores and by genome-wide SNPs. *Transl Psychiatry.* 2016;6:e731.
12. Hanna GL, Veenstra-Vanderweele J, Cox NJ, et al. Evidence for a susceptibility locus on chromosome 10p15 in early-onset obsessive-compulsive disorder. *Biol Psychiatry.* 2007;62:856–862.
13. Grisham JR, Anderson TM, Sachdev PS. Genetic and environmental influences on obsessive-compulsive disorder. *Eur Arch Psychiatry Clin Neurosci.* 2008;258:107–116.
14. Samuels J, Shugart YY, Grados MA, et al. Significant linkage to compulsive hoarding on chromosome 14 in families with obsessive-compulsive disorder: results from the OCD Collaborative Genetics Study. *Am J Psychiatry.* 2007;164:493–499.
15. Murphy DL, Moya PR, Fox MA, et al. Anxiety and affective disorder comorbidity related to serotonin and other neurotransmitter systems: obsessive-compulsive disorder as an example of overlapping clinical and genetic heterogeneity. *Philos Trans R Soc Lond B Biol Sci.* 2013;368:20120435.
16. Pittenger C, Bloch MH. Pharmacological treatment of obsessive-compulsive disorder. *Psychiatr Clin North Am.* 2014;37:375–391.

17. Taylor S. Disorder-specific genetic factors in obsessive-compulsive disorder: a comprehensive meta-analysis. *Am J Med Genet B Neuropsychiatr Genet.* 2016;171B:325–332.

18. Melo-Felippe FB, de Salles Andrade JB, Giori IG, et al. Catechol-O-methyltransferase gene polymorphisms in specific obsessive-compulsive disorder patients' subgroups. *J Mol Neurosci.* 2016;58:129–136.

19. Ting JT, Feng G. Glutamatergic synaptic dysfunction and obsessive-compulsive disorder. *Curr Chem Genomics.* 2008;2:62–75.

20. Wu K, Hanna GL, Rosenberg DR, et al. The role of glutamate signaling in the pathogenesis and treatment of obsessive-compulsive disorder. *Pharmacol Biochem Behav.* 2012;100:726–735.

21. Zhu Y, Fan Q, Han X, et al. Decreased thalamic glutamate level in unmedicated adult obsessive-compulsive disorder patients detected by proton magnetic resonance spectroscopy. *J Affect Disord.* 2015;178:193–200.

22. Pittenger C, Bloch MH, Williams K. Glutamate abnormalities in obsessive compulsive disorder: neurobiology, pathophysiology, and treatment. *Pharmacol Ther.* 2011;132:314–332.

23. Arnold PD, Sicard T, Burroughs E, et al. Glutamate transporter gene *SLC1A1* associated with obsessive-compulsive disorder. *Arch Gen Psychiatry.* 2006;63:769–776.

24. Stewart SE, Mayerfeld C, Arnold PD, et al. Meta-analysis of association between obsessive-compulsive disorder and the 3' region of neuronal glutamate transporter gene *SLC1A1*. *Am J Med Genet B Neuropsychiatr Genet.* 2013;162B:367–379.

25. Su AI, Cooke MP,Ching KA, et al. Large-scale analysis of the human and mouse transcriptomes. *Proc Natl Acad Sci USA.* 2002;99:4465–4470.

26. Arnold PD, Macmaster FP, Richter MA, et al. Glutamate receptor gene (*GRIN2B*) associated with reduced anterior cingulate glutamatergic concentration in pediatric obsessive-compulsive disorder. *Psychiatry Res.* 2009;172:136–139.

27. Alonso P, Gratacos M, Segalas C, et al. Association between the NMDA glutamate receptor GRIN2B gene and obsessive-compulsive disorder. *J Psychiatry Neurosci.* 2012;37:273–281.

28. Wu K, Hanna GL, Easter P, et al. Glutamate system genes and brain volume alterations in pediatric obsessive-compulsive disorder: a preliminary study. *Psychiatry Res.* 2013;211:214–220.

29. Kohlrausch FB, Giori IG, Melo-Felippe FB, et al. Association of GRIN2B gene polymorphism and obsessive compulsive disorder and symptom dimensions: a pilot study. *Psychiatry Res.* 2016;243:152–155.

30. Saxena S, Rauch SL. Functional neuroimaging and the neuroanatomy of obsessive-compulsive disorder. *Psychiatr Clin North Am.* 2000;23:563–586.

31. Stewart SE, Yu D, Scharf JM, et al. Genome-wide association study of obsessive-compulsive disorder. *Mol Psychiatry.* 2013;18:788–798.

32. Mattheisen M, Samuels JF, Wang Y, et al. Genome-wide association study in obsessive-compulsive disorder: results from the OCGAS. *Mol Psychiatry.* 2015;20:337–344.

33. Pe'er I, Yelensky R, Altshuler D, et al. Estimation of the multiple testing burden for genomewide association studies of nearly all common variants. *Genet Epidemiol.* 2008;32:381–385.

34. Dudbridge F, Gusnanto A. Estimation of significance thresholds for genomewide association scans. *Genet Epidemiol.* 2008;32:227–234.

35. Costas J, Carrera N, Alonso P, et al. Exon-focused genome-wide association study of obsessive-compulsive disorder and shared polygenic risk with schizophrenia. *Transl Psychiatry.* 2016;6:e768.

36. Cappi C, Brentani H, Lima L, et al. Whole-exome sequencing in obsessive-compulsive disorder identifies rare mutations in immunological and neurodevelopmental pathways. *Transl Psychiatry.* 2016;6:e764.

37. Ripke S, O'Dushlaine C, Chambert K, et al. Genome-wide association analysis identifies 13 new risk loci for schizophrenia. *Nat Genet.* 2013;45:1150–1159.

38. Jones CA, Watson DJ, Fone KC. Animal models of schizophrenia. *Br J Pharmacol.* 2011;164:1162–1194.

39. Burguiere E, Monteiro P, Mallet L, et al. Striatal circuits, habits, and implications for obsessive-compulsive disorder. *Curr Opin Neurobiol.* 2015;30:59–65.

40. Feusner JD, Hembacher E, Phillips KA. The mouse who couldn't stop washing: pathologic grooming in animals and humans. *CNS Spectr.* 2009;14:503–513.

41. Grados M, Prazak M, Saif A, et al. A review of animal models of obsessive-compulsive disorder: a focus on developmental, immune, endocrine and behavioral models. *Expert Opin Drug Discov.* 2016;11:27–43.

42. Greer JM, Capecchi MR. Hoxb8 is required for normal grooming behavior in mice. *Neuron.* 2002;33:23–34.

43. Capecchi MR. Hox genes and mammalian development. *Cold Spring Harb Symp Quant Biol.* 1997;62:273–281.

44. Zike I, Xu T, Hong N, et al. Rodent models of obsessive compulsive disorder: evaluating validity to interpret emerging neurobiology. *Neuroscience.* 2017;345:256–273.

45. Welch JM, Lu J, Rodriguiz RM, et al. Cortico-striatal synaptic defects and OCD-like behaviours in Sapap3-mutant mice. *Nature.* 2007;448:894–900.

46. Menzies L, Chamberlain SR, Laird AR, et al. Integrating evidence from neuroimaging and neuropsychological studies of obsessive-compulsive disorder: the orbitofronto-striatal model revisited. *Neurosci Biobehav Rev.* 2008;32:525–549.

47. Wan Y, Ade KK, Caffall Z, et al. Circuit-selective striatal synaptic dysfunction in the Sapap3 knockout mouse model of obsessive-compulsive disorder. *Biol Psychiatry.* 2014;75:623–630.

48. Burguiere E, Monteiro P, Feng G, et al. Optogenetic stimulation of lateral orbitofronto-striatal pathway suppresses compulsive behaviors. *Science.* 2013;340:1243–1246.

49. Shmelkov SV, Hormigo A, Jing D, et al. Slitrk5 deficiency impairs corticostriatal circuitry and leads to obsessive-compulsive-like behaviors in mice. *Nat Med.* 2010;16:598–602, 1p following 02.

50. Peghini P, Janzen J, Stoffel W. Glutamate transporter EAAC-1-deficient mice develop dicarboxylic aminoaciduria and behavioral abnormalities but no neurodegeneration. *EMBO J.* 1997;16:3822–3832.

51. Schizophrenia Working Group of the Psychiatric Genomics Consortium. Biological insights from 108 schizophrenia-associated genetic loci. *Nature.* 2014;511:421–427.

52. O'Donovan MC. What have we learned from the Psychiatric Genomics Consortium. *World Psychiatry.* 2015;14:291–293.

53. Pigott TA, Seay SM. A review of the efficacy of selective serotonin reuptake inhibitors in obsessive-compulsive disorder. *J Clin Psychiatry.* 1999;60:101–106.

54. Brandl EJ, Muller DJ, Richter MA. Pharmacogenetics of obsessive-compulsive disorders. *Pharmacogenomics.* 2012;13:71–81.

55. Zai G, Brandl EJ, Muller DJ, et al. Pharmacogenetics of antidepressant treatment in obsessive-compulsive disorder: an update and implications for clinicians. *Pharmacogenomics.* 2014;15:1147–1157.

56. Qin H, Samuels JF, Wang Y, et al. Whole-genome association analysis of treatment response in obsessive-compulsive disorder. *Mol Psychiatry.* 2016;21:270–276.

57. Goldstein DB, Need AC, Singh R, et al. Potential genetic causes of heterogeneity of treatment effects. *Am J Med.* 2007;120:S21–S25.

58. Billett EA, Richter MA, King N, et al. Obsessive compulsive disorder, response to serotonin reuptake inhibitors and the serotonin transporter gene. *Mol Psychiatry.* 1997;2:403–406.

59. Denys D, Van Nieuwerburgh F, Deforce D, et al. Association between serotonergic candidate genes and specific phenotypes of obsessive compulsive disorder. *J Affect Disord.* 2006;91:39–44.

60. Di Bella D, Erzegovesi S, Cavallini MC, et al. Obsessive-Compulsive Disorder, 5-HTTLPR polymorphism and treatment response. *Pharmacogenomics J.* 2002;2:176–181.

61. Grunblatt E, Tschakarjan S, Brezinka V, et al. Extraordinarily fast response to low-dose sertraline in a child with severe obsessive-compulsive disorder and high functioning serotonin transporter genotype. *J Child Adolesc Psychopharmacol.* 2014;24:102–104.

62. McDougle CJ, Epperson CN, Price LH, et al. Evidence for linkage disequilibrium between serotonin transporter protein gene (SLC6A4) and obsessive compulsive disorder. *Mol Psychiatry.* 1998;3:270–273.

63. Miguita K, Cordeiro Q, Shavitt RG, et al. Association study between genetic monoaminergic polymorphisms and OCD response to clomipramine treatment. *Arq Neuropsiquiatr.* 2011;69:283–287.

64. Zhang L, Liu X, Li T, et al. Molecular pharmacogenetic studies of drug responses to obsessive-compulsive disorder and six functional genes. *Zhonghua Yi Xue Yi Chuan Xue Za Zhi.* 2004;21:479–481.

65. Corregiari FM, Bernik M, Cordeiro Q, et al. Endophenotypes and serotonergic polymorphisms associated with treatment response in obsessive-compulsive disorder. *Clinics (Sao Paulo).* 2012;67:335–340.

66. Denys D, Van Nieuwerburgh F, Deforce D, et al. Prediction of response to paroxetine and venlafaxine by serotonin-related genes in obsessive-compulsive disorder in a randomized, double-blind trial. *J Clin Psychiatry.* 2007;68:747–753.

67. Sallee FR, DeVane CL, Ferrell RE. Fluoxetine-related death in a child with cytochrome P-450 2D6 genetic deficiency. *J Child Adolesc Psychopharmacol.* 2000;10:27–34.

68. Baumann P, Barbe R, Vabre-Bogdalova A, et al. Epileptiform seizure after sertraline treatment in an adolescent experiencing obsessive-compulsive disorder and presenting a rare pharmacogenetic status. *J Clin Psychopharmacol.* 2006;26:679–681.

69. Brandl EJ, Tiwari AK, Zhou X, et al. Influence of CYP2D6 and CYP2C19 gene variants on antidepressant response in obsessive-compulsive disorder. *Pharmacogenomics J.* 2014;14:176–181.

70. Van Nieuwerburgh FC, Denys DA, Westenberg HG, et al. Response to serotonin reuptake inhibitors in OCD is not influenced by common CYP2D6 polymorphisms. *Int J Psychiatry Clin Pract.* 2009;13:345–348.

71. Muller DJ, Brandl EJ, Hwang R, et al. The AmpliChip(R) CYP450 test and response to treatment in schizophrenia and obsessive compulsive disorder: a pilot study and focus on cases with abnormal CYP2D6 drug metabolism. *Genet Test Mol Biomarkers.* 2012;16:897–903.

72. Mostafavi Abdolmaleky H. Horizons of psychiatric genetics and epigenetics: where are we and where are we heading? *Iran J Psychiatry Behav Sci.* 2014;8:1–10.

73. Weinhold B. Epigenetics: the science of change. *Environ Health Perspect.* 2006;114:A160–A167.

74. Mostafavi-Abdolmaleky H, Glatt ST. Epigenetics in psychiatry. In Roach HI, Bronner F, Oreffo RO, eds., *Epigenetic Aspects of Chronic Diseases.* London: Springer; 2011: 163–174.

75. Abdolmaleky HM, Nohesara S, Ghadirivasfi M, et al. DNA hypermethylation of serotonin transporter gene promoter in drug naive patients with schizophrenia. *Schizophr Res.* 2014;152:373–380.

76. Aberg KA, McClay JL, Nerella S, et al. Methylome-wide association study of schizophrenia: identifying blood biomarker signatures of environmental insults. *JAMA Psychiatry.* 2014;71:255–264.

77. Liu J, Chen J, Ehrlich S, et al. Methylation patterns in whole blood correlate with symptoms in schizophrenia patients. *Schizophr Bull.* 2014;40:769–776.

78. Wockner LF, Noble EP, Lawford BR, et al. Genome-wide DNA methylation analysis of human brain tissue from schizophrenia patients. *Transl Psychiatry.* 2014;4:e339.

79. Sanders AR, Goring HH, Duan J, et al. Transcriptome study of differential expression in schizophrenia. *Hum Mol Genet.* 2013;22:5001–5014.

80. Glatt SJ, Stone WS, Nossova N, et al. Similarities and differences in peripheral blood gene-expression signatures of individuals with schizophrenia and their first-degree biological relatives. *Am J Med Genet B Neuropsychiatr Genet.* 2011;156B:869–887.

81. Banigan MG, Kao PF, Kozubek JA, et al. Differential expression of exosomal microRNAs in prefrontal cortices of schizophrenia and bipolar disorder patients. *PLoS One.* 2013;8:e48814.

82. Beveridge NJ, Gardiner E, Carroll AP, et al. Schizophrenia is associated with an increase in cortical microRNA biogenesis. *Mol Psychiatry.* 2010;15:1176–1189.

83. Perkins DO, Jeffries CD, Jarskog LF, et al. microRNA expression in the prefrontal cortex of individuals with schizophrenia and schizoaffective disorder. *Genome Biol.* 2007;8:R27.

84. Glatt SJ, Cohen OS, Faraone SV, et al. Dysfunctional gene splicing as a potential contributor to neuropsychiatric disorders. *Am J Med Genet B Neuropsychiatr Genet.* 2011;156B:382–392.

85. Zhang Y, Bertolino A, Fazio L, et al. Polymorphisms in human dopamine D2 receptor gene affect gene expression, splicing, and neuronal activity during working memory. *Proc Natl Acad Sci USA.* 2007;104:20552–20557.

86. Zhao C, Xu Z, Wang F, et al. Alternative-splicing in the exon-10 region of GABA(A) receptor beta(2) subunit gene: relationships between novel isoforms and psychotic disorders. *PLoS One.* 2009;4:e6977.

Chapter 5

The Role of Environmental Factors in the Pathogenesis of Obsessive-Compulsive and Related Disorders

Catarina Raposo-Lima and Pedro Morgado

Introduction

Obsessive-compulsive disorder (OCD) is a common and debilitating mental disorder characterized by the presence of obsessions (intrusive and repetitive thoughts, images and/or urges that cause intense anxiety) and compulsions (repetitive motor or mental behaviors driven by the subject to reduce the anxiety triggered by obsessions). OCD is a heterogeneous chronic disease which typically establishes during adolescence or young adulthood. Although OCD was once thought to be primarily psychogenic in origin [1], available evidence indicates that it has a genetic basis [2]. Efforts to search for genes are in progress and many candidate genes have been studied, but results to date have been disappointing and current evidence makes clear that OCD is only moderately heritable. In this chapter, we review what is known about the relative contribution of environmental factors to the etiology of OCD and which factors have been implicated.

Recent Research Findings

Prenatal and Perinatal Factors

Prenatal and perinatal stresses have been advanced as potential risk factors for a number of psychiatric disorders such as schizophrenia, autism, depression and addictive disorder [3,4,5,6]. Although the mechanism remains unknown, this hypothesis has been supported by evidence from animal studies. For example, some studies show that prenatal stress/corticosteroids results in adult behavioral impairments in the progeny of rats, including anhedonia, anxiety-like behavior and drug-seeking [7,8].

Many prenatal and perinatal complications have been studied as potential risk factors for the development of OCD in humans. Examples of these include birth trauma, the use of forceps, prolonged labor, history of illness during pregnancy and lower birth weight, all of which have been associated with an increased risk of OCD [9,10,11]. However, most of these reports are based on small clinical samples and reveal some methodological issues. Advanced parental age, large family size, birth order and birth seasonality have also been studied as potential risk factors for OCD. So far, a clear association between these variables and increased risk of disease has not been established [12,13,14,15,16].

The influence of the reproductive cycle in the onset of OCD has been appraised by a significant amount of studies. OCD onset related to menarche was identified by Alpak and Karamustafalioglu [17] and Labad and colleagues [18,19], with approximately 22% of patients reporting OCD onset in the same year as menarche [18,19]. Most of these findings, however, are based on retrospective self-reported data from small clinical samples. Of note, a study by Gugliemi et al. with a sample of 542 women with OCD found that only 13% of all participants reported the same association [20].

Numerous authors have tackled pregnancy and its relation with the onset of OCD or influence on symptom expression. Retrospective reports of OCD onset during pregnancy vary significantly in number (2.2–39% of participants), mostly at the cost of selection criteria applied and number of participants in the studies [17,18,19,20,21,22,23,24]. Regarding symptom severity during pregnancy in previously diagnosed OCD patients, findings are conflicting: while some authors found pre-existing obsessive-compulsive symptoms (OCS) to worsen during pregnancy, others state an improvement or no change at all [17,18,19,20,21,22,23,24,25].

Considerable evidence shows that recent pregnancy could significantly increase the risk for OCD [26]. Several studies addressing this topic found OCD onset in the postpartum to be frequently reported by participants [17,18,19,20,23,27,28], but only one involved a large clinical sample ($n = 542$) and found this association to be present in only 4.7% of participants [20]. With a sample of 400 non-clinical postpartum women, Zambaldi and colleagues reported that 9% of participants met the criteria for OCD, with approximately 2% having disease onset in the postpartum period [29].

A prospective cohort study by Uguz and colleagues involving 302 women with no prior history of OCD reported a 4% incidence of OCD at six weeks postpartum (12 of 302 participants). Follow-up one year later showed that most of these women had not sought any psychiatric treatment and, of those, 88.9% still met the criteria for OCD [30]. Although these observations resulted from a very small sample (only 11 participants), this may suggest OCS arising postpartum may persist if not treated, which is concurrent with the view of OCD as a chronic disease [31]. Similarly to pregnancy studies, the postpartum period and its impact on symptom severity have also been evaluated [17,18,20,32]. Exacerbation of symptoms was frequently reported by participants, although improvement and no change were also stated.

Little is known about the impact of miscarriage in the onset of OCD [23,33,34]. While some authors reported an increased risk for OCD in women after miscarriage [33], others have found no significant association between these variables [34]. Similarly, limited information exists regarding the prevalence of OCD during menopause. Few retrospective cross-sectional studies based on self-reports indicate prevalence rates of 2.2–9.0% [17,18,20,35].

Thus far, perinatal complications seem to be the most important perinatal factor contributing to increased risk of OCD, though uncertainties remain. Further work is needed to establish solid conclusions and cause–effect associations and future studies should invest effort on gathering larger samples, the use of matched control groups, adequate diagnostic procedures and detailed description of the risk factors under study and its biological consequences; for instance, cerebral anoxia.

Parental Styles

Multiple studies have focused on how distinct parenting styles may influence the risk of developing OCD. Aspects assessed include poor parental care, rejection and overprotection, among others [36,37,38,39]. Although a few authors found an association between some of these characteristics and increased risk of OCD, others report no significant relation between variables.

Parental accommodation to OCD symptomatology (i.e., facilitation by parents of ritualistic behaviors) has also been a line of study, mostly focusing on its relationship with OCS severity and response to treatment. These studies have reported family accommodation to be highly prevalent and to be correlated with symptom severity and functional impairment and to mediate the relation between the two [40,41]. Additionally, family accommodation has been linked to poorer familial functioning and other negative family outcomes [42,43] and to increased incidence of parental psychopathology (mostly OCS) [43,44].

Evidence is so far insufficient to support an association between parenting styles and the risk of OCD, since the majority of studies in this particular field are based on self-reported retrospective data and mostly small non-representative samples. Despite these limitations, the most consistent findings concern parental accommodation and its impact in symptom severity and response to treatment.

Sociodemographic Factors

Studies examining the relationship between socioeconomic status and risk of OCD have conveyed mixed and inconsistent results. While some have found a positive association between low income status and OCD [14,45,46], yet others reached contradictory results, reporting high socioeconomic status to be related with increased risk of OCD [47]. Additionally, some authors have found no significant association between variables [48]. Interestingly, the study by Lihua and colleagues reported an association between higher educational level and lower socioeconomic status and OCD [46]. Other authors, however, have reached different conclusions, reporting lower education and unemployment to be significantly associated with OCD [49].

Stress and Traumatic Life Events

There is a considerable amount of evidence supporting an important contribution of stress in the pathophysiology of neuropsychiatric disorders such as depression, anxiety and addictive disorders [50,51]. The deleterious effect of chronic stress over brain function has been consistently reported by numerous animal studies, describing both structural and chemical abnormalities in a variety of brain structures [52,53,54]. Additionally, stress is known to produce significant behavioral changes in humans and rodents, manifested as memory and behavioral flexibility deficits, hyperanxious states and depressive-like symptoms [54,55,56,57,58].

Systematic research on the role of stress in the pathophysiology of OCD began several decades ago. Up to this date, many studies have reported a positive association between OCD and history of stressful life events [47,59,60]. These may be broadly defined as occurrences likely to result in readjustment, requiring changes in people's usual activities and may include marital separation, family disruption, bereavement, illness or unemployment [61]. Following this line of work, several authors have found OCD onset to be related with an increased number of stressful life events occurring either six or twelve months prior to symptom development [62,63]. On the contrary, one small case–control retrospective study has found no significant difference in the number of previous stressful events in OCD patients relative to controls [27].

History of traumatic events or post-traumatic stress disorder (PTSD) and their association with OCD have also been the focus of numerous studies. Case series on this subject have suggested a link between both disorders [64,65]. Many other studies have pointed in the same direction, by finding elevated rates of OCD and OCS in patients with PTSD [66] or a significant association between OCD and history of childhood trauma [67,68], including sexual abuse [68]. Conversely, results from other research point to an increased rate of PTSD or history of traumatic events in patient with OCD [69], including in a subset of treatment-resistant individuals with OCD [70].

In a cross-sectional study assessing the clinical characteristics of OCD in patients developing the disorder either before or after diagnosis of PTSD, or without PTSD, Fontenelle and colleagues found post-traumatic OCD to be independently related with specific features; for instance, later onset of disease, increased frequency of impulse control disorders (self-mutilation and compulsive buying disorder), history of suicidal thoughts and panic disorder with agoraphobia [71]. Real et al. also reported patients with OCD who experience stressful events at symptom onset to present a distinctive clinical pattern; in this case, a later onset of OCS was found to occur in these individuals compared with participants with OCD and no prior record of stressful events [59].

Regarding symptom severity, some authors have found a positive association with a history of stressful or traumatic events [72], while others have not reached the same conclusion [73]. The literature is scarce on the treatment response in patients with OCD with or without a history of trauma or PTSD, and it remains to be defined whether the findings by Shavitt and colleagues, for instance, who reported no differences in treatment response between groups [74], will be replicated.

Despite all the work in this field, the relationship between OCD and PTSD is not straightforward, given the inconsistency of findings across studies and the limitations of most study designs. Indeed, some authors have reported no significant association between history of trauma and OCD onset [75] nor significantly elevated frequency of traumatic events in adult [76] or pediatric patients with OCD [39], including past history of sexual assault [66]. In this vein, Huppert and colleagues have investigated the relationship between OCD and PTSD symptoms in a sample including healthy controls and patients with PTSD, OCD and other anxiety disorders. The authors found symptoms to be related in all samples and highlighted the hypothesis of a possible overlap in symptoms, which may contribute to inflate the association between OCD and PTSD [77].

There is, however, a considerable number of animal studies that support the notion of stress being an important risk factor for the development of OCD. For instance, chronic stress is able to induce impairments on decision-making processes, biasing behavior toward the adoption of habits in detriment of goal-directed actions, and these effects are associated with a structural reorganization of neuronal circuits involving the medial prefrontal cortex, the orbitofrontal cortex and the dorsal striatum [78,79]. These structures are involved in the control of action selection and decision making processes, and impairments in these areas have been observed in disorders such as drug addiction, impulse-control disorders and OCD [80].

A tendency to shift from a goal-directed to a habit-based pattern of decision making has also been noted in healthy humans exposed to chronic stress [81]. Other experiments have showed that rats exposed to a prolonged period of stress develop a risk-aversive pattern of choices on a rat gambling task [82]. Hence, this stress-induced bias toward habits and the risk-aversive propensity may be important factors in the pathophysiology of compulsivity, a key feature of OCD [83,84].

In summary, results from human studies assessing the role of stress in the pathophysiology of OCD are insufficient to support a clear cause–effect relationship between both variables. More work is needed in this area; specifically, prospective studies involving large representative samples with information regarding treatment status, severity of symptoms, clear and detailed histories of stressful life events and the presence of a control group, to cite a few. Animal models of OCD and studies on the impact of stress on behavior have so far produced interesting and rather consistent results. These studies will be important to clarify the pathophysiological mechanisms and neuronal changes behind OCD and the interplay between specific environmental factors and genetic background.

Brain Injury

Acquired brain injury may present in various forms; for instance, stroke, infection, trauma, tumors, or may result from toxic or metabolic causes [85]. Neuropsychiatric impairments such as anxiety symptoms [86,87], major depression [86,87,88] and attention-deficit/hyperactivity disorder [89], have been described following brain injury, but little is known about the relationship of OCD with brain injury. Most evidence suggesting a link between the two is based on case reports or small case series, especially when considering stroke or brain tumors [90].

Insufficient and inconsistent evidence exists regarding the association between traumatic brain injury and the development of OCD [91]. Most studies have based their findings on retrospective data (some self-reported) and involved relatively small clinical samples. While some authors described a positive association between traumatic brain injury and OCS [78] or new-onset OCD [92], Deb and colleagues found the prevalence of OCD in the traumatic brain injury cohort to be no different than that in the general population [93].

Thus far, there is little information on the association between lesions of specific brain regions and the development of OCD. Grados and colleagues have tried to address this issue and reported medial prefrontal and temporal lesions to be related with new onset OCD in children and adolescents after severe traumatic brain injury [94].

Critically, care must be taken when identifying patients with OCD after traumatic brain injury, since diagnosis may be complicated by other comorbidities such as memory and executive deficits, which may help explain repetitive or perseverative behaviors [95]. Other variables such as severity of injury, type and location of lesion, comorbidities, previous history of OCS, are aspects that need to be included in the analysis, so that cause–effect associations may be more accurately assessed. Accurate diagnosis is key. The *Diagnostic and Statistical Manual of Mental Disorders*, fifth edition, includes the category Obsessive-Compulsive and Related Disorders Due to Another Medical Condition [96], under which these cases may be filed.

Vitamin Deficiency

Vitamin B12 and Folate

Vitamin B12 and folate play important roles in brain metabolism and deficiency of either of these vitamins is known to be associated with a variety of neuropsychiatric manifestations [97]. Unlike other psychiatric disorders, the role of vitamin B12 and folate deficiency in OCD pathology has been insufficiently studied and results in this field have been somewhat inconsistent. Following this line of research, Atmaca and colleagues evaluated serum folate and homocysteine levels in 23 patients with OCD and controls and correlated these with Yale-Brown Obsessive Compulsive Scale (Y-BOCS) scores [98]. Authors found patients with OCD to exhibit lower folate and higher homocysteine levels compared with controls. Serum folate concentrations negatively correlated with Y-BOCS score, while the opposite was described for homocysteine concentration [98].

In another small case–control study, Türksoy and colleagues found elevated homocysteine levels and a higher rate of vitamin B12 deficiency in some patients with OCD. However, the authors of both studies assumed that the small sample size limited well-founded assumptions on the association between vitamin B12, folate or homocysteine levels and OCD [99]. In addition, while data on vitamin B12 and homocysteine levels is consistent between studies [98,99,100], conflicting results regarding serum concentrations of folate in patients with OCD further complicate the picture [100].

Vitamin D

A considerable number of studies have suggested a role for low levels of vitamin D in the pathophysiology of psychiatric disorders such as schizophrenia, autism, depression and anxiety disorders [101,102,103,104]. So far, only one small case–control study has addressed this issue involving pediatric patients with OCD [100]. The authors reported lower vitamin D levels in patients with OCD relative to controls and a significant correlation between these levels and Y-BOCS score. However, the low number of participants and lack of control for other variables limit the ability to generalize conclusions drawn from this work [100]. The role of vitamin D deficiency in the pathophysiology of OCD thus remains to be defined.

Substance Use

OCD is frequently comorbid with other psychiatric disorders, such as depression and anxiety [105], but little is known about comorbidity with substance use disorders and how substance use may increase the risk or influence the clinical course of OCD. A few studies focusing on this matter have reported substance users to be more likely than healthy controls to have OCD [106], while others have found a higher prevalence of substance use disorders among patients with OCD [107]. Despite the large samples involved in most of these studies, the majority are retrospective in nature and thus susceptible to recall bias and some included only patients with substance use disorders, limiting the ability to apply findings to the general population.

Most importantly, considerable quantities of evidence and theories on addiction neurobiology suggest common mechanisms and overlapping neuronal circuits involved in both the pathophysiology of addictive behaviors and OCD [108,109]. It is thus possible that patients with substance use disorders present features of both disorders, such as high levels of impulsivity, and compulsive, repetitive behaviors, while not meeting the criteria for full-blown OCD.

Infections and Immunity

To date, there is a growing number of studies suggesting a possible link between streptococcal infections and the development of OCD and tic disorders in children. This proposed OCD subtype – pediatric autoimmune neuropsychiatric disorders associated with streptococcal infections – was first described by Swedo and colleagues in 1989 and is characterized by a relapse–remitting course of sudden onset and/or exacerbation of OCS associated with neurological dysfunction in children following group A β-hemolytic streptococcal (GABHS) infection [110,111]. The pathological mechanism behind this syndrome is believed to involve cross-reactivity of anti-streptococcal antibodies with basal ganglia tissue (particularly the caudate and putamen) and the rising of anti-streptolysin O levels [112,113].

A variety of studies have focused on the relationship between GABHS infection and OCD. Retrospective studies involving children and adolescents with GABHS infection have found a positive association between history of streptococcal infection and OCD or OCS [114,115]. On the contrary, many other authors have found no significant association between OCD onset or exacerbation of symptoms and GABHS infection [116,117] nor a higher frequency of GABHS infection anteceding OCD development [118,119].

Based on observations suggesting a higher frequency of family history of autoimmune disease in some pediatric neuropsychiatric disorders, Murphy and colleagues have explored the presence of various autoimmune disorders in 107 mothers of children with OCD and reported a higher prevalence of these among study mothers (17.8%) [120]. Despite the limitations of this study – for instance, the absence of a control group and the limited access to medical records – further work focusing on a better characterization of familial history of specific autoimmune diseases may contribute to a better understanding of the impact of maternal autoimmunity on pediatric OCD.

Until now, studies in the field of immunology and OCD have focused on a variety of immunological parameters including the temporal relation with newly acquired GABHS infection, cytokine and chemokine levels, T cell function, the presence of anti-streptococcal and anti-neuronal antibodies, and expression of D8/17 surface antigen on lymphocytes, in an effort to uncover a potential biological marker that could help in identification of cases. Most have produced conflicting results [121,122]. Data regarding plasma or cerebrospinal fluid levels of cytokines are inconsistent, with authors finding either elevated [123,124], lower [125] or normal [126,127] levels compared with controls. The same is true for research assessing T cell function [127,128]. Studies that have explored the presence of anti-streptococcal and anti-basal ganglia antibodies in patients with OCD also led to inconclusive results [129,130].

In conclusion, the existing studies have produced conflicting and inconsistent results, thus not allowing a firm association between infection and risk of OCD.

Cross-Diagnostic Approaches and Their Implications for Classification and Diagnosis

Obsessive-compulsive related disorders (OCRDs) share a neurocognitive model involving endophenotypic deficits in behavioral inhibition underpinned by abnormalities in corticostriatothalamic loops and monoamine (serotonin, dopamine) transmission [83,131]. Development of these brain circuits occurs during the prenatal period and childhood and is influenced by several environmental factors.

Studies on the impact of environmental insults on the pathophysiology of OCRDs, namely pathological skin picking, trichotillomania, body dysmorphic disorder (BDD) and hoarding disorder, are scarce. However, given the clinical observations that stress and anxiety may contribute to an exacerbation of symptoms, most research on this matter has focused on the relationship between the presence of stressful or traumatic events and the development of OCRDs.

In this vein, several authors have described patients with trichotillomania and pathological skin picking to report a higher number of childhood traumatic or negative events compared with healthy individuals [132,133] and studies on hoarding disorder have found past traumatic experiences and hoarding to co-occur commonly [134,135,136]. Studies on BDD are scarce, although the existent literature seems to point in the same direction as to other OCRDs [137].

Regarding disease onset or severity, there is some evidence suggesting a relationship with stressful events in hoarding disorder [135,138,139] and trichotillomania [132].

So far, there is little evidence for shared environmental factors between OCD and OCRDs, and the contribution of other environmental influences in the pathophysiology of OCRDs, such as those we have described in this chapter for OCD, have not been consistently studied. Nevertheless, it is interesting to note how stressful events seem to be related with the emergence of OCD and other OCRDs.

It seems reasonable to hypothesize that stress may act by altering specific brain circuits, most notably the corticostriatothalamic circuits (already implicated in the pathophysiology of OCD), thus contributing to the expression of common symptomatology, such as compulsive, repetitive behavior [78]. It remains to be defined, however, whether there is in fact a common neurobiological mechanism behind OCS in different pathologies, since features such as obsessionality, harm avoidance and compulsive behaviors are shared but differently expressed across these disorders.

Given the symptom fluctuation that is known to occur in OCD, it is possible that other OCRDs may in fact constitute a group of heterogeneous manifestations of a common basic dysfunction. It is thus critical to uncover how genetic vulnerability and environmental insults interact to understand how shared neurobiological models result in different pathologies. On the other hand, OCRDs represent a constellation of exacerbated, otherwise normal, behaviors, suggesting that behavioral responses initially settled as part of a coping mechanism eventually evolve to maladaptive, pathological manifestations. In line with this hypothesis is the finding of features of trichotillomania and pathological skin picking, such as duration or severity of illness, to be negatively correlated with the presence of post-traumatic stress symptoms in patients with those disorders [132,133]. However, how the transition to maladaptive, compulsive behavior occurs, and what exactly is the relationship between stressful events and the development of such self-harming behaviors remain to be defined.

Ultimately, a transdiagnostic approach would allow us to consider not only trichotillomania, pathological skin picking, hoarding disorder and BDD as OCRDs, but also other entities that are characterized by compulsivity, altered behavioral inhibition as well as dysfunctional corticostriatothalamic circuits, namely behavioral addictions such as gambling disorder, compulsive buying behavior, Internet and sexual addictions [131,140].

Clinical Implications of Cross-Diagnostic Approaches for Treatment and Prevention

Bearing in mind the prospect of a common neurobiological basis for OCD and OCRDs, it is reasonable to assume that treatment strategies that successfully control OCD symptomatology could be useful in the management of OCRDs. However, while the use of selective serotonin reuptake inhibitors (SSRIs) has presented somewhat disappointing results in this regard, psychotherapeutic techniques have shown promising outcomes in many OCRDs [141,142,143].

It is possible to hypothesize environmental etiological factors such as chronic stress and traumatic events to be critical in producing important neurobiological dysfunctions, namely over the corticostriatothalamic loops, and that the effects of psychotherapeutic approaches on these circuits are distinct from those produced by pharmacological agents, thus explaining the differences in treatment effectiveness.

Additionally, SSRIs have been the cornerstone in the treatment of OCD but have led to unsatisfactory results in the management of a number of OCRDs [141,142,143]. It could be that exploring novel treatment options, such as modulation of circuits with dopaminergic agents, which have proven interestingly useful in animal models of the disorder, may be the common pathway in the treatment of OCD and OCRDs [82].

Future Directions

There is substantial empirical evidence that several environmental factors contribute to the etiology and pathogenesis of OCRDs. However, as the existing studies have produced conflicting and inconsistent results, more research is needed in this field, particularly prospective studies with clear inclusion criteria and refined methodological approaches. Future animal and clinical studies should combine risk variants of susceptibility genes with several environmental factors such as prenatal and perinatal insults, inflammation and chronic stress. These studies could be useful to identify brain mechanisms involved in the pathophysiology of OCD and OCRDs and may provide novel approaches for prevention and treatment of OCD and related disorders.

References

1. Freud S. *Three Case Histories*. New York, NY: Macmillan; 1909.
2. Taylor S. Etiology of obsessions and compulsions: a meta-analysis and narrative review of twin studies. *Clin Psychol Rev.* 2011;31(8):1361–1372.
3. Koenig JI, Kirkpatrick B, Lee P. Glucocorticoid hormones and early brain development in schizophrenia. *Neuropsychopharmacology.* 2002;27:309–318.
4. Nestler EJ, Barrot M, DiLeone RJ, et al. Neurobiology of depression. *Neuron.* 2002;34:13–25.
5. Gillott A, Standen PJ. Levels of anxiety and sources of stress in adults with autism. *J Intellect Disabil.* 2007;11:359–370.
6. Koob GF. Addiction is a reward deficit and stress surfeit disorder. *Front Psychiatry.* 2013;4:72.
7. Li Y, Li GY, Li LJ, et al. Subsequently enhanced CPP to morphine following chronic but not acute footshock stress associated with corticosterone mechanism in rats. *Int J Neurosci.* 2007;117(9):1237–1255.
8. Rodrigues AJ, Leão P, Pêgo JM, et al. Mechanisms of initiation and reversal of drug-seeking behavior induced by prenatal exposure to glucocorticoids. *Mol Psychiatry.* 2012;17(12):1295–1305.
9. Geller DA, Wieland N, Carey K, et al. Perinatal factors affecting expression of obsessive-compulsive disorder in children and adolescents. *J Child Adolesc Psychopharmacol.* 2008;18:373–379.
10. Cath DC, van Grootheest DS, Willemsen G, et al. Environmental factors in obsessive-compulsive behavior: evidence from discordant and concordant monozygotic twins. *Behav Genet.* 2008;38:108–120.
11. Brander G, Rydell M, Kuja-Halkola R, et al. Association of perinatal risk factors with obsessive-compulsive disorder: a population-based birth cohort, sibling control study. *JAMA Psychiatry.* 2016;73(11):1135–1144.
12. Steinhausen HC, Bisgaard C, Munk-Jørgensen P, et al. Family aggregation and risk factors of obsessive-compulsive disorders in a nationwide three-generation study. *Depress Anxiety.* 2013;30:1177–1184.
13. Chudal R, Leivonnen S, Rintala H, et al. Parental age and the risk of obsessive-compulsive disorder and Tourette syndrome/chronic tic disorder in a nationwide population-based sample. *J Affect Disord.* 2017;223:101–105.
14. Heyman I, Fombonne E, Simmons H, et al. Prevalence of obsessive-compulsive disorder in the British nationwide survey of child mental health. *Br J Psychiatry.* 2001;179:324–329.
15. Brynska A, Wolanczyk T. Epidemiology and phenomenology of obsessive-compulsive disorder in non-referred young adolescents. *Eur Child Adolesc Psychiatry.* 2005;14(6):319–327.
16. Atladóttir HO, Parner ET, Schendel D, et al. Variation in incidence of neurodevelopmental disorders with season of birth. *Epidemiology.* 2007;18(2):240–245.
17. Alpak G, Karamustafalioglu O. Female reproductive cycle events in symptom worsening and onset of obsessive-compulsive disorder. *Eur Neuropsychopharmacol.* 2009;19:S592.

18. Labad J, Menchón JM, Alonso P, et al. Female reproductive cycle and obsessive-compulsive disorder. *J Clin Psychiatry.* 2005;66(4):428–435.

19. Labad J, Alonso P, Segalas C, et al. Distinct correlates of hoarding and cleaning symptom dimensions in relation to onset of obsessive-compulsive disorder at menarche or the perinatal period. *Arch Women's Ment Health.* 2010;13(1):75–81.

20. Guglielmi V, Vulink NC, Denys D, et al. Obsessive-compulsive disorder and female reproductive cycle events: results from the OCD and reproduction collaborative study. *Depress Anxiety.* 2014;31(12):979–987.

21. Williams KE, Koran LM. Obsessive-compulsive disorder in pregnancy, the puerperium, and the pre-menstruum. *J Clin Psychiatry.* 1997;58(7):330–334.

22. Uguz F, Gezginc K, Zeytinci IE, et al. Obsessive-compulsive disorder in pregnant women during the third trimester of pregnancy. *Compr Psychiatry.* 2007;48(5):441–445.

23. Forray A, Focseneanu M, Pittman B, et al. Onset and exacerbation of obsessive-compulsive disorder in pregnancy and the postpartum period. *J Clin Psychiatry.* 2010;71(8):1061–1068.

24. Frydman I, do Brasil PE, Torres AR, et al. Late-onset obsessive-compulsive disorder: risk factors and correlates. *J Psychiatr Res.* 2014;49:68–74.

25. Uguz F, Kaya V, Gezginc K, et al. Clinical correlates of worsening in obsessive-compulsive symptoms during pregnancy. *Gen Hosp Psychiatry.* 2011;33(2):197–199.

26. Russell EJ, Fawcett JM, Mazmanian D. Risk of obsessive-compulsive disorder in pregnant and postpartum women: a meta-analysis. *J Clin Psychiatry.* 2013;74(4):377–385.

27. Maina G, lbert U, Bogetto F, et al. Recent life events and obsessive-compulsive disorder (OCD): the role of pregnancy/delivery. *Psychiatry Res.* 1999;89(1):49–58.

28. Wenzel A, Haugen EN, Jackson LC, et al. Anxiety symptoms and disorders at eight weeks postpartum. *J Anxiety Disord.* 2005;19(3):295–311.

29. Zambaldi CF, Cantilino A, Montenegro AC, et al. Postpartum obsessive-compulsive disorder: prevalence and clinical characteristics. *Compr Psychiatry.* 2009;50(6):503–509.

30. Uguz F, Akman C, Kaya N, et al. Postpartum-onset obsessive-compulsive disorder: incidence, clinical features, and related factors. *J Clin Psychiatry.* 2007;68(1):132–138.

31. Fontenelle LF, Marques C, Mendlowicz MV, Versiani M. Early- and late-onset obsessive-compulsive disorder in adult patients: an exploratory clinical and therapeutic study. *J Psychiatr Res.* 2003;37:127–133.

32. House SJ, Tripathi SP, Knight BT, et al. Obsessive-compulsive disorder in pregnancy and the post-partum period: course of illness and obstetrical outcome. *Arch Women's Ment Health.* 2016;19(1):3–10.

33. Geller PA, Klier CM, Neugebauer R. Anxiety disorders following miscarriage. *J Clin Psychiatry.* 2001;62(6):432–438.

34. Gold KJ, Boggs ME, Muzik M, et al. Anxiety disorders and obsessive-compulsive disorder 9 months after perinatal loss. *Gen Hosp Psychiatry.* 2014;36:650–654.

35. Uguz F, Sahingoz M, Gezginc K, et al. Obsessive-compulsive disorder in postmenopausal women: prevalence, clinical features, and comorbidity. *Aust N Z J Psychiatry.* 2010;44(2):183–187.

36. Aycicegi A, Harris CL, Dinn WM. Parenting style and obsessive-compulsive symptoms and personality traits in a student sample. *Clin Psychol Psychother.* 2002;9(6):406–417.

37. Alonso P, Menchón JM, Mataix-Cols D, et al. Perceived parental rearing style in obsessive-compulsive-disorder: relation to symptom dimensions. *Psychiatry Res.* 2004;127(3):267–278.

38. Yoshida T, Taga C, Matsumoto Y, et al. Paternal overprotection in obsessive-compulsive disorder and depression with obsessive traits. *Psychiatry Clin Neurosci.* 2005;59(5):533–538.

39. Ivarsson T, Saavedra F, Granqvist P, et al. Traumatic and adverse attachment childhood experiences are not characteristic of OCD but of depression in adolescents. *Child Psychiatry Hum Dev.* 2015;47(2):270–280.

40. Bipeta R, Yerramilli SSRR, Pingali S, et al. A cross-sectional study of insight and family accommodation in pediatric obsessive-compulsive disorder. *Child Adolesc Psychiatry Ment Health.* 2013;7:20.

41. Gomes JB, Van Noppen B, Pato M, et al. Patient and family factors associated with family accommodation in obsessive-compulsive disorder. *Psychiatry and Clin Neurosci.* 2014;66(8):621–630.

42. Ferrão YA, Shavitt RG, Bedin NR, et al. Clinical features associated to refractory obsessive–compulsive disorder. *J Affect Disord.* 2006;94(1–3):199–209.

43. Albert U, Bogetto F, Maina G, et al. Family accommodation in obsessive-compulsive disorder: relation to symptom dimensions, clinical and family characteristics. *Psychiatry Res.* 2010;179(2):204–211.

44. Calvo R, Lazaro L, Castro-Fornieles J, et al. Obsessive-compulsive personality disorder traits and personality dimensions in parents of children with obsessive-compulsive disorder. *Eur Psychiatry.* 2009;24:201–206.

45. Moreso NV, Hernández-Martinez C, Val AV, et al. Socio-demographic and psychopathological

risk factors in obsessive-compulsive disorder: epidemiologic study of school population. *Int J Clin Health Psychol.* 2013;13(2):118–126.

46. Lihua M, Tao Z, SiYong H, et al. Obsessive-compulsive disorder in general hospital outpatients: prevalence, correlates, and comorbidity in Lanzhou, China. *Asia Pac Psychiatry.* 2014;6(3):308–318.
47. Valleni-Basile LA, Garrison CZ, Waller JL, et al. Incidence of obsessive-compulsive disorder in a community sample of young adolescents. *J Am Acad Child Adolesc Psychiatry.* 1996;35(7):898–906.
48. Yoldascan E, Ozenli Y, Kutlu O, et al. Prevalence of obsessive-compulsive disorder in Turkish university students and assessment of associated factors. *BMC Psychiatry.* 2009;9:40.
49. Alghamdi HM, Awadalla AW. Sociodemographic and quality of life of patients with obsessive-compulsive disorder: a comparison within Saudi Arabia's population. *Int Neuropsychiatr Dis J.* 2016;6(3):1–15.
50. de Kloet ER, Joëls M, Holsboer F. Stress and the brain: from adaptation to disease. *Nat Rev Neurosci.* 2005;6(6):463–475.
51. Sinha R. Chronic stress, drug use, and vulnerability to addiction. *Ann N Y Acad Sci.* 2008;1141:105–130.
52. Sousa N, Almeida OF, Holsboer F, et al. Maintenance of hippocampal cell numbers in young and aged rats submitted to chronic unpredictable stress: comparison with the effects of corticosterone treatment. *Stress.* 1998;2(4):237–249.
53. Mitra R, Jadhav S, McEwen BS, et al. Stress duration modulates the spatiotemporal patterns of spine formation in the basolateral amygdala. *Proc Natl Acad Sci USA.* 2005;102(26):9371–9376.
54. Cerqueira JJ, Mailliet F, Almeida OF, et al. The prefrontal cortex as a key target of the maladaptive response to stress. *J Neurosci.* 2007;27(11):2781–2787.
55. Mizoguchi K, Yuzurihara M, Ishige A, et al. Chronic stress induces impairment of spatial working memory because of prefrontal dopaminergic dysfunction. *J Neurosci.* 2010;20(4):1568–1574.
56. McEwen BS. Protection and damage from acute and chronic stress: allostasis and allostatic overload and relevance to the pathophysiology of psychiatric disorders. *Ann N Y Acad Sci.* 2004;1032:1–7.
57. Bessa JM, Mesquita AR, Oliveira M, et al. A trans-dimensional approach to the behavioral aspects of depression. *Front Behav Neurosci.* 2009;3:1.
58. Pêgo JM, Morgado P, Pinto LG, et al. Dissociation of the morphological correlates of stress-induced anxiety and fear. *Eur J Neurosci.* 2008;27(6):1503–1516.
59. Real E, Labad J, Alonso P, et al. Stressful life events at onset of obsessive-compulsive disorder are associated with a distinct clinical pattern. *Depress Anxiety.* 2011;28(5):367–376.
60. Rosso G, Albert U, Asinari GF, et al. Stressful life events and obsessive-compulsive disorder: clinical features and symptom dimensions. *Psychiatry Res.* 2012;197(3):259–264.
61. Dohrenwend BP. Inventorying stressful life events as risk factors for psychopathology: toward resolution of the problem of intracategory variability. *Psychological Bulletin.* 2006;132(3):477–495.
62. Khanna S, Rajendra PN, Channabasavanna SM. Life events and onset of obsessive-compulsive disorder. *Int J Soc Psychiatry.* 1988;34(4):305–309.
63. Sarkhel S, Praharaj SK, Sinha VK, et al. Role of life events in obsessive-compulsive disorder. *Isr J Psychiatry Relat Sci.* 2011;48(3):182–185.
64. Sasson Y, Dekel S, Nacasch N, et al. Post-traumatic obsessive-compulsive disorder: a case series. *Psychiatry Res.* 2005;135(2):145–152.
65. Fostick L, Nacasch N, Zohar J. Acute obsessive-compulsive disorder (OCD) in veterans with post-traumatic stress disorder (PTSD). *World J Biol Psychiatry.* 2012;13(4):312–315.
66. Nacasch N, Fostick L, Zohar J. High prevalence of obsessive-compulsive disorder among posttraumatic stress disorder patients. *Eur Neuropsychopharmacol.* 2011;21(12):876–879.
67. Carpenter L, Chung, MC. Childhood trauma in obsessive-compulsive disorder: the roles of alexithymia and attachment. *Psychol Psychother.* 2011;84(4):367–388.
68. Grisham JR, Fullana MA, Mataix-Cols D, et al. Risk factors prospectively associated with adult obsessive-compulsive symptom dimensions and obsessive-compulsive disorder. *Psychol Med.* 2011;41(12):2495–2506.
69. Lafleur DL, Petty C, Mancuso E, et al. Traumatic events and obsessive-compulsive disorder in children and adolescents: is there a link? *J Anxiety Disord.* 2011;25(4):513–519.
70. Gershuny BS, Baer L, Parker H, et al. Trauma and posttraumatic stress disorder in treatment-resistant obsessive-compulsive disorder. *Depress Anxiety.* 2008;25(1):69–71.
71. Fontenelle LF, Cocchi L, Harrison BJ, et al. Towards a post-traumatic subtype of obsessive-compulsive disorder. *J Anxiety Disord.* 2012;26(2):377–383.
72. Vidal-Ribas P, Stringaris A, Rück C, et al. Are stressful life events causally related to the severity of obsessive-compulsive symptoms? A monozygotic twin difference study. *European Psychiatry.* 2015;30(5):309–316.

73. Landau D, Iervolino AC, Pertusa A, et al. Stressful life events and material deprivation in hoarding disorder. *J Anxiety Disord.* 2011;25(2):192–202.

74. Shavitt RG, Valério C, Fossaluza V, et al. The impact of trauma and post-traumatic stress disorder on the treatment response of patients with obsessive-compulsive disorder. *Eur Arch Psychiatry Clin Neurosci.* 2010;260(2):91–99.

75. Grabe HJ, Ruhrmann S, Spitzer C, et al. Obsessive-compulsive disorder and posttraumatic stress disorder. *Psychopathology.* 2008;41(2):129–134.

76. Fontenelle LF, Domingues AM, Souza WF, et al. History of trauma and dissociative symptoms among patients with obsessive-compulsive disorder and social anxiety disorder. *Psychiatr Q.* 2007;78(3):241–250.

77. Huppert JD, Moser JS, Gershuny BS, et al. The relationship between obsessive-compulsive and posttraumatic stress symptoms in clinical and non-clinical samples. *J Anxiety Disord.* 2005;19(1):127–136.

78. Dias-Ferreira E, Sousa JC, Melo I, et al. Chronic stress causes frontostriatal reorganization and affects decision-making. *Science.* 2009;325(5940):621–625.

79. Taylor SB, Anglin JM, Paode PR, et al. Chronic stress may facilitate the recruitment of habit- and addiction-related neurocircuitries through neuronal restructuring of the striatum. *Neuroscience.* 2014;280:231–242.

80. Torregrossa MM, Quinn JJ, Taylor JC. Impulsivity, compulsivity, and habit: the role of orbitofrontal cortex revisited. *Biol Psychiatry.* 2008;63(3):253–255.

81. Soares JM, Sampaio A, Ferreira LM, et al. Stress-induced changes in human decision-making are reversible. *Transl Psychiatry.* 2012;2:e131.

82. Morgado P, Marques F, Ribeiro B, et al. Stress induced risk-aversion is reverted by D2/D3 agonist in the rat. *Eur Neuropsychopharmacol.* 2015;25(10):1744–1752.

83. Burguière E, Monteiro P, Mallet L, et al. Striatal circuits, habits, and implications for obsessive-compulsive disorder. *Curr Opin Neurobiol.* 2015;30:59–65.

84. Gillan CM, Robbins TW, Sahakian BJ, et al. The role of habit in compulsivity. *Eur Neuropsychopharmacol.* 2016;26(5):828–840.

85. Royal College of Physicians and British Society of Rehabilitation Medicine. In Turner L, editor. *Rehabilitation following acquired brain injury: National clinical guidelines.* London: RCP, BSRM, 2003.

86. Schonberger M, Ponsford J, Gould KR, et al. The temporal relationship between depression, anxiety, and functional status after traumatic brain injury: a cross-lagged analysis. *J Int Neuropsychol Soc.* 2011;17(5):781–787.

87. Shafiei E, Fakharian E, Omidi A, et al. Effect of mild traumatic brain injury and demographic factors on psychological outcome. *Arch Trauma Res.* 2016;5(2):e29729.

88. Jorge RE, Robinson RG, Moser D, et al. Major depression following traumatic brain injury. *Arch Gen Psychiatry.* 2004;61(1):42–50.

89. Levin H, Hanten G, Max J, et al. Symptoms of attention-deficit/hyperactivity disorder following traumatic brain injury in children. *J Dev Behav Pediatr.* 2007;28:108–118.

90. Coetzer BR. Obsessive-compulsive disorder following traumatic brain injury: a review. *Int J Psychiatry in Medicine.* 2004;34:363–377.

91. Grados MA. Obsessive-compulsive disorder after traumatic brain injury. *Int Rev Psychiatry.* 2003;15(4):350–358.

92. Silver JM, Kramer R, Greenwald S, et al. The association between head injuries and psychiatric disorders: findings from the New Haven NIMH epidemiologic catchment area study. *Brain Inj.* 2001;15(11):935–945.

93. Deb S, Lyons I, Koutzoukis C, et al. Rate of psychiatric illness 1 year after traumatic brain injury. *Am J Psychiatry.* 1999;156(3):374–378.

94. Grados MA, Vasa RA, Riddle MA, et al. New onset obsessive-compulsive symptoms in children and adolescents with severe traumatic brain injury. *Depress Anxiety.* 2008;25(5):398–407.

95. Coetzer BR, Stein DJ. Obsessive-compulsive disorder after traumatic brain injury: diagnostic issues. *J Cogn Rehabil.* 2003;4:4–8.

96. American Psychiatric Association. *Diagnostic and Statistical Manual of Mental Disorders.* 5th ed. Washington, DC: APA; 2013.

97. Reynolds E. Vitamin B12, folic acid, and the nervous system. *Lancet Neurol.* 2006;5(11):949–960.

98. Atmaca M, Tezcan E, Kuloglu M, et al. Serum folate and homocysteine levels in patients with obsessive-compulsive disorder. *Psychiatry Clin Neurosci.* 2005;59(85):616–620.

99. Türksoy N, Bilici R, Yalçıner A, et al. Vitamin B12, folate, and homocysteine levels in patients with obsessive–compulsive disorder. *Neuropsychiatr Dis Treat.* 2014;10:1671–1675.

100. Esnafoğlu E, Yaman E. Vitamin B12, folic acid, homocysteine and vitamin D levels in children and adolescents with obsessive-compulsive disorder. *Psychiatry Res.* 2017;254:232–237.

101. Crews M, Lally J, Gardner-Sood P, et al. Vitamin D deficiency in first episode psychosis: a case-control study. *Schizophr Res.* 2013;150(2–3):533–537.

102. Mazahery H, Camargo CA Jr, Conlon C, et al. Vitamin D and autism spectrum disorder: a literature review. *Nutrients.* 2016;8(4):236.

103. Anglin RE, Samaan Z, Walter SD, et al. Vitamin D deficiency and depression in adults: systematic review and meta-analysis. *Br J Psychiatry.* 2013;202:100–107.

104. Bičíková M, Dušková M, Vítků J, et al. Vitamin D in anxiety and affective disorders. *Physiol Res.* 2015;64(Suppl 2):S101–S103.

105. Denys D, Tenney N, van Megen HJ, et al. Axis I and II comorbidity in a large sample of patients with obsessive-compulsive disorder. *J Affect Disord.* 2004;80(2–3):155–162.

106. Crum RM, Anthony JC. Cocaine use and other suspected risk factors for obsessive-compulsive disorder: a prospective study with data from the Epidemiologic Catchment Area surveys. *Drug Alcohol Depend.* 1993;31(3):281–295.

107. Blom RM, Koeter M, van den Brink W, et al. Co-occurrence of obsessive-compulsive disorder and substance use disorder in the general population. *Addiction.* 2011;106(12):2178–2185.

108. Fontenelle LF, Oostermeijer S, Harrison BJ, et al. Obsessive-compulsive disorder, impulse-control disorders and drug addiction. *Drugs.* 2011;71(7):827–840.

109. Everitt BJ, Robbins TW. Drug addiction: updating actions to habits to compulsions ten years on. *Annu Rev Psychol.* 2016;67:8.1–8.28.

110. Swedo SE, Rapoport JL, Cheslow DL, et al. High prevalence of obsessive-compulsive symptoms in patients with Sydenham's chorea. *Am J Psychiatry.* 1989;146(2):246–249.

111. Swedo SE, Leonard HL, Garvey M, et al. Pediatric autoimmune neuropsychiatric disorders associated with streptococcal infections: clinical description of the first 50 cases. *Am J Psychiatry.* 1998;155:264–271.

112. Snider LA, Swedo SE. Post-streptococcal autoimmune disorders of the central nervous system. *Curr Opin Neurol.* 2003;16:359–365.

113. Cutforth T, DeMille MM, Agalliu I, et al. CNS autoimmune disease after *Streptococcus pyogenes* infections: animal models, cellular mechanisms and genetic factors. *Future Neurol.* 2016;11(1):63–76.

114. Abadi O, Nazik H, Gurkan K, et al. Group A beta-hemolytic streptococcal infections and obsessive-compulsive symptoms in a Turkish pediatric population. *Psychiatry Clin Neurosci.* 2006;60(1):103–105.

115. Cox CJ, Zuccolo AJ, Edwards EV, et al. Anti-neuronal antibodies in a heterogeneous group of youth and young adults with tics and obsessive-compulsive disorder. *J Child Adolesc Psychopharmacol.* 2015;25(1):76–85.

116. Luo F, Leckman JF, Katsovich L, et al. Prospective longitudinal study of children with tic disorders and/or obsessive-compulsive disorder: relationship of symptom exacerbations to newly acquired streptococcal infections. *Pediatrics.* 2004;113:e578–e585.

117. Leckman JF, King RA, Gilbert DL, et al. Streptococcal upper respiratory tract infections and exacerbations of tic and obsessive-compulsive symptoms: a prospective longitudinal study. *J Am Acad Child Adolesc Psychiatry.* 2011;50:108–118.

118. Mell LK, Davis RL, Owens D. Association between streptococcal infection and obsessive-compulsive disorder, Tourette's syndrome, and tic disorder. *Pediatrics.* 2005;116:56–60.

119. Schrag A, Gilbert R, Giovannoni G, et al. Streptococcal infection, Tourette syndrome, and OCD: is there a connection? *Neurology.* 2009;73(16):1256–1263.

120. Murphy TK, Storch EA, Turner A, et al. Maternal history of autoimmune disease in children presenting with tics and/or obsessive-compulsive disorder. *J Neuroimmunol.* 2010;229(1–2):243–247.

121. Swedo SE, Leonard HL, Mittleman BB, et al. Identification of children with pediatric autoimmune neuropsychiatric disorders associated with streptococcal infections by a marker associated with rheumatic fever. *Am J Psychiatry.* 1997;154:110–112.

122. Inoff-Germain G, Rodriguez RS, Torres-Alcantara S, et al. An immunological marker (D8/17) associated with rheumatic fever as a predictor of childhood psychiatric disorders in a community sample. *J Child Psychol Psychiatry.* 2003;44:782–790.

123. Rao NP, Venkatasubramanian G, Ravi V, et al. Plasma cytokine abnormalities in drug-naïve, comorbidity-free obsessive-compulsive disorder. *Psychiatry Res.* 2015;229(3):949–952.

124. Şimşek Ş, Yüksel T, Çim A, et al. Serum cytokine profiles of children with obsessive-compulsive disorder shows the evidence of autoimmunity. *Int J Neuropsychopharmacol.* 2016;19(8):pyw027.

125. Brambilla F, Perna G, Bellodi L, et al. Plasma interleukin-1 beta and tumor necrosis factor concentrations in obsessive-compulsive disorders. *Biol Psychiatry.* 1997;42:976–981.

126. Carpenter LL, Heninger GR, McDougle CJ, et al. Cerebrospinal fluid interleukin-6 in obsessive–compulsive disorder and trichotillomania. *Psychiatry Res.* 2002;112:257–262.

127. Denys D, Fluitman S, Kavelaars A, et al. Decreased TNF-α and NK activity in obsessive–compulsive disorder. *Psychoneuroendocrinology.* 2004;29:945.

128. Barber Y, Toren P, Achiron A, et al. T cell subsets in obsessive–compulsive disorder. *Neuropsychobiology.* 1996;34:63–66.

129. Dale RC, Heyman I, Giovannoni G, et al. Incidence of anti-brain antibodies in children with obsessive–compulsive disorder. *Br J Psychiatry.* 2005;187:314–319.

130. Gause C, Morris C, Vernekar S, et al. Anti-neuronal antibodies in OCD: comparisons in children with OCD-only, OCD + chronic tics and OCD+PANDAS. *J Neuroimmunol.* 2009;214(1–2):118–124.

131. Robbins TW, Gillan CM, Smith DG, et al. Neurocognitive endophenotypes of impulsivity and compulsivity: towards dimensional psychiatry. *Trends Cogn Sci.* 2012;16(1):81–91.

132. Gershuny BS, Keuthen NJ, Gentes EL, et al. Current post-traumatic stress disorder and history of trauma in trichotillomania. *J Clin Psychol.* 2006;62(12):1521–1529.

133. Özten E, Sayar GH, Eryılmaz G, et al. The relationship of psychological trauma with trichotillomania and skin picking. *Neuropsychiatr Dis Treat.* 2015;11:1203–1210.

134. Hartl TL, Duffany SR, Allen GJ, et al. Relationships among compulsive hoarding, trauma, and attention-deficit/hyperactivity disorder. *Behav Res Ther.* 2005;43(2):269–276.

135. Landau D, Iervolino AC, Pertusa A, et al. Stressful life events and material deprivation in hoarding disorder. *J Anxiety Disord.* 2011;25(2):192–202.

136. Shaw MA, Witcraft SM, Timpano KR. The relationship between traumatic life events and hoarding symptoms: a multi-method approach. *Cogn Behav Ther.* 2016;45(1):49–59.

137. Didie ER, Tortolani CC, Pope CG, et al. Childhood abuse and neglect in body dysmorphic disorder. *Child Abuse Negl.* 2006;30(10):1105–1115.

138. Cromer KR, Schmidt NB, Murphy DL. Do traumatic events influence the clinical expression of compulsive hoarding? *Behav Res Ther.* 2007;45(11):2581–2592.

139. Tolin DF, Meunier SA, Frost RO, et al. Course of compulsive hoarding and its relationship to life events. *Depress Anxiety.* 2010;27(9):829–838.

140. Potenza MN. Neurobiology of gambling behaviors. *Curr Opin Neurobiol.* 2013;23(4):660–667.

141. Walther MR, Ricketts EJ, Conelea CA, et al. Recent advances in the understanding and treatment of trichotillomania. *J Cogn Psychother.* 2010;24(1):46–64.

142. Wetterneck CT, Teng EJ, Stanley MA. Current issues in the treatment of OC-spectrum conditions. *Bull Menninger Clin.* 2010;74(2):141–166.

143. Lochner C, Roos A, Stein DJ. Excoriation (skin-picking) disorder: a systematic review of treatment options. *Neuropsychiatr Dis Treat.* 2017;13:1867–1872.

Chapter 6

Immunology of Obsessive-Compulsive and Related Disorders

Antonio L. Teixeira, Natalia P. Rocha and Andrea H. Marques

Introduction

The role of immune dysfunction in the pathogenesis and pathophysiology of obsessive-compulsive disorder (OCD) has been investigated since the 1980s, when a high frequency of obsessive-compulsive symptoms, tics and other behavioral changes was reported in children with rheumatic (or Sydenham) chorea [1], the neurologic form of rheumatic fever. Rheumatic fever is a well-known autoimmune disorder that develops after children had been infected with the group A beta-hemolytic Streptococcus (GABHS).

Although the most common manifestation of rheumatic fever is carditis, some patients can develop arthritis or chorea: involuntary non-rhythmic movements affecting limb and axial muscles. The mechanism proposed for rheumatic fever pathogenesis is that the immune response against GABHS ultimately damages the heart, the synovia and/or the basal ganglia, due to molecular mimicry between epitopes from these structures and the bacteria.

In the 1990s and early 2000s, there was a great enthusiasm with the autoimmune hypothesis of OCD related to streptococcal infection, and the term "PANDAS", an acronym for *pediatric autoimmune neuropsychiatric disorders associated with streptococcal infection*, was coined. The definition of PANDAS encompasses acute prepubertal onset of OCD and/or tic disorders, possibly related to GABHS, and with a fluctuating course.

Later, when clinical trials with antibiotics and immune-modulatory strategies delivered disappointing results, the interest in the immune basis of OCD decreased. Ironically, at the same time, a growing interest ensued in the investigation of immune mechanisms in other psychiatric disorders, mainly schizophrenia and bipolar disorder [2,3]. This chapter discusses the evidence for immune system involvement in OCD and related disorders, and how this can be translated into clinical practice. First, a brief review on the functioning of the immune system is presented, highlighting a range of physiological roles played by immune mechanisms.

Overview of the Immune System: From a Defense to a Homeostatic System

The immune system is traditionally regarded as a host defense system that protects the individual from invading organisms. In recent years, a great attention has been paid to the role played by the immune system in a series of physiological and pathological conditions not involving protection against infectious agents. Among these conditions, it has been largely recognized that immune mechanisms participate in central nervous system functioning and, as a consequence, in the pathophysiology of neuropsychiatric disorders. This led to the reconceptualization of the immune system as a homeostatic system that works with other regulatory pathways to keep homeostasis.

The immune system is composed of a highly complex network of cells and molecules that are distributed throughout the body. These cells and molecules can be found in lymphoid organs (lymph nodes, thymus, spleen, bone marrow) or circulating in the blood, from where they can reach virtually all organs or structures of the body. The immune response is didactically divided in innate and adaptive. Lymphocytes are major cellular components of the adaptive immune response. They are capable of displaying powerful effector mechanisms that are essential in combating infections. By the same token, lymphocyte activity must be continuously regulated to avoid self-tissue damage.

Lymphocytes originate from hematopoietic cells in the bone marrow and differentiate into distinct lymphocyte types in primary lymphoid organs, expressing different cell receptors. In mammals, B cells are developed in the bone marrow, while T cell progenitors migrate to the thymus to generate mature T lymphocytes. The main populations of mature T lymphocytes are recognized as $CD4^+$ (T helper, Th) or $CD8^+$ (T cytotoxic) T cells.

Lymphocytes expressing receptors with high affinity to self-antigens either suffer programmed cell death or differentiate into regulatory T cells (Treg). Conversely, mature lymphocytes expressing a diverse repertoire of binding potential migrate to secondary lymphoid organs where they are exposed to antigens directly or through antigen-presenting cells. Once stimulated by antigens, lymphocytes may be activated to generate effector responses involving B cell antibody production and/or T cell proliferation and further activation [4]. When activated through the interaction with antigen-presenting cells and their secreted cytokines, $CD4^+$ or T helper lymphocytes can differentiate into independent subsets with distinct effector functions, named Th1, Th2 and Th17 cells.

For many years the brain was regarded as an immune privileged site, meaning that immune responses never or very rarely happened in the brain. However, this view changed significantly with the recognition that immune-associated mechanisms occur in the brain not only as a defense to infection or injury but also contribute to important physiological functions of the central nervous system. Microglia are myeloid cells with phagocytic activity resident in the central nervous system, and have traditionally been seen as innate immune cells mediating inflammatory responses following infection or cellular damage in the brain. Recently, microglia functions have also been recognized to be important for homeostasis maintenance.

The physiological roles played by microglia depend on a dynamic crosstalk among microglia, other glia cell types and neurons, and include synaptic plasticity and neurogenesis. Microglia are key players in the process of eliminating neurons during development as they enter programmed cell death, phagocytizing dead or dying neurons and associated debris. In contrast to their role in promoting cell death, microglia also promote neuronal proliferation and survival. In addition, peripheral immune cells as well as their inflammatory mediators, mainly cytokines, can shape microglia response, influencing their functioning [5,6].

Recent Research Findings

Diathesis–Stress Model: Immune Mechanisms as Mediators of Obsessive-Compulsive Symptoms

The so-called diathesis–stress model, which proposes that the interaction of genetic and environmental factors leads to the development of OCD, is probably the most classic model to explain the disease pathogenesis. Although simplistic and applicable to other major psychiatric disorders, this model provides a framework to test whether different pathogenic factors are involved in OCD. In this context, a dysregulated immune function, either genetically determined or environmentally elicited, could play a role in the emergence of OCD [7].

A 2013 meta-analysis evaluating a total of 230 polymorphisms from 113 genetic-association studies reported that OCD was mainly associated with neurotransmitter-related polymorphisms [8]. Secondary analysis of these data found that other candidate polymorphisms were associated with trophic factors and an immunologic factor, *TNFA* (rs361525) [8]. Interestingly, this single nucleotide polymorphism in the tumor necrosis factor alpha (TNF-α) gene has been linked to OCD and a wide variety of inflammatory conditions [9]. The TNF-α polymorphism was also associated with structural brain changes (i.e., smaller hippocampal volumes) in healthy people [10]. A 2017 study found a higher frequency of HLA-DR4 alleles in early-onset OCD in comparison with healthy subjects, suggesting a role of the immune system in the pathophysiological model of this OCD subgroup [11]. It is worth mentioning that there is considerable amount of evidence indicating different neurobiological underpinnings of early- compared with late-onset OCD. Accordingly, it is possible that immune mechanisms could play a more relevant role in early-onset OCD.

The immune system could also mediate the role played by environmental factors, such as infections, in the pathogenesis of OCD. In the late 1980s, Susan Swedo et al., at the National Institute of Mental Health, observed increased frequency of obsessive-compulsive symptoms in children and adolescents with rheumatic fever [1], a finding that was independently confirmed by other groups [12]. Moreover, OCD and related disorders aggregate more frequently in first-degree relatives of rheumatic fever probands than in healthy controls [13,14]. Polymorphisms of the promoter region of the TNF-α gene have been associated with OCD and rheumatic fever [15,16], indicating that both conditions may share common genetic vulnerability mediated by genes relevant for immune response.

Rheumatic fever is an inflammatory autoimmune disease caused by GABHS. Based on the association between GABHS infection with OCD, an autoimmune model for childhood-onset neuropsychiatric disorders was proposed by Swedo [1,17]. She argued that a subset of childhood OCD and/or tic disorders would be causally related to GABHS infection outside the context of rheumatic fever, the so-called PANDAS. In other words, PANDAS could be regarded as a variant of Sydenham chorea with a unique psychiatric profile and absence of chorea.

However, the concept of PANDAS has been questioned, and its validity is debatable. For instance, patients with PANDAS do not have rheumatic cardiac disease while patients with Sydenham chorea frequently do [18]. Some studies failed to find autoantibodies against the basal ganglia in children with PANDAS [19,20,21]. Regarding the psychiatric profile, OCD and tics can be comorbid, but they are different from both clinical and biological perspectives.

The central feature of PANDAS (i.e., the temporal association between the onset or exacerbation of OCD/tics and a GABHS infection) is even more complicated. A prospective case–control study of children who met diagnostic criteria for PANDAS found that most psychiatric exacerbations in these patients could not be linked to GABHS infection [22]. A second prospective case–control study containing 31 patients with PANDAS and 53 patients with OCD or Tourette's disorder without PANDAS found no group differences in the number of GABHS infections or the number of clinical exacerbations [23]. Moreover, studies with chronic antibiotic prophylaxis against GABHS infection and tonsillectomy/adenoidectomy failed to show significant clinical improvement of either OCD or tics in the context of PANDAS [24]. A recent clinical trial failed to demonstrate superiority of intravenous immunoglobulin therapy over placebo in treating PANDAS [25]. Together, these studies cast doubt on the PANDAS hypothesis.

In a 2015 study, Swedo et al. reviewed 140 cases of PANDAS, showing the predominance of males over females by two to one, early (around 7 years old) and acute onset of OCD symptoms and multiple neuropsychiatric comorbidities, including separation anxiety (more than 85%), sleep problems (more than 70%) and tics (more than 60%) [26]. It is worth noting a subtle change in the way PANDAS were defined with OCD as a core condition, while tics were considered comorbid. More than 20% of the cases from community clinics failed to document GABHS infection, not fulfilling PANDAS criteria, but meeting criteria for "*pediatric acute-onset neuropsychiatric syndrome*" (PANS) [27].

The PANS construct was proposed to encompass a larger category of childhood acute-onset of neuropsychiatric syndromes, not requiring evidence of GABHS infection, and that could have multiple causes (infectious, rheumatologic, neurologic, endocrine, among others). By definition, PANS is characterized by an abrupt onset of OCD or eating disorder (i.e., severely restricted food intake), followed by a series of behavioral symptoms including anxiety, irritability, emotional lability, behavioral regression, and deterioration in school performance [27].

On the basis of conflicting evidence for PANDAS and in line with the concept of PANS, an independent group proposed a broader and alternative concept of "*childhood acute neuropsychiatric symptoms*" (CANS) [24]. In contrast to the PANS definition, a broad list of behavioral symptoms, including obsessive-compulsive symptoms, could indicate CANS. In both cases, PANS and CANS, there is the recognition that acute-onset OCD might have multiple causes beyond GABHS infection.

Other infectious agents have been associated with OCD, such as Borna disease virus and *Toxoplasma gondii*. These infectious agents could determine either direct neuronal and glial damage or activation of an immune response leading to an indirect damage to the brain. *T. gondii* is a ubiquitous protozoan that has been implicated in the pathogenesis of other psychiatric disorders [28]. This parasite has a strong tropism for the central nervous system, especially the basal ganglia.

Miman et al. [29] evaluated the seropositivity for anti-*Toxoplasma* immunoglobulin G antibodies in 42 patients with OCD and 100 matched controls. Seropositivity was significantly higher in OCD (47.6%) in comparison with controls (19%). A cross-sectional study involving 7471 patients confirmed the association between toxoplasmosis and OCD [30]. In this study, patients with positive serology for toxoplasmosis had approximately 2.5 times higher odds of being diagnosed with OCD. Even when the full picture of OCD was not present, the infected patients scored higher on a scale assessing obsessive-compulsive symptoms [30].

Linking Immune Dysfunction to Obsessive-Compulsive Symptoms

Different approaches have investigated whether there is immune dysfunction in OCD, including the study of autoimmunity, the assessment of levels of immune molecules and cells in the blood and in cerebrospinal fluid (CSF), and the study of microglial activity.

Besides emerging in the context of rheumatic fever, OCD seems to be associated with other autoimmune diseases, such as multiple sclerosis and systemic lupus erythematosus (reviewed in Perez-Vigil et al. [31]). However, the evidence linking autoimmunity to OCD is relatively weak, derived mainly from cross-sectional studies with limited sample size and frequently without control groups.

A series of studies has investigated the levels of circulating cytokines in patients with OCD in comparison with controls, with mixed and sometimes opposing results. A meta-analysis of proinflammatory cytokines reported that circulating levels of interleukin 1-beta (IL-1β) are decreased in patients with OCD, while no difference was found in IL-6 and TNF-α levels [32]. In stratified subgroup analysis, moderating effects of age, pharmacological treatment and comorbid mood disorders were noticed. For example, IL-6 levels were high in drug-free adults with OCD, while IL-6 levels were low in children with OCD taking psychotropic drugs. Conversely, IL-2, IL-17A and TNF-α levels were reported to be significantly higher in non-medicated children with OCD compared with age-matched controls [33]. Other psychiatric conditions in children and adolescents, such as mood disorders and schizophrenia, are also associated with altered levels of inflammatory cytokines, undermining the specificity of these findings [34].

Our group showed that adult patients with OCD exhibit increased plasma levels of soluble receptors of TNF-α type 1 (sTNFR1) and type 2 (sTNFR2), and the chemokines CXCL8/IL-8 and CCL3/MIP-1α in comparison with controls [35]. Plasma levels of sTNFR1 (an inflammatory marker highly associated with TNF-α activity) correlated positively with the severity of washing symptoms in our OCD sample, while CCL24/eotaxin-2 (a chemokine commonly released in the context of Th2 skewed immune response) levels correlated negatively with the severity of hoarding.

Very few studies have investigated levels of cytokines in the CSF in OCD, again with mixed results. While Carpenter et al. [36] did not find significant difference in CSF IL-6 levels between adult patients with OCD and controls, Mittleman et al. [37] reported a relative skewing of CSF cytokines toward a Th1 profile in patients with OCD.

Studies evaluating immune cell phenotypes in OCD are also scarce. Marazziti et al. [38,39] reported that patients with OCD show a significant increase of $CD8^+$ (T cytotoxic) and decrease of $CD4^+$ (T helper) T lymphocytes when compared with controls. These changes reversed with clinical improvement after selective serotonin reuptake inhibitor treatment. Accordingly, it was proposed that immunophenotype changes would be state-dependent biomarkers (i.e., markers of the ongoing psychological stress).

Indeed, stress can activate the hypothalamic–pituitary–adrenal (HPA) axis with subsequent release of catecholamines and glucocorticoids capable of modulating the number and function of immune cells. To better understand the involvement of autoimmunity and/or immune dysfunction in OCD, a more comprehensive characterization of phenotype and functioning of immune cells, especially those directly involved in autoimmunity as Treg and Th1/Th17, is needed.

The most studied immune markers in OCD were antibodies, mainly anti-streptolysin O (ASO) and anti-basal ganglia antibodies (ABGA) [40]. For instance, a case–control study comprising 74 patients with OCD and 44 controls with major depression found a higher percentage of positive ASO titers in OCD (16.3 vs. 2.3%), but comparable levels of other autoantibodies, including anti-nuclear, anti-neutrophil cytoplasmic and anti-thyroglobulin [41]. Interestingly, four out of 74 patients with OCD while none of the controls were found to be positive for ABGA. These results led the authors to conclude that the majority of adults with OCD do not seem to have any immune dysfunction [41]. Nevertheless, immune dysfunction could be present in a small subgroup of patients. Corroborating this hypothesis, another study found a higher positivity rate for ABGA (19/96, 19.8%) in patients with OCD in comparison with a group composed of patients with depression and schizophrenia (2/50, 4%). There was no difference in the rates of positivity for ASO between OCD and control groups [42]. Accordingly, ABGA positivity would be a specific finding in a subgroup of OCD in which immune mechanisms could play a pathogenic role.

A meta-analysis of seven case–control studies totaling 844 participants confirmed that a significantly greater proportion of those with OCD were ABGA seropositive compared with various controls (odds ratio, OR, 4.97; 95% CI 2.88–8.55), and remained significant after controlling for different variables such as age, gender, disease severity and duration, among others [43]. Moreover, one study evaluating CSF reported a significantly higher proportion of ABGA positivity in patients with OCD in comparison with healthy controls (OR 5.60; 95% CI 1.04–30.20) [44].

It remains to be established whether ABGA play a direct pathogenic role, are a marker of autoimmunity secondary to basal ganglia lesion or are merely an epiphenomenon found in OCD samples. Another concern is the lack of standardization of laboratory protocols for measuring ABGA, which is partly due to the mixed nature of the basal ganglia antigens implicated in autoimmunity, including lysogangliosides, tubulin, dopamine receptors and neuronal glycolytic enzymes.

While microglia have been implicated in the pathogenesis of animal models of OCD, data addressing its role specifically in human OCD are still scarce [45]. A positron emission tomography (PET) imaging study with [11C]-(R)-(2-chlorophenyl)-N-methyl-N-(1-methylpropyl)-3-isoquinoline-carboxamide ([11C]-(R)-PK11195), a ligand to the translocator protein receptor that is expressed by activated microglia, showed increased binding in bilateral caudate nuclei in Tourette's disorder patients in comparison with controls [46]. Using another translocator protein-binding PET radiotracer, F-18–labeled N-(2-(2-fluoroethoxy)benzyl)-N-(4-phenoxypyridin-3-yl) acetamide ([18F]FEPPA), a study found increased translocator protein distribution volume in the dorsal caudate, orbitofrontal cortex, thalamus, ventral striatum and dorsal putamen of patients with OCD in comparison with controls [47].

The same study [46] also assessed children with PANDAS, reporting increased binding in bilateral caudate and bilateral lentiform nuclei. However, clinical data on these later cases are lacking, being unclear whether they had OCD, Tourette's disorder, or both clinical phenotypes. *Postmortem* analysis of gene expression in the brain from patients with Tourette's disorder confirmed the activation of microglia in the striatum [48]. Further evaluation of microglial activation is definitely warranted in the context of OCD, as this can be regarded as more direct evidence of neuroinflammation.

Cross-Diagnostic Approach and its Potential Implication for Classification

With the considerable amount of evidence of immune involvement in OCD pathogenesis and pathophysiology, the scarcity of studies exploring this subject in OCD-related conditions such as body dysmorphia, hair-pulling (trichotillomania), excoriation and hoarding disorders is surprising. In one of the very few available studies, Carpenter et al. (2002) failed to show altered CSF levels of IL-6 in 26 patients with OCD and 9 patients with trichotillomania in comparison with 26 matched controls [36].

It remains to be established whether obsessions and compulsions – not necessarily fulfilling the diagnostic criteria for OCD or PANDAS – are associated with immune dysfunction. Only a few studies have investigated this possibility.

As discussed above, our group showed that sTNFR1 levels correlated positively with the severity of washing symptoms, while CCL24/eotaxin2 levels correlated negatively with the severity of hoarding in patients with OCD. The interpretation of these results is rather complex, but might suggest that certain subsets of patients with OCD would be more associated with immune dysfunction than others, and different immune mechanisms could be involved. Furthermore, the severity of depression was inversely correlated with CCL3/MIP-1α, CXCL9/MIG and CXCL10/IP-10 levels [35]. Oglodek et al. showed that the chemokines CCL5/RANTES, CCL-2/MCP-1 and CXCL-12/SDF-1 were elevated in patients with anxiety and personality disorders, including obsessive-compulsive personality disorder, in comparison with controls [50].

Tics were related to Sydenham chorea and PANDAS [51,52]. Interestingly, a 2009 study showed that only patients with Tourette's disorder and obsessive-compulsive symptoms, but not the group with Tourette's disorder without these symptoms, had increased plasma levels of IL-12 when compared with controls. In addition, the Tourette's disorder group with obsessive-compulsive symptoms had higher IL-2 levels than the Tourette's disorder group without obsessive-compulsive symptoms [53]. Another study failed to confirm immune activation in children with tic disorders, since serum concentrations of several cytokines and soluble adhesion molecules did not differ between patients and controls. However, serum IL-2 levels were positively correlated with tic severity, while IL-12 levels were negatively correlated with the severity of obsessive-compulsive symptoms [54]. In sum, the issues of the association of obsessive-compulsive symptoms and immune dysfunction/markers, and the validity of an immune subtype of OCD, are still open. If confirmed, immune-based strategies could be indicated for selected cases.

Therapeutic Implications

Immunomodulatory strategies have been investigated for the treatment of OCD. The first trial was conducted by Perlmutter et al. (1999), who enrolled 30 children with severe, infection-triggered exacerbations of OCD or tic disorders (possibly fulfilling PANDAS criteria, which were not available at the time) in a randomized treatment study with plasma exchange (five single-volume exchanges over 2 weeks), intravenous immunoglobulin (IVIG; 1 g/kg daily on 2 consecutive days) or placebo (saline solution given in the same manner as IVIG). At 1 month, the IVIG and plasma exchange groups showed significant improvement in obsessive-compulsive symptoms, anxiety and overall functioning, while plasma exchange also improved tics. Treatment gains were maintained at 1 year [55]. After this controlled trial, several case reports and series confirmed therapeutic benefits of IVIG and plasmapheresis for OCD in the context of PANDAS.

In a 2016 trial, 35 children meeting criteria for PANDAS and moderate to severe OCD were enrolled in a randomized double-blind, placebo-controlled, 6-week trial of IVIG (1 g/kg/day on 2 consecutive days), followed by open-label treatment for non-responders, with follow-up at 12 and 24 weeks [25]. During the double-blind phase, there was a non-statistically significant reduction of the severity of the obsessive-compulsive symptoms in the IVIG group. However, there was a very noticeable improvement of symptoms in the open-label phase, which could be ascribed to expectation bias, the natural course of the condition, or immunomodulatory properties of IVIG [25]. These mixed results indicate the need of a larger trial to evaluate the role of IVIG in the treatment of PANDAS-related OCD. Owing to the equivocal nature of PANDAS, it is important to define diagnostic and prognostic biomarkers able to identify the immune-related OCD subgroup and to predict response to immunotherapy, respectively [49].

On the assumption that unexplained sudden and severe onset of OCD and related disorders may be secondary to infectious agents, a double-blind pilot study assessed the efficacy of azithromycin in the treatment of OCD and associated symptoms in children with PANS. The study found a greater reduction in OCD severity in the azithromycin group compared with the placebo group, with greater tic severity being associated with enhanced treatment response. These results suggest that azithromycin may be helpful in treating children and adolescents meeting the PANS diagnosis, especially those with elevated levels of both OCD and tic symptoms [56].

The efficacy of beta-lactam antibiotics in reducing OCD and/or tic severity was also evaluated. Children with new-onset symptoms receiving cefdinir exhibited notable, albeit non-statistically significant, improvement in tic and obsessive-compulsive symptoms compared with the placebo group. A fully powered study is still warranted to explore the efficacy of cefdinir as a therapeutic tool for CANS/PANS [57].

The use of the cyclooxygenase-inhibitor celecoxib in addition to antibiotic prophylaxis was associated with improvement of tics and pathological behaviors, such as aggression and social withdrawal in a patient suffering from Tourette's disorder. The withdrawal of celecoxib resulted in a marked worsening of symptoms while the reintroduction had positive therapeutic effects [58].

A 2017 retrospective chart review study showed that the oral use of corticosteroids hastened symptom improvement or resolution in patients with new-onset and relapsing–remitting PANS and PANDAS. In addition, when corticosteroids were given earlier in a flare, symptoms improved more quickly and patients achieved clinical remission sooner. Longer courses of corticosteroids resulted in more sustainable responses [59]. These results are in line with previous reports showing that long-term use of corticosteroids was associated with reduction of severity and duration of symptoms in Sydenham chorea [60,61,62]. Not only corticosteroids, but also non-steroidal anti-inflammatory drugs were associated with reduced neuropsychiatric symptom duration in patients with new-onset and relapsing–remitting PANS and PANDAS, when given prophylactically or within 30 days of flare onset [63]. Randomized, placebo-controlled trials are warranted to evaluate both non-steroidal anti-inflammatory drugs and corticosteroids efficacy on PANS symptoms.

Future Directions

Different approaches have shown changes in immune parameters in OCD. The first challenge is to understand the biological meaning of these findings. It is still uncertain whether they represent an inherited or acquired vulnerability, a direct pathogenic player, a reaction to the stressful experience of obsessive-compulsive symptoms, or an epiphenomenon. Genetic studies reported that immune-related genes are associated with OCD, while rheumatic fever provides compelling evidence for the link between OCD and acquired autoimmunity.

As described for other major psychiatric disorders, HPA axis activation due to psychological stress can influence immune function, leading to changes observed across psychiatric diagnoses, especially low-grade inflammation (i.e., increased levels of proinflammatory cytokines, such as IL-6 and TNF-α). If a pathogenic role is confirmed, it is more likely that immune mechanisms are relevant for a subset of OCD. Based on ABGA results, it is reasonable to hypothesize that around 20% of patients with OCD would be part of this immune-related OCD subset. It remains to be established, however, whether this subset differs from other OCD subgroups based on the type (contamination/washing plus symmetry plus harm/checking plus hoarding plus sexual or religious obsessions) or severity of obsessive-compulsive symptoms, and psychiatric and neurological comorbidity. It is possible that early-onset or pediatric patients with OCD would be more represented in this immune-related subset. It is also uncertain whether subclinical obsessive-compulsive symptoms are more related to immune dysfunction/biomarkers than other symptomatic dimensions, such as depression, mania or psychosis.

Besides ABGA – which have several methodological problems with their measurement – other immune biomarkers, such as proinflammatory cytokines and C-reactive protein, could be used for identifying these immune-related patients with OCD. This would be a true step forward in precision medicine for OCD. A related move would be the evaluation of these patients' clinical outcomes after standard pharmacological and psychological treatments, and their eligibility for immune-based strategies.

Approximately 40–65% of patients with OCD have a response to a selective serotonin reuptake inhibitor or clomipramine, a number that can increase with cognitive behavioral therapy. Early-onset OCD, coexisting tics and hoarding symptoms have been associated with a poor response to pharmacological treatment [64]. Interestingly, two of these conditions (i.e., early onset and tic comorbidity) are present in the PANDAS hypothesis, and are possibly overrepresented in an immune-related OCD subset, as suggested above. Other OCD related disorders also deserve further investigation.

References

1. Swedo SE, Rapoport JL, Cheslow DL, et al. High prevalence of obsessive-compulsive symptoms in patients with Sydenham's chorea. *Am J Psychiatry.* 1989;146(2):246–249.
2. Barbosa IG, Machado-Vieira R, Soares JC, Teixeira AL. The immunology of bipolar disorder. *Neuroimmunomodulation.* 2014;21(2–3):117–122.
3. Khandaker GM, Dantzer R, Jones PB. Immunopsychiatry: important facts. *Psychol Med.* 2017:1–9.
4. Olsen Saraiva Camara N, Lepique AP, Basso AS. Lymphocyte differentiation and effector functions. *Clin Dev Immunol.* 2012;2012:510603.
5. Ziv Y, Ron N, Butovsky O, et al. Immune cells contribute to the maintenance of neurogenesis and spatial learning abilities in adulthood. *Nat Neurosci.* 2006;9(2):268–275.
6. de Miranda AS, Zhang CJ, Katsumoto A, Teixeira AL. Hippocampal adult neurogenesis: does the immune system matter? *J Neurol Sci.* 2017;372:482–495.
7. Teixeira AL, Rodrigues DH, Marques AH, Miguel EC, Fontenelle LF. Searching for the immune basis of obsessive-compulsive disorder. *Neuroimmunomodulation.* 2014;21(2–3):152–158.
8. Taylor S. Molecular genetics of obsessive-compulsive disorder: a comprehensive meta-analysis of genetic association studies. *Mol Psychiatry.* 2013;18(7):799–805.
9. Jia Y, Qin HJ, Zhang JX, Liu XL, Li LJ. Association of the tumour necrosis factor-alpha polymorphisms rs361525 and rs1800629 with susceptibility to psoriasis: a meta-analysis. *Clin Exp Dermatol.* 2013;38(8):836–844.

10. Baune BT, Konrad C, Grotegerd D, et al. Tumor necrosis factor gene variation predicts hippocampus volume in healthy individuals. *Biol Psychiatry.* 2012;72(8):655–662.

11. Rodriguez N, Morer A, Gonzalez-Navarro EA, et al. Human-leukocyte antigen class II genes in early-onset obsessive-compulsive disorder. *World J Biol Psychiatry.* 2017:1–7.

12. Maia DP, Teixeira AL, Jr, Quintao Cunningham MC, Cardoso F. Obsessive compulsive behavior, hyperactivity, and attention deficit disorder in Sydenham chorea. *Neurology.* 2005;64(10):1799–1801.

13. Hounie AG, Pauls DL, do Rosario-Campos MC, et al. Obsessive-compulsive spectrum disorders and rheumatic fever: a family study. *Biol Psychiatry.* 2007;61(3):266–272.

14. Seixas AA, Hounie AG, Fossaluza V, et al. Anxiety disorders and rheumatic fever: is there an association? *CNS Spectr.* 2008;13(12):1039–1046.

15. Ramasawmy R, Fae KC, Spina G, et al. Association of polymorphisms within the promoter region of the tumor necrosis factor-alpha with clinical outcomes of rheumatic fever. *Mol Immunol.* 2007;44(8):1873–1878.

16. Hounie AG, Cappi C, Cordeiro Q, et al. TNF-alpha polymorphisms are associated with obsessive-compulsive disorder. *Neurosci Lett.* 2008;442(2):86–90.

17. Swedo SE, Leonard HL, Rapoport JL. The pediatric autoimmune neuropsychiatric disorders associated with streptococcal infection (PANDAS) subgroup: separating fact from fiction. *Pediatrics.* 2004;113(4):907–911.

18. Snider LA, Sachdev V, Mackaronis JE, St Peter M, Swedo SE. Echocardiographic findings in the PANDAS subgroup. *Pediatrics.* 2004;114(6): e748–e751.

19. Singer HS, Hong JJ, Yoon DY, Williams PN. Serum autoantibodies do not differentiate PANDAS and Tourette syndrome from controls. *Neurology.* 2005;65(11):1701–1707.

20. Brilot F, Merheb V, Ding A, Murphy T, Dale RC. Antibody binding to neuronal surface in Sydenham chorea, but not in PANDAS or Tourette syndrome. *Neurology.* 2011;76(17):1508–1513.

21. Morris CM, Pardo-Villamizar C, Gause CD, Singer HS. Serum autoantibodies measured by immunofluorescence confirm a failure to differentiate PANDAS and Tourette syndrome from controls. *J Neurol Sci.* 2009;276(1–2):45–48.

22. Kurlan R, Johnson D, Kaplan EL. Tourette Syndrome Study G. Streptococcal infection and exacerbations of childhood tics and obsessive-compulsive symptoms: a prospective blinded cohort study. *Pediatrics.* 2008;121(6):1188–1197.

23. Leckman JF, King RA, Gilbert DL, et al. Streptococcal upper respiratory tract infections and exacerbations of tic and obsessive-compulsive symptoms: a prospective longitudinal study. *J Am Acad Child Adolesc Psychiatry.* 2011;50(2):108–118.e3.

24. Singer HS, Gilbert DL, Wolf DS, Mink JW, Kurlan R. Moving from PANDAS to CANS. *J Pediatr.* 2012;160(5):725–731.

25. Williams KA, Swedo SE, Farmer CA, et al. Randomized, controlled trial of intravenous immunoglobulin for pediatric autoimmune neuropsychiatric disorders associated with streptococcal infections. *J Am Acad Child Adolesc Psychiatry.* 2016;55(10):860–867.e2.

26. Swedo SE, Seidlitz J, Kovacevic M, et al. Clinical presentation of pediatric autoimmune neuropsychiatric disorders associated with streptococcal infections in research and community settings. *J Child Adolesc Psychopharmacol.* 2015;25(1):26–30.

27. Chang K, Frankovich J, Cooperstock M, et al. Clinical evaluation of youth with pediatric acute-onset neuropsychiatric syndrome (PANS): recommendations from the 2013 PANS Consensus Conference. *J Child Adolesc Psychopharmacol.* 2015;25(1):3–13.

28. de Barros JL, Barbosa IG, Salem H, et al. Is there any association between *Toxoplasma gondii* infection and bipolar disorder? A systematic review and meta-analysis. *J Affect Disord.* 2017;209:59–65.

29. Miman O, Mutlu EA, Ozcan O, Atambay M, Karlidag R, Unal S. Is there any role of *Toxoplasma gondii* in the etiology of obsessive-compulsive disorder? *Psychiatry Res.* 2010;177(1–2):263–265.

30. Flegr J, Horacek J. Toxoplasma-infected subjects report an obsessive-compulsive disorder diagnosis more often and score higher in obsessive-compulsive inventory. *Eur Psychiatry.* 2017;40:82–87.

31. Perez-Vigil A, Fernandez de la Cruz L, Brander G, Isomura K, Gromark C, Mataix-Cols D. The link between autoimmune diseases and obsessive-compulsive and tic disorders: a systematic review. *Neurosci Biobehav Rev.* 2016;71:542–562.

32. Gray SM, Bloch MH. Systematic review of proinflammatory cytokines in obsessive-compulsive disorder. *Curr Psychiatry Rep.* 2012;14(3):220–228.

33. Simsek S, Yuksel T, Cim A, Kaya S. Serum cytokine profiles of children with obsessive-compulsive disorder shows the evidence of autoimmunity. *Int J Neuropsychopharmacol.* 2016;19(8):pii: pyw027.

34. Mitchell RH, Goldstein BI. Inflammation in children and adolescents with neuropsychiatric disorders: a systematic review. *J Am Acad Child Adolesc Psychiatry.* 2014;53(3):274–296.

35. Fontenelle LF, Barbosa IG, Luna JV, de Sousa LP, Abreu MN, Teixeira AL. A cytokine study of adult patients with obsessive-compulsive disorder. *Compr Psychiatry.* 2012;53(6):797–804.

36. Carpenter LL, Heninger GR, McDougle CJ, Tyrka AR, Epperson CN, Price LH. Cerebrospinal fluid interleukin-6 in obsessive-compulsive disorder and trichotillomania. *Psychiatry Res.* 2002;112(3):257–262.

37. Mittleman BB, Castellanos FX, Jacobsen LK, Rapoport JL, Swedo SE, Shearer GM. Cerebrospinal fluid cytokines in pediatric neuropsychiatric disease. *J Immunol.* 1997;159(6):2994–2999.

38. Marazziti D, Presta S, Pfanner C, et al. Immunological alterations in adult obsessive-compulsive disorder. *Biol Psychiatry.* 1999;46(6):810–814.

39. Marazziti D, Mungai F, Masala I, et al. Normalisation of immune cell imbalance after pharmacological treatments of patients suffering from obsessive-compulsive disorder. *J Psychopharmacol.* 2009;23(5):567–573.

40. da Rocha FF, Correa H, Teixeira AL. Obsessive-compulsive disorder and immunology: a review. *Prog Neuropsychopharmacol Biol Psychiatry.* 2008;32(5):1139–1146.

41. Maina G, Albert U, Bogetto F, et al. Anti-brain antibodies in adult patients with obsessive-compulsive disorder. *J Affect Disord.* 2009;116(3):192–200.

42. Nicholson TR, Ferdinando S, Krishnaiah RB, et al. Prevalence of anti-basal ganglia antibodies in adult obsessive-compulsive disorder: cross-sectional study. *Br J Psychiatry.* 2012;200(5):381–386.

43. Pearlman DM, Vora HS, Marquis BG, Najjar S, Dudley LA. Anti-basal ganglia antibodies in primary obsessive-compulsive disorder: systematic review and meta-analysis. *Br J Psychiatry.* 2014;205(1):8–16.

44. Bhattacharyya S, Khanna S, Chakrabarty K, Mahadevan A, Christopher R, Shankar SK. Anti-brain autoantibodies and altered excitatory neurotransmitters in obsessive-compulsive disorder. *Neuropsychopharmacology.* 2009;34(12):2489–2496.

45. Frick L, Pittenger C. Microglial dysregulation in OCD, Tourette syndrome, and PANDAS. *J Immunol Res.* 2016;2016:8606057.

46. Kumar A, Williams MT, Chugani HT. Evaluation of basal ganglia and thalamic inflammation in children with pediatric autoimmune neuropsychiatric disorders associated with streptococcal infection and Tourette syndrome: a positron emission tomographic (PET) study using 11C-[R]-PK11195. *J Child Neurol.* 2015;30(6):749–756.

47. Attwells S, Setiawan E, Wilson AA, et al. Inflammation in the neurocircuitry of obsessive-compulsive disorder. *JAMA Psychiatry.* 2017;74(8):833–840.

48. Lennington JB, Coppola G, Kataoka-Sasaki Y, et al. Transcriptome analysis of the human striatum in Tourette syndrome. *Biol Psychiatry.* 2016;79(5):372–382.

49. Ebrahimi Taj F, Noorbakhsh S, Ghavidel Darestani S, Shirazi E, Javadinia S. Group A beta-hemolytic streptococcal infection in children and the resultant neuro-psychiatric disorder; a cross sectional study; Tehran, Iran. *Basic Clin Neurosci.* 2015;6(1):38–43.

50. Oglodek EA, Szota AM, Just MJ, Mos DM, Araszkiewicz A. The MCP-1, CCL-5 and SDF-1 chemokines as pro-inflammatory markers in generalized anxiety disorder and personality disorders. *Pharmacol Rep.* 2015;67(1):85–89.

51. Kawikova I, Leckman JF, Kronig H, et al. Decreased numbers of regulatory T cells suggest impaired immune tolerance in children with Tourette syndrome: a preliminary study. *Biol Psychiatry.* 2007;61(3):273–278.

52. Leckman JF, Katsovich L, Kawikova I, et al. Increased serum levels of interleukin-12 and tumor necrosis factor-alpha in Tourette's syndrome. *Biol Psychiatry.* 2005;57(6):667–673.

53. Gabbay V, Coffey BJ, Guttman LE, et al. A cytokine study in children and adolescents with Tourette's disorder. *Prog Neuropsychopharmacol Biol Psychiatry.* 2009;33(6):967–971.

54. Bos-Veneman NG, Bijzet J, Limburg PC, Minderaa RB, Kallenberg CG, Hoekstra PJ. Cytokines and soluble adhesion molecules in children and adolescents with a tic disorder. *Prog Neuropsychopharmacol Biol Psychiatry.* 2010;34(8):1390–1395.

55. Perlmutter SJ, Leitman SF, Garvey MA, et al. Therapeutic plasma exchange and intravenous immunoglobulin for obsessive-compulsive disorder and tic disorders in childhood. *Lancet.* 1999;354(9185):1153–1158.

56. Murphy TK, Brennan EM, Johnco C, et al. A double-blind randomized placebo-controlled pilot study of azithromycin in youth with acute-onset obsessive-compulsive disorder. *J Child Adolesc Psychopharmacol.* 2017;27(7):640–651.

57. Murphy TK, Parker-Athill EC, Lewin AB, Storch EA, Mutch PJ. Cefdinir for recent-onset pediatric neuropsychiatric disorders: a pilot randomized trial. *J Child Adolesc Psychopharmacol.* 2015;25(1):57–64.

58. Muller N. Anti-inflammatory therapy with a COX-2 inhibitor in Tourette's syndrome. *Inflammopharmacology.* 2004;12(3):271–275.

59. Brown K, Farmer C, Farhadian B, Hernandez J, Thienemann M, Frankovich J. Pediatric acute-onset neuropsychiatric syndrome response to oral corticosteroid bursts: an observational study of patients in an academic community-based PANS clinic. *J Child Adolesc Psychopharmacol.* 2017;27(7):629–639.

60. Barash J, Margalith D, Matitiau A. Corticosteroid treatment in patients with Sydenham's chorea. *Pediatr Neurol.* 2005;32(3):205–207.

61. Paz JA, Silva CA, Marques-Dias MJ. Randomized double-blind study with prednisone in Sydenham's chorea. *Pediatr Neurol.* 2006;34(4):264–269.

62. Walker AR, Tani LY, Thompson JA, Firth SD, Veasy LG, Bale JF, Jr. Rheumatic chorea: relationship to systemic manifestations and response to corticosteroids. *J Pediatr.* 2007;151(6):679–683.

63. Brown KD, Farmer C, Freeman GM, Jr, et al. Effect of early and prophylactic nonsteroidal anti-inflammatory drugs on flare duration in pediatric acute-onset neuropsychiatric syndrome: an observational study of patients followed by an academic community-based pediatric acute-onset neuropsychiatric syndrome clinic. *J Child Adolesc Psychopharmacol.* 2017;27(7):619–628.

64. Grant JE. Clinical practice: obsessive-compulsive disorder. *N Engl J Med.* 2014;371(7):646–653.

Chapter 7

Neurocognitive Basis of Compulsivity

Martijn Figee, Judy Luigjes, Anneke Goudriaan, Ingo Willuhn and Damiaan Denys

Introduction

Compulsivity in obsessive-compulsive disorder (OCD) is related to the feelings of limited voluntary control and being compelled to perform repetitious, self-defeating behaviors [1,2]. Based on analogies between the compulsive characteristics of OCD and substance-use disorders, some researchers have proposed to view OCD as a behavioral addiction [3,4], together with pathological gambling, compulsive computer use, compulsive sexual behavior and compulsive buying [3,5]. Compulsivity is the central theme in the newly delineated class of obsessive-compulsive and related disorders of the fifth edition of the *Diagnostic and Statistical Manual of Mental Disorders* (DSM-5) [6], that groups OCD together with body dysmorphic disorder (BDD), trichotillomania, skin-picking disorder and hoarding disorder. Finally, compulsivity related to eating and body weight is characteristic for anorexia nervosa, bulimia nervosa and binge eating disorder. The study of different aspects of compulsivity and their neural correlates in these disorders may help to define shared brain networks that can help identifying appropriate prevention and treatment targets.

Compulsivity may be decomposed into various factors with a mainly cognitive, affective or motivational nature. First, compulsivity, as engagement in self-defeating repetitive behaviors, hints at impaired reward and/or punishment processing. Second, the diminished ability to stop or divert unwanted ideas and actions suggests the presence of cognitive and behavioral inflexibility. Third, habitual responding and diminished goal-directed control suggests excessive habit-learning. In this chapter, we study the neural overlap of these different aspects of compulsivity in OCD, substance-use disorders, behavioral addictions and eating disorders, using findings from human imaging studies, animal models of compulsive behavior and associated neurotransmitters. We use these data to define which neural processes are central to compulsivity and to use this knowledge for the identification of transdiagnostic interventions.

Recent Research Findings

Reward Processing

Compulsivity may be explained by dysfunctional brain reward systems, driving the development of a restricted behavioral repertoire at the cost of healthy rewarding actions. Indeed, patients with OCD displayed attenuated monetary reward anticipation activity in the ventral striatum compared to controls in some studies [7,8], which matches blunted reward anticipation signals of the ventral striatum in alcohol [9], nicotine [10] and cannabis dependence [11], and in a behavioral addiction like pathological gambling [12,13]. In a meta-analysis, blunted striatal activation during reward anticipation was found across 643 individuals with various drug addictions or pathological gambling compared with 609 healthy individuals as controls [14]. In OCD, blunted striatal activity in response to natural (monetary) rewards is paralleled by increased striatal activity in response to symptom-provoking stimuli [15], which appears to be analogous to ventral striatal hyperactivation associated with disorder-specific stimuli in drug addiction [16,17].

In eating disorders, a similar pattern of ventral striatal hyper-responsivity to disease-specific stimuli is observed (i.e., to body stimuli and food in anorexia nervosa [18], over-eating and bulimia nervosa [19,20]). This striatal activation correlates with compulsive over-eating scores in individuals who are overweight exposed to personally relevant high-calorie cues [21]. Similar to other disorders of compulsivity, striatal hyperresponsivity to disease-specific stimuli in eating disorders is paralleled by aberrant processing of natural rewards. However, opposite responses have been suggested in individuals with over-eating compared with food restriction. Over-eating or binge-eating is associated with blunted striatal monetary reward responses [22,23], comparable with findings in addictions and OCD. On the contrary, increased rather than blunted ventral striatal responses to money or pleasant taste are found in anorexia nervosa [23]. This indicates a hyperresponsivity to both pathological and natural rewards in anorexia nervosa which may be explained by an ability of a patient with anorexia nervosa to cognitively compensate for blunted reward processing. In coherence with this notion, excessive capacity to delay reward has been associated to perfectionistic and rigid personality traits that are also typical for anorexia nervosa [24], which is opposite to diminished delay reward responding in over-eating [25] and addiction [26]. In support of an overlapping reward deficiency, patients with anorexia nervosa, when in a hungry state, failed to show striatal reward activation compared with controls [27].

Together, this suggests that the ventral striatum may be less responsive when recruited for healthy reward processing due to its bias toward drugs in addiction, and in parallel, due to its bias to disease-specific stimuli in OCD, behavioral addictions and eating disorders.

Punishment Sensitivity

Individuals engaged in compulsive behaviors may be less capable of noticing its self-damaging consequences, which suggests impairment of (neural processes underlying) sensitivity to punishment. Although studies in OCD confirm dysfunctional processing of punishments, the results are diverging, with brain activity during monetary loss anticipation in patients with OCD being either normal [7] or increased in the medial prefrontal cortex [28], or decreased in the ventral striatum [29]. The latter finding suggests decreased striatal sensitivity to punishment in OCD, which matches with decreased striatal loss-anticipation signals in pathological gambling [30] but not in alcohol addiction [31].

The study by Choi et al. [30] also found that pathological gamblers and patients with OCD share decreased loss-anticipation signals in the insula. The insula is involved in the mediation of bodily interoceptive signals for processing negative cues, and this region has also been associated with drug craving [32]. Therefore, we speculate that insula dysfunction may be involved in compulsivity in OCD and addictive behaviors contributing to a diminished ability to weigh the negative consequences of compulsive actions. Similar to OCD and addiction, decreased striatal sensitivity to punishment is also suggested in obese individuals with binge eating disorder compared with individuals without the disorder who are obese [22]. In contrast, patients with anorexia nervosa show increased striatal responses to monetary losses [33], and increased punishment sensitivity associated with increased striatal and insular responses during monetary reward prediction errors [34,35].

In summary, compulsive drug seeking and craving may be associated with attenuated neural processing of punished behavior in ventral corticostriatal pathways and insula, with some evidence suggesting similar impairments underlying compulsivity in OCD, pathological gambling and binge eating. Diminished punishment sensitivity may in part explain why these patients have difficulties stopping compulsive behaviors despite their self-damaging consequences. However, anorexia nervosa is associated with excessive rather than diminished punishment processing, which together with excessive reward processing, might suggest a diverging origin of compulsivity in this group.

Negative Reinforcement

Compulsive behaviors may be performed to avoid aversive or anxiety-inducing outcomes. Indeed, a prominent theory in addiction research emphasizes the increasingly important role of negative reinforcement when drug taking becomes more compulsive over time [36]. In many patients, drug taking is initially driven by its pleasurable effects; however, over time, the motivation seems to shift, with an increased role for negative reinforcement that accompanies the development of compulsive drug use. Negative reinforcement that can drive drug use includes removal of an aversive state, whether this is physical withdrawal symptoms or a negative emotional state such as anxiety, stress or depression. There are even addicted patients who report never to have experienced pleasure and for whom negative reinforcement was their main drive throughout the course of drug use [37].

Recruitment of anti-reward brain systems associated with aversive or stress-like states may underlie negative reinforcement in compulsive drug use. An important region implicated in these anti-reward systems is the extended amygdala (bed nucleus of the stria terminalis, BNST) and the lateral habenula [38]. Adaptations of these systems may persist during and beyond drug abstinence, creating a condition of chronic dysphoria and increasing the likelihood of relapse in a compulsive attempt to self-medicate this unwanted condition [39]. In addition, medial prefrontal–amygdala circuits involved in fear conditioning have been implicated in persistent drug-seeking behavior [40,41]. Similarly, in problem gambling, excessive responses in the amygdala and insula have been linked to craving elicited by gambling pictures [42], suggesting that negative reinforcement circuits could also have a role in compulsivity in behavioral addictions.

Negative reinforcement may promote compulsions in patients with OCD from the start of the disorder. Traditionally, OCD has been viewed as an anxiety disorder, and for many patients, the need to reduce anxiety or stress contributes to the persistence of the compulsions as supported by experiments that show decreases in anxiety or discomfort when patients are allowed to execute compulsive behaviors after being exposed to symptom-provoking situations [43]. However, contrary to findings in drug addiction, brain anti-reward systems such as the BNST or lateral habenula have not yet been directly linked to OCD. Nevertheless, schedule-induced polydipsia in rats, which is assumed to model aspects of human compulsivity, is associated with changes in the firing behavior of BNST neurons [44].

Also, note that not all patients with OCD report anxiety or stress and that negative reinforcement may contribute differently to the compulsions of these patients. In some cases of OCD, compulsive behaviors may start with anxiety and harm avoidance but gradually evolve into more habitual or impulsive responding with progression of the disease [45]. In other cases, OCD may develop first as a propensity to compulsive behaviors, followed by anxiety and obsessive thoughts in response to these compulsive urges [2]. In line with the latter notion, structural and functional imaging studies in OCD and case studies of acquired OCD after brain injuries have often failed to demonstrate clear pathology of the limbic system such as found in anxiety disorders, but rather indicate that compulsivity may primarily stem from basal ganglia–prefrontal dysfunction [11,46,47]. Akin to OCD and addictions, individuals with eating disorders may overconsume or restrict foods in an effort to regulate negative emotions [48]; however, research is lacking examining shared neural correlates of negative affect.

In summary, compulsivity in addiction, OCD and eating disorders may be driven by negative reinforcement (i.e., avoidance or relief of dysphoria, stress, anxiety or other negative emotions), with underlying abnormalities in brain anti-reward and anxiety circuits involving the BST, amygdala, habenula and medial prefrontal cortex.

Cognitive and Behavioral Flexibility

Cognitive and behavioral inflexibility represent core features of compulsivity in OCD [2,49], substance-use disorders [50], and some behavioral addictions [51,52]. Contingency-related flexibility refers to the adaptation of behavior or cognitive strategies after positive or negative contingencies. Contingency-related flexibility has been linked to the orbitofrontal cortex [53]. Abundant evidence implicates abnormalities of the orbitofrontal cortex in OCD, such as decreased volume and increased symptom-related activity. Probabilistic reversal-learning tasks tap into the construct of contingency-related flexibility, and patients with OCD compared with controls demonstrate defective orbitofrontal cortex recruitment during these tasks [54,55].

Similarly, substance-use disorders have been associated with reduced orbitofrontal cortex volume [56], hyperactivation during drug taking and dysfunctional reversal-learning responses [57]. Moreover, a study directly comparing OCD and stimulant-dependent individuals showed that compulsive symptom scores were significantly correlated with reduced orbitofrontal connectivity in both groups [57]. Diminished reversal learning speed along with dysfunctional orbitofrontal cortex responses during reversal learning have also been found in individuals with pathological gambling [52,58]. Finally, behavioral inflexibility measured as slower reversal learning was demonstrated in alcohol dependence, pathological video gaming, binge eating disorder [59] and anorexia nervosa [60]. Behavioral inflexibility and its associated neural impairments in anorexia nervosa may be linked to compulsive food restriction, as these impairments were not found in women of normal weight who had recovered from anorexia nervosa [60].

Cognitive flexibility can also be measured with attentional set-shifting tasks in which attention is required to switch between multiple stimuli or tasks, requiring activation of the ventrolateral prefrontal cortex [61]. Impaired set-shifting may promote perseveration and compulsive actions [62]. Set-shifting is found to be impaired in adult patients with OCD [63] and in pediatric OCD, which was associated with decreased frontostriatal activation [64]. Comparable set-shifting impairments have also been found in individuals with gambling problems [51,65] and higher set-shifting errors discriminated pathological gamblers from problem or recreational gamblers [66]. On the other hand, set-shifting was intact in individuals with compulsive buying [67]. Finally, impaired set-shifting was reported in individuals with opioid [68], stimulant [69] and alchol use disorders [70], and in individuals with binge eating disorder [59,70,71] and anorexia nervosa [72]. No set-shifting impairment was found in adolescents with anorexia nervosa [73], suggesting that cognitive inflexibility may develop at a later stage, secondary to compulsive behaviors. In individuals with binge eating disorder, poor set-shifting correlated with feelings of loss of control over eating [71].

In summary, cognitive and behavioral inflexibility appear to be shared aspects of compulsivity in OCD, addiction and eating disorders, reflecting corticostriatal dysfunction, in particular impaired top-down control of orbitofrontal and ventrolateral prefrontal cortices. There is some evidence that this inflexibility develops over time when compulsivity progresses and becomes uncontrollable.

Habit Learning

Habits can be defined as automatic, inflexible behaviors performed regardless of their consequences. Although it has long been speculated that habits may be a hallmark of OCD, excessive habits were first demonstrated in animal models of addiction in association with defective goal-directed behaviors that are mediated by frontostriatal mechanisms [74,75]. These animal studies suggest a gradual progression from hedonic to habitual drug use over time associated with a shift from recruitment of ventral to more dorsal regions of the striatum (e.g., Belin and Everitt [76]; Willuhn et al. [77]). One imaging study in humans suggested some indirect support for this ventral to dorsal shift by showing increased cue-induced activity in the ventral striatum in social drinkers and increased cue-induced activity in the dorsal striatum in heavy drinkers [39].

The first study directly investigating habits in addicted humans confirmed the presence of an imbalance between goal-directed and habitual control and between ventral and dorsal frontostriatal recruitment [78]. Patients with alcohol dependence compared with healthy controls showed a decrease in goal-directed learning associated with decreased activity in the ventromedial prefrontal cortex and the anterior putamen and an increase in habit learning associated with increased activity in the posterior putamen. Moreover, ventromedial prefrontal cortex activation during goal-directed learning was negatively associated with alcohol dependence duration.

Excessive habit learning was also demonstrated in OCD [79]. However, contrary to addiction, neuroimaging data from 2014 do not support a ventral to dorsal transition underlying habit formation in OCD, but rather hyperactivation of the ventral striatum (caudate) leading to impaired goal-directed control over behavior [80]. In accordance with a shared dysfunction of these motivational brain systems in various disorders of compulsivity, lower gray-matter volumes of the caudate and medial orbitofrontal cortex were associated with excessive habit formation in patients with OCD, as well as in individuals with stimulant addiction and those with binge eating disorder [81]. Contrary to OCD, addictions and binge eating disorder, no evidence for excessive appetitive or avoidance habits and no correlation with compulsivity scores were found in women with anorexia nervosa.

In summary, habitual behaviors that are performed regardless of their consequences may be central to compulsivity in OCD, addiction and over-eating, reflecting imbalances between ventral and dorsal frontostriatal recruitment. As of yet, compulsivity in anorexia nervosa has not been found to be dependent on habit learning.

Cross-Diagnostic Approaches and Their Implications for Classification and Diagnosis

Unlike traditional diagnoses based on the DSM, the transdiagnostic neurocognitive aspects of compulsivity reviewed here are more directly linked to neurobiological processes. Diagnostic classification of these neurocognitive aspects may therefore enable identification of more targeted treatments than currently possible. However, before such a novel transdiagnostic system could be clinically applied, further research is needed assessing these neurocognitive aspects of compulsivity in mixed diagnostic groups. Examples of transdiagnostic compulsivity questionnaires that can be used in these studies are the Dutch Dimensional Obsessive Compulsive Scale (unpublished), the DSM-5 obsessive–compulsive spectrum scale [82] or the Padua Inventory [83]. Examples of self-report questionnaires for reward and punishment sensitivity are the Behavioral Inhibition/Activation System [84] and the Sensitivity to Punishment and Sensitivity to Reward Questionnaire [85]. Using these questionnaires, reward and punishment sensitivity have been linked to self-reported compulsivity on the Padua Inventory in healthy and addicted individuals [86], and together, these measures correlated with blunted ventral–striatal activation during reward processing [87]. These findings suggest that the association between compulsivity and sensitivities to reward and punishment can be classified with self-report questionnaires in addicted individuals, and a similar approach could be investigated in OCD, behavioral addiction and eating disorders. Other neurocognitive aspects of compulsivity, such as inflexibility or excessive habit learning, may be less easily captured in questionnaires. However, a 2017 study successfully applied an online task in a large community sample to demonstrate habitual tendencies (deficits in goal-directed learning) that were associated with self-reported compulsivity on the Padua Inventory across individuals with symptoms of OCD, addiction and eating disorders [88].

Clinical Implications of Cross-Diagnostic Approaches for Treatment and Prevention

Dopaminergic Treatment Targets

The impaired sensitivity for natural or drug rewards underlying compulsivity may stem from impaired striatal dopamine function [89]. Indeed, OCD, addiction and over-eating are associated with decreased striatal availability of dopamine D_1 and D_2-like receptors, coupled with blunted dopamine release [90,91,92,93]. Drug and food taking is associated with dopamine release and decreased D_2-availability is related to greater craving responses in addiction [91]. Thus, compulsive behaviors in addiction, OCD and eating disorders may serve to overcome negative feelings and discomfort associated with dopamine dysfunction, suggesting some potential for dopamine agonists in the treatment of compulsivity.

Indeed, in stimulant-dependent individuals, dopaminergic enhancement with the dopamine D_2-like agonist pramipexole reversed abnormal perseverative responding and associated caudate dysfunction. However, no perseverative abnormalities or pramipexole-induced changes were observed in patients with OCD [94]. On the contrary, the dopamine D_2-like receptor antagonist sulpiride has been found to remediate quinpirole-induced compulsive-like behavior [95] and D_2-antagonists are effective for OCD when added to serotonergic agents [96].

Contrary to the attenuated natural reward responses in most disorders of compulsivity, including compulsive over-eating, a general hyperresponsivity of brain reward circuits in anorexia nervosa suggests a hypersensitive dopamine system in these patients. In agreement, treatment with the dopamine partial agonist aripiprazole 1–5 mg, which is assumed to downregulate dopamine D_2 receptor activity and stabilize dopaminergic tone, was associated with weight gain in anorexia nervosa [97]. Low-dose aripiprazole was also shown to block reinstatement of cocaine seeking in rats [98].

Lisdexamfetamine, which is able to induce dopamine release, is one of the few efficacious treatments for binge eating disorder [99,100]. It must be noted that dopamine-agonizing agents, when used for Parkinson's disease, are also known to induce compulsivity, such as binge eating, pathological gambling or compulsive sexual behavior, suggesting that the effect of dopamine agonists on compulsivity may depend on baseline dopamine levels. Finally, opioid antagonists, such as naltrexone and nalmefene, can modulate dopamine in the ventral tegmental area and have been found effective in case studies for compulsive sexual behavior, alcohol dependency and compulsive buying.

Serotonergic Treatment Targets

OCD is associated with decreased presynaptic serotonin transporter availability in thalamic and midbrain–pons regions, together with increased postsynaptic serotonin (5-HT_{2A}) receptor availability in cortical areas, indicating diminished serotonergic input into frontosubcortical circuits (for review, see Figee et al. [89]). Compulsive drug seeking in rats was reversed by the facilitating of serotonin transmission using a serotonin reuptake inhibitor or a 5-HT_{2C} receptor agonist [101], and 5-HT_{2C} agonistic agents are also investigated for obesity. Currently available drugs with 5-HT_{2C} agonistic properties include aripiprazole. There is preclinical evidence that habitual aspects of compulsivity may respond to selective serotonin reuptake inhibitors (SSRIs). SSRIs in rats were able to reduce compulsive lever pressing in response to extinguished food signals [102]. Also, animal models suggest that behavioral inflexibility (reversal learning impairments) may be linked to dysfunction of serotonin in the orbitofrontal cortex [103], with SSRIs (citalopram) rescuing behavioral flexibility via normalization of the serotonergic tone of the orbitofrontal cortex [104]. SSRIs are first-line drugs for OCD [105], with some support for its use in bulimia nervosa [106]. Though SSRIs have not been found efficacious in addictions or anorexia nervosa, a promising avenue might be to test these drugs transdiagnostically with habit learning or behavioral inflexibility as primary outcomes. Cognitive therapy may be able to reverse impaired cognitive inflexibility (set-shifting) and its underlying impairment of frontostriatal activity, as was suggested in patients with anorexia nervosa [72,107].

Gamma-Aminobutyric Acid and Glutamate

It has been suggested that the development of compulsive drug taking is mediated by impaired γ-aminobutyric acid (GABA)-ergic inhibition of drug-related dopamine release [108,109]. Indeed, $GABA_B$-agonizing agents such as baclofen are able to inhibit reinforcing effects of drugs and are promising treatment candidates for addictions [110]. Impairment of GABA-ergic systems has also been found in OCD; for example, decreased plasma GABA [111] and decreased GABA in the medial prefrontal cortex as measured with proton magnetic resonance spectroscopy [112]. Moreover, similar to the potential efficacy of GABA-agonistic agents for addictions, recent animal models indicate that selective GABA release in the striatum may be responsible for the efficacy of DBS for OCD [113,114].

Glutamatergic signaling is important for prefrontal top-down control over striatal dopamine [115]. Converging evidence suggests aberrant frontostriatal glutamatergic signaling in OCD [116]. Moreover, electrophysiological animal work indicates that the efficacy of ventral striatal deep brain stimulation for OCD may depend on restored glutamatergic orbitofrontal cortex control over striatal regions [117,118], which might also explain the anti-compulsive effects of glutamatergic agents such as ketamine [119]. It was hypothesized in 2015 that glutamatergic frontostriatal changes may also be critical for the transition from regular to compulsive drug use [120]. Gabapentin and pregabalin may diminish craving for drugs or gambling and affect cognitive inflexibility by reducing glutamate signaling [121]. The glutamatergic antagonists topiramate and memantine have shown beneficial effects in OCD [122,123], and are also tested in drug dependence, pathological gambling and over-eating [124]. N-acetylcysteine is another drug that may reduce glutamate release, which has shown efficacy for compulsive hair pulling and skin picking [125,126], and has also been tested in OCD, pathological gambling and drug addiction [127,128].

Neuromodulation

Many of the reviewed neurocognitive aspects of compulsivity are associated with dysregulated frontostriatal network activity, which can be targeted with neuromodulation. Frontostriatal connectivity can be normalized with deep brain stimulation of the ventral striatum and with repetitive transcranial magnetic stimulation (rTMS) of the medial prefrontal cortex, and these normalizations correlate with obsessive-compulsive symptom improvement [8,129]. Preliminary evidence suggests that the effects of deep brain stimulation and rTMS in individuals with substance-use disorders depend on similar changes in frontostriatal connectivity [130,131].

Another potential transdiagnostic target for neuromodulation in compulsivity is the reward circuit. Deep brain stimulation of the ventral striatum for OCD has been related to a normalization of anticipatory reward responses in the ventral striatum [8]. Deep brain stimulation using a similar target has shown preliminary effects in drug and food addiction [132] and is currently being investigated in anorexia nervosa [133]. Of interest, activation of the reward pathway from the ventral tegmental area to the ventral striatum using a dual viral strategy normalized food intake in rat models of anorexia nervosa [134].

Preclinical lesioning and deep brain stimulation studies have indicated that quinpirole (dopamine-agonist) induced repetitive checking involves the ventral striatum and subthalamic nucleus [135,136], and deep brain stimulation using these two targets is effective for OCD [137,138]. Quinpirole-induced compulsive lever pressing correlated with diminished dopamine neuron activity in the ventral tegmental area, which was proposed to reflect lower baseline dopamine burst-firing as a characteristic of compulsivity [139]. This might explain why effective ventral striatum deep brain stimulation in patients with OCD enhanced dopaminergic neurotransmission [140]. Finally, overreliance on negative reinforcement in compulsivity may be targeted with deep brain stimulation of brain anti-reward systems such as the extended amygdala, BST or lateral habenula [34]. BNST deep brain stimulation is currently being investigated for OCD [141,142] and was reported effective in a patient with anorexia nervosa [143]. Habenula deep brain stimulation was effective in addiction animal models [144].

Future Directions

We reviewed the neurocognitive overlap of compulsivity in OCD, substance-use disorders, behavioral addictions and eating disorders, to determine the processes that are central to compulsivity and may serve as transdiagnostic treatment targets. First, the available data suggest that compulsivity is related to impaired reward and punishment processing in the ventral striatum and associated attenuated dopamine release, and with negative reinforcement in limbic and anti-reward systems, which may at least partly explain the presence of repetitive self-defeating behaviors at the cost of healthy rewards. Second, compulsivity entails cognitive and behavioral inflexibility, which may be rooted in a shared impairment of ventromedial prefrontal top-down regulation, together with prefrontal serotonergic defects. Finally, habitual responding regardless of its consequences is an aspect of compulsivity that might be related to imbalances between ventral and dorsal frontostriatal recruitment. Although these neurocognitive aspects of compulsivity greatly overlap in OCD, addictions and over-eating, divergent findings are often noted in anorexia nervosa.

Apart from the reviewed similarities between neurocognitive aspects and treatment targets of compulsivity in OCD, addictions and eating disorders, there are noticeable differences in pharmacotherapy. For example, SSRIs show efficacy for OCD but not for addiction and anorexia nervosa, and opioid receptor antagonists show efficacy for multiple addictions [145], but generally not for OCD, where opioid agonists (such as morphine) rather than antagonists may have some efficacy [146]. It must be noted, though, that pharmacotherapy may not be highly suitable for targeted treatment of compulsivity, owing to its rather non-specific mechanism of action. In contrast, the reviewed compulsivity aspects and their neural correlates represent promising transdiagnostic targets for neuromodulation. For example, deep brain stimulation of the ventral striatum is able to improve compulsivity in OCD via a restoration of ventral striatal reward processing and reduction of frontostriatal over-connectivity [8] with similar changes suggested for deep brain stimulation in addiction [131], and potentially also eating disorders [147]. Likewise, cortical neuromodulation (e.g., rTMS of the medial prefrontal cortex) may change compulsivity in OCD and addiction through similar frontostriatal connectivity changes [130,131,148]. Therefore, future studies of compulsivity and its neural correlates have great potential to advance neuromodulation for psychiatry.

Taken together, these findings suggest that transdiagnostic measures of compulsivity warrant additional study in substance and behavioral addictions, as well as in OCD and other conditions (skin picking, trichotillomania. binge eating/obesity, compulsive shopping, compulsive sexual behaviors, problematic Internet use), with the hope that such studies may identify appropriate targets for prevention and treatment initiatives.

References

1. Denys D. Obsessionality and compulsivity: a phenomenology of obsessive-compulsive disorder. *Philos Ethics Humanit Med.* 2011;6(3):1–7.
2. Robbins TW, Gillan CM, Smith DG, et al. Neurocognitive endophenotypes of impulsivity and compulsivity: towards dimensional psychiatry. *Trends Cogn Sci.* 2012;16(1):81–91.
3. Holden C, "Behavioral" addictions: do they exist? *Science.* 2001;294:980–982.
4. Denys D, van der Wee N, Janssen J, et al. Low level of dopaminergic D2 receptor binding in obsessive-compulsive disorder. *Biol Psychiatry.* 2002;55:1041–1045.
5. Grant JE, Brewer JA, Potenza MN. The neurobiology of substance and behavioral addictions. *CNS Spectr.* 2006;12:924–930.

6. American Psychiatric Association. *Diagnostic and Statistical Manual of Mental Disorders* (5th ed.). Washington, DC: APA; 2013.
7. Figee M, Vink M, de Geus F, et al. Dysfunctional reward circuitry in obsessive-compulsive disorder. *Biol Psychiatr.* 2011;69(9):867–874.
8. Figee M, Luigjes J, Smolders R, et al. Deep brain stimulation restores frontostriatal network activity in obsessive-compulsive disorder. *Nat Neurosci.* 2014;17(9):1286.
9. Wrase J, Schlagenhauf F, Kienast T, et al. Dysfunction of reward processing correlates with alcohol craving in detoxified alcoholics. *Neuroimage.* 2007;35(2):787–794.
10. Buhler M, Vollstadt-Klein S, Kobiella A, et al. Nicotine dependence is characterized by disordered reward processing in a network driving motivation. *Biol Psychiatry.* 2009;67:745–752.
11. Van Hell HH, Vink M, Ossewaarde L, et al. Chronic effects of cannabis use on the human reward system: an fMRI study. *Eur Neuropsychopharmacol.* 2010;20(3):153–163.
12. Reuter J, Raedler T, Rose M, et al. Pathological gambling is linked to reduced activation of the mesolimbic reward system. *Nat Neurosci.* 2005;8:147–148.
13. De Greck M, Enzi, B, Prösch U, et al. Decreased neuronal activity in reward circuitry of pathological gamblers during processing of personal relevant stimuli. *Hum Brain Mapp.* 2010;31:1802–1812.
14. Luijten M, Schellekens AF, Kühn S, et al. Disruption of reward processing in addiction: an image-based meta-analysis of functional magnetic resonance imaging studies. *JAMA Psychiatry.* 2017;74(4):387–398.
15. Rotge J, Guehl D, Dilharreguy B, et al. Provocation of obsessive–compulsive symptoms: a quantitative voxel-based meta-analysis of functional neuroimaging studies. *J Psychiatry Neurosci.* 2008;33:405–412.
16. Diekhof EK, Falkai P, Gruber O. Functional neuroimaging of reward processing and decision-making: a review of aberrant motivational and affective processing in addiction and mood disorders. *Brain Res Rev.* 2008;59:164–184.
17. Zhu Y, Hu X, Wang J, Chen J, et al. Processing of food, body and emotional stimuli in anorexia nervosa: a systematic review and meta-analysis of functional magnetic resonance imaging studies. *Eur Eat Disord Rev.* 2012;20(6):439–450.
18. Gearhardt AN, Yokum S, Orr PT, et al. Neural correlates of food addiction. *Arch Gen Psychiatry.* 2011;68(8):808–816.
19. García-García I, Horstmann A, Jurado MA, et al. Reward processing in obesity, substance addiction and non-substance addiction. *Obes Rev.* 2014;15(11):853–869.
20. Wierenga CE, Bischoff-Grethe A, Melrose AJ, et al. Hunger does not motivate reward in women remitted from anorexia nervosa. *Biol Psychiatry.* 2015;77(7):642–652.
21. Filbey FM, Myers US, Dewitt S. Reward circuit function in high BMI individuals with compulsive overeating: similarities with addiction. *Neuroimage.* 2012;63:1800–1806.
22. Balodis IM, Kober H, Worhunsky PD, et al. Monetary reward processing in obese individuals with and without binge eating disorder. *Biol Psychiatry.* 2013;73:877–886.
23. Frank GK, Reynolds JR, Shott ME, et al. Anorexia nervosa and obesity are associated with opposite brain reward response. *Neuropsychopharmacology.* 2012;37(9):2031–2046.
24. Pinto A, Steinglass JE, Greene AL, et al. Capacity to delay reward differentiates obsessive-compulsive disorder and obsessive compulsive personality disorder. *Biol Psychiatry.* 2014;75(8):653–659.
25. Steinglass JE, Lempert KM, Choo TH, et al. Temporal discounting across three psychiatric disorders: anorexia nervosa, obsessive compulsive disorder, and social anxiety disorder. *Depress Anxiety.* 2017;34(5):463–470.
26. Kekic M, Bartholdy S, Cheng J, et al. Increased temporal discounting in bulimia nervosa. *Int J Eat Disord.* 2016;49(12):1077–1081.
27. Amlung M, Vedelago L, Acker J, et al. Steep delay discounting and addictive behavior: a meta-analysis of continuous associations. *Addiction.* 2017;112(1):51–62.
28. Kaufmann C, Beucke, JC, Preuße, et al. Medial prefrontal brain activation to anticipated reward and loss in obsessive–compulsive disorder. *Neuroimage Clin.* 2013;2:212–220.
29. Jung WH, Kang D-H, Han JY, et al. Aberrant ventral striatal responses during incentive processing in unmedicated patients with obsessive–compulsive disorder. *Acta Psychiatr Scand.* 2011;123(5):376–386.
30. Choi JS, Shin YC, Jung WH, et al. Altered brain activity during reward anticipation in pathological gambling and obsessive–compulsive disorder. *PloS One.* 2012;7(9):e45938.
31. van Holst RJ, Clark L, Veltman DJ, et al. Enhanced striatal responses during expectancy coding in alcohol dependence. *Drug Alcohol Depend.* 2014;142:204–208.
32. Naqvi NH, Rudrauf D, Damasio H, Bechara A. Damage to the insula disrupts addiction to cigarette smoking. *Science.* 2007;315(5811):531–534.

33. Wagner A, Aizenstein H, Venkatraman VK, et al. Altered reward processing in women recovered from anorexia nervosa. *Am J Psychiatry.* 2007;164(12):1842–1849.

34. DeGuzman M, Shott ME, Yang TT, et al. Association of elevated reward prediction error response with weight gain in adolescent anorexia nervosa. *Am J Psychiatry.* 2017;174(6):557–565.

35. Frank GK, Collier S, Shott ME, et al. Prediction error and somatosensory insula activation in women recovered from anorexia nervosa. *J Psychiatry Neurosci.* 2016;41(5):304–311.

36. Koob GF. The dark side of emotion: the addiction perspective. *Eur J Pharmacol.* 2015;753:73–87.

37. Kennett J, Matthews S, Snoek A. Pleasure and addiction. *Front Psychiatry.* 2013;4:117.

38. Root DH, Mejias-Aponte CA, Qi J, et al. Role of glutamatergic projections from ventral tegmental area to lateral habenula in aversive conditioning. *J Neurosci.* 2014;34(42):13906–13910.

39. Vollstädt-Klein S, Wichert S, Rabinstein J, et al. Initial, habitual and compulsive alcohol use is characterized by a shift of cue processing from ventral to dorsal striatum. *Addiction.* 2010;105(10):1741–1749.

40. Peters J, Kalivas PW, Quirk GJ. Extinction circuits for fear and addiction overlap in prefrontal cortex. *Learn Mem.* 2009;16(5):279–288.

41. Crunelle CL, Kaag AM, van den Munkhof HE, et al. Dysfunctional amygdala activation and connectivity with the prefrontal cortex in current cocaine users. *Hum Brain Mapp.* 2015;36(10):4222–4230.

42. Goudriaan AE, de Ruiter MB, van den Brink W, et al. Brain activation patterns associated with cue reactivity and craving in abstinent problem gamblers, heavy smokers and healthy controls: an fMRI study. *Addict Biol.* 2010;15(4):491–503.

43. Rachman S, de Silva P, Roper G. The spontaneous decay of compulsive urges. *Behav Res Ther.* 1976;14:445–453.

44. Welkenhuysen M, Gligorijevic I, Ameye L, et al. Neuronal activity in the bed nucleus of the stria terminalis in a rat model for obsessive–compulsive disorder. *Behav Brain Res.* 2013;240:52–59.

45. Kashyap H, Fontenelle LF, Miguel EC, et al. "Impulsive compulsivity" in obsessive–compulsive disorder: a phenotypic marker of patients with poor clinical outcome. *J Psychiatr Res.* 2012;46:1146–1152.

46. Whiteside SP, Port JD, Abramowitz JS. A meta-analysis of functional neuroimaging in obsessive–compulsive disorder. *Psychiatry Res.* 2004;132(1):69–79.

47. Radua J, van den Heuvel OA, Surguladze S, Mataix-Cols D. Meta-analytical comparison of voxel-based morphometry studies in obsessive–compulsive disorder vs other anxiety disorders. *Arch Gen Psychiatry.* 2010;67(7):701–711.

48. Schulte EM, Grilo CM, Gearhardt AN. Shared and unique mechanisms underlying binge eating disorder and addictive disorders. *Clin Psychol Rev.* 2016;44:125–139.

49. Chamberlain SR, Fineberg NA, Blackwell AD, et al. Motor inhibition and cognitive flexibility in obsessive–compulsive disorder and trichotillomania. *Am J Psychiatry.* 2006;163:1282–1284.

50. Izquierdo A, Jentsch JD. Reversal learning as a measure of impulsive and compulsive behavior in addictions. *Psychopharmacology (Berl).* 2012;219(2):607–620.

51. Goudriaan AE, Oosterlaan J, de Beurs E. et al. Neurocognitive functions in pathological gambling: a comparison with alcohol dependence, Tourette syndrome and normal controls. *Addiction.* 2006;101:534–547.

52. Vanes LD, van Holst RJ, Jansen JM, et al. Contingency learning in alcohol dependence and pathological gambling: learning and unlearning reward contingencies. *Alcohol Clin Exp Res.* 2014;38(6):1602–1610.

53. Bechara A, Damasio H, Damasio AR. Emotion, decision-making and the orbitofrontal cortex. *Cereb Cortex.* 2000;10:295–307.

54. Remijnse PL, Nielen MM, van Balkom AJ, et al. Reduced orbitofrontal-striatal activity on a reversal learning task in obsessive–compulsive disorder. *Arch Gen Psychiatry.* 2006;63(11):1225–1236.

55. Chamberlain SR, Menzies L, Hampshire A, et al. Orbitofrontal dysfunction in patients with obsessive–compulsive disorder and their unaffected relatives. *Science.* 2008;321:421–422.

56. Franklin TR, Acton PD, Maldjian JA, et al. Decreased gray matter concentration in the insular, orbitofrontal, cingulate, and temporal cortices of cocaine patients. *Biol Psychiatry.* 2002;51(2):134–142.

57. Meunier D, Ersche KD, Craig KJ, et al. Brain functional connectivity in stimulant drug dependence and obsessive–compulsive disorder. *NeuroImage.* 2012;59(2):1461–1468.

58. de Ruiter MB, Veltman DJ, Goudriaan AE, et al. Response perseveration and ventral prefrontal sensitivity to reward and punishment in male problem gamblers and smokers. *Neuropsychopharmacology.* 2009;34:1027–1038.

59. Banca P, Harrison NA, Voon V. Compulsivity across the pathological misuse of drug and non-drug rewards. *Front Behav Neurosci.* 2016;10:154.

60. Hildebrandt T, Grotzinger A, Reddan M, et al. Testing the disgust conditioning theory of food-avoidance in adolescents with recent onset anorexia nervosa. *Behav Res Ther.* 2015;71:131–138.

61. Hampshire A, Owen AM. Fractionating attentional control using event-related fMRI. *Cereb Cortex.* 2006;16:1679–1689.

62. Stalnaker TA, Takahashi Y, Roesch MR, et al. Neural substrates of cognitive inflexibility after chronic cocaine exposure. *Neuropharmacology.* 2009;56(Suppl 1):S63–S72.

63. Watkins LH, Sahakian BJ, Robertson MM, et al. Executive function in Tourette's syndrome and obsessive–compulsive disorder. *Psychol Med.* 2005;35:571–582.

64. Britton JC, Rauch SL, Rosso IM, et al. Cognitive inflexibility and frontal-cortical activation in pediatric obsessive–compulsive disorder. *J Am Acad Child Adolesc Psychiatry.* 2010;49:944–953.

65. Odlaug BL, Chamberlain SR, Kim SW, et al. A neurocognitive comparison of cognitive flexibility and response inhibition in gamblers with varying degrees of clinical severity. *Psychol Med.* 2011;41:2111–2119.

66. Chamberlain SR, Stochl J, Redden SA, et al. Latent class analysis of gambling subtypes and impulsive/compulsive associations: time to rethink diagnostic boundaries for gambling disorder? *Addict Behav.* 2017;72:79–85.

67. Derbyshire KL, Chamberlain SR, Odlaug BL, et al. Neurocognitive functioning in compulsive buying disorder. *Ann Clin Psychiatry.* 2014;26:57–63.

68. Ornstein TJ, Iddon JL, Baldacchino AM, et al. Profiles of cognitive dysfunction in chronic amphetamine and heroin abusers. *Neuropsychopharmacology.* 2000;23:113–126.

69. Woicik PA, Urban C, Alia-Klein N, et al. A pattern of perseveration in cocaine addiction may reveal neurocognitive processes implicit in the Wisconsin card sorting test. *Neuropsychologia.* 2011;49(7):1660–1669.

70. Banca P, Harrison NA, Voon V. Compulsivity across the pathological misuse of drug and non-drug rewards. *Front Behav Neurosci.* 2016;10:154.

71. Dingemans AE, Visser H, Paul L, et al. Set-shifting abilities, mood and loss of control over eating in binge eating disorder: an experimental study. *Psychiatry Res.* 2015;230(2):242–248.

72. Zastrow A, Kaiser S, Stippich C, et al. Neural correlates of impaired cognitive-behavioral flexibility in anorexia nervosa. *Am J Psychiatry.* 2009;166(5):608–616.

73. Fitzpatrick KK, Darcy A, Colborn D, et al. Set-shifting among adolescents with anorexia nervosa. *Int J Eat Disord.* 2012;45:909–912.

74. Everitt BJ, Robbins TW. Neural systems of reinforcement for drug addiction: from actions to habits to compulsion. *Nat Neurosci.* 2005;8:1481–1489.

75. Everitt BJ, Belin D, Economidou D, et al. Neural mechanisms underlying the vulnerability to develop compulsive drug-seeking habits and addiction. *Philos Trans R Soc Lond B Biol Sci.* 2008;363(1507):3125–3135.

76. Belin D, Everitt BJ. Cocaine seeking habits depend upon dopamine-dependent serial connectivity linking the ventral with the dorsal striatum. *Neuron.* 2008;57:432–441.

77. Willuhn I, Burgeno LM, Everitt BJ, et al. Hierarchical recruitment of phasic dopamine signaling in the striatum during the progression of cocaine use. *Proc Natl Acad Sci USA.* 2012;109:20703–20708.

78. Sjoerds Z, de Wit S, van den Brink W, et al. Behavioral and neuroimaging evidence for overreliance on habit learning in alcohol-dependent patients. *Transl Psychiatry.* 2013;3:e337.

79. Gillan CM, Papmeyer M, Morein–Zamir S, et al. Disruption in the balance between goal-directed behavior and habit learning in obsessive–compulsive disorder. *Am J Psychiatry.* 2011;168(7):718–726.

80. Gillan CM, Morein-Zamir S, Urcelay GP, et al. Enhanced avoidance habits in obsessive–compulsive disorder. *Biol Psychiatry.* 2014;75(8):631–638.

81. Voon V, Derbyshire K, Ruck C, et al. Disorders of compulsivity: a common bias towards learning habits. *Mol Psychiatry.* 2015;20(3):345–352.

82. LeBeau RT, Mischel ER, Simpson HB, et al. Preliminary assessment of obsessive–compulsive spectrum disorder scales for DSM-5. *J Obsess Compuls Relat Disord.* 2013;2(2):114–118.

83. Sternberger LG, Burns GL. Obsessions and compulsions: psychometric properties of the Padua Inventory with an American college population. *Behav Res Ther.* 1990;28(4):341–345.

84. Carver CS, White TL. Behavioral inhibition, behavioral activation, and affective responses to impending reward and punishment: the BIS/BAS Scales. *J Personality Social Psychol.* 1994;67(2):319–333.

85. Torrubia R, Avila C, Molto J, et al. The Sensitivity to Punishment and Sensitivity to Reward Questionnaire (SPRSQ) as a measure of Gray's anxiety and impulsivity dimensions. *Personality Individual Diff.* 2001;31(6):837–862.

86. Meda SA, Stevens MC, Potenza MN, et al. Investigating the behavioral constructs of impulsivity domains using principal component analysis. *Behav Pharmacol.* 2009;20:390–399.

87. Andrews MA, Meda SA, Thomas AD, et al. Individuals family history positive for alcoholism show fMRI abnormalities in reward sensitivity that are related to impulsivity factors. *Biol Psychiatry.* 2011; 69:675–683.

88. Gillan CM, Fineberg NA, Robbins TW. A trans-diagnostic perspective on obsessive-compulsive disorder. *Psychol Med.* 2017;47(9):1528–1548.

89. Figee, M., Booij, J., Denys, D. Molecular imaging of obsessive compulsive disorder. In: Shenton ME, Turetsky BI, eds. *Understanding Neuropsychiatric Disorders: Insights from Neuroimaging.* Cambridge University Press; 2010:260–273.

90. Brambilla F, Bellodi L, Perna G, et al. Dopamine function in obsessive–compulsive disorder: growth hormone response to apomorphine stimulation. *Biol Psychiatry.* 1997;42(10):889–897.

91. Volkow ND, Fowler JS, Wang GJ, et al. Imaging dopamine's role in drug abuse and addiction. *Neuropharmacology.* 2009;56(Suppl 1):3–8.

92. Wang GJ, Volkow ND, Logan J, et al. Brain dopamine and obesity. *Lancet.* 2001;357(9253):354–357.

93. De Weijer BA, van de Giessen E, van Amelsvoort TA, et al. Lower striatal dopamine D2/3 receptor availability in obese compared with non-obese subjects. *EJNMMI Res.* 2011;16:37.

94. Ersche KD, Roiser JP, Abbott S, et al. Response perseveration in stimulant dependence is associated with striatal dysfunction and can be ameliorated by a D(2/3) receptor agonist. *Biol Psychiatry.* 2011;70(8):754–762.

95. Eagle DM, Noschang C, d'Angelo LS, et al. The dopamine D2/D3 receptor agonist quinpirole increases checking-like behaviour in an operant observing response task with uncertain reinforcement: a novel possible model of OCD. *Behav Brain Res.* 2014;264:207–229.

96. Vulink NC, Figee M, Denys D. Review of atypical antipsychotics in anxiety. *Eur Neuropsychopharmacol.* 2011;21(6):429–449.

97. Frank GK, Shott ME, Hagman JO, et al. The partial dopamine D2 receptor agonist aripiprazole is associated with weight gain in adolescent anorexia nervosa. *Int J Eat Disord.* 2017;50(4):447–450.

98. Feltenstein MW, Altar CA, See RE. Aripiprazole blocks reinstatement of cocaine seeking in an animal model of relapse. *Biol Psychiatry.* 2007;61(5):582–590.

99. Citrome L. Lisdexamfetamine for binge eating disorder in adults: a systematic review of the efficacy and safety profile for this newly approved indication – what is the number needed to treat, number needed to harm and likelihood to be helped or harmed? *Int J Clin Pract.* 2015;69(4):410–421.

100. Hudson JI, McElroy SL, Ferreira-Cornwell MC, et al. Efficacy of lisdexamfetamine in adults with moderate to severe binge-eating disorder: a randomized clinical trial. *JAMA Psychiatry.* 2017;74(9):903–910.

101. Pelloux Y, Dilleen R, Economidou D, et al. Reduced forebrain serotonin transmission is causally involved in the development of compulsive cocaine seeking in rats. *Neuropsychopharmacology.* 2012; 37(11):2505–2514.

102. Joel D, Ben-Amir E, Doljansky J, et al. "Compulsive" lever-pressing in rats is attenuated by the serotonin re-uptake inhibitors paroxetine and fluvoxamine but not by the tricyclic antidepressant desipramine or the anxiolytic diazepam. *Behav Pharmacol.* 2004;15:241–252.

103. Clarke HF, Dalley JW, Crofts HS, Robbins TW, Roberts AC. Cognitive inflexibility after prefrontal serotonin depletion. *Science.* 2004;304:878–880.

104. Barlow RL, Alsiö J, Jupp B, et al. Markers of serotonergic function in the orbitofrontal cortex and dorsal raphé nucleus predict individual variation in spatial-discrimination serial reversal learning. *Neuropsychopharmacology.* 2015;40(7):1619–1630.

105. Fineberg NA, Brown A, Reghunandanan SP, et al. Evidence-based pharmacotherapy of obsessive-compulsive disorder. *Int J Neuropsychopharmacol.* 2012;15:1173–1191.

106. Hay PJ, Claudino AM. Clinical psychopharmacology of eating disorders: a research update. *Int J Neuropsychopharmacol.* 2012;15(2):209–222.

107. Brockmeyer T, Walther S, Ingenerf K, et al. Brain effects of computer-assisted cognitive remediation therapy in anorexia nervosa: a pilot fMRI study. *Psychiatry Res.* 2016;249:52–56.

108. Goodman A. Neurobiology of addiction. An integrative review. *Biochem Pharmacol.* 2008;75(1):266–322.

109. Vlachou S, Markou A. GABAB receptors in reward processes. *Adv Pharmacol.* 2010;58:315–371.

110. Filip M, Frankowska M, Sadakierska-Chudy A, et al. GABA-B receptors as a therapeutic strategy in substance use disorders: focus on positive allosteric modulators. *Neuropharmacology.* 2015;88C:36–47.

111. Russo AJ, Pietsch SC. Decreased hepatocyte growth factor (HGF) and gamma aminobutyric acid

(GABA) in individuals with obsessive–compulsive disorder (OCD). *Biomark Insights.* 2013;8:107–114.

112. Simpson HB, Shungu DC, Bender Jr J, et al. Investigation of cortical glutamate–glutamine and γ-aminobutyric acid in obsessive–compulsive disorder by proton magnetic resonance spectroscopy. *Neuropsychopharmacology.* 2012;37(12):2684–2692.

113. Burguiere E, Monteiro P, Feng G, et al. Optogenetic stimulation of lateral orbitofronto-striatal pathway suppresses compulsive behaviors. *Science.* 2013;340:1243–1246.

114. Xie Y, Heida T, Stegenga J. High-frequency electrical stimulation suppresses cholinergic accumbens interneurons in acute rat brain slices through GABAB receptors. *Eur J Neurosci.* 2014;40(11):3653–3662.

115. Arnsten AF, Wang M, Paspalas CD. Dopamine's actions in primate prefrontal cortex: challenges for treating cognitive disorders. *Pharmacol Rev.* 2015;67(3):681–696.

116. Wu K, Hanna GL, Rosenberg DR, et al. The role of glutamate signaling in the pathogenesis and treatment of obsessive–compulsive disorder. *Pharmacol Biochem Behav.* 2012;100(4):726–735.

117. McCracken CB, Grace AA. High-frequency deep brain stimulation of the nucleus accumbens region suppresses neuronal activity and selectively modulates afferent drive in rat orbitofrontal cortex in vivo. *J Neurosci.* 2007;27:12601–12610.

118. Yan N, Chen N, Zhu H, et al. High-frequency stimulation of nucleus accumbens changes in dopaminergic reward circuit. *PloS One.* 2013;8(11):e79318.

119. Rodriguez CI, Kegeles LS, Levinson, et al. Randomized controlled crossover trial of ketamine in obsessive–compulsive disorder: proof-of-concept. *Neuropsychopharmacology.* 2013;38(12):2475–2483.

120. Van Huijstee AN, Mansvelder HD. Glutamatergic synaptic plasticity in the mesocorticolimbic system in addiction. *Front Cell Neurosci.* 2015;8:466.

121. Pettorruso M, De Risio L, Martinotti GD, et al. Targeting the glutamatergic system to treat pathological gambling: current evidence and future perspectives. *BioMed Res Int.* 2014;109786.

122. Berlin HA, Koran LM, Jenike MA, et al. Double-blind, placebo-controlled trial of topiramate augmentation in treatment-resistant obsessive-compulsive disorder. *J Clin Psychiatry.* 2011;72(5):716–721.

123. Aboujaoude E, Barry JJ, Gamel N. Memantine augmentation in treatment-resistant obsessive-compulsive disorder: an open-label trial. *J Clin Psychopharmacol.* 2009;29(1):51–5.

124. Pettorruso M, De Risio L, Martinotti G, et al. Targeting the glutamatergic system to treat pathological gambling: current evidence and future perspectives. *Biomed Res Int.* 2014;2014:109786.

125. Grant JE, Odlaug BL, Kim SW. N-acetylcysteine, a glutamate modulator, in the treatment of trichotillomania: a double-blind, placebo-controlled study. *Arch Gen Psychiatry.* 2009;66(7):756–763.

126. Grant JE, Chamberlain SR, Redden SA, et al. N-Acetylcysteine in the treatment of excoriation disorder: a randomized clinical trial. *JAMA Psychiatry.* 2016;73(5):490–496.

127. Oliver G, Dean O, Camfield D, et al. N-acetyl cysteine in the treatment of obsessive compulsive and related disorders: a systematic review. *Clin Psychopharmacol Neurosci.* 2015;13(1):12–24.

128. Nocito Echevarria MA, Andrade Reis T, Ruffo Capatti G, et al. N-acetylcysteine for treating cocaine addiction – a systematic review. *Psychiatry Res.* 2017;251:197–203.

129. Dunlop K, Woodside B, Olmsted M, et al. Reductions in cortico-striatal hyperconnectivity accompany successful treatment of obsessive-compulsive disorder with dorsomedial prefrontal rTMS. *Neuropsychopharmacology.* 2016;41(5):1395–1403.

130. De Ridder D, Vanneste S, Kovacs, et al. Transient alcohol craving suppression by rTMS of dorsal anterior cingulate: an fMRI and LORETA EEG study. *Neurosci Lett.* 2011;496:5–10.

131. Valencia-Alfonso CE, Luigjes J, Smolders R, et al. Effective deep brain stimulation in heroin addiction: a case report with complementary intracranial electroencephalogram. *Biol Psychiatry.* 2012;71(8):e35–e37.

132. Mantione M, van de Brink W, Schuurman PR, et al. Smoking cessation and weight loss after chronic deep brain stimulation of the nucleus accumbens: therapeutic and research implications: case report. *Neurosurgery.* 2010;66(1):E218.

133. Graat I, Figee M, Denys D. The application of deep brain stimulation in the treatment of psychiatric disorders. *Int Rev Psychiatry.* 2017;29(2):178–190.

134. Foldi CJ, Milton LK, Oldfield BJ. The role of mesolimbic reward neurocircuitry in prevention and rescue of the activity-based anorexia (ABA) phenotype in rats. *Neuropsychopharmacology.* 2017;42(12):2292–2300.

135. Mundt A, Klein J, Joel D, et al. High-frequency stimulation of the nucleus accumbens core and shell reduces quinpirole-induced compulsive checking in rats. *Eur J Neurosci.* 2009;29(12):2401–2412.

136. Winter C, Mundt A, Jalali R, et al. High frequency stimulation and temporary inactivation of the subthalamic nucleus reduce quinpirole-induced compulsive checking behavior in rats. *Exp Neurol.* 2008;210(1):217–218.

137. Mallet L, Polosan M, Jaafari N, et al. Subthalamic nucleus stimulation in severe obsessive-compulsive disorder. *N Engl J Med.* 2008;359(20):2121–2134.

138. Denys D, Mantione M, Figee M, et al. Deep brain stimulation of the nucleus accumbens for treatment-refractory obsessive-compulsive disorder. *Arch Gen Psychiatry.* 2010;67(10):1061–1068.

139. Sesia T, Bizup B, Grace AA. Evaluation of animal models of obsessive–compulsive disorder: correlation with phasic dopamine neuron activity. *Int J Neuropsychopharmacol.* 2013;16(6):1295–1307.

140. Figee M, de Koning P, Klaassen S, et al. Deep brain stimulation induces striatal dopamine release in obsessive-compulsive disorder. *Biol Psychiatry.* 2014;75(8):647–652.

141. Nuttin B, Gielen F, van Kuyck K, et al. Targeting bed nucleus of the stria terminalis for severe obsessive–compulsive disorder: more unexpected lead placement in obsessive–compulsive disorder than in surgery for movement disorders. *World Neurosurg.* 2013;80(3–4):S30.e11–S30.e16.

142. Raymaekers S, Vansteelandt K, Luyten L, et al. Long-term electrical stimulation of bed nucleus of stria terminalis for obsessive-compulsive disorder. *Mol Psychiatry.* 2017;22(6):931–934.

143. Blomstedt P, Naesström M, Bodlund O. Deep brain stimulation in the bed nucleus of the stria terminalis and medial forebrain bundle in a patient with major depressive disorder and anorexia nervosa. *Clin Case Rep.* 2017;5(5):679–684.

144. Luigjes J, van den Brink W, Feenstra M, et al. Deep brain stimulation in addiction: a review of potential brain targets. *Mol Psychiatry.* 2012;17(6):572–583.

145. Potenza MN, Koran LM, Pallanti S. The relationship between obsessive–compulsive and impulse control disorders: a current understanding and future research directions. *Psychiatry Res.* 2009;170:22–31.

146. Koran LM, Aboujaoude E, Bullock KD. Double-blind treatment with oral morphine in treatment-resistant obsessive–compulsive disorder. *J Clin Psychiatry.* 2005;66(3):353–359.

147. Oudijn MS, Storosum JG, Nelis E, et al. Is deep brain stimulation a treatment option for anorexia nervosa? *BMC Psychiatry.* 2013;13:277.

148. Kravitz AV, Tomasi D, LeBlanc KH, et al. Cortico-striatal circuits: novel therapeutic targets for substance use disorders. *Brain Res.* 2015;1628(Pt A):186–198.

Chapter 8

Structural Brain Imaging of Obsessive-Compulsive and Related Disorders

Carles Soriano-Mas and Ben J. Harrison

Introduction

The first assessments of brain structural alterations in obsessive-compulsive disorder (OCD) used x-ray technology to explore structures such as the basal ganglia and the ventricular system, which were relatively easy to identify with computed tomography, to provide the first evidence of subtle neuroanatomical alterations in patients suffering from the disorder [1]. Other studies took a more clinical perspective and employed computed tomography to associate neuroradiological findings, like basal ganglia calcifications, with OCD [2]. Since then, magnetic resonance imaging (MRI) has prevailed over other imaging approaches, because of both the lower invasiveness of the approach and its superior spatial resolution. Although some early studies also used MRI to explore the association between particular neuroradiological signs and OCD symptoms [3], most research in the field has subsequently described "group level" as opposed to "case level" findings, which are the focus of this chapter. Importantly, while a large number of such studies have been published, which has facilitated the development and refinement of neurobiological models of OCD [4,5], the ultimate causes of structural brain alterations in this disorder (i.e., changes in the neuropil, synapse or glial cell number) and the precise nature of the relationship between brain alterations and clinical manifestations remain current topics of research enquiry and debate.

Structural imaging studies are capable of assessing both regional changes across the whole brain or evaluating specific regions of interest. The main difference between these two approaches is that the whole-brain approach does not require *a-priori* hypotheses about the regions to evaluate, whereas the latter approach is based on the specific targeting of brain regions of interest based on existing hypotheses and models. In recent years, there has also been an increasing number of studies performed at the meta- or mega-analytic level, which relates to pooling together the results (meta-analyses) or the raw data (mega-analyses) from numerous independent studies, in an attempt to confirm what are the most robust and reliable findings across them. The results of these analyses are discussed below.

Structural brain alterations may be quantified with different outcome variables. Indeed, there is substantial methodological variability across studies, related to the use of different image pre-processing and analysis algorithms. Most studies use T1-weighted images, which offer an excellent contrast between gray and white matter, to quantify changes in cortical and subcortical gray matter regions. Such assessments may include estimations of regional volumes, including voxel-wise quantifications throughout the brain (as in voxel-based morphometry) and volume valuations of specific subcortical structures (as in the assessments of striatal and limbic volumes in FreeSurfer approaches). FreeSurfer approaches also provide thickness estimations for the cortical mantle, which may be obtained for each surface vertex or for a series of predefined cortical parcellations. Other measurements such as surface area, folding or tissue density are sometimes also reported. Notably, only some of these measurements (i.e., voxel-wise volumes or density) can be also obtained for white matter. However, in recent years, the analysis of white matter alterations has become more closely aligned with the use of a distinct imaging modality – diffusion weighted imaging. This MRI modality is based on the quantification of the movement of water molecules, which is used to infer the integrity of white-matter tracts. Studies using diffusion-weighted imaging typically report regional anisotropy and diffusivity estimates. These are two complementary indexes that refer to the preference of water molecules to diffuse in one predominant direction inside white-matter tracts. In general, a high anisotropic diffusion and a low diffusivity rate are expected within healthy white-matter tracts.

Recent Research Findings

Gray-Matter Findings

Overall, research findings in this domain suggest that patients with OCD demonstrate gray-matter volume increases in specific subcortical structures and gray-matter volume decreases in related cortical areas. These changes are frequently observed in the corticostriatal-thalamic-cortical (CSTC) circuits or loops, but also occur in regions outside these circuits.

Exploratory whole-brain assessments in adults with OCD have consistently detected volume increases in the lenticular nucleus. Interestingly, in studies using voxel-wise approaches, such increases are typically located in the putamen [6,7,8,9], while whole-volume assessment methods have typically localized volume changes in the globus pallidus [10]. These apparently discrepant findings, most likely explained by methodological factors (i.e., the difficulties of voxel-wise approaches to discriminate between gray and white matter tissue intensities in some subcortical structures), do not undermine the observation that volume increases in lenticular nuclei have been one of the most consistently reported findings in patients with OCD. Outside the CSTC loops, volume increases have been also reported in regions such as the anterior and posterior cerebellum, although less consistently [6,8,11].

Voxel-wise whole-brain studies have also shown that subcortical volume increases are typically accompanied by gray-matter volume decreases in cortical regions of the CSTC loops, such as the ventral and dorsal medial prefrontal cortices (typically including the anterior cingulate cortex), and the inferior frontal gyrus [7,11]. Similar findings have been reported on the basis of cortical thickness measurements, although the pattern of cortical thinning is typically more widespread than voxel-wise volume reductions, encompassing also the motor cortices, medial and lateral parietal regions (including the posterior cingulate cortex and the angular gyri) and caudal temporal regions [12,13].

Results from studies assessing gray-matter changes in samples of children or adolescents with OCD are in partial agreement with the findings of adult samples. Voxel-wise analyses have indicated similar volume increases in the lenticular nuclei, as well as the caudate nucleus [7]. These findings, however, have not been replicated with FreeSurfer volume evaluations of specific subcortical nuclei, which have mainly detected volume increases in the thalamus [10]. As in adult samples, volume decreases have been also detected in the cortex of children and adolescents with OCD, although medial wall alterations have been typically circumscribed to dorsal regions [7]. The inferior frontal gyrus has been additionally reported to be decreased in volume, and volume decreases have also been noted in posterior cerebral regions, such as the lateral occipital cortex [7].

White-Matter Findings

Although results to date have been notably varied across studies, some consistent findings can be highlighted. Anterior midline tracts (encompassing parts of the cingulate bundle and the corpus callosum) appear to demonstrate decreased fractional anisotropy in patients with OCD [14,15]. Interestingly, in a multimodal meta-analysis of white matter alterations in OCD – evaluating both diffusion imaging and white-matter volume assessments [16] – decreased fractional anisotropy in anterior midline tracts was accompanied by white-matter volume increases, suggesting that white-matter tracts were probably not damaged per se but disorganized, with an increased number of fibers crossing in diverse directions. Since these fibers are supposed to convey signals within the CSTC circuits, these findings have been interpreted within the neurobiological models of CSTC dysfunction in OCD [4].

Conversely, other tracts linking regions of the CSTC, such as the anterior limb of the internal capsule, have shown increased fractional anisotropy in OCD [15,16], which has been interpreted as the structural connectivity underpinning of the orbitofrontal-striatal hyperactivity and increased functional connectivity characteristically reported in patients with OCD [17]. This finding may also be linked to the symptomatic reduction observed in patients with OCD who are undergoing psychosurgery treatments aimed at this region [18]. Likewise, the decreased fractional anisotropy reported in tracts linking anterior and posterior brain regions, such as the inferior fronto-occipital fasciculus or the superior and inferior longitudinal tracts [15,16], may help to integrate cortical alterations observed in posterior brain regions, connected with frontal cortical and subcortical structures throughout these tracts, in prevailing models of CSTC dysfunction.

Regarding children and adolescent samples, it is difficult to draw firm conclusions about white-matter alterations, owing to the comparatively fewer studies available and their smaller sample sizes. Existing results, however, suggest that children and adolescents with OCD show increased fractional anisotropy in some regions where adult patients have shown decreased fractional anisotropy (i.e., corpus callosum, cingulate bundle, and the inferior fronto-occipital and longitudinal fasciculi) [14]. Such results may be suggestive of an accelerated white-matter maturation in subjects with OCD [19,20], which may lead to enduring morphometric alterations in adulthood.

Factors Modulating Brain Morphometry Features

There are a number of clinical and sociodemographic variables that have been described to interact with the structural brain alterations described in OCD. Age and years of evolution of the disorder have been shown to interact with gray-matter volume increases in the putamen [8], with larger increases being more evident in older compared with younger subjects. In a mega-analysis assessing a very large cohort of patients with a wide age range [11], gray-matter volume increases in the putamen were not detected when assessing the whole dataset, although an interaction between gray-matter volume and age (i.e., gray-matter loss with increasing age in healthy controls vs. gray-matter preservation in patients with OCD) was evident in this location. On the basis of these findings, gray-matter volume increases in the putamen have been interpreted to be the result of structural plasticity stemming from the prolonged history of functional hyperactivity of the region [11], although other studies have noted volume increases in the putamen in pediatric and adolescent samples [20,21,22]. In a recent meta-analysis of voxel-wise gray-matter assessments in OCD [7], medication status has been also shown to modulate volume increases in the left putamen. On the other hand, Cheng et al. [23] have reported increased putamen volumes in treatment-naïve children with a first episode of OCD. Clearly, the issue of medication effects on putamen volume in OCD requires further direct study.

Comorbidity with depression, which occurs in up to approximately 60% of patients with OCD, has also been shown to contribute to the structural alterations described in OCD samples. Volume reductions in the hippocampus of patients with OCD have been linked, at least partially, to comorbid depressive symptoms [10,24]. Such hippocampal alterations are also observed in other psychiatric disorders, such as major depression [25], schizophrenia [26] and bipolar disorder [27], and have been suggested to be associated with the "neurotoxic" effects of chronic stress [28]. Likewise, gray-matter volume decreases in the medial orbitofrontal cortex have been described to be more marked in patients with history of comorbid depression [24], indicating that both groups of symptoms may additively contribute to the pattern of structural alterations described in OCD samples.

Regarding the morphometric correlates of the different OCD symptom dimensions, results to date have been inconsistent and difficult to reconcile across studies, potentially due to the varied sample compositions and sizes across studies [29,30,31,32,33,34,35]. Early reports suggested that harm/checking-related symptoms could be associated with specific volume reductions in the amygdala [8], but more recent studies have failed to replicate this finding. Other studies have attempted to describe the structural underpinnings of specific obsessive-compulsive symptoms beyond symptom dimensions. For example, volume increases in the sensorimotor cortex have been observed in patients with sensory phenomena [36]. Similarly, the presence of obsessive-compulsive dysfunctional beliefs has been associated with volume reductions in the temporal pole [37], and, interestingly, patients with autogenous obsessions, characterized, among other features, by the predominant presence of obsessive-compulsive dysfunctional beliefs (i.e., thought-action fusion and control over thoughts), have also been shown to present reduced temporal pole volumes [38]. Moreover, this subgroup of patients appears to not present the volumetric increases in the lenticular nucleus typically observed in OCD samples [38], which may align with another clinical feature of this group of patients, such as their increased rate of mental compared with overt or motor compulsions.

Cross-Diagnostic Approaches and Their Implications for Classification and Diagnosis

Some of the structural alterations reviewed above have been also observed in samples of healthy people in association with more general compulsivity traits.

Specifically, ventral striatal volumes (including the ventral putamen) were reported to be correlated with compulsivity traits in a community sample of adolescents [39]. Similar results involving the putamen nucleus have been also reported for subclinical obsessive-compulsive symptoms in a sample of healthy young adults [40]. These results suggest that such structural features could be also observed in other clinical populations with prominent compulsivity traits. For instance, cocaine dependent individuals display morphological features resembling those observed in patients with OCD, with gray-matter increases in the striatum [41]. Similar volume increases in the putamen or ventral striatum have also been observed in obesity [42] and non-substance addictions [43]. Other studies, however, have reported decreased caudate volumes in subjects with substance addictions [44]. One suggestion is that the caudate and putamen are potentially linked to opposing behavioral patterns (i.e., flexible goal directed behavior and habit formation bias) [45,46], and thus compulsive behaviors could potentially be observed both in the context of decreased dorsal caudate volumes or increased ventral striatal/lenticular volumes. This notion is in agreement with classical functional models indicating that compulsivity disorders show hyperactivated ventral corticostriatal circuits in combination with hypoactivated dorsal circuits [47].

At the cortical level, some of the most prominent features of OCD are also observed in other compulsivity disorders. Decreased lateral and medial orbitofrontal volumes have been observed in cannabis [48] and cocaine dependent individuals [41], binge eating disorder [45], and obsessive-compulsive related disorders, including body dysmorphic disorder [49,50]. Such volume reductions in medial and lateral orbitofrontal cortices seem to be associated with different functional impairments. Lateral orbitofrontal alterations have been typically associated with disrupted motor response inhibition [51], while medial orbitofrontal alterations may relate to the deployment of habit-like patterns of behavior [45]. Importantly, patients with trichotillomania present an important discordance in relation to other compulsivity and obsessive-compulsive spectrum disorders, since they display increases in cortical thickness in the lateral orbitofrontal cortex [52,53]. At the neurocognitive level, patients exhibit deficits typical of compulsivity spectrum disorders [53], which indicates that similar functional impairments may be associated with opposite patterns of structural alteration.

Similar to compulsivity disorders, attention deficit and hyperactivity disorder (ADHD) has also been associated with gray-matter reductions in medial and lateral orbitofrontal cortices [54,55], which may account for the behavioral similarities between these disorders (e.g., impaired motor inhibition). Nevertheless, in contrast with compulsivity disorders, patients with ADHD typically show decreased striatal volumes [54]. This pattern of decreases in prefrontal cortex volume, in combination with reduced striatal volumes, is also observed in autism spectrum disorder (ASD), another neurodevelopmental disorder with some clinical and phenomenological overlap with OCD. Contrary to ADHD, however, reductions in prefrontal cortex volume in ASD do not encompass the orbitofrontal regions, but rather the dorsomedial prefrontal cortex [56]. In OCD and ASD, dorsomedial prefrontal cortex reductions encompass alterations in rostral/dorsal anterior cingulate, and, in addition to these two disorders, these reductions have been also described in body dysmorphic disorder [50] and other compulsivity disorders [57].

Importantly, dorsomedial prefrontal cortex reductions have also been characteristically observed in depression and anxiety disorders [58]. Indeed, in a meta-analysis of volume alterations in OCD and anxiety disorders, volume decreases in dorsomedial prefrontal cortex were described in both type of disorders [59]. In patients with OCD, these observations have also been shown to be more pronounced in those with comorbid anxiety or depressive disorders [11]. Such volume decreases in the dorsomedial prefrontal cortex have been suggested to underpin alterations in emotion regulation processes, which may be commonly altered in compulsivity, ASD, depressive and anxiety disorders [11]. Nevertheless, since dorsomedial prefrontal cortex activity has been related to different psychological processes (i.e., threat appraisal, catastrophizing or worrying) [60], volume decreases in this brain region may be associated with different behavioral features across different diagnoses.

OCD and other anxiety disorders differ in relation to volume decreases in the amygdala, which have been consistently reported in panic, social anxiety and post-traumatic stress disorders (reviewed in Bandelow et al. [61]), but scarcely reported in OCD [62], despite amygdala and amygdala circuit functional alterations having been suggested as being central to OCD pathophysiology [5]. However, other studies of OCD have shown decreases in amygdala volume specifically in treatment refractory OCD [63], and in patients with prominent harm/checking symptoms [8]. Altered structural connectivity of the amygdala has recently been reported in OCD, with results indicating that it is more strongly, although less efficiently, connected to neighboring regions [64]. This result may provide a neurostructural underpinning to ideas stemming from functional neuroimaging research, suggesting that, in OCD, the amygdala exerts an increased control on information flow in other brain areas [65].

The incidence of tic disorders is increased in patients with OCD [66], with the structural imaging correlates of tic disorders (Gilles de la Tourette) and OCD also demonstrating some relevant overlap. Similarly to children with OCD, children with Tourette's disorder show volume increases in bilateral putamen and the corpus callosum [67], although somewhat surprisingly, these results were not observed in other studies assessing children and adults with Tourette and comorbid obsessive-compulsive symptoms, who instead showed reduced lenticular volumes [68]. Another study attempted to identify different neurostructural patterns associated with specific phenotypes within Tourette's disorder [69]. While patients with simple and complex tics were characterized by cortical thinning in (pre)motor and prefrontal regions, OCD symptom severity in patients with comorbid OCD was correlated with premotor cortex thickness. Draganski et al. [70] provided further insight into the issue by reporting that the intensity of premonitory sensations in patients with Tourette's disorder was associated with increases in sensorimotor cortex volume. Taken together, these results agree with findings showing that patients with OCD who have sensory phenomena, the bodily sensations and urges frequently preceding compulsions, show increases in volume in the sensorimotor cortex [36]. Sensorimotor gray-matter volume increases therefore seem to be a common mechanism underlying the presence of premonitory sensations in Tourette's disorder and OCD, possibly as a consequence of the structural plasticity induced by the increased demand in somatosensory processing. Overall, these findings support a growing emphasis on the contribution of sensorimotor corticostriatal circuits in OCD pathophysiology [71], which have been the target of some therapeutic neurostimulation approaches [72]. Interestingly, neuromodulation of the premotor cortex has also been shown to be effective for patients with Tourette's disorder, and specifically in patients with comorbid OCD [73].

Clinical Implications of Cross-Diagnostic Approaches for Treatment and Prevention

The findings reported in this chapter suggest that there may be different treatment targets underpinning a variety of altered processes, to which modulation might be effective for ameliorating obsessive-compulsive and related symptoms across different disorders. However, results from the few reports of the effects of medication on alterations in brain anatomy in OCD have been notably heterogenous. Treatment with selective serotonin reuptake inhibitors (SSRIs) has been shown to "normalize" pretreatment structural alterations in white matter (i.e., fractional anisotropy alterations in the corpus callosum and internal capsule of "drug-naïve" adult patients) [74], or to increase initially decreased left putamen volumes [75]. In pediatric patients, SSRIs have been shown to "normalize" pretreatment increased thalamic volumes [76]. Cognitive behavioral therapy (CBT; i.e., exposure with response prevention) has also been shown to modify brain structure in pediatric patients. Specifically, gray-matter volumes in the orbitofrontal cortex were observed to increase in children with OCD after CBT [77], with these effects being particularly apparent in younger children (8–12 years) [78]. Such CBT-induced changes, however, have not been observed in adult populations [75].

Other studies have used structural magnetic resonance imaging to predict treatment response. While the studies described could provide insight about the mechanisms of action of treatments, studies aiming to predict treatment response may allow the development of optimized and personalized treatment strategies on the basis of pretreatment neuroimaging information. Although results have been mixed, these studies have identified some regions in which the relationship with treatment response may deserve further research. Notably, Hoexter et al. [79] reported that treatment with SSRIs or CBT could be predicted by different morphometric features. In this study, symptom improvement after fluoxetine was predicted by smaller pretreatment gray-matter volume within the right ventrolateral cortex. Conversely, symptom improvement after CBT was predicted by larger pre-treatment gray-matter volumes in the subgenual cingulate cortex. These findings are of interest for a number of reasons. First, because the study identified two different brain regions as potential targets for two different treatments. Second, because the region predicting fluoxetine response partially overlaps the inferior frontal gyri clusters consistently described to be decreased in volume in OCD. Third, because the subgenual cingulate cortex, predictor of CBT response, has been the center of much attention in previous years as one of the neuromodulation targets of interest for mood disorders [80,81], and its volume has also been found to correlate with the response to CBT in other disorders [82,83].

The ventromedial prefrontal cortex, a relatively large region that encompasses the subgenual anterior cingulate cortex, the rostral anterior cingulate cortex and the medial orbitofrontal cortex, has been consistently observed to be decreased in volume in OCD. Basic research has shown that this region is associated with fear extinction recall – an associative learning process linked to the mechanism of action of CBT [84,85]. Other studies have found that other parts of the ventromedial prefrontal cortex, such as the rostral anterior cingulate cortex, are also associated with response to CBT in OCD [86], although, in this study, the authors found that a good response to CBT was predicted by decreased cortical thickness. In any case, these results seem to indicate that morphometric features of ventromedial prefrontal cortex may predict response to CBT, which is probably related to the regulation that this part of the prefrontal cortex exerts over subcortical (e.g., amygdalal) activity. A study assessing structural covariance (i.e., volume correlation across distant structures) between ventromedial prefrontal cortex and amygdala volumes found an increased coupling between these structures in a large sample of patients with OCD, which was interpreted as a consequence of impaired cortical regulation of limbic activity in these subjects [87]. Control of amygdala activity, however, may not depend solely on the ventromedial prefrontal cortex, since volume reductions in other prefrontal regions of the cortex, such as the dorsolateral prefrontal region, have been also associated with poor outcome from CBT in OCD [88].

Structural neuroimaging has been also used in conjunction with neuromodulation techniques. Cecconi et al. [89] showed that gamma ventral capsulotomy resulted in an increase in gray-matter volume in the right inferior frontal gyri. More recently, Makris et al. [90] used diffusion magnetic resonance imaging to study the variability within the region of the ventral capsule/ventral striatum, a typical target of deep brain stimulation treatments for OCD. Results suggest that the morphology of individual orbitofrontothalamic fibers should be taken into account when planning deep brain stimulation interventions. The combination of structural and functional neuroimaging will definitely help in developing more personalized and efficient approaches to deep brain stimulation.

Finally, it should be acknowledged that structural neuroimaging, to date, has contributed little to the development and implementation of prevention strategies for OCD and related disorders. In a 2018 study, however, Suñol et al. [91] assessed a large series of healthy children and correlated the intensity of subclinical obsessive-compulsive symptoms with gray- and white-matter volumes. The authors observed that different symptom dimensions were associated with specific morphometric features. Thus, ordering symptoms were negatively related to gray-matter volumes in the ventral caudate, and obsessing symptoms correlated negatively with gray- and white-matter volumes in the right temporal pole. Conversely, hoarding symptoms were positively associated with gray- and white-matter volumes in the left inferior frontal gyrus. Since subclinical obsessive-compulsive symptoms may be a precursor to OCD [92], these findings may be considered as neural signatures of risk for developing OCD or other mental health disorders, and could significantly contribute to the identification of at-risk individuals, which is crucial for developing targeted interventions aimed at preventing the development or minimizing the impact of obsessive-compulsive symptoms. In this sense, there are some reports suggesting that CBT may be useful in individuals with subclinical OCD symptoms for preventing the development of a full-blown disorder [93].

Future Directions

In the future, it is anticipated that imaging hardware and software developments will allow for the assessment of more refined structural alterations in OCD and related disorders. These new approaches will probably provide new and unanticipated evidence that will generate more comprehensive neurobiological models of OCD. Here, we present a list of ideas that may help in the development of such models.

First, it is clear that disease models will not be constructed exclusively on the basis of structural brain imaging data. Functional alterations and behavioral impairments are only partially reflected in structural alterations, so we need to integrate structural findings with information from functional and metabolic imaging to be able to draw meaningful conclusions. The integration of imaging findings with those from other levels of analysis (from genes to behavior) is also indispensable, as is developing cross-species research approaches to integrate the valuable information that may be derived from animal models (i.e., more robust mechanistic explanations).

Second, we need to understand the precise neurobiological correlates of the structural outcome measurements used in most studies. There is currently much confusion about the neurobiological meaning and functional relevance of volume, cortical thickness or surface changes. That is, more basic research is needed to elucidate the precise neurobiological processes that underpin such measurements. Progress in this domain will undoubtedly facilitate more accurate models of the disorder.

Third, we need to perform sufficiently powered studies. Since it is typically very expensive and time consuming to recruit a large enough sample of patients and control subjects from the same center, multicenter approaches, such as the Enhancing Neuro Imaging Genetics through Meta-Analysis consortium, which has working groups on OCD, ADHD, autism, addiction and anxiety, represent one approach to addressing the issue of replicability across studies. These "big-data" initiatives to date largely represent the amalgamation of existing datasets across imaging sites, and therefore also present limitations with regard to methodological and design consistency across studies. For these reasons, new large-scale multisite investigations, to which imaging, clinical and other assessment protocols are standardized across sites, likely represent an important collaborative path in the study of OCD and related disorders.

Fourth, we need to develop novel methods to understand and characterize the clear heterogeneity of psychiatric disorders, such as OCD. It stands to reason that patients with different clinical phenotypes will in part demonstrate different patterns of underlying neurobiological alteration. New conceptual approaches may be required to account for the heterogeneity of OCD, in turn, stimulating lines of neurobiological research. Recent proposals such as the Research Domain Criteria initiative may represent a relevant starting point, since the focus of the research will move from specific diagnoses to core domains of alteration (e.g., compulsivity).

Finally, the translation of neuroimaging and other research findings to clinical practice remains an important pursuit, especially given the lack of valid biological markers that exist for psychiatric disorders, such as OCD. Machine learning and artificial intelligence methods (i.e., multivariate statistical methods to classify groups of patients or to predict their responses) will likely play a major role in this effort. Structural imaging information is relatively easy to obtain and, therefore, may be available for a large number of patients. It is important to make use of these data to optimize management of these conditions. Structural imaging data may also be used in those at-risk individuals (e.g., offspring of patients with subclinical symptoms) to identify alterations in specific brain circuits that may preventively be targeted with non-invasive treatment approaches.

References

1. Luxenberg JS, Swedo SE, Flament MF, et al. Neuroanatomical abnormalities in obsessive-compulsive disorder detected with quantitative X-ray computed tomography. *Am J Psychiatry.* 1988;145:1089–1093.
2. López-Villegas D, Kulisevsky J, Deus J, et al. Neuropsychological alterations in patients with computed tomography-detected basal ganglia calcification. *Arch Neurol.* 1996;53:251–256.
3. Berthier ML, Kulisevsky J, Gironell A, et al. Obsessive-compulsive disorder and traumatic brain injury: behavioral, cognitive, and neuroimaging findings. *Neuropsychiatry Neuropsychol Behav Neurol.* 2001;14:23–31.
4. Menzies L, Chamberlain SR, Laird AR, et al. Integrating evidence from neuroimaging and neuropsychological studies of obsessive-compulsive disorder: the orbitofronto-striatal model revisited. *Neurosci Biobehav Rev.* 2008;32:525–549.
5. Milad MR, Rauch SL. Obsessive-compulsive disorder: beyond segregated cortico-striatal pathways. *Trends Cogn Sci.* 2012;16:43–51.
6. Eng GK, Sim K, Chen SH. Meta-analytic investigations of structural grey matter, executive domain-related

functional activations, and white matter diffusivity in obsessive compulsive disorder: an integrative review. *Neurosci Biobehav Rev.* 2015;52:233–257.

7. Hu X, Du M, Chen L, et al. Meta-analytic investigations of common and distinct grey matter alterations in youths and adults with obsessive-compulsive disorder. *Neurosci Biobehav Rev.* 2017;78:91–103.
8. Pujol J, Soriano-Mas C, Alonso P, et al. Mapping structural brain alterations in obsessive-compulsive disorder. *Arch Gen Psychiatry.* 2004;61:720–730.
9. Radua J, Mataix-Cols D. Voxel-wise meta-analysis of grey matter changes in obsessive-compulsive disorder. *Br J Psychiatry.* 2009;195:393–402.
10. Boedhoe PS, Schmaal L, Abe Y, et al. Distinct subcortical volume alterations in pediatric and adult OCD: a worldwide meta- and mega-analysis. *Am J Psychiatry.* 2017;174:60–69.
11. de Wit SJ, Alonso P, Schweren L, et al. Multicenter voxel-based morphometry mega-analysis of structural brain scans in obsessive-compulsive disorder. *Am J Psychiatry.* 2014;171:340–349.
12. Fouche JP, du Plessis S, Hattingh C, et al. Cortical thickness in obsessive-compulsive disorder: multisite mega-analysis of 780 brain scans from six centres. *Br J Psychiatry.* 2017;210:67–74.
13. Boedhoe PS, Schmaal L, Abe Y, et al. Cortical abnormalities associated with pediatric and adult obsessive-compulsive disorder: findings from the ENIGMA obsessive-compulsive disorder working group. *Am J Psychiatry.* 2018;175:453–462.
14. Koch K, Reess TJ, Rus OG, et al. Diffusion tensor imaging (DTI) studies in patients with obsessive-compulsive disorder (OCD): a review. *J Psychiatr Res.* 2014;54:26–35.
15. Piras F, Piras F, Caltagirone C, et al. Brain circuitries of obsessive compulsive disorder: a systematic review and meta-analysis of diffusion tensor imaging studies. *Neurosci Biobehav Rev.* 2013;37:2856–2877.
16. Radua J, Grau M, van den Heuvel OA, et al. Multimodal voxel-based meta-analysis of white matter abnormalities in obsessive-compulsive disorder. *Neuropsychopharmacology.* 2014;39:1547–1557.
17. Harrison BJ, Soriano-Mas C, Pujol J, et al. Altered corticostriatal functional connectivity in obsessive-compulsive disorder. *Arch Gen Psychiatry.* 2009;66:1189–1200.
18. Alonso P, Cuadras D, Gabriëls L, et al. Deep brain stimulation for obsessive-compulsive disorder: a meta-analysis of treatment outcome and predictors of response. *PLoS One.* 2015;10:e0133591.
19. Gruner P, Vo A, Ikuta T, et al. White matter abnormalities in pediatric obsessive-compulsive disorder. *Neuropsychopharmacology.* 2012;37:2730–2739.
20. Zarei M, Mataix-Cols D, Heyman I, et al. Changes in gray matter volume and white matter microstructure in adolescents with obsessive-compulsive disorder. *Biol Psychiatry.* 2011;70:1083–1090.
21. Gilbert AR, Keshavan MS, Diwadkar V, et al. Gray matter differences between pediatric obsessive-compulsive disorder patients and high-risk siblings: a preliminary voxel-based morphometry study. *Neurosci Lett.* 2008;435:45–50.
22. Szeszko PR, Christian C, Macmaster F, et al. Gray matter structural alterations in psychotropic drug-naive pediatric obsessive-compulsive disorder: an optimized voxel-based morphometry study. *Am J Psychiatry.* 2008;165:1299–1307.
23. Cheng B, Cai W, Wang X, et al. Brain gray matter abnormalities in first-episode, treatment-naive children with obsessive-compulsive disorder. *Front Behav Neurosci.* 2016;10:141.
24. Cardoner N, Soriano-Mas C, Pujol J, et al. Brain structural correlates of depressive comorbidity in obsessive-compulsive disorder. *Neuroimage.* 2007;38:413–421.
25. Schmaal L, Veltman DJ, van Erp TG, et al. Subcortical brain alterations in major depressive disorder: findings from the ENIGMA major depressive disorder working group. *Mol Psychiatry.* 2016;21:806–812.
26. van Erp TG, Hibar DP, Rasmussen JM, et al. Subcortical brain volume abnormalities in 2028 individuals with schizophrenia and 2540 healthy controls via the ENIGMA consortium. *Mol Psychiatry.* 2016;21:585.
27. Hibar DP, Westlye LT, van Erp TG, et al. Subcortical volumetric abnormalities in bipolar disorder. *Mol Psychiatry.* 2016;21:1710–1716.
28. Kassem MS, Lagopoulos J, Stait-Gardner T, et al. Stress-induced grey matter loss determined by MRI is primarily due to loss of dendrites and their synapses. *Mol Neurobiol.* 2013;47:645–661.
29. Alvarenga PG, do Rosário MC, Batistuzzo MC, et al. Obsessive-compulsive symptom dimensions correlate to specific gray matter volumes in treatment-naïve patients. *J Psychiatr Res.* 2012;46:1635–1642.
30. Glahn A, Prell T, Grosskreutz J, et al. Obsessive-compulsive disorder is a heterogeneous disorder: evidence from diffusion tensor imaging and magnetization transfer imaging. *BMC Psychiatry.* 2015;15:135.

31. Hirose M, Hirano Y, Nemoto K, et al. Relationship between symptom dimensions and brain morphology in obsessive-compulsive disorder. *Brain Imaging Behav.* 2017;11:1326–1333.
32. Lázaro L, Calvo A, Ortiz AG, et al. Microstructural brain abnormalities and symptom dimensions in child and adolescent patients with obsessive-compulsive disorder: a diffusion tensor imaging study. *Depress Anxiety.* 2014;31:1007–1017.
33. Okada K, Nakao T, Sanematsu H, et al. Biological heterogeneity of obsessive-compulsive disorder: a voxel-based morphometric study based on dimensional assessment. *Psychiatry Clin Neurosci.* 2015;69:411–421.
34. van den Heuvel OA, Remijnse PL, Mataix-Cols D, et al. The major symptom dimensions of obsessive-compulsive disorder are mediated by partially distinct neural systems. *Brain.* 2009;132:853–868.
35. Yagi M, Hirano Y, Nakazato M, et al. Relationship between symptom dimensions and white matter alterations in obsessive-compulsive disorder. *Acta Neuropsychiatr.* 2017;29:153–163.
36. Subirà M, Sato JR, Alonso P, et al. Brain structural correlates of sensory phenomena in patients with obsessive-compulsive disorder. *J Psychiatry Neurosci.* 2015;40:232–240.
37. Alonso P, Orbegozo A, Pujol J, et al. Neural correlates of obsessive-compulsive related dysfunctional beliefs. *Prog Neuropsychopharmacol Biol Psychiatry.* 2013;47:25–32.
38. Subirà M, Alonso P, Segalàs C, et al. Brain structural alterations in obsessive-compulsive disorder patients with autogenous and reactive obsessions. *PLoS One.* 2013;8:e75273.
39. Montigny C, Castellanos-Ryan N, Whelan R, et al. A phenotypic structure and neural correlates of compulsive behaviors in adolescents. *PLoS One.* 2013;8:e80151.
40. Kubota Y, Sato W, Kochiyama T, et al. Putamen volume correlates with obsessive compulsive characteristics in healthy population. *Psychiatry Res.* 2016;249:97–104.
41. Ersche KD, Barnes A, Jones PS, et al. Abnormal structure of frontostriatal brain systems is associated with aspects of impulsivity and compulsivity in cocaine dependence. *Brain.* 2011;134:2013–2024.
42. Zhang B, Tian X, Tian D, et al. Altered regional gray matter volume in obese men: a structural MRI study. *Front Psychol.* 2017;8:125.
43. Cai C, Yuan K, Yin J, et al. Striatum morphometry is associated with cognitive control deficits and symptom severity in internet gaming disorder. *Brain Imaging Behav.* 2016;10:12–20.
44. Morales AM, Lee B, Hellemann G, et al. Gray-matter volume in methamphetamine dependence: cigarette smoking and changes with abstinence from methamphetamine. *Drug Alcohol Depend.* 2012;125:230–238.
45. Voon V, Derbyshire K, Rück C, et al. Disorders of compulsivity: a common bias towards learning habits. *Mol Psychiatry.* 2015;20:345–352.
46. Wunderlich K, Dayan P, Dolan RJ. Mapping value based planning and extensively trained choice in the human brain. *Nat Neurosci.* 2012;15:786–791.
47. Phillips ML, Drevets WC, Rauch SL, et al. Neurobiology of emotion perception II: implications for major psychiatric disorders. *Biol Psychiatry.* 2003;54:515–528.
48. Chye Y, Solowij N, Suo C, et al. Orbitofrontal and caudate volumes in cannabis users: a multi-site mega-analysis comparing dependent versus non-dependent users. *Psychopharmacology (Berl).* 2017;234:1985–1995.
49. Atmaca M, Bingol I, Aydin A, et al. Brain morphology of patients with body dysmorphic disorder. *J Affect Disord.* 2010;123:258–263.
50. Buchanan B, Rossell S, Maller JJ, et al. Regional brain volumes in body dysmorphic disorder compared to controls. *Aust N Z J Psychiatry.* 2014;48:654–662.
51. van den Heuvel OA, van Wingen G, Soriano-Mas C, et al. Brain circuitry of compulsivity. *Eur Neuropsychopharmacol.* 2016;26:810–827.
52. Chamberlain SR, Harries M, Redden SA, et al. Cortical thickness abnormalities in trichotillomania: international multi-site analysis. *Brain Imaging Behav.* 2018;12:823–828.
53. Odlaug BL, Chamberlain SR, Derbyshire KL, et al. Impaired response inhibition and excess cortical thickness as candidate endophenotypes for trichotillomania. *J Psychiatr Res.* 2014;59:167–173.
54. Norman LJ, Carlisi C, Lukito S, et al. Structural and functional brain abnormalities in attention-deficit/hyperactivity disorder and obsessive-compulsive disorder: a comparative meta-analysis. *JAMA Psychiatry.* 2016;73:815–825.
55. Villemonteix T, De Brito SA, Slama H, et al. Structural correlates of COMT Val158Met polymorphism in childhood ADHD: a voxel-based morphometry study. *World J Biol Psychiatry.* 2015;16:190–199.
56. Carlisi CO, Norman LJ, Lukito SS, et al. Comparative multimodal meta-analysis of structural and functional brain abnormalities in autism spectrum disorder and obsessive-compulsive disorder. *Biol Psychiatry* 2017;82:83–102.
57. Zois E, Kiefer F, Lemenager T, et al. Frontal cortex gray matter volume alterations in pathological gambling

occur independently from substance use disorder. *Addict Biol.* 2017;22:864–872.

58. van Tol MJ, van der Wee NJ, van den Heuvel OA, et al. Regional brain volume in depression and anxiety disorders. *Arch Gen Psychiatry.* 2010;67:1002–1011.

59. Radua J, van den Heuvel OA, Surguladze S, et al. Meta-analytical comparison of voxel-based morphometry studies in obsessive-compulsive disorder vs other anxiety disorders. *Arch Gen Psychiatry.* 2010;67:701–711.

60. Kalisch R, Gerlicher AM. Making a mountain out of a molehill: on the role of the rostral dorsal anterior cingulate and dorsomedial prefrontal cortex in conscious threat appraisal, catastrophizing, and worrying. *Neurosci Biobehav Rev.* 2014;42:1–8.

61. Bandelow B, Baldwin D, Abelli M, et al. Biological markers for anxiety disorders, OCD and PTSD – a consensus statement. Part I: neuroimaging and genetics. *World J Biol Psychiatry.* 2016;17:321–365.

62. Szeszko PR, Robinson D, Alvir JM, et al. Orbital frontal and amygdala volume reductions in obsessive-compulsive disorder. *Arch Gen Psychiatry.* 1999;56:913–919.

63. Atmaca M, Yildirim H, Ozdemir H, et al. Hippocampus and amygdalar volumes in patients with refractory obsessive-compulsive disorder. *Prog Neuropsychopharmacol Biol Psychiatry.* 2008;32:1283–1286.

64. Reess TJ, Rus OG, Schmidt R, et al. Connectomics-based structural network alterations in obsessive-compulsive disorder. *Transl Psychiatry.* 2016;6:e882.

65. de Vries FE, de Wit SJ, Cath DC, et al. Compensatory frontoparietal activity during working memory: an endophenotype of obsessive-compulsive disorder. *Biol Psychiatry.* 2014;76:878–887.

66. Ivarsson T, Melin K, Wallin L. Categorical and dimensional aspects of co-morbidity in obsessive-compulsive disorder (OCD). *Eur Child Adolesc Psychiatry.* 2008;17:20–31.

67. Roessner V, Overlack S, Schmidt-Samoa C, et al. Increased putamen and callosal motor subregion in treatment-naïve boys with Tourette syndrome indicates changes in the bihemispheric motor network. *J Child Psychol Psychiatry.* 2011;52:306–314.

68. Peterson BS, Thomas P, Kane MJ, et al. Basal Ganglia volumes in patients with Gilles de la Tourette syndrome. *Arch Gen Psychiatry.* 2003;60:415–424.

69. Worbe Y, Gerardin E, Hartmann A, et al. Distinct structural changes underpin clinical phenotypes in patients with Gilles de la Tourette syndrome. *Brain.* 2010;133:3649–3660.

70. Draganski B, Martino D, Cavanna AE, et al. Multispectral brain morphometry in Tourette syndrome persisting into adulthood. *Brain.* 2010;133:3661–3675.

71. Cano M, Alonso P, Martínez-Zalacaín I, et al. Altered functional connectivity of the subthalamus and the bed nucleus of the stria terminalis in obsessive-compulsive disorder. *Psychol Med.* 2018;48:919–928.

72. Mantovani A, Rossi S, Bassi BD, et al. Modulation of motor cortex excitability in obsessive-compulsive disorder: an exploratory study on the relations of neurophysiology measures with clinical outcome. *Psychiatry Res.* 2013;210:1026–1032.

73. Bloch Y, Arad S, Levkovitz Y. Deep TMS add-on treatment for intractable Tourette syndrome: a feasibility study. *World J Biol Psychiatry.* 2016;17:557–561.

74. Yoo SY, Jang JH, Shin YW, et al. White matter abnormalities in drug-naïve patients with obsessive-compulsive disorder: a diffusion tensor study before and after citalopram treatment. *Acta Psychiatr Scand.* 2007;116:211–219.

75. Hoexter MQ, de Souza Duran FL, D'Alcante CC, et al. Gray matter volumes in obsessive-compulsive disorder before and after fluoxetine or cognitive-behavior therapy: a randomized clinical trial. *Neuropsychopharmacology.* 2012;37:734–745.

76. Gilbert AR, Moore GJ, Keshavan MS, et al. Decrease in thalamic volumes of pediatric patients with obsessive-compulsive disorder who are taking paroxetine. *Arch Gen Psychiatry.* 2000;57:449–456.

77. Huyser C, van den Heuvel OA, Wolters LH, et al. Increased orbital frontal gray matter volume after cognitive behavioural therapy in paediatric obsessive compulsive disorder. *World J Biol Psychiatry.* 2013;14:319–331.

78. Huyser C, van den Heuvel OA, Wolters L, et al. A longitudinal VBM study in paediatric obsessive-compulsive disorder at 2-year follow-up after cognitive behavioural therapy. *World J Biol Psychiatry.* 2014;15:443–452.

79. Hoexter MQ, Dougherty DD, Shavitt RG, et al. Differential prefrontal gray matter correlates of treatment response to fluoxetine or cognitive-behavioral therapy in obsessive-compulsive disorder. *Eur Neuropsychopharmacol.* 2013;23:569–580.

80. Berlim MT, McGirr A, Van den Eynde F, et al. Effectiveness and acceptability of deep brain stimulation (DBS) of the subgenual cingulate cortex for treatment-resistant depression: a systematic review and exploratory meta-analysis. *J Affect Disord.* 2014;159:31–38.

81. Redlich R, Opel N, Grotegerd D, et al. Prediction of individual response to electroconvulsive therapy via machine learning on structural magnetic resonance imaging data. *JAMA Psychiatry.* 2016;73:557–564.

82. Bryant RA, Felmingham K, Whitford TJ, et al. Rostral anterior cingulate volume predicts treatment response to cognitive-behavioural therapy for posttraumatic stress disorder. *J Psychiatry Neurosci.* 2008;33:142–146.

83. Seminowicz DA, Shpaner M, Keaser ML, et al. Cognitive-behavioral therapy increases prefrontal cortex gray matter in patients with chronic pain. *J Pain.* 2013;14:1573–1584.

84. Milad MR, Quinn BT, Pitman RK, et al. Thickness of ventromedial prefrontal cortex in humans is correlated with extinction memory. *Proc Natl Acad Sci USA.* 2005;102:10706–10711.

85. Quirk GJ, Mueller D. Neural mechanisms of extinction learning and retrieval. *Neuropsychopharmacology.* 2008;33:56 72.

86. Fullana MA, Cardoner N, Alonso P, et al. Brain regions related to fear extinction in obsessive-compulsive disorder and its relation to exposure therapy outcome: a morphometric study. *Psychol Med.* 2014;44:845–856.

87. Subirà M, Cano M, de Wit SJ, et al. Structural covariance of neostriatal and limbic regions in patients with obsessive-compulsive disorder. *J Psychiatry Neurosci.* 2016;41:115–123.

88. Tsuchiyagaito A, Hirano Y, Asano K, et al. Cognitive-behavioral therapy for obsessive-compulsive disorder with and without autism spectrum disorder: gray matter differences associated with poor outcome. *Front Psychiatry.* 2017;8:143.

89. Cecconi JP, Lopes AC, Duran FL, et al. Gamma ventral capsulotomy for treatment of resistant obsessive-compulsive disorder: a structural MRI pilot prospective study. *Neurosci Lett.* 2008;447:138–142.

90. Makris N, Rathi Y, Mouradian P, et al. Variability and anatomical specificity of the orbitofrontothalamic fibers of passage in the ventral capsule/ventral striatum (VC/VS): precision care for patient-specific tractography-guided targeting of deep brain stimulation (DBS) in obsessive compulsive disorder (OCD). *Brain Imaging Behav.* 2016;10:1054–1067.

91. Suñol M, Contreras-Rodríguez O, Macià D, et al. Brain structural correlates of subclinical obsessive-compulsive symptoms in healthy children. *J Am Acad Child Adolesc Psychiatry.* 2018;57:41–47.

92. Fullana MA, Mataix-Cols D, Caspi A, et al. Obsessions and compulsions in the community: prevalence, interference, help-seeking, developmental stability, and co-occurring psychiatric conditions. *Am J Psychiatry.* 2009;166:329–336.

93. Zucker BG, Craske MG, Blackmore MA, et al. A cognitive behavioral workshop for subclinical obsessions and compulsions. *Behav Res Ther.* 2006;44:289–304.

Chapter 9

Functional Magnetic Resonance Imaging Studies of Obsessive-Compulsive and Related Disorders

Jaewook Han and Jun Soo Kwon

Recent Research Findings

Since the 1980s, a large number of functional neuroimaging studies using positron emission tomography (PET), single-photon emission computed tomography (SPECT) and functional magnetic resonance imaging (fMRI) in obsessive-compulsive disorder (OCD) have identified abnormal hyperactivity throughout the frontal and subcortical regions, such as the orbitofrontal cortex, anterior cingulate cortex (ACC), caudate nucleus and thalamus. Although little work has been done on obsessive-compulsive and related disorders (OCRDs) other than OCD, some fMRI studies have investigated neurobiological abnormalities in hoarding disorder, body dysmorphic disorder (BDD), trichotillomania and skin-picking disorder. In this chapter, we review fMRI findings on OCRDs and discuss their implications. We have classified the studies and present summarizing tables depending on the paradigms and objectives (Tables 9.1–9.5). In this section, we focus on OCD as the prototype of OCRDs, on which a host of studies have been done. We extend to other OCRDs and mental disorders in a transdiagnostic view, and discuss its implication on classification, diagnosis, treatment and prevention in the following sections.

fMRI studies have demonstrated aberrant activation of related brain regions during symptom provocation in OCD. In the first fMRI study using the symptom provocation paradigm in OCD, Breiter and Rauch used provocative stimulus in terms of the sensory, motor and cognitive components; for example, exposure to tissue soaked in toilet water [20]. They reported increased activation in the orbitofrontal, lateral frontal, anterior temporal, anterior cingulate and insular cortex, as well as caudate, lenticulate and amygdala in patients. Other studies reported increased activation of the insula, frontal area and other brain regions during exposure to disgust-inducing pictures [14,17]. While some findings suggest that there is no difference in neural activation between patients with OCD and healthy controls during the processing of threat-inducing pictures, which indicates that sensitivity to negative stimuli in OCD is restricted to disgust, not fear [15,17,19], discrepant reports also exist [6,7].

There have also been approaches to address distinct neural correlates across symptom dimensions. Phillips and colleagues used neutral, normally disgusting, and washer-relevant pictures for patients with OCD with symptoms that predominantly concerned washing (washers) and checking (checkers), and for healthy controls [19]. All three groups showed activation of the insula and visual regions implicated in the perception of aversive stimuli. However, only the washers had similar regions activated by washer-relevant pictures. In line with this, following fMRI studies demonstrated discrete neural activation across symptom dimensions in OCD, during cognitive tasks or in a resting state, as well as in symptom-provoking conditions [4,12,103]. Together, these findings suggest that a distinct neural mechanism is involved in mediation of each obsessive-compulsive symptom. In this respect, a transdiagnostic dimensional approach using functional neuroimaging can possibly provide better understanding of individual variance in phenomenology and neurobiology among patients with OCD.

Previous fMRI studies using symptom-provocation paradigms in patients with OCD have shown increased activity most consistently in the orbitofrontal cortex, cingulate cortex and caudate which are components of the corticostriatothalamocortical (CSTC) circuit. Based on these findings, the CSTC model has been postulated as a neurobiological model of OCD that mediates symptomatic expressions. In this model, it has been suggested that an imbalance of activity in excitatory (direct) and inhibitory (indirect) pathways within the CSTC circuit produces hyperactivation in

Table 9.1 Functional magnetic resonance imaging studies using symptom provocation paradigms.

Year	Authors [reference]	Sample	Task	Findings
2016	Beucke et al. [1]	28 BDD, 28 HC	Face matching task (HSF, NSF or LSF)	Reduced local amygdalar connectivity. BDD-Y-BOCS scores correlated with connectivity of OFC.
2015	Moody et al. [2]	20 AN, 20 BDD, 20 HC	Face matching task (HSF, NSF or LSF)	Increased FC between occipital and fusiform face areas, associated with symptom severity in BDD.
2014	Via et al. [3]	67 OCD, 67 HC	Emotional face matching task	Greater amygdalar activation, associated with severity of aggression/checking and sexual/religious symptom dimensions in response to fearful face stimuli.
2014	Jhung et al. [4]	26 OCD (13 with and 13 without contamination/washing symptoms), 18 HC	Symptom provocation by augmented reality	Altered FC between VS and insula in those with contamination/washing symptoms, correlated with contamination/washing symptom severity.
2014	Simon et al. [5]	21 OCD, 21 HC	Distraction task during symptom provocation	Amygdala hyperactivation across symptom dimensions. Dampening of amygdala hyperactivity during distraction.
2013	Milad et al. [6]	21 OCD, 21 HC	Fear conditioning and extinction recall	Reduced activation in caudate and hippocampus during fear conditioning, as well as in cerebellum, PCC and putamen during extinction recall.
2012	Weygandt et al. [7]	10 OCD, 10 HC	Disgust/fear-inducing and neutral pictures	Altered activation of OFC and caudate.
2012	Bohon et al. [8]	17 BDD, 16 HC	Own-face, familiar-face and oval images	Activity in left ventral visual stream was associated with anxiety, stronger for own-face versus familiar-face stimuli.
2011	Feusner et al. [9]	14 BDD, 14 HC	Matching task (photographs of house of HSF, NSF or LSF)	Lesser activity in parahippocampal and lingual gyrus, and precuneus for LSF images. Lesser activity in dorsal occipital cortex and vlPFC for HSF and NSF images associated with greater symptom severity.
2010	Lee et al. [10]	9 pediatric TTM, 10 HC	Symptom provocation of VO or VT	Greater activation in temporal cortex, PCC and putamen during VO session. Higher activity in precuneus and PCC during VT condition.
2009	An et al. [11]	29 OCD (13 with and 16 without prominent hoarding symptoms), 21 HC	Hoarding-related and symptom-unrelated anxiety provoking pictures	Greater activation in vmPFC in response to hoarding-related anxiety provocation in patients with prominent hoarding symptoms.

2007	Lawrence et al. [12]	17 OCD, 19 HC	Emotional face stimuli (fear or disgust)	Greater activation in vlPFC but reduced activation in thalamus to facial expressions of disgust. Increased vlPFC activation in female patients with high washing symptoms.
2007	Feusner et al. [13]	12 BDD, 13 HC	Face matching task (HSF, NSF or LSF)	Greater activity in lateral PFC and temporal cortex for all face tasks and ACC for LSF task.
2005	Schienle et al. [14]	10 OCD, 10 HC	Disgust/fear-inducing pictures	Greater activation in PFC, insula, supramarginal gyrus, caudate and thalamus to OCD-relevant pictures. Greater activation in insula to OCD-irrelevant disgust/fear-inducing pictures.
2004	Mataix-Cols et al. [15]	16 OCD, 17 HC	Symptom-related and -unrelated emotional pictures	Distinct pattern of activation associated with each symptom dimension: vmPFC and caudate (washing); putamen and thalamus (checking); precentral gyrus and OFC (hoarding).
2004	Cannistraro et al. [16]	10 OCD, 10 HC	Emotional face stimuli (fearful and happy)	Reduced activation of amygdala across all face conditions.
2003	Shapira et al. [17]	8 OCD, 8 HC	Disgust/threat-inducing pictures	Greater increases in insula, IFG and parahippocampal region during disgust-inducing condition.
2000	Adler et al. [18]	7 OCD	Individually tailored provocative stimuli	Activation in OFC, DLPFC, ACC, superior frontal and temporal cortices.
2000	Phillips et al. [19]	14 OCD (7 washers and 7 checkers), 14 HC	Normally disgusting- and washer-relevant pictures	All subjects showed activation of visual regions and insula. Only washers had similar regions activated by washer-relevant pictures.
1996	Breiter et al. [20]	10 OCD, 5 HC	Symptom provocation task	Greater activation in OFC, ACC, insula, caudate, temporal cortex, lenticulate and amygdala.

ACC, anterior cingulate cortex; AN, anorexia nervosa; BDD, body dysmorphic disorder; BDD-Y-BOCS, Yale-Brown obsessive compulsive scale modified for body dysmorphic disorder; DLPFC, dorsolateral prefrontal cortex; FC, functional connectivity; HC, healthy controls; HSF, high spatial frequency; IFG, inferior frontal gyrus; LSF, low spatial frequency; NSF, normal spatial frequency; OCD, obsessive-compulsive disorder; OFC, orbitofrontal cortex; PCC, posterior cingulate cortex; PFC, prefrontal cortex; STN, subthalamic nucleus; TTM, trichotillomania; vlPFC, ventrolateral prefrontal cortex; vmPFC, ventromedial prefrontal cortex; VO, visual only; VT, visual and tactile; VS, ventral striatum.

Table 9.2 Functional magnetic resonance imaging studies using cognitive activation paradigms.

Year	Author [reference]	Sample	Task	Findings
2016	Hough et al. [21]	17 OCD, 15 HD, 25 HC	Go/no-go task, Stroop task	In HD, greater activity in ACC and DLPFC during conflict monitoring and response inhibition compared with HC, and greater activity in DLPFC compared with OCD.
2016	Morein-Zamir et al. [22]	19 OCD, 19 HC	Combined stop-shift task	Reduced activation across frontal-parietal areas for shifting but not stopping. Abnormal caudate and thalamus activation.
2016	Odlaug et al. [23]	18 SPD, 15 HC	Tower of London task	Underactivation in DS (maximal in caudate), ACC and right medial frontal regions.
2016	Han et al. [24]	20 OCD, 21 HC	Delayed-response working memory task	Connectivity from DLPFC to OFC was negatively modulated by negative emotional distraction.
2016	Weidt et al. [25]	18 OCD, 18 SAD, 18 HC	Emotional anticipation and perception task	Increased activation in amygdala, caudate, PFC and OFC while anticipating unspecific emotional stimuli in both patient groups. Decreased rACC activation in OCD patients during perception, but no differences in anticipation phase.
2015	van Velzen et al. [26]	41 OCD, 17 unaffected first-degree relatives, 37 HC	Stop-signal task	Altered connectivity between IFG and amygdala during response inhibition in patients and their unaffected relatives.
2015	Marsh et al. [27]	33 OCD, 33 HC	Reward-based learning task	Abnormal recruitment of mesolimbic, ventral striatal circuitry.
2015	Gillan et al. [28]	37 OCD, 33 HC	Avoidance training and habit test	Excessive habit formation which was associated with hyperactivation in caudate. Hyperactivation in medial OFC during acquisition of avoidance; however this did not relate directly to habit formation.
2015	Rotge et al. [29]	14 OCD, 14 HC	Checking task	Error signals increased OFC activations, whereas checking behaviors decreased these activations in HC. No such modulation was observed in patients.
2014	Tolin et al. [30]	24 OCD, 24 HD, 24 HC	Go/no-go task	Greater precentral gyrus activation in HD, whereas greater OFC activation in OCD during response inhibition.
2014	Marsh et al. [31]	22 OCD, 22 HC	Simon spatial incompatibility task	Increased activity in response to conflict-laden stimuli in frontostriatal regions, specifically a right hemisphere cluster encompassing putamen, insula and IFG.
2014	de Vries et al. [32]	43 OCD, 17 unaffected siblings, 37 HC	Visuospatial n-back task	Compensatory task-related frontoparietal hyperactivity in patients and siblings.
2014	Agam et al. [33]	21 OCD, 20 HC	Antisaccade task	Abnormal adjustments in post- vs. pre-error trial. Increased default network activation including in rACC.
2013	Kang et al. [34]	18 OCD, 18 HC	Modified version of stop-signal task	Lower activation in cingulate cortex and BG during response inhibition. Increased FC of caudate during resting state.

2013	White et al. [35]	21 TTM, 14 HC	Monetary incentive delay task	Decreased NAc activation to reward anticipation, but over-activity of NAc to both gain and loss outcomes.
2013	Jung et al. [36]	19 OCD, 18 HC	Monetary incentive delay task	Increased FC between NAc and OFC during resting state. Reduced FC between NAc and limbic areas during incentive processing.
2013	Stern et al. [37]	25 OCD, 29 HC	Decision making task	Greater activation in vmPFC, OFC, temporal cortex, insula, parahippocampus and amygdala.
2012	de Wit et al. [38]	41 OCD, 17 unaffected siblings, 37 HC	Stop-signal task	Greater activity in presupplementary motor area during inhibition in patients and siblings.
2012	Tolin et al. [39]	31 OCD, 43 HD, 33 HC	Decision making task	Increased ACC and insula activity in HD compared with OCD and HC during decision making.
2012	Harrison et al. [40]	73 OCD, 73 HC	Moral dilemma task	Increased OFC activation and more robust activation in DLPFC and MTG.
2012	Cocchi et al. [41]	17 OCD, 19 HC	Multisource interference task	Differences in FC were most pronounced during rest-task transitions and mainly involved dACC and insula.
2011	van den Heuvel et al. [42]	22 OCD, 14 panic disorder, 14 hypochondriasis, 22 HC	Tower of London task	Decreased activation in precuneus, caudate nucleus and thalamus in all patients. State anxiety and task performance correlated with dorsal frontal-striatal activation in all patients.
2011	Jung et al. [43]	20 OCD, 20 HC	Monetary incentive delay task	Increased VS activation in no-loss minus loss outcome but not in gain anticipation.
2011	Stern et al. [44]	39 OCD, 33 HC	Error-eliciting interference task	Reduced vmPFC activation and greater insula activation during errors. Increased FC between vmPFC and insula and thalamus.
2011	Figee et al. [45]	18 OCD, 19 HC	Monetary incentive delay task	Attenuated reward anticipation activity in NAc.
2010	Rubia et al. [46]	10 OCD, 18 ADHD, 20 HC	Stop-signal task, switch task	Both patient groups shared brain dysfunction in OFC and DLPFC during inhibition. ADHD-specific dysfunction was observed in BG, inferior prefrontal and cingulate cortices.
2010	Schlösser et al. [47]	21 OCD, 21 HC	Stroop task	Increased activation in fronto-cingulate system during incongruent task condition. Stronger dACC-DLPFC modulation of effective connectivity.
2010	Fitzgerald et al. [48]	18 pediatric OCD, 18 HC	Multisource interference task	Increased dACC-ventral MFG connectivity during task, and decreased dACC-right anterior operculum and ventral MFG-posterior cingulate connectivity during rest.
2009	Remijnse et al. [49]	20 OCD, 20 MDD, 27 HC	Reversal learning task	Blunted responsiveness of OFC-striatal loop during reward, and in OFC and insula during affective switching.
2009	Nakao et al. [50]	40 OCD, 25 HC	N-back task	Greater activation in DLPFC, STG, insula and cuneus. Right OFC activity positively correlated with Y-BOCS scores.

(*continued*)

Table 9.2 *(cont.)*

Year	Author [reference]	Sample	Task	Findings
2008	Woolley et al. [51]	10 pediatric OCD, 9 HC	Stop task, motor Stroop task and switch task	Reduced activation in OFC, thalamus and BG during stop task.
2008	Chamberlain et al. [52]	14 OCD, 12 unaffected first-degree relatives, 15 HC	Reversal learning task, set-shifting task	Reduced activation in cortical regions including OFC during reversal learning in patients and their relatives.
2008	Gu et al. [53]	21 OCD, 21 HC	Task-switching paradigm	Decreased activation in OFC, DLPFC, ACC, vmPFC, and caudate during task-switching. Task performances correlated with activation of OFC and ACC.
2007	Yücel et al. [54]	19 OCD, 19 HC	Multisource interference task	Greater activation of supplementary motor area and deactivation of rACC during high- vs. low-conflict trials. Reduced levels of neuronal N-acetylaspartate in dACC, which negatively correlated with BOLD activation of the region.
2007	Roth et al. [55]	12 OCD, 14 HC	Go/no-go task	Less activation in several right-hemisphere regions during response inhibition including IFG.
2007	Rauch et al. [56]	10 TTM, 10 HC	Serial reaction time task	No significant differences in implicit learning or in activation within striatum, hippocampus or other brain regions.
2007	Rauch et al. [57]	12 OCD, 12 HC	Serial reaction time task	Increased hippocampus and OFC activation during implicit sequence learning. Inverse correlation between striatal activation and specific symptom factors.
2006	Remijnse et al. [58]	20 OCD, 27 HC	Reversal learning task	Reduced responsiveness in OFC, and caudate on reward outcome. Reduced activity in OFC, insula, DLPFC and anterior PFC during affective switching.
2005	Maltby et al. [59]	14 OCD, 14 HC	Go/no-go task	Only correctly rejected, high-conflict trials produced excessive activation in both action monitoring (ACC, lateral PFC) and frontal striatal regions (OFC, caudate, and thalamus)..
2005	van den Heuvel et al. [60]	22 OCD, 22 HC	Tower of London task	Reduced DLPFC and caudate nucleus activation during planning.
2005	Fitzgerald et al. [61]	8 OCD, 7 HC	Flanker interference task	Greater error-related activation of ACC. This activity positively correlated with symptom severity.
2005	Viard et al. [62]	12 OCD, 15 HC	Conflict task	Increased activation in ACC and parietal lobe.
2003	Ursu et al. [63]	11 OCD, 13 HC	Continuous performance task	Increased ACC activation during high-conflict trials.

ACC, anterior cingulate cortex; ADHD, attention deficit and hyperactivity disorder; BG, basal ganglia; BOLD, blood oxygen level dependent; dACC, dorsal anterior cingulate cortex; DLPFC, dorsolateral prefrontal cortex; DS, dorsal striatum; FC, functional connectivity; HC, healthy controls; HD, hoarding disorder; IFG, inferior frontal gyrus; MDD, major depression disorder; MFG, medial frontal gyrus; MTG, middle temporal gyrus; NAc, nucleus accumbens; OCD, obsessive-compulsive disorder; OFC, orbitofrontal cortex; PFC, prefrontal cortex; rACC, rostral anterior cingulate cortex; SAD, social anxiety disorder; SPD, skin picking disorder; STG, superior temporal gyrus; TTM, trichotillomania; vmPFC, ventromedial prefrontal cortex; VS, ventral striatum; Y-BOCS, Yale-Brown obsessive compulsive scale.

Table 9.3 Functional magnetic resonance imaging studies related to the effects of treatments.

Year	Author	Sample	Treatment	Findings
2017	Zhao et al. [64]	31 OCD, 25 HC	cognitive-coping therapy with or without pharmacotherapy	Difference of ALFF in frontal, temporal, parietal and other areas between patients and HC disappeared after relief of symptoms.
2016	Dunlop et al. [65]	20 OCD, 40 HC	rTMS	Reduction in dmPFC-VS connectivity correlated to improvement on Y-BOCS.
2015	Yang et al. [66]	22 OCD, 22 HC	CBT	Improvement of OCD symptoms correlated with reduction of ReHo in OFC and cerebellum.
2015	de Wit et al. [67]	43 OCD, 38 HC	rTMS	Real vs. sham DLPFC stimulation differentially modulated frontal-amygdala connectivity during emotion regulation.
2014	Morgiève et al. [68]	35 OCD	CBT	Anxiety ratings and hemodynamic response in ACC but not OFC decreased with symptom improvement.
2014	Shin et al. [69]	25 OCD, 23 HC	SSRI	Decreased baseline small-world efficiency, modular organization and connectivity degree elevated after effective treatment.
2013	Figee et al. [70]	16 OCD, 13 HC	DBS	DBS targeted at NAc normalized activity, reduced excessive connectivity between NAc and PFC, and decreased frontal low-frequency oscillations during symptom provocation.
2012	Tolin et al. [71]	6 HD, 6 HC	CBT	Baseline differences in hemodynamic activity between HD and HC disappeared after CBT.
2011	Han et al. [72]	10 OCD, 20 HC	pharmacotherapy	After treatment, activation deficit partially normalized not in dorsal frontoparietal regions but in ventral frontal–striatal circuit.
2011	Freyer et al. [73]	10 OCD, 10 HC	CBT	Increased activity in caudate head during strategy change within a reversal learning task after CBT compared with baseline.
2008	Lázaro et al. [74]	12 pediatric OCD, 12 HC	fluoxetine and behavioral counseling	Higher activation in MFG. Activation in insula and putamen decreased after effective treatment.
2008	Nabeyama et al. [75]	11 OCD, 19 HC	BT	Less activation in ACC and cerebellum. Following clinical improvement, cerebellum and parietal lobe showed increased activation, and OFC, MFG, and temporal regions showed decreased activation during Stroop task.
2007	van der Wee et al. [76]	14 OCD	paroxetine or venlafaxine	Performance (n-back task) improved only in responders and was associated with a change in overall pattern of brain activity during task.
2005	Nakao et al. [77]	10 OCD	fluvoxamine or BT	After symptom improvement, provocation–related activation in OFC, DLPFC and ACC decreased, whereas Stroop task–related activation in parietal cortex and cerebellum increased.

ACC, anterior cingulate cortex; ALFF, amplitude of low frequency fluctuations; BT, behavior therapy; CBT, cognitive behavioral therapy; DBS, deep brain stimulation; DLPFC, dorsolateral prefrontal cortex; dmPFC, dorsomedial prefrontal cortex; HC, healthy controls; HD, hoarding disorder; MFG, medial frontal gyrus; NAc, nucleus accumbens; OCD, obsessive-compulsive disorder; OFC, orbitofrontal cortex; PFC, prefrontal cortex; ReHo, regional homogeneity; rTMS, repetitive transcranial magnetic stimulation; SSRI, selective serotonin reuptake inhibitors; VS, ventral striatum; Y-BOCS, Yale-Brown Obsessive Compulsive Scale.

Table 9.4 Functional magnetic resonance imaging studies on the prediction of treatment response.

Year	Author	Subjects	Treatment	Findings
2015	Feusner et al. [78]	17 OCD	CBT	Small-worldness and clustering coefficient increased after treatment. Decreases in modularity correlated with symptom improvement.
2015	Göttlich et al. [79]	17 OCD, 19 HC	CBT	Lower degree centrality of amygdala. Degree centrality of right basolateral nuclei group of amygdala positively correlated with CBT response.
2014	Olatunji et al. [80]	12 OCD	CBT	Baseline activity in temporal pole and amygdala during symptom provocation was associated with better response to CBT.
2010	Sanematsu et al. [81]	17 OCD	Fluvoxamine	Pretreatment activation in cerebellum and STG positively correlated with improvement in Y-BOCS scores after treatment.

CBT, cognitive behavioral therapy; HC, healthy controls; OCD, obsessive-compulsive disorder; STG, superior temporal gyrus; Y-BOCS, Yale-Brown Obsessive Compulsive Scale.

the whole circuit to generate OCD symptomatology [112]. Abnormal activation of the insula is often reported as well. The insula is known as the part of the gustatory cortex that processes unpleasant tastes and smells mediating the disgust response [113,114]. Accordingly, abnormal activation of the insula during symptom provocation suggests that patients with OCD may be prone to experiencing disgust and may show an exaggerated neural response to related stimuli.

On the other hand, various cognitive activation paradigms have been used in fMRI research to examine the neurobiological underpinning of cognitive deficits in OCD. Impaired response inhibition has long been theorized to be a model for OCD symptoms. Behavioral, event-related potential and neuroimaging studies have inferred impaired response inhibition in patients with OCD from the motor response inhibition in stop-signal or go/no-go tasks and cognitive inhibition in the Stroop or negative priming task [115,116,117,118]. Maltby and colleagues used the go/no-go task in which participants were instructed to respond as quickly as possible with a button press to "go" stimuli and to inhibit responding to a "no-go" stimulus during fMRI [59]. Under the no-go condition, when the participants needed a strong response inhibition, participants with OCD showed increased activation in the anterior cingulate, prefrontal, and orbitofrontal cortices, caudate, and thalamus compared with healthy controls. In contrast, other fMRI studies reported hypoactivation of these areas during response inhibition [34,51,55]. Aberrant brain activity during inhibition was also observed in close relatives of patients with OCD. De Wit and colleagues compared the stop-signal reaction time (SSRT) and regional brain activity of patients with OCD, their unaffected siblings and healthy controls [38]. In that study, both patients and siblings showed greater activity in the left presupplementary motor area during successful inhibition compared with healthy controls, which negatively correlated with the SSRT. Another study by van Velzen and colleagues also reported an increased SSRT in patients with OCD, but not in siblings, compared with healthy controls, with altered connectivity between the inferior frontal gyrus and the amygdala during response inhibition [26]. These discrepancies among studies may be attributed to different task designs, heterogeneity of the study participants or the effects of medication.

Previous neurocognitive studies have also reported impaired cognitive flexibility in patients with OCD and their unaffected close relatives [58,118,119]. Among various tasks, reversal learning and task-switching paradigm have been used to evaluate dysfunctional brain activation regarding cognitive flexibility in OCD. The orbitofrontal cortex has long been known to be important in reversal learning, which has a role in altering behavior flexibly after negative feedback [120,121]. fMRI studies have identified impaired performance and aberrant orbitofrontal cortex activation during reversal learning in patients with OCD. Using the reversal learning paradigm, Remijnse and colleagues reported

Table 9.5 Other resting-state functional magnetic resonance imaging studies.

Year	Author	Sample	Approach	Findings
2017	Jung et al. [82]	61 OCD, 61 HC	Unsupervised clustering and multilevel FC techniques	Disruption of small-world properties and FC in orbito-fronto-striato-thalamic circuit.
2017	Posner et al. [83]	30 OCD, 32 HC	Seed-based connectivity	Reduced inverse DMN-SN connectivity was associated with increased symptom severity and decreased sustained attention.
2017	Vaghi et al. [84]	44 OCD, 43 HC	Seed-based connectivity, ICA	Reduced FC between caudate and vlPFC was associated with reduced cognitive flexibility. Goal-directed performance was related to reduced FC between putamen and DLPFC, as well as to symptom severity.
2017	Xie et al. [89]	68 OCD, 33 HC	Granger causality analysis	Enhanced functional coupling in reward circuits and weakened functional coupling in cognitive control system.
2016	Armstrong et al. [85]	21 pediatric OCD, 20 HC	Graph theoretical analysis	Disruption of small-worldness, modularity and higher clustering coefficients in frontopolar site.
2016	Chen et al. [86]	30 OCD, 30 HC	Voxel-based FC analysis	Reduced FC within CSTC circuitry. Decreased caudate-thalamus connectivity within CSTC circuitry positively correlated with illness duration.
2016	Tang et al. [87]	18 OCD, 16 HC	ALFF, VBM	Overactivation of cerebellum and parietal lobe and reduced activation of cingulate gyrus, putamen and caudate.
2016	Tian et al. [88]	29 OCD, 29 HC	Graph theoretical analysis	Increased FC in CSTC circuit and additionally parietal, occipital, temporal and cerebellar regions. Affected FC strength in cerebellum, OFC and occipital cortex correlated with symptom severity.
2016	Zhu et al. [90]	28 OCD, 28 HC	ALFF	Increased ALFF in frontopolar cortex and OFC, with decreased ALFF in insula. Insular intrinsic activity correlated with Y-BOCS score.
2016	Bernstein et al. [91]	15 pediatric OCD, 13 HC	Seed-based connectivity	Lower FC between putamen and right cortical areas including OFC, IFG, insula and operculum.
2015	Abe et al. [92]	37 OCD, 38 HC	Granger causality analysis	Hyperinfluence of OFC over VS, which was not mediated by another brain area within striatum.
2014	Beucke et al. [93]	46 OCD, 46 HC	Seed-based connectivity	Reduced connectivity within dmPFC self-subsystem, and increased connectivity between self-subsystem and salience and attention networks.
2014	Hou et al. [94]	39 OCD, 20 unaffected first-degree relatives, 39 HC	Graph theoretical analysis	Increased FC within CSTC circuits and decreased FC in occipital, temporal cortices and cerebellum in patients. Patients and relatives exhibited overlapping increased FC in caudate, OFC and MTG.
2014	Anticevic et al. [95].	27 OCD 66 HC	GBC	Reduced FC in PFC and increased FC in putamen and cerebellum. Increased GBC in DS and thalamus, which was reduced in patients on medication.

(continued)

Table 9.5 *(cont.)*

Year	Author	Sample	Approach	Findings
2014	Peng et al. [96]	15 OCD, 15 unaffected siblings, 28 HC	Seed-based connectivity	Reduced strength of default network FC with PCC, and increased FC in inferior frontal lobe, insula, superior parietal cortex and STG. Unaffected siblings only showed reduced local connectivity in PCC.
2014	Gruner et al. [97]	23 pediatric OCD, 23 HC	ALFF, ICA	Reduced IC expression in visual network. Higher IC expression in ACC/PCC network correlated with greater severity of compulsions.
2014	Posner et al. [98]	23 OCD, 20 HC	Seed-based connectivity	Unmedicated OCD subjects showed reduced connectivity within limbic CSTC loop, which correlated with symptom severity.
2014	Weber et al. [99]	11 pediatric OCD, 9 HC	ICA	Reduced connectivity in BA 8 and BA 40 in cingulate network in OCD and increased connectivity in BA 43 of auditory network.
2013	Beucke et al. [100]	46 OCD (23 unmedicated), 46 HC	Voxel-wise whole-brain correlation analysis	Greater distant connectivity in OFC and STN and greater local connectivity in OFC and putamen. Distant connectivity of OFC and putamen positively correlated with symptom severity. Medicated patients showed reduced local connectivity of VS compared with unmedicated patients.
2013	Cheng et al. [101]	23 OCD, 23 HC	ALFF, ICA	Reduced ALFF in PCC and increased ALFF in ACC.
2013	Hou et al. [102]	33 OCD, 33 HC	Seed voxel correlation approach	Abnormal functional integration in CSTC circuits and DMN. Increased FC within CSTC circuits positively correlated with Y-BOCS score.
2013	Harrison et al. [103]	74 OCD, 74 HC	Seed-based connectivity	Common connectivity alteration involving VS and OFC that predicted illness severity. Distinct anatomical relationships between severity of symptom dimensions and striatal FC.
2012	Hou et al. [104]	23 OCD, 23 HC	ALFF	Increased ALFF in OFC, ACC as well as decreased ALFF in cerebellum and parietal cortex. ALFF in OFC positively correlated with total Y-BOCS scores.
2012	Meunier et al. [105]	18 OCD, 18 stimulant dependent individuals, 18 HC	Nodal connectivity analysis	Reduced FC in OFC. Compulsive symptom severity was associated with greater reductions of OFC connectivity.
2012	Stern et al. [106]	30 OCD (17 unmedicated) and 32 HC	Seed-based connectivity	Altered connectivity between FPN seeds and several regions of DMN including PCC, MFG, posterior inferior parietal lobule and parahippocampus. Greater positive connectivity between FPN and regions outside DMN, including thalamus, lateral frontal cortex and somatosensory/motor regions.

2011	Fitzgerald et al. [107]	60 OCD, 61 HC	Seed-based connectivity	Youngest patients showed reduced connectivity of DS and medial dorsal thalamus to rACC and dACC, respectively. Increased connectivity of DS to ventral MFG was observed in patients at all developmental stages.
2011	Sakai et al. [108]	20 OCD, 23 HC	Seed-based connectivity	Increased FC with VS to OFC, vmPFC and DLPFC.
2011	Zhang et al. [109]	18 OCD, 16 HC	Graph theoretical analysis	Decreased FC in posterior temporal regions and increased FC in cingulate, precuneus, thalamus and cerebellum. Higher local clustering, implying abnormal functional organization in control network.
2010	Jang et al. [110]	22 OCD, 22 HC	Seed-based connectivity	Decreased FC within DMN in ACC, MFG and putamen.
2009	Harrison et al. [111]	21 OCD, 21 HC	Seed-based connectivity	Increased FC along a ventral corticostriatal axis, implicating OFC and surrounding areas. Reduced FC of DS and lateral PFC, and of VS with region of midbrain VTA.

ACC, anterior cingulate cortex; ALFF, amplitude of low frequency fluctuations; BA, Brodmann area; CSTC, corticostriatothalamocortical; dACC, dorsal anterior cingulate cortex; DLPFC, dorsolateral prefrontal cortex; DMN, default mode network; dmPFC, dorsomedial prefrontal cortex; DS, dorsal striatum; FC, functional connectivity; FPN, fronto-parietal network; GBC, global brain connectivity; HC, healthy controls; IC, independent component; ICA, Independent component analysis; IFG, inferior frontal gyrus; MFG, middle frontal gyrus; MTG, middle temporal gyrus; OCD, obsessive-compulsive disorder: OFC, orbitofrontal cortex; PCC, posterior cingulate cortex; PFC, prefrontal cortex; rACC, rostral anterior cingulate cortex; ReHo, regional homogeneity; SN, salience network; STG, superior temporal gyrus; STN, subthalamic nucleus; VBM, voxel-based morphometry; vlPFC, ventrolateral prefrontal cortex; vmPFC, ventromedial prefrontal cortex; VS, ventral striatum; VTA, ventral tegmental area; Y-BOCS, Yale-Brown Obsessive Compulsive Scale.

that patients with OCD showed reduced activation in the orbitofrontal, dorsolateral prefrontal, and anterior prefrontal cortices, and insula when they successfully adapted their response to the negative feedback [58]. Chamberlain and colleagues also used the reversal learning paradigm and reported reduced activation in the orbitofrontal, lateral prefrontal and parietal cortices in patients with OCD and their unaffected close relatives [52]. Gu and colleagues adopted the task-switching paradigm, which requires the ability to disengage attention from a previous task, resolve interference from previous stimuli or task sets and update new task sets [53]. In this study, the OCD group showed a higher error rate and decreased activation in the orbitofrontal, dorsolateral prefrontal, anterior cingulate, ventromedial prefrontal cortices and caudate during task switching compared with healthy controls. Furthermore, the orbitofrontal and ventromedial prefrontal cortices were activated only slightly in healthy controls at the switch minus repeat contrast, while these areas in the OCD group were activated during the repeat condition or hypoactivated. This finding supports the hypothesis of an imbalance between ventral and dorsal frontostriatal system in OCD pathophysiology, resulting in a hyperactivated ventral and an inhibited dorsal frontostriatal system. Other fMRI studies using the task-switching paradigm also reported underactivation of the frontostriatal and frontoparietal areas during task switching [22,72].

Previous electrophysiological studies on OCD have additionally shown an exaggerated error-related negativity [122,123,124]. Several fMRI studies have also reported error-related hyperactivity of the ACC in patients with OCD [59,61,63]. Applying dynamic causal modeling, Schlösser and colleagues reported enhanced activation in the frontocingulate system in patients with OCD during error processing elicited by an incongruent condition of the Stroop task [47]. Based on event-related potential and fMRI findings to date, it is suggested that excessive error signals generated by the frontocingulate system, especially the ACC, may be associated with patients' difficulty suppressing an emotional response to aversive, unexpected events or mistakes.

Deficits in executive function, such as planning and working memory, have also been reported in patients with OCD and their unaffected relatives [125,126,127,128]. In line with these findings, fMRI studies have reported impaired performance and aberrant activation in the dorsolateral prefrontal and orbitofrontal cortices, caudate and frontoparietal network during n-back or Tower of London (ToL) tasks in patients with OCD [32,50,60,129]. In addition, fMRI studies reported that patients with OCD exhibit altered activity and functional connectivity in the corticostriatal–limbic regions including the prefrontal area, nucleus accumbens and amygdala during reward processing [27,36,43,45].

Recently, various resting-state fMRI analytic methods including functional connectivity and graph theory-based approaches have been applied. These approaches have enabled researchers to assess the regional connectivity of resting-state and task-free brain activity, thus increasing our understanding of the complex brain network. Despite some discrepancies, convergent findings from resting-state fMRI studies in OCD have indicated altered functional connectivity in the CSTC circuit, with findings most often focused on the orbitofrontal and cingulate cortices and the striatum [70,94,100,103,108,111]. Moreover, not a few recent resting-state fMRI studies on OCD have reported disruption in a large-scale brain network including temporal, parietal, occipital cortices and cerebellum, which suggests pathophysiology beyond the CSTC circuit [64,66,87,88,94,95,96,104,106,109].

Cross-Diagnostic Approaches and Their Implications for Classification and Diagnosis

Functional neuroimaging has led to a greater understanding of the pathophysiology of mental disorders, providing neurobiological bases for classification of mental disorders with similar and overlapping phenomenology. To date, a number of functional neuroimaging studies have demonstrated the dysfunction of the fear network, particularly amygdalar hyperactivity in response to fearful or negative stimuli in anxiety disorders such as post-traumatic stress disorder (PTSD), panic disorder, specific phobia, social anxiety disorder and generalized anxiety disorder [130,131,132,133,134,135]. On the other hand, several studies reported activation of the prefrontal cortex during fear extinction, suggesting a regulating effect of the prefrontal cortex on the amygdalar fear reaction [136,137]. Furthermore, despite some discrepancy, functional neuroimaging studies on PTSD reported hypoactivity of the medial prefrontal cortex (mPFC) during symptom provocation [138,139,140,141,142], and decrease of amygdalar activity, as well as increased activity of the mPFC following effective treatments [143,144,145]. Taken together, convergent functional neuroimaging findings give insight that the fear network, including the amygdala and prefrontal cortex, may serve central roles in fear conditioning and extinction. Further, dysfunction of the same network is suggested to be the neurobiological underpinning of anxiety disorders, reflecting a heightened fear response and impaired top-down regulation of fear.

Conversely, there is limited evidence for a prominent role for the amygdala in the pathophysiology of OCD [3,5,146]. As already discussed, findings of functional neuroimaging studies in OCD have focused on disturbances in the frontostriatal circuit. Moreover, in a fMRI study by Cannistraro and colleagues, patients with OCD exhibited even attenuated amygdalar response to fearful faces compared with healthy controls [16]. Simon and colleagues investigated brain activation during individually tailored symptom provocation [146]. They observed increased activation of frontostriatal areas in response to OCD-related stimuli in patients with OCD compared with healthy controls, contrasted with neutral and generally aversive but symptom-unrelated stimuli. Interestingly, amygdala hyperactivation in the OCD group was found during presentation of unrelated aversive stimuli as well as during OCD-related symptom provocation. Thus, the authors suggested that amygdalar hyperactivation in OCD might reflect general emotional hyperarousal rather than OCD-related anxiety. Taken together, it is suggested that the disruption of the frontostriatal circuit may be involved in the pathophysiology of OCD, while the dysfunction of the fear network, including the amygdala and the prefrontal cortex, may mediate an exaggerated fear reaction in anxiety disorders. In this light, the transdiagnostic approach using functional neuroimaging may provide useful information for the differential diagnosis between anxiety disorders and OCD.

On the other hand, there is evidence that the disruption of the frontostriatal circuit may be the neurobiological underpinning of compulsivity, as shown not only in OCD but also in substance use disorders, both of which share a compulsive nature [147,148]. Moreover, preliminary evidence suggests that neuromodulation such as repetitive transcranial magnetic stimulation (rTMS) or deep brain stimulation exerts therapeutic effects through a similar mechanism in OCD and substance use disorders, by modulating frontostriatal connectivity [65,70,149,150]. fMRI studies have also elucidated similar pattern of altered brain activation during reward processing across various mental disorders which share common phenomenology of compulsivity. Altered activity or connectivity of the ventral striatum during reward processing was found in trichotillomania [35], substance use disorders [151,152,153,154,155], behavioral addictions including pathological gambling [154,156,157,158,159,160] and eating disorders [161,162], as well as in OCD [27,36,43,45,70]. As described earlier in this chapter, patients with OCD show deficits in cognitive flexibility and aberrant brain activity in the prefrontal cortex during reversal learning tasks or task switching. In line with this, fMRI studies have also identified impaired cognitive flexibility and decreased recruitment of the prefrontal cortex during reversal learning or set shifting in pathological gambling, substance use disorders [163,164] and eating disorders [165]. Taken together, albeit with some discrepancies, convergent evidence from fMRI research suggests the dysfunction of frontostriatal circuit or impaired prefrontal control over the striatum may be a common neurobiological underpinning of compulsivity in various mental disorders.

Of note, functional neuroimaging research has reported discrete neural correlates of hoarding compared with other kinds of obsessive-compulsive symptoms. In an early PET study, Saxena and colleagues reported that compared with non-hoarding patients with OCD, hoarders exhibited lower metabolism in the dorsal anterior cingulate cortex, which negatively correlated with hoarding severity [166]. An and colleagues compared OCD patients with and without hoarding symptoms in a fMRI study using a symptom provocation paradigm [11]. The patients with prominent hoarding symptoms showed greater activation in response to hoarding-related but not to hoarding-unrelated anxiety in the bilateral ventromedial prefrontal cortex (vmPFC) compared with those without hoarding symptoms and with healthy controls. Neuropsychological and behavioral studies have reported that patients with OCD gather more evidence to reach a decision and have an impaired decision making ability compared with healthy controls, despite some inconsistencies in the results [118,167,168]. Hoarding disorder shares this phenotype of OCD, in that the disorder is characterized by marked avoidance of decision making about possessions. Stern and colleagues reported that the OCD group showed greater activation in the prefrontal, temporal, limbic and paralimbic regions, including the orbitofrontal cortex, insula and amygdala, during decision making compared with healthy controls [37]. Rotge and colleagues reported a different pattern of activation in the orbitofrontal cortex during the decision making process elicited by a checking task in patients with OCD compared with healthy controls [29]. Tolin and colleagues compared neural activity among patients with hoarding disorder, patients with OCD and healthy control participants, during decisions to keep or discard possessions [39]. During decision making about items belonging to them, the hoarding group showed greater activity in the ACC and insula compared with the OCD group and healthy controls. Taken together, these findings suggest both OCD and hoarding disorder exhibit altered activation in brain regions related to decision making in a distinct manner. In addition, two studies examined the difference in brain activation using fMRI under a response inhibition condition elicited by the go/no-go task in patients with hoarding disorder, patients with OCD and healthy controls. Hough and colleagues demonstrated that individuals with hoarding disorder showed greater activity in the ACC and right DLPFC than did healthy controls, and greater right DLPFC activity compared with those with the OCD group [21]. They also observed differences in activity between the hoarding and healthy control groups, and between the hoarding and OCD groups in regions (ACC, insula, orbitofrontal cortex and striatum) involved in evaluating stimulus–response–reward associations, or the personal and task-relevant value of stimuli and behavioral responses to stimuli. Another study by Tolin and colleagues reported that the hoarding group showed greater precentral gyrus activation, whereas the OCD group exhibited elevated orbitofrontal cortex activation during successful response inhibition [30]. During response inhibition failures, the OCD group but not the hoarding group showed excessive activity in the bilateral orbitofrontal cortex. Despite discrepancies in the results, these preliminary findings support the neurobiological distinction between hoarding disorder and OCD. In other words, obsessive-compulsive symptoms other than hoarding are mediated by a dysfunctional frontostriatal circuit involving the orbitofrontal cortex and striatum, whereas hoarding symptom seems to be mediated by a distinct neural circuit involving the cingulate cortex, vmPFC and limbic structures [11,21,30,39].

fMRI studies on BDD have focused on abnormal pattern of brain activation during face processing, indicating aberrant visual processing as a neurobiological underpinning of the disorder. Feusner and colleagues observed hyperactivity in the orbitofrontal cortex and striatum in patients with BDD when being presented with their own face compared with a familiar face [169]. As mentioned previously, abnormal hyperactivity in these regions during symptom provocation is well known and has been replicated in OCD. This overlap suggests that similarities in symptom expression in OCD and BDD, such as obsessive thoughts and compulsive behaviors, may attribute to the abnormality of common brain circuitry. Other fMRI studies using face-processing or face-matching tasks, or viewing neutral, non-symptom-related stimuli, such as pictures of houses, have reported abnormal activation patterns of several brain regions in BDD [1,2,8,9,13,170]. These regions include not only the prefrontal area and amygdala but also the ventral visual stream. These findings suggest that the pathophysiology of BDD, while seemingly related to obsession and compulsion on physical appearance, may be more involved in brain regions related to visual information processing compared with OCD.

Regarding the neurobiology of trichotillomania and skin-picking disorder, limited knowledge is available and few neuroimaging studies have been done. Lee and colleagues examined the pattern of brain activation in pediatric patients with trichotillomania during symptom provocation elicited by visual and/or tactile stimuli [10]. The trichotillomania group exhibited greater activation in the temporal, dorsal posterior cingulate cortex, putamen and precuneus compared with healthy controls during symptom provocation. Previous fMRI studies using symptom provocation paradigms in patients with OCD have also reported abnormal activation in temporal, cingulate and striatal regions [18,171]. In addition, as mentioned previously, altered activity of the nucleus accumbens during reward processing was observed in both trichotillomania and OCD [35]. Although preliminary, these findings suggest that trichotillomania shares some neurobiological overlap with OCD. Odlaug and colleagues reported in 2016 that patients with skin-picking disorder showed underactivation in the dorsal striatum, anterior cingulate and medial frontal regions during a ToL task [23]. Based on this finding, they suggested that the area of dysfunction extends from the medial to the lateral prefrontal networks in OCD, whereas it may be more restricted to the medial sectors of this circuitry in skin-picking disorder.

In summary, fMRI research to date has demonstrated both shared and distinct neurobiological underpinnings across OCRDs and other mental disorders of a compulsive nature, indicating disruption of the frontostriatal circuit as a neural basis for compulsivity. The controversy over whether OCRDs actually share neurobiological overlap and dysfunction in the common neural circuit still exists and further investigation is needed. Nonetheless, fMRI research has provided neurobiological bases for classification of OCRDs, distinguishing them from other diagnostic entities.

Clinical Implications of Cross-Diagnostic Approaches for Treatment and Prevention

Early studies using PET or SPECT reported a reduction in metabolism or regional cerebral blood flow in the caudate, frontal areas including the orbitofrontal and anterior cingulate cortices, and thalamus during or after effective treatment in OCD patients, supporting the CSTC model of OCD [172,173,174,175,176,177,178, 179,180,181]. Over the past two decades, fMRI has also been used to investigate the effects of treatments in OCRDs. Nakao and colleagues reported changes in brain activation during the Stroop and symptom provocation tasks in patients with OCD before and after 12 weeks of either pharmacotherapy with fluvoxamine or behavioral therapy [77]. After symptom improvement, symptom provocation-related activation in the orbitofrontal cortex, DLPFC and ACC decreased, whereas Stroop task-related activation in the temporal and parietal cortices, cerebellum, DLPFC and ACC increased. Van der Wee and colleagues examined changes in working memory performance (n-back task) and brain activation patterns during the task before and after 12 weeks of pharmacological treatment in patients with OCD [76]. Only in treatment responders did performance improve, which was associated with changes in the overall pattern of brain activity during the task. Shin and colleagues used the graph theory approach to examine the change in the topological properties of the brain network using resting-state fMRI after selective serotonin reuptake inhibitor (SSRI) treatment in patients with OCD (Figure 9.1) [69]. The OCD group showed a decreased small-world efficiency and functional association between the default-mode and frontoparietal modules, as well as widespread altered connectivity degrees in many brain areas compared with healthy controls at the baseline. After 16 weeks of SSRI treatment which resulted in clinical improvement, small-world efficiency, modular organization and connectivity degree were significantly elevated. Furthermore, a significant correlation was observed between the improvement of obsessive-compulsive symptoms and the changes in connectivity degree in the right ventral frontal cortex in patients with OCD after treatment. These findings suggest that the symptomatic expression of OCD may be the outcome of the disturbed optimal balance in the brain networks and that symptom improvement with SSRI treatment is accompanied by reinstatement of this balance.

Nabeyama and colleagues examined the effects of behavioral therapy alone using fMRI during the Stroop test. After 12 weeks of behavioral therapy, a significant improvement was achieved in obsessive-compulsive symptoms and the performance of the task. The OCD group showed increased activation in the cerebellum and parietal lobe, whereas decreased activation was observed in the orbitofrontal cortex, middle frontal gyrus and temporal regions during the task after treatment [75]. Freyer and colleagues reported that patients with OCD exhibited increased activity of the caudate head during strategy change within a reversal learning task after cognitive behavioral therapy (CBT) compared with baseline [73]. Morgiéve and colleagues adopted a more elaborate design to demonstrate the effect of CBT during an exposure task using personalized obsession-inducing images [68]. To investigate the dynamics of the treatment response, they conducted a systematic clinical and fMRI evaluation immediately before the start of a three-month course of CBT and then halfway through and at the end of the course, as well as six months after the course. They reported that the baseline hemodynamic response to personalized obsession-inducing images in the anterior cingulate and orbitofrontal cortices progressively decreased with symptom improvement across the four time points. In resting-state fMRI research by Yang and colleagues, the improvement of obsessive-compulsive symptoms in response to CBT was found to correlate with the reduction of regional

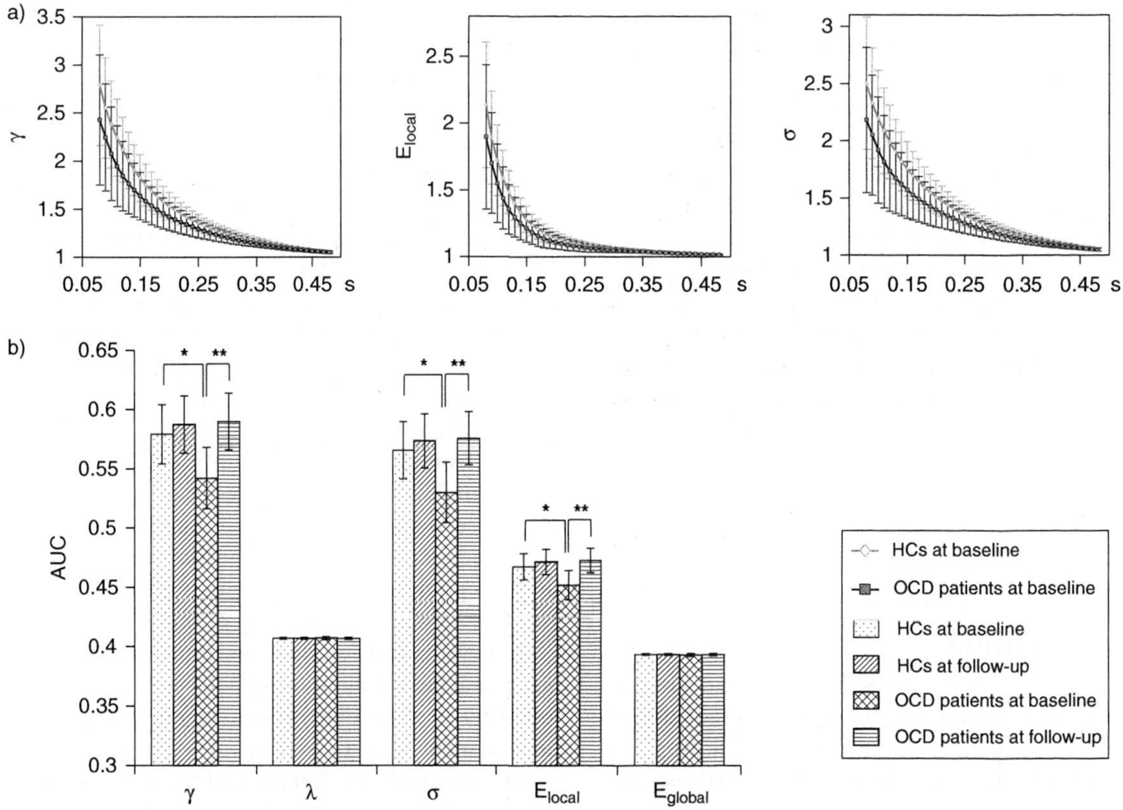

Figure 9.1 (a) Between- and within-group differences in the area under the curves. Patients with OCD showed significantly decreased clustering coefficient, small-worldness and local efficiency, all of which were significantly improved after 16 weeks of SSRI treatment. (b) The mean correlation matrix for each group demonstrated that altered modular organization of patients with OCD have been significantly alleviated after the treatment. AUC, area under curves; HCs, healthy controls; OCD, obsessive-compulsive disorder; SSRI, selective serotonin reuptake inhibitor; E_{global}, normalized global efficiency; E_{local}, normalized local efficiency; γ, normalized clustering coefficient; λ,normalized characteristic path length; s, sparsity threshold; σ, normalized small-world. *$P < .05$, with permutation test; **$P < .05$, with paired permutation test. Adapted with permission from Shin et al., 2014 [69].

homogeneity in the orbitofrontal cortex and the cerebellum [66].

In summary, despite some discrepancies in the results, previous fMRI studies regarding treatment effects in OCD have generally reported baseline abnormal activity or connectivity in the frontostriatal regions, which normalized following effective treatment accompanied by improvement of symptoms and/or cognitive functions. The most frequently reported region to be associated with treatment effect is the orbitofrontal cortex, while some evidence has also been shown for the ACC, DLPFC, putamen, parietal and temporal cortices, and cerebellum. The various analytic methods for fMRI, in addition to the research paradigms used and the heterogeneity of patients with respect to symptom dimensions, duration of illness and comorbidity, may be responsible for the inconsistencies in the results, as well as the diversity of the treatment modalities. In that patients with OCRDs often have poor insight and hide their obsessive-compulsive symptoms, these preliminary findings suggest that fMRI can be employed in diagnosis as an objective state marker of symptom severity or for the evaluation of treatment effect. Further investigation is needed to delineate neural mechanisms of pharmacotherapy and CBT, which will provide better understanding of the process of each treatment modality at the neural circuit level. Also, as mentioned previously, recent fMRI findings suggest that neuromodulation such as rTMS and deep brain stimulation may lead to symptom remediation by normalizing the disrupted corticostriatal circuit in

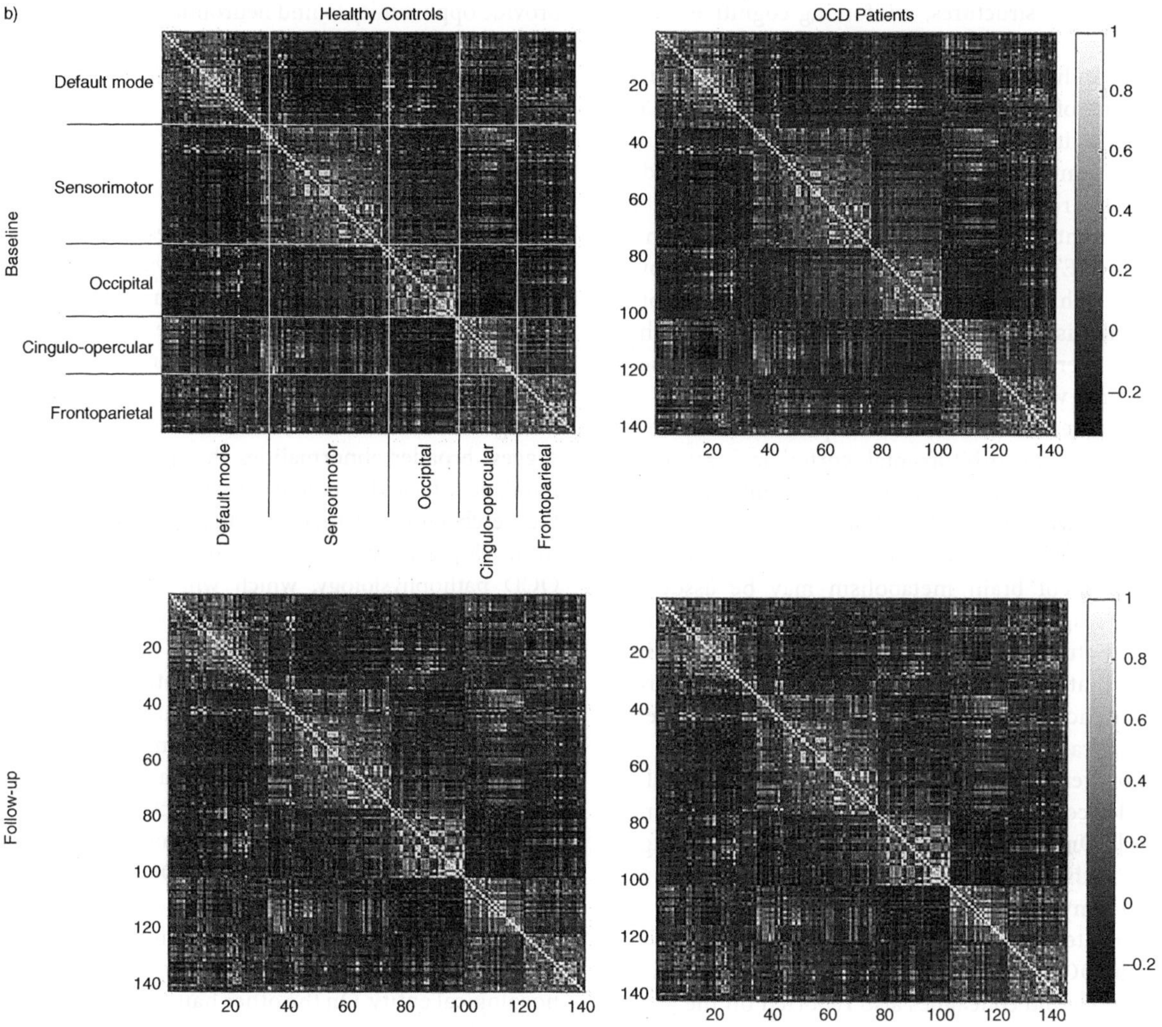

Figure 9.1 *(cont.)*

a similar manner in OCD and substance use disorder. Future research in this field will extend our knowledge of the neural mechanism of neuromodulation, and will provide useful information for the decision of target region or parameter of neuromodulation in a transdiagnostic fashion.

There has been a paucity of neuroimaging research into the effects of treatment in OCRDs other than OCD. There is a preliminary study by Tolin and colleagues regarding CBT response in hoarding disorder [71]. In that study, six patients with hoarding disorder and six healthy controls underwent an fMRI task in which they made simulated decisions about whether to acquire or discard a variety of objects. Those with hoarding disorder then received 16 sessions of CBT and then repeated the same fMRI decision making tasks. Before treatment, hyperactivity of diffuse areas including the medial frontal gyrus, parietal, temporal and occipital areas, cingulate, insula, putamen, caudate, precuneus, lingual gyrus, cuneus, hippocampus and cerebellum was observed in patients with hoarding disorder compared with healthy controls during acquiring and discarding decisions, which no longer differed significantly after CBT, suggesting normalization of neural function. Brook and Stein reviewed fMRI studies examining the neural bases of CBT in anxiety disorders [182]. They concluded that despite somewhat different neural circuitry, CBT may act in a similar way to increase prefrontal control of subcortical structures, reinforcing cognitive regulation of emotion. In light of these findings, preliminary indications are that CBT may lead to a similar pattern of change in brain activity in hoarding disorder as in OCD and anxiety disorders.

Recently, fMRI has been attempted to identify neuroimaging biomarkers for predicting the treatment response in patients with OCD. In an early PET study, Brody and colleagues showed that a higher pretreatment orbitofrontal cortex metabolism predicted a better response to behavioral therapy and worse response to fluoxetine in patients with OCD [183]. Consistently, Saxena and colleagues found that a lower pretreatment metabolism in the orbitofrontal cortex was associated with a greater improvement in patients with OCD treated with paroxetine [174]. Taken together, the findings of these PET studies suggest that particular patterns of brain metabolism may be associated with response to specific treatment modality. In an fMRI study using symptom provocation paradigm, Sanematsu and colleagues reported that pretreatment activation in the cerebellum and superior temporal gyrus positively correlated with the improvement in Yale-Brown Obsessive Compulsive Scale score after 12 weeks of fluvoxamine treatment [81]. On the other hand, Olatunji and colleagues found that the baseline activity in the temporal pole and amygdala during symptom provocation was associated with a better response to CBT in patients with OCD [80]. Applying graph theory analysis, Göttlich and colleagues also reported on the abnormality of the amygdala [79]. They assessed whole-brain resting-state functional connectivity prior to CBT in unmedicated patients with OCD and healthy controls and found that the pretreatment resting-state functional connectivity of the amygdala positively correlated with the response to CBT. Feusner and colleagues also applied graph theory analysis to resting-state fMRI data from patients with OCD prior to and following CBT [78]. They observed that small-worldness and clustering coefficient increased after CBT. Furthermore, a higher pretreatment small-world connectivity was associated with relapse after CBT. These discrepancies in results may be attributed to the heterogeneity of patients, diversity of analytic methods and treatment modalities.

There is also a paucity of research on OCRDs other than OCD. Future investigations in this field will provide opportunity to find neuroimaging biomarkers on the prediction of onset, relapse and treatment response, enabling individually tailored treatment in patients with OCRDs.

Future Directions

In summary, various fMRI approaches have enabled investigation into abnormal brain activations not only during symptom provocation and various cognitive tasks but also during the resting state in individuals with OCD. Previous reports have emphasized the frontostriatal circuit as being central to the neurobiological model of OCD, while recent fMRI studies suggest broader abnormalities that involve the temporal, parietal and occipital cortex, limbic regions and the cerebellum. Further investigations are required to develop a fully integrated model of circuit-based OCD pathophysiology, which will enable a better understanding of the neurobiology of obsession, compulsion and related phenomena.

Although there has been a relative paucity of research regarding OCRDs other than OCD, some fMRI studies have also shown neurobiological abnormalities in individuals with hoarding disorder, BDD, trichotillomania or skin-picking disorder. These studies have elucidated the neurobiological overlap and distinction between OCD and other OCRDs, thus providing a better conceptualization of OCRD as a heterogenous group of multiple, potentially overlapping phenotypes rather than a unitary nosological entity. On the other hand, fMRI research has indicated abnormalities of different neural circuits between OCD and anxiety disorders, with a prominent role for the fear network, including the amygdala in the latter. fMRI studies on substance use disorders, behavioral addictions and eating disorders, which share compulsivity and overlapping cognitive deficits with OCD, have demonstrated common involvement of the frontostriatal circuit across these disorders. Based on these findings, it is suggested that the aberration of the frontostriatal circuit may be the neurobiological underpinning of compulsivity, which mediates deficits in cognitive flexibility and reward processing, as well as compulsive behaviors. Taken together, these findings have provided a neurobiological basis for the classification of OCRDs and other diagnostic entities, with a better understanding of compulsivity as a transdiagnostic concept.

In addition, fMRI research has presented the neural bases of the therapeutic effect of pharmacotherapy, CBT and neuromodulation. Further investigation is needed to delineate the neural mechanism of each treatment modality. Preliminary evidence that neuromodulation, such as rTMS and deep brain stimulation, exerts a therapeutic effect in OCD and substance use disorders by similar mechanisms suggests that application of these modalities across disorders in a transdiagnostic manner might be valid. There has also been research using fMRI to predict treatment response in OCD. Future research in this field will provide opportunities to find transdiagnostic biomarkers to predict the onset, relapse and response to treatment, enabling individually tailored treatment.

However, there are also limitations and obstacles. There have been few neuroimaging studies of OCRDs other than OCD with small sizes of samples. Moreover, most neuroimaging studies were of cross-sectional design, which does not ensure a direct causal inference. The heterogeneity of patients, comorbidities and medication effects can also work as confounders. In addition, the diversity of paradigms and analytic methods applied in neuroimaging research may result in inconsistent findings. On a technical aspect, susceptibility artifacts and the limited spatial resolution of fMRI are challenging as well. Finally, whether the altered brain activation is primarily caused by the pathophysiology of the disorder, or is the result of compensatory activation also remains to be further elucidated. Thus, studies with large samples and of longitudinal, experimental design that directly compare various mental disorders and that encompass genetic, neuroimaging, neuropsychological and clinical approaches are recommended. Future investigations in this field are warranted and will expand our knowledge of common and distinct neurobiology across OCRDs, enabling a transdiagnostic approach encompassing diagnosis, treatment and prevention in clinical practice.

Acknowledgments

We thank Seoyeon Kwak and Taek wan Kim, PhD candidates, for reviewing and summarizing previous studies. We also thank Youngwoo Bryan Yoon and Dahye Bae, PhD candidates, Kang Ik Kevin Cho, PhD, as well as Solhee Kim, BS, for editing the tables.

References

1. Beucke JC, Sepulcre J, Buhlmann U, Kathmann N, Moody T, Feusner JD. Degree connectivity in body dysmorphic disorder and relationships with obsessive and compulsive symptoms. *Eur Neuropsychopharmacol.* 2016;26(10):1657–1666.
2. Moody TD, Sasaki MA, Bohon C, et al. Functional connectivity for face processing in individuals with body dysmorphic disorder and anorexia nervosa. *Psychol Med.* 2015;45(16):3491–3503.
3. Via E, Cardoner N, Pujol J, et al. Amygdala activation and symptom dimensions in obsessive-compulsive disorder. *Br J Psychiatry.* 2014;204(1):61–68.
4. Jhung K, Ku J, Kim SJ, et al. Distinct functional connectivity of limbic network in the washing type obsessive-compulsive disorder. *Prog Neuropsychopharmacol Biol Psychiatry.* 2014;53:149–155.
5. Simon D, Adler N, Kaufmann C, Kathmann N. Amygdala hyperactivation during symptom provocation in obsessive–compulsive disorder and its modulation by distraction. *Neuroimage Clin.* 2014;4:549–557.
6. Milad MR, Furtak SC, Greenberg JL, et al. Deficits in conditioned fear extinction in obsessive-compulsive disorder and neurobiological changes in the fear circuit. *JAMA Psychiatry.* 2013;70(6):608–618.
7. Weygandt M, Blecker CR, Schäfer A, et al. fMRI pattern recognition in obsessive-compulsive disorder. *Neuroimage.* 2012;60(2):1186–1193.
8. Bohon C, Hembacher E, Moller H, Moody TD, Feusner JD. Nonlinear relationships between anxiety and visual processing of own and others' faces in body dysmorphic disorder. *Psychiatry Res.* 2012;204(2–3):132–139.
9. Feusner JD, Hembacher E, Moller H, Moody TD. Abnormalities of object visual processing in body dysmorphic disorder. *Psychol Med.* 2011;41(11):2385–2397.
10. Lee JA, Kim CK, Jahng GH, et al. A pilot study of brain activation in children with trichotillomania during a visual-tactile symptom provocation task: a functional magnetic resonance imaging study. *Prog Neuropsychopharmacol Biol Psychiatry.* 2010;34(7):1250–1258.
11. An SK, Mataix-Cols D, Lawrence NS, et al. To discard or not to discard: the neural basis of hoarding symptoms in obsessive-compulsive disorder. *Mol Psychiatry.* 2009;14(3):318–331.
12. Lawrence NS, An SK, Mataix-Cols D, Ruths F, Speckens A, Phillips ML. Neural responses to facial expressions of disgust but not fear are modulated

by washing symptoms in OCD. *Biol Psychiatry*. 2007;61(9):1072–1080.

13. Feusner JD, Townsend J, Bystritsky A, Bookheimer S. Visual information processing of faces in body dysmorphic disorder. *Arch Gen Psychiatry*. 2007;64(12):1417–1425.
14. Schienle A, Schafer A, Stark R, Walter B, Vaitl D. Neural responses of OCD patients towards disorder-relevant, generally disgust-inducing and fear-inducing pictures. *Int J Psychophysiol*. 2005;57(1):69–77.
15. Mataix-Cols D, Wooderson S, Lawrence N, Brammer MJ, Speckens A, Phillips ML. Distinct neural correlates of washing, checking, and hoarding symptom dimensions in obsessive-compulsive disorder. *Arch Gen Psychiatry*. 2004;61(6):564–576.
16. Cannistraro PA, Wright CI, Wedig MM, et al. Amygdala responses to human faces in obsessive-compulsive disorder. *Biol Psychiatry*. 2004;56(12):916–920.
17. Shapira NA, Liu Y, He AG, et al. Brain activation by disgust-inducing pictures in obsessive-compulsive disorder. *Biol Psychiatry*. 2003;54(7):751–756.
18. Adler CM, McDonough-Ryan P, Sax KW, Holland SK, Arndt S, Strakowski SM. fMRI of neuronal activation with symptom provocation in unmedicated patients with obsessive compulsive disorder. *J Psychiatr Res*. 2000;34(4–5):317–324.
19. Phillips ML, Marks IM, Senior C, et al. A differential neural response in obsessive-compulsive disorder patients with washing compared with checking symptoms to disgust. *Psychol Med*. 2000;30(5):1037–1050.
20. Breiter HC, Rauch SL, Kwong KK, et al. Functional magnetic resonance imaging of symptom provocation in obsessive-compulsive disorder. *Arch Gen Psychiatry*. 1996;53(7):595–606.
21. Hough CM, Luks TL, Lai K, et al. Comparison of brain activation patterns during executive function tasks in hoarding disorder and non-hoarding OCD. *Psychiatry Res*. 2016;255:50–59.
22. Morein-Zamir S, Voon V, Dodds CM, et al. Divergent subcortical activity for distinct executive functions: stopping and shifting in obsessive compulsive disorder. *Psychol Med*. 2016;46(4):829–840.
23. Odlaug BL, Hampshire A, Chamberlain SR, Grant JE. Abnormal brain activation in excoriation (skin-picking) disorder: evidence from an executive planning fMRI study. *Br J Psychiatry*. 2016;208(2):168–174.
24. Han HJ, Jung WH, Yun JY, et al. Disruption of effective connectivity from the dorsolateral prefrontal cortex to the orbitofrontal cortex by negative emotional distraction in obsessive-compulsive disorder. *Psychol Med*. 2016;46(5):921–932.
25. Weidt S, Lutz J, Rufer M, et al. Common and differential alterations of general emotion processing in obsessive-compulsive and social anxiety disorder. *Psychol Med*. 2016;46(7):1427–1436.
26. van Velzen LS, de Wit SJ, Ćurĉić-Blake B, et al. Altered inhibition-related frontolimbic connectivity in obsessive-compulsive disorder. *Hum Brain Mapp*. 2015;36(10):4064–4075.
27. Marsh R, Tau GZ, Wang Z, et al. Reward-based spatial learning in unmedicated adults with obsessive-compulsive disorder. *Am J Psychiatry*. 2015;172(4):383–392.
28. Gillan CM, Apergis-Schoute AM, Morein-Zamir S, et al. Functional neuroimaging of avoidance habits in obsessive-compulsive disorder. *Am J Psychiatry*. 2015;172(3):284–293.
29. Rotge JY, Langbour N, Dilharreguy B, et al. Contextual and behavioral influences on uncertainty in obsessive-compulsive disorder. *Cortex*. 2015;62:1–10.
30. Tolin DF, Witt ST, Stevens MC. Hoarding disorder and obsessive-compulsive disorder show different patterns of neural activity during response inhibition. *Psychiatry Res*. 2014;221(2):142–148.
31. Marsh R, Horga G, Parashar N, Wang Z, Peterson BS, Simpson HB. Altered activation in fronto-striatal circuits during sequential processing of conflict in unmedicated adults with obsessive-compulsive disorder. *Biol Psychiatry*. 2014;75(8):615–622.
32. de Vries FE, de Wit SJ, Cath DC, et al. Compensatory frontoparietal activity during working memory: an endophenotype of obsessive-compulsive disorder. *Biol Psychiatry*. 2014;76(11):878–887.
33. Agam Y, Greenberg JL, Isom M, et al. Aberrant error processing in relation to symptom severity in obsessive-compulsive disorder: a multimodal neuroimaging study. *Neuroimage Clin*. 2014;5:141–151.
34. Kang DH, Jang JH, Han JY, et al. Neural correlates of altered response inhibition and dysfunctional connectivity at rest in obsessive-compulsive disorder. *Prog Neuropsychopharmacol Biol Psychiatry*. 2013;40:340–346.
35. White MP, Shirer WR, Molfino MJ, Tenison C, Damoiseaux JS, Greicius MD. Disordered reward processing and functional connectivity in trichotillomania: a pilot study. *J Psychiatr Res*. 2013;47(9):1264–1272.
36. Jung WH, Kang DH, Kim E, Shin KS, Jang JH, Kwon JS. Abnormal corticostriatal-limbic functional connectivity in obsessive-compulsive disorder during reward processing and resting-state. *Neuroimage Clin*. 2013;3:27–38.
37. Stern ER, Welsh RC, Gonzalez R, Fitzgerald KD, Abelson JL, Taylor SF. Subjective uncertainty and

limbic hyperactivation in obsessive-compulsive disorder. *Hum Brain Mapp*. 2013;34(8):1956–1970.

38. de Wit SJ, de Vries FE, van der Werf YD, et al. Presupplementary motor area hyperactivity during response inhibition: a candidate endophenotype of obsessive-compulsive disorder. *Am J Psychiatry*. 2012;169(10):1100–1108.

39. Tolin DF, Stevens MC, Villavicencio AL, et al. Neural mechanisms of decision making in hoarding disorder. *Arch Gen Psychiatry*. 2012;69(8):832–841.

40. Harrison BJ, Pujol J, Soriano-Mas C, et al. Neural correlates of moral sensitivity in obsessive-compulsive disorder. *Arch Gen Psychiatry*. 2012;69(7):741–749.

41. Cocchi L, Harrison BJ, Pujol J, et al. Functional alterations of large-scale brain networks related to cognitive control in obsessive-compulsive disorder. *Hum Brain Mapp*. 2012;33(5):1089–1106.

42. van den Heuvel OA, Mataix-Cols D, Zwitser G, et al. Common limbic and frontal-striatal disturbances in patients with obsessive compulsive disorder, panic disorder and hypochondriasis. *Psychol Med*. 2011;41(11):2399–2410.

43. Jung WH, Kang DH, Han JY, et al. Aberrant ventral striatal responses during incentive processing in unmedicated patients with obsessive-compulsive disorder. *Acta Psychiatr Scand*. 2011;123(5):376–386.

44. Stern ER, Welsh RC, Fitzgerald KD, et al. Hyperactive error responses and altered connectivity in ventromedial and frontoinsular cortices in obsessive-compulsive disorder. *Biol Psychiatry*. 2011;69(6):583–591.

45. Figee M, Vink M, de Geus F, et al. Dysfunctional reward circuitry in obsessive-compulsive disorder. *Biol Psychiatry*. 2011;69(9):867–874.

46. Rubia K, Cubillo A, Smith AB, Woolley J, Heyman I, Brammer MJ. Disorder-specific dysfunction in right inferior prefrontal cortex during two inhibition tasks in boys with attention-deficit hyperactivity disorder compared to boys with obsessive-compulsive disorder. *Hum Brain Mapp*. 2010;31(2):287–299.

47. Schlösser RG, Wagner G, Schachtzabel C, et al. Fronto-cingulate effective connectivity in obsessive compulsive disorder: a study with fMRI and dynamic causal modeling. *Hum Brain Mapp*. 2010;31(12):1834–1850.

48. Fitzgerald KD, Stern ER, Angstadt M, et al. Altered function and connectivity of the medial frontal cortex in pediatric obsessive-compulsive disorder. *Biol Psychiatry*. 2010;68(11):1039–1047.

49. Remijnse PL, Nielen MM, van Balkom AJ, et al. Differential frontal-striatal and paralimbic activity during reversal learning in major depressive disorder and obsessive-compulsive disorder. *Psychol Med*. 2009;39(9):1503–1518.

50. Nakao T, Nakagawa A, Nakatani E, et al. Working memory dysfunction in obsessive-compulsive disorder: a neuropsychological and functional MRI study. *J Psychiatr Res*. 2009;43(8):784–791.

51. Woolley J, Heyman I, Brammer M, Frampton I, McGuire PK, Rubia K. Brain activation in paediatric obsessive compulsive disorder during tasks of inhibitory control. *Br J Psychiatry*. 2008;192(1):25–31.

52. Chamberlain SR, Menzies L, Hampshire A, et al. Orbitofrontal dysfunction in patients with obsessive-compulsive disorder and their unaffected relatives. *Science*. 2008;321(5887):421–422.

53. Gu BM, Park JY, Kang DH, et al. Neural correlates of cognitive inflexibility during task-switching in obsessive-compulsive disorder. *Brain*. 2008;131(Pt 1):155–164.

54. Yücel M, Harrison BJ, Wood SJ, et al. Functional and biochemical alterations of the medial frontal cortex in obsessive-compulsive disorder. *Arch Gen Psychiatry*. 2007;64(8):946–955.

55. Roth RM, Saykin AJ, Flashman LA, Pixley HS, West JD, Mamourian AC. Event-related functional magnetic resonance imaging of response inhibition in obsessive-compulsive disorder. *Biol Psychiatry*. 2007;62(8):901–909.

56. Rauch SL, Wright CI, Savage CR, et al. Brain activation during implicit sequence learning in individuals with trichotillomania. *Psychiatry Res*. 2007;154(3):233–240.

57. Rauch SL, Wedig MM, Wright CI, et al. Functional magnetic resonance imaging study of regional brain activation during implicit sequence learning in obsessive-compulsive disorder. *Biol Psychiatry*. 2007;61(3):330–336.

58. Remijnse PL, Nielen MM, van Balkom AJ, et al. Reduced orbitofrontal-striatal activity on a reversal learning task in obsessive-compulsive disorder. *Arch Gen Psychiatry*. 2006;63(11):1125–1136.

59. Maltby N, Tolin DF, Worhunsky P, O'Keefe TM, Kiehl KA. Dysfunctional action monitoring hyperactivates frontal-striatal circuits in obsessive-compulsive disorder: an event-related fMRI study. *Neuroimage*. 2005;24(2):495–503.

60. van den Heuvel OA, Veltman DJ, Groenewegen HJ, et al. Frontal-striatal dysfunction during planning in obsessive-compulsive disorder. *Arch Gen Psychiatry*. 2005;62(3):301–309.

61. Fitzgerald KD, Welsh RC, Gehring WJ, et al. Error-related hyperactivity of the anterior cingulate cortex in obsessive-compulsive disorder. *Biol Psychiatry*. 2005;57(3):287–294.

62. Viard A, Flament MF, Artiges E, et al. Cognitive control in childhood-onset obsessive-compulsive

disorder: a functional MRI study. *Psychol Med.* 2005;35(7):1007–1017.

63. Ursu S, Stenger VA, Shear MK, Jones MR, Carter CS. Overactive action monitoring in obsessive-compulsive disorder: evidence from functional magnetic resonance imaging. *Psychol Sci.* 2003;14(4):347–353.

64. Zhao HZ, Wang CH, Gao ZZ, et al. Effectiveness of cognitive-coping therapy and alteration of resting-state brain function in obsessive-compulsive disorder. *J Affect Disord.* 2017;208:184–190.

65. Dunlop K, Woodside B, Olmsted M, Colton P, Giacobbe P, Downar J. Reductions in cortico-striatal hyperconnectivity accompany successful treatment of obsessive-compulsive disorder with dorsomedial prefrontal rTMS. *Neuropsychopharmacology.* 2016;41(5):1395–1403.

66. Yang XY, Sun J, Luo J, et al. Regional homogeneity of spontaneous brain activity in adult patients with obsessive-compulsive disorder before and after cognitive behavioural therapy. *J Affect Disord.* 2015;188:243–251.

67. de Wit SJ, van der Werf YD, Mataix-Cols D, et al. Emotion regulation before and after transcranial magnetic stimulation in obsessive compulsive disorder. *Psychol Med.* 2015;45(14):3059–3073.

68. Morgieve M, N'Diaye K, Haynes WI, et al. Dynamics of psychotherapy-related cerebral haemodynamic changes in obsessive compulsive disorder using a personalized exposure task in functional magnetic resonance imaging. *Psychol Med.* 2014;44(7):1461–1473.

69. Shin DJ, Jung WH, He Y, et al. The effects of pharmacological treatment on functional brain connectome in obsessive-compulsive disorder. *Biol Psychiatry.* 2014;75(8):606–614.

70. Figee M, Luigjes J, Smolders R, et al. Deep brain stimulation restores frontostriatal network activity in obsessive-compulsive disorder. *Nat Neurosci.* 2013;16(4):386–387.

71. Tolin DF, Stevens MC, Nave A, Villavicencio AL, Morrison S. Neural mechanisms of cognitive behavioral therapy response in hoarding disorder: a pilot study. *J Obsessive Compuls Relat Disord.* 2012;1(3):180–188.

72. Han JY, Kang DH, Gu BM, et al. Altered brain activation in ventral frontal-striatal regions following a 16-week pharmacotherapy in unmedicated obsessive-compulsive disorder. *J Korean Med Sci.* 2011;26(5):665–674.

73. Freyer T, Kloppel S, Tuscher O, et al. Frontostriatal activation in patients with obsessive-compulsive disorder before and after cognitive behavioral therapy. *Psychol Med.* 2011;41(1):207–216.

74. Lázaro L, Caldú X, Junqué C, et al. Cerebral activation in children and adolescents with obsessive-compulsive disorder before and after treatment: a functional MRI study. *J Psychiatr Res.* 2008;42(13):1051–1059.

75. Nabeyama M, Nakagawa A, Yoshiura T, et al. Functional MRI study of brain activation alterations in patients with obsessive-compulsive disorder after symptom improvement. *Psychiatry Res.* 2008;163(3):236–247.

76. van der Wee NJ, Ramsey NF, van Megen HJ, Denys D, Westenberg HG, Kahn RS. Spatial working memory in obsessive-compulsive disorder improves with clinical response: a functional MRI study. *Eur Neuropsychopharmacol.* 2007;17(1):16–23.

77. Nakao T, Nakagawa A, Yoshiura T, et al. Brain activation of patients with obsessive-compulsive disorder during neuropsychological and symptom provocation tasks before and after symptom improvement: a functional magnetic resonance imaging study. *Biol Psychiatry.* 2005;57(8):901–910.

78. Feusner JD, Moody T, Lai TM, et al. Brain connectivity and prediction of relapse after cognitive-behavioral therapy in obsessive-compulsive disorder. *Front Psychiatry.* 2015;6:74.

79. Göttlich M, Krämer UM, Kordon A, Hohagen F, Zurowski B. Resting-state connectivity of the amygdala predicts response to cognitive behavioral therapy in obsessive compulsive disorder. *Biol Psychol.* 2015;111:100–109.

80. Olatunji BO, Ferreira-Garcia R, Caseras X, et al. Predicting response to cognitive behavioral therapy in contamination-based obsessive-compulsive disorder from functional magnetic resonance imaging. *Psychol Med.* 2014;44(10):2125–2137.

81. Sanematsu H, Nakao T, Yoshiura T, et al. Predictors of treatment response to fluvoxamine in obsessive-compulsive disorder: an fMRI study. *J Psychiatr Res.* 2010;44(4):193–200.

82. Jung WH, Yücel M, Yun JY, et al. Altered functional network architecture in orbitofronto-striato-thalamic circuit of unmedicated patients with obsessive-compulsive disorder. *Hum Brain Mapp.* 2017;38(1):109–119.

83. Posner J, Song I, Lee S, et al. Increased functional connectivity between the default mode and salience networks in unmedicated adults with obsessive-compulsive disorder. *Hum Brain Mapp.* 2017;38(2):678–687.

84. Vaghi MM, Vertes PE, Kitzbichler MG, et al. Specific frontostriatal circuits for impaired cognitive flexibility and goal-directed planning in obsessive-compulsive disorder: evidence from resting-state functional connectivity. *Biol Psychiatry.* 2017;81(8):708–717.

85. Armstrong CC, Moody TD, Feusner JD, et al. Graph-theoretical analysis of resting-state fMRI in pediatric obsessive-compulsive disorder. *J Affect Disord.* 2016;193:175–184.

86. Chen Y, Juhas M, Greenshaw AJ, et al. Abnormal resting-state functional connectivity of the left caudate nucleus in obsessive-compulsive disorder. *Neurosci Lett.* 2016;623:57–62.

87. Tang W, Zhu Q, Gong X, Zhu C, Wang Y, Chen S. Cortico-striato-thalamo-cortical circuit abnormalities in obsessive-compulsive disorder: a voxel-based morphometric and fMRI study of the whole brain. *Behav Brain Res.* 2016;313:17–22.

88. Tian L, Meng C, Jiang Y, et al. Abnormal functional connectivity of brain network hubs associated with symptom severity in treatment-naive patients with obsessive-compulsive disorder: a resting-state functional MRI study. *Prog Neuropsychopharmacol Biol Psychiatry.* 2016;66:104–111.

89. Xie C, Ma L, Jiang N, et al. Imbalanced functional link between reward circuits and the cognitive control system in patients with obsessive-compulsive disorder. *Brain Imaging Behav.* 2017;11(4):1099–1109.

90. Zhu Y, Fan Q, Zhang H, et al. Altered intrinsic insular activity predicts symptom severity in unmedicated obsessive-compulsive disorder patients: a resting state functional magnetic resonance imaging study. *BMC Psychiatry.* 2016;16:104.

91. Bernstein GA, Mueller BA, Schreiner MW, et al. Abnormal striatal resting-state functional connectivity in adolescents with obsessive-compulsive disorder. *Psychiatry Res.* 2016;247:49–56.

92. Abe Y, Sakai Y, Nishida S, et al. Hyper-influence of the orbitofrontal cortex over the ventral striatum in obsessive-compulsive disorder. *Eur Neuropsychopharmacol.* 2015;25(11):1898–1905.

93. Beucke JC, Sepulcre J, Eldaief MC, Sebold M, Kathmann N, Kaufmann C. Default mode network subsystem alterations in obsessive-compulsive disorder. *Br J Psychiatry.* 2014;205(5):376–382.

94. Hou JM, Zhao M, Zhang W, et al. Resting-state functional connectivity abnormalities in patients with obsessive-compulsive disorder and their healthy first-degree relatives. *J Psychiatry Neurosci.* 2014;39(5):304–311.

95. Anticevic A, Hu S, Zhang S, et al. Global resting-state functional magnetic resonance imaging analysis identifies frontal cortex, striatal, and cerebellar dysconnectivity in obsessive-compulsive disorder. *Biol Psychiatry.* 2014;75(8):595–605.

96. Peng ZW, Xu T, He QH, et al. Default network connectivity as a vulnerability marker for obsessive compulsive disorder. *Psychol Med.* 2014;44(7):1475–1484.

97. Gruner P, Vo A, Argyelan M, et al. Independent component analysis of resting state activity in pediatric obsessive-compulsive disorder. *Hum Brain Mapp.* 2014;35(10):5306–5315.

98. Posner J, Marsh R, Maia TV, Peterson BS, Gruber A, Simpson HB. Reduced functional connectivity within the limbic cortico-striato-thalamo-cortical loop in unmedicated adults with obsessive-compulsive disorder. *Hum Brain Mapp.* 2014;35(6):2852–2860.

99. Weber AM, Soreni N, Noseworthy MD. A preliminary study of functional connectivity of medication naive children with obsessive-compulsive disorder. *Prog Neuropsychopharmacol Biol Psychiatry.* 2014;53:129–136.

100. Beucke JC, Sepulcre J, Talukdar T, et al. Abnormally high degree connectivity of the orbitofrontal cortex in obsessive-compulsive disorder. *JAMA Psychiatry.* 2013;70(6):619–629.

101. Cheng Y, Xu J, Nie B, et al. Abnormal resting-state activities and functional connectivities of the anterior and the posterior cortexes in medication-naive patients with obsessive-compulsive disorder. *PLoS One.* 2013;8(6):e67478.

102. Hou J, Song L, Zhang W, et al. Morphologic and functional connectivity alterations of corticostriatal and default mode network in treatment-naive patients with obsessive-compulsive disorder. *PLoS One.* 2013;8(12):e83931.

103. Harrison BJ, Pujol J, Cardoner N, et al. Brain corticostriatal systems and the major clinical symptom dimensions of obsessive-compulsive disorder. *Biol Psychiatry.* 2013;73(4):321–328.

104. Hou J, Wu W, Lin Y, et al. Localization of cerebral functional deficits in patients with obsessive-compulsive disorder: a resting-state fMRI study. *J Affect Disord.* 2012;138(3):313–321.

105. Meunier D, Ersche KD, Craig KJ, et al. Brain functional connectivity in stimulant drug dependence and obsessive-compulsive disorder. *Neuroimage.* 2012;59(2):1461–1468.

106. Stern ER, Fitzgerald KD, Welsh RC, Abelson JL, Taylor SF. Resting-state functional connectivity between fronto-parietal and default mode networks in obsessive-compulsive disorder. *PLoS One.* 2012;7(5):e36356.

107. Fitzgerald KD, Welsh RC, Stern ER, et al. Developmental alterations of frontal-striatal-thalamic connectivity in obsessive-compulsive disorder. *J Am Acad Child Adolesc Psychiatry.* 2011;50(9):938–948.

108. Sakai Y, Narumoto J, Nishida S, et al. Corticostriatal functional connectivity in non-medicated patients

with obsessive-compulsive disorder. *Eur Psychiatry.* 2011;26(7):463–469.

109. Zhang T, Wang J, Yang Y, et al. Abnormal small-world architecture of top-down control networks in obsessive-compulsive disorder. *J Psychiatry Neurosci.* 2011;36(1):23–31.

110. Jang JH, Kim JH, Jung WH, et al. Functional connectivity in fronto-subcortical circuitry during the resting state in obsessive-compulsive disorder. *Neurosci Lett.* 2010;474(3):158–162.

111. Harrison BJ, Soriano-Mas C, Pujol J, et al. Altered corticostriatal functional connectivity in obsessive-compulsive disorder. *Arch Gen Psychiatry.* 2009;66(11):1189–1200.

112. Saxena S, Rauch SL. Functional neuroimaging and the neuroanatomy of obsessive-compulsive disorder. *Psychiatr Clin North Am.* 2000;23(3):563–86

113. Phillips ML, Young AW, Senior C, et al. A specific neural substrate for perceiving facial expressions of disgust. *Nature.* 1997;389(6550):495–498.

114. Sprengelmeyer R, Rausch M, Eysel UT, Przuntek H. Neural structures associated with recognition of facial expressions of basic emotions. *Proc Biol Sci.* 1998;265(1409):1927–1931.

115. Chamberlain SR, Fineberg NA, Blackwell AD, Robbins TW, Sahakian BJ. Motor inhibition and cognitive flexibility in obsessive-compulsive disorder and trichotillomania. *Am J Psychiatry.* 2006;163(7):1282–1284.

116. Penadés R, Catalán R, Rubia K, Andrés S, Salamero M, Gastó C. Impaired response inhibition in obsessive compulsive disorder. *Eur Psychiatry.* 2007;22(6):404–410.

117. Menzies L, Achard S, Chamberlain SR, et al. Neurocognitive endophenotypes of obsessive-compulsive disorder. *Brain.* 2007;130(Pt 12):3223–3236.

118. Chamberlain SR, Fineberg NA, Menzies LA, et al. Impaired cognitive flexibility and motor inhibition in unaffected first-degree relatives of patients with obsessive-compulsive disorder. *Am J Psychiatry.* 2007;164(2):335–338.

119. Veale DM, Sahakian BJ, Owen AM, Marks IM. Specific cognitive deficits in tests sensitive to frontal lobe dysfunction in obsessive-compulsive disorder. *Psychol Med.* 1996;26(6):1261–1269.

120. Dias R, Robbins TW, Roberts AC. Dissociation in prefrontal cortex of affective and attentional shifts. *Nature.* 1996;380(6569):69–72.

121. Hornak J, O'Doherty J, Bramham J, et al. Reward-related reversal learning after surgical excisions in orbito-frontal or dorsolateral prefrontal cortex in humans. *J Cogn Neurosci.* 2004;16(3):463–478.

122. Endrass T, Schuermann B, Kaufmann C, Spielberg R, Kniesche R, Kathmann N. Performance monitoring and error significance in patients with obsessive-compulsive disorder. *Biol Psychol.* 2010;84(2):257–263.

123. Johannes S, Wieringa BM, Nager W, et al. Discrepant target detection and action monitoring in obsessive-compulsive disorder. *Psychiatry Res.* 2001;108(2):101–110.

124. Carrasco M, Harbin SM, Nienhuis JK, Fitzgerald KD, Gehring WJ, Hanna GL. Increased error-related brain activity in youth with obsessive-compulsive disorder and unaffected siblings. *Depress Anxiety.* 2013;30(1):39–46.

125. Purcell R, Maruff P, Kyrios M, Pantelis C. Neuropsychological deficits in obsessive-compulsive disorder: a comparison with unipolar depression, panic disorder, and normal controls. *Arch Gen Psychiatry.* 1998;55(5):415–423.

126. Chamberlain SR, Fineberg NA, Blackwell AD, Clark L, Robbins TW, Sahakian BJ. A neuropsychological comparison of obsessive-compulsive disorder and trichotillomania. *Neuropsychologia.* 2007;45(4):654–662.

127. Kashyap H, Kumar JK, Kandavel T, Reddy YC. Neuropsychological functioning in obsessive-compulsive disorder: are executive functions the key deficit? *Compr Psychiatry.* 2013;54(5):533–540.

128. Delorme R, Goussé V, Roy I, et al. Shared executive dysfunctions in unaffected relatives of patients with autism and obsessive-compulsive disorder. *Eur Psychiatry.* 2007;22(1):32–38.

129. van der Wee NJ, Ramsey NF, Jansma JM, et al. Spatial working memory deficits in obsessive compulsive disorder are associated with excessive engagement of the medial frontal cortex. *Neuroimage.* 2003;20(4):2271–2280.

130. Rauch SL, Whalen PJ, Shin LM, et al. Exaggerated amygdala response to masked facial stimuli in posttraumatic stress disorder: a functional MRI study. *Biol Psychiatry.* 2000;47(9):769–776.

131. Schneider F, Weiss U, Kessler C, et al. Subcortical correlates of differential classical conditioning of aversive emotional reactions in social phobia. *Biol Psychiatry.* 1999;45(7):863–871.

132. Stein MB, Goldin PR, Sareen J, Zorrilla LT, Brown GG. Increased amygdala activation to angry and contemptuous faces in generalized social phobia. *Arch Gen Psychiatry.* 2002;59(11):1027–1034.

133. Tillfors M, Furmark T, Marteinsdottir I, et al. Cerebral blood flow in subjects with social phobia

during stressful speaking tasks: a PET study. *Am J Psychiatry*. 2001;158(8):1220–1226.

134. Nitschke JB, Sarinopoulos I, Oathes DJ, et al. Anticipatory activation in the amygdala and anterior cingulate in generalized anxiety disorder and prediction of treatment response. *Am J Psychiatry*. 2009;166(3):302–310.

135. McClure EB, Monk CS, Nelson EE, et al. Abnormal attention modulation of fear circuit function in pediatric generalized anxiety disorder. *Arch Gen Psychiatry*. 2007;64(1):97–106.

136. Quirk GJ, Likhtik E, Pelletier JG, Paré D. Stimulation of medial prefrontal cortex decreases the responsiveness of central amygdala output neurons. *J Neurosci*. 2003;23(25):8800–8807.

137. Sotres-Bayon F, Cain CK, LeDoux JE. Brain mechanisms of fear extinction: historical perspectives on the contribution of prefrontal cortex. *Biol Psychiatry*. 2006;60(4):329–336.

138. Shin LM, Wright CI, Cannistraro PA, et al. A functional magnetic resonance imaging study of amygdala and medial prefrontal cortex responses to overtly presented fearful faces in posttraumatic stress disorder. *Arch Gen Psychiatry*. 2005;62(3):273–281.

139. Williams LM, Kemp AH, Felmingham K, et al. Trauma modulates amygdala and medial prefrontal responses to consciously attended fear. *Neuroimage*. 2006;29(2):347–357.

140. Britton JC, Phan KL, Taylor SF, Fig LM, Liberzon I. Corticolimbic blood flow in posttraumatic stress disorder during script-driven imagery. *Biol Psychiatry*. 2005;57(8):832–840.

141. Lindauer RJ, Booij J, Habraken JB, et al. Cerebral blood flow changes during script-driven imagery in police officers with posttraumatic stress disorder. *Biol Psychiatry*. 2004;56(11):853–861.

142. Phan KL, Britton JC, Taylor SF, Fig LM, Liberzon I. Corticolimbic blood flow during nontraumatic emotional processing in posttraumatic stress disorder. *Arch Gen Psychiatry*. 2006;63(2):184–192.

143. Peres JF, Newberg AB, Mercante JP, et al. Cerebral blood flow changes during retrieval of traumatic memories before and after psychotherapy: a SPECT study. *Psychol Med*. 2007;37(10):1481–1491.

144. Seedat S, Warwick J, van Heerden B, et al. Single photon emission computed tomography in posttraumatic stress disorder before and after treatment with a selective serotonin reuptake inhibitor. *J Affect Disord*. 2004;80(1):45–53.

145. Felmingham K, Kemp A, Williams L, et al. Changes in anterior cingulate and amygdala after cognitive behavior therapy of posttraumatic stress disorder. *Psychol Sci*. 2007;18(2):127–129.

146. Simon D, Kaufmann C, Müsch K, Kischkel E, Kathmann N. Fronto-striato-limbic hyperactivation in obsessive-compulsive disorder during individually tailored symptom provocation. *Psychophysiology*. 2010;47(4):728–738.

147. Upadhyay J, Maleki N, Potter J, et al. Alterations in brain structure and functional connectivity in prescription opioid-dependent patients. *Brain*. 2010;133(Pt 7):2098–2114.

148. Hu Y, Salmeron BJ, Gu H, Stein EA, Yang Y. Impaired functional connectivity within and between frontostriatal circuits and its association with compulsive drug use and trait impulsivity in cocaine addiction. *JAMA Psychiatry*. 2015;72(6):584–592.

149. De Ridder D, Vanneste S, Kovacs S, Sunaert S, Dom G. Transient alcohol craving suppression by rTMS of dorsal anterior cingulate: an fMRI and LORETA EEG study. *Neurosci Lett*. 2011;496(1):5–10.

150. Valencia-Alfonso CE, Luigjes J, Smolders R, et al. Effective deep brain stimulation in heroin addiction: a case report with complementary intracranial electroencephalogram. *Biol Psychiatry*. 2012;71(8):e35–e37.

151. Wrase J, Schlagenhauf F, Kienast T, et al. Dysfunction of reward processing correlates with alcohol craving in detoxified alcoholics. *Neuroimage*. 2007;35(2):787–794.

152. Bühler M, Vollstädt-Klein S, Kobiella A, et al. Nicotine dependence is characterized by disordered reward processing in a network driving motivation. *Biol Psychiatry*. 2010;67(8):745–752.

153. Becker A, Kirsch M, Gerchen MF, Kiefer F, Kirsch P. Striatal activation and frontostriatal connectivity during non-drug reward anticipation in alcohol dependence. *Addict Biol*. 2017;22(3):833–843.

154. Luijten M, Schellekens AF, Kühn S, Machielse MW, Sescousse G. Disruption of reward processing in addiction: an image-based meta-analysis of functional magnetic resonance imaging studies. *JAMA Psychiatry*. 2017;74(4):387–398.

155. Martz ME, Trucco EM, Cope LM, et al. Association of marijuana use with blunted nucleus accumbens response to reward anticipation. *JAMA Psychiatry*. 2016;73(8):838–844.

156. Reuter J, Raedler T, Rose M, Hand I, Gläscher J, Büchel C. Pathological gambling is linked to reduced activation of the mesolimbic reward system. *Nat Neurosci*. 2005;8(2):14708.

157. de Greck M, Enzi B, Prösch U, Gantman A, Tempelmann C, Northoff G. Decreased neuronal

activity in reward circuitry of pathological gamblers during processing of personal relevant stimuli. *Hum Brain Mapp*. 2010;31(11):1802–1812.

158. Balodis IM, Kober H, Worhunsky PD, Stevens MC, Pearlson GD, Potenza MN. Diminished frontostriatal activity during processing of monetary rewards and losses in pathological gambling. *Biol Psychiatry*. 2012;71(8):749–757.

159. Choi JS, Shin YC, Jung WH, et al. Altered brain activity during reward anticipation in pathological gambling and obsessive-compulsive disorder. *PLoS One*. 2012;7(9):e45938.

160. Romanczuk-Seiferth N, Koehler S, Dreesen C, Wüstenberg T, Heinz A. Pathological gambling and alcohol dependence: neural disturbances in reward and loss avoidance processing. *Addict Biol*. 2015;20(3):557–569.

161. Balodis IM, Kober H, Worhunsky PD, et al. Monetary reward processing in obese individuals with and without binge eating disorder. *Biol Psychiatry*. 2013;73(9):877–886.

162. Cha J, Ide JS, Bowman FD, Simpson HB, Posner J, Steinglass JE. Abnormal reward circuitry in anorexia nervosa: a longitudinal, multimodal MRI study. *Hum Brain Mapp*. 2016;37(11):3835–3846.

163. de Ruiter MB, Veltman DJ, Goudriaan AE, Oosterlaan J, Sjoerds Z, van den Brink W. Response perseveration and ventral prefrontal sensitivity to reward and punishment in male problem gamblers and smokers. *Neuropsychopharmacology*. 2009;34(4):1027–1038.

164. Verdejo-Garcia A, Clark L, Verdejo-Román J, et al. Neural substrates of cognitive flexibility in cocaine and gambling addictions. *Br J Psychiatry*. 2015;207(2):158–164.

165. Sato Y, Saito N, Utsumi A, et al. Neural basis of impaired cognitive flexibility in patients with anorexia nervosa. *PLoS One*. 2013;8(5):e61108.

166. Saxena S, Brody AL, Maidment KM, et al. Cerebral glucose metabolism in obsessive-compulsive hoarding. *Am J Psychiatry*. 2004;161(6):1038–1048.

167. Starcke K, Tuschen-Caffier B, Markowitsch HJ, Brand M. Dissociation of decisions in ambiguous and risky situations in obsessive-compulsive disorder. *Psychiatry Res*. 2010;175(1–2):114–120.

168. Erhan C, Bulut GÇ, Gökçe S, et al. Disrupted latent decision processes in medication-free pediatric OCD patients. *J Affect Disord*. 2017;207:32–37.

169. Feusner JD, Moody T, Hembacher E, et al. Abnormalities of visual processing and frontostriatal systems in body dysmorphic disorder. *Arch Gen Psychiatry*. 2010;67(2):197–205.

170. Li W, Lai TM, Bohon C, et al. Anorexia nervosa and body dysmorphic disorder are associated with abnormalities in processing visual information. *Psychol Med*. 2015;45(10):2111–2122.

171. Rotge JY, Guehl D, Dilharreguy B, et al. Provocation of obsessive-compulsive symptoms: a quantitative voxel-based meta-analysis of functional neuroimaging studies. *J Psychiatry Neurosci*. 2008;33(5):405–412.

172. Baxter LRJ, Schwartz JM, Bergman KS, et al. Caudate glucose metabolic rate changes with both drug and behavior therapy for obsessive-compulsive disorder. *Arch Gen Psychiatry*. 1992;49(9):681–689.

173. Benkelfat C, Nordahl TE, Semple WE, King AC, Murphy DL, Cohen RM. Local cerebral glucose metabolic rates in obsessive-compulsive disorder. Patients treated with clomipramine. *Arch Gen Psychiatry*. 1990;47(9):840–848.

174. Saxena S, Brody AL, Maidment KM, et al. Localized orbitofrontal and subcortical metabolic changes and predictors of response to paroxetine treatment in obsessive-compulsive disorder. *Neuropsychopharmacology*. 1999;21(6):683–693.

175. Saxena S, Brody AL, Ho ML, et al. Differential cerebral metabolic changes with paroxetine treatment of obsessive-compulsive disorder vs major depression. *Arch Gen Psychiatry*. 2002;59(3):250–261.

176. Schwartz JM, Stoessel PW, Baxter LRJ, Martin KM, Phelps ME. Systematic changes in cerebral glucose metabolic rate after successful behavior modification treatment of obsessive-compulsive disorder. *Arch Gen Psychiatry*. 1996;53(2):109–113.

177. Swedo SE, Pietrini P, Leonard HL, et al. Cerebral glucose metabolism in childhood-onset obsessive-compulsive disorder. Revisualization during pharmacotherapy. *Arch Gen Psychiatry*. 1992;49(9):690–694.

178. Kang DH, Kwon JS, Kim JJ, et al. Brain glucose metabolic changes associated with neuropsychological improvements after 4 months of treatment in patients with obsessive-compulsive disorder. *Acta Psychiatr Scand*. 2003;107(4):291–297.

179. Ho Pian KL, van Megen HJ, Ramsey NF, et al. Decreased thalamic blood flow in obsessive-compulsive disorder patients responding to fluvoxamine. *Psychiatry Res*. 2005;138(2):89–97.

180. Rubin RT, Ananth J, Villanueva-Meyer J, Trajmar PG, Mena I. Regional 133xenon cerebral blood flow and cerebral 99mTc-HMPAO uptake in patients with

obsessive-compulsive disorder before and during treatment. *Biol Psychiatry*. 1995;38(7):429–437.

181. Hoehn-Saric R, Schlaepfer TE, Greenberg BD, McLeod DR, Wong SH. Cerebral blood flow in obsessive-compulsive patients with major depression: effect of treatment with sertraline or desipramine on treatment responders and non-responders. *Psychiatry Res*. 2001;108(2):89–100.

182. Brooks SJ, Stein DJ. A systematic review of the neural bases of psychotherapy for anxiety and related disorders. *Dialogues Clin Neurosci*. 2015;17(3):261–279.

183. Brody AL, Saxena S, Schwartz JM, et al. FDG-PET predictors of response to behavioral therapy and pharmacotherapy in obsessive compulsive disorder. *Psychiatry Res*. 1998;84(1):1–6.

Chapter 10

Epidemiology of Obsessive-Compulsive Disorder

Roselind Lieb, Patrizia D. Hofer and Karina Wahl

Introduction

Epidemiology is the scientific discipline that explores the distribution of health phenomena (e.g., mental disorders or physical diseases) in defined populations, as well as factors that influence this distribution [1]. Research in epidemiology is crucial for understanding many aspects of health phenomena. For instance, knowledge about the burden of a disorder (e.g., its prevalence or incidence) in a given population is critical for planning health services. Other aspects include the natural course (e.g., risk period for first manifestation), the prognosis and the identification of factors involved in the etiology and development of the course of the disorder or disease. A greater understanding of these aspects could enhance the development of new modes of prevention or intervention.

Epidemiology can be roughly divided into *descriptive* and *analytic* epidemiology. *Descriptive* epidemiology explores mainly the description of health phenomena, their natural course and the evaluation of health services. *Analytic* epidemiology addresses mainly questions about risk or causal factors. Epidemiological research is an important supplement to clinical research because clinical results are not usually generalizable to non-clinical samples. For instance, epidemiological community surveys have demonstrated that not all individuals affected by a mental disorder receive treatment [2]. Therefore, affected individuals under treatment cannot be considered as being fully representative of the characteristics of the disorder in the general population. Epidemiological studies that include community samples without regard to whether the subjects have sought treatment are therefore necessary to complete the clinically based knowledge of disorders.

This chapter focuses on basic epidemiological knowledge of obsessive-compulsive disorder (OCD). We first provide information on its prevalence in the general population, followed by insights into the age of onset of OCD in affected individuals, as well as aspects of treatment seeking and impairment. After these mostly descriptive epidemiological contributions, we focus on comorbidity; that is, on the relation of OCD with other mental disorders, as well as on the temporal patterns of comorbidity. We close this chapter by addressing the risk factors that have so far been evaluated by epidemiological research.

Recent Research Findings

Prevalence

Motivated by the development of reliable diagnostic criteria and standardized diagnostic instruments for their assessment, systematic research on the epidemiological aspects of OCD began in the 1980s, with the first epidemiological survey that provided information about the prevalence of OCD in the general population by using standardized diagnostic criteria, the *Diagnostic and Statistical Manual of Mental Disorders*, third edition (DSM-III) [3], being the Epidemiological Catchment Area (ECA) Program developed by the US National Institute of Mental Health [4]. Since then, a number of population-based surveys have been performed using highly structured or standardized diagnostic instruments that reliably assess diagnostic criteria according to the DSM-III [4], DSM-III-R [5], DSM-IV [6] or ICD-10 [7].

Prevalence studies generally determine two estimates: lifetime and 12-month prevalence. Lifetime prevalence is an estimate of the proportion of people in a population at a point in time who either have the disorder or have had it over their lifetime up to the time of the estimation. In terms of the lifetime prevalence of OCD among adults, results from community surveys that have used standardized instruments suggest that between 0.3% and 3.5% of the adult population meet diagnostic criteria for OCD at least once in their lifetime (for a review see Fontenelle et al. [8] and Somers et al. [9]; for more recent studies see, e.g., Caraveo-Anduaga and Bermudez [10], de Bruijn et al. [11] and Ruscio et al. [12]). On the basis of the prevalence findings of 14 community-based studies all over the world, Somers et al. [9] derived a pooled "best estimate" of 1.3% (95% confidence interval, CI, 0.86–1.8%].

The 12-month prevalence is an estimate of the proportion of individuals with the disorder in the 12 months before the time of the estimation. The 12-month prevalence of OCD that have been reported vary between 0.1% and 3.6% (for a review see Fontenelle et al. [8] and Somers et al. [9]; for more recent studies see, e.g., de Bruijn et al. [11], Ruscio et al. [12], Kessler et al. [13], Crino et al. [14], Jacobi et al. [15], Adam et al. [16], Kessler et al. [17]). The pooled "best estimate" determined by Somers et al. [9] on the basis of nine community studies was 0.54% (95% CI 0.28–0.86%). As shown, the prevalence estimates vary greatly between the reported findings. Heterogeneity among estimates for OCD may be a function of assessment instrument, country studied and response rate [9].

Epidemiological studies have further demonstrated that OCD can already be observed in childhood and adolescence. Studies that used standardized instruments revealed lifetime estimates between 0.5% and 2.6% and 12-month estimates between 0.0% and 4.0% for children and adolescents (for review see Fontenelle et al. [8] and Fullana et al. [19]). In the German Early Developmental Stages of Psychopathology (EDSP) study, in which more than 3000 adolescents and young adults (14–24 years) were followed over 10 years, 0.7% fulfilled lifetime DSM-IV criteria for OCD at baseline, and 0.6% in the past 12 months [18]. In New Zealand, the prospective Dunedin Multidisciplinary Health and Development Study of an unselected birth cohort found that 2.3% of the respondents fulfilled DSM-IV criteria for OCD at age 26, and 1.8% at age 32 [19].

Epidemiological studies have additionally suggested that forms, which by definition do not fulfill all of the diagnostic criteria of a given diagnosis, seem to be common. For such subthreshold forms of OCD, lifetime prevalence between 2.0% and 8.7% have been reported [11,16,20,21]. Moving to the symptom level, the American National Comorbidity Survey Replication (NCS-R) found that 28.2% of the respondents reported experiencing obsessions or compulsions at some time in their lives [12].

Comparable high rates of OCD at the symptomatic level were reported from the Dunedin Multidisciplinary Health and Development Study [19]. This study estimated that 21–25% of individuals from the general population endorse obsessions and/or compulsions as defined by the DSM-IV, but without meeting full diagnostic criteria. In the German National Health Interview and Examination Survey – Mental Health Survey (GHS-MHS), 13.5% of the respondents reported having experienced at least one obsessive-compulsive symptom in the 12 months before the assessment [16]. These and data from other surveys (e.g., Wittchen et al. [22] and Valleni-Basile et al. [23]) support the conclusion that subclinical OCD on the symptomatic or subthreshold level may be experienced by far more people in the general population than would be expected by the prevalence estimates of full diagnoses.

Age of Onset

As shown by the prevalence findings described above, OCD can already be observed during childhood. Several community epidemiological surveys have collected retrospective data on the age of onset of OCD and have demonstrated that specifically the second and third decades in life seem to be the most critical periods for first onset. Partially dependent on the age range in the study sample, mean ages of onset for OCD reported from cross-sectional studies in adult samples ranged between 19 and 35.5 years [20,21,24,25,26,27,28].

Using more sophisticated life table survival analysis (a method that analyzes the time until the occurrence of a certain event; e.g., the age of onset of a certain mental disorder, such as OCD) the ECA study reported highest risk for first manifestation of OCD between ages 15 and 39 years. The median age of onset of OCD was 23 years [29], which was the highest median among the assessed DSM-III anxiety disorders. Using the same method, the NCS-R [12] and a longitudinal study conducted in Zurich [30] reported a mean age of onset of 19.5 years. In the NCS-R, age of onset curves revealed highest risks for both males and females in the second and third decades (see Figure 10.1). This steepest increase in first onset of OCD between the ages of 10 and 30 years was convincingly replicated in the Zurich study [30].

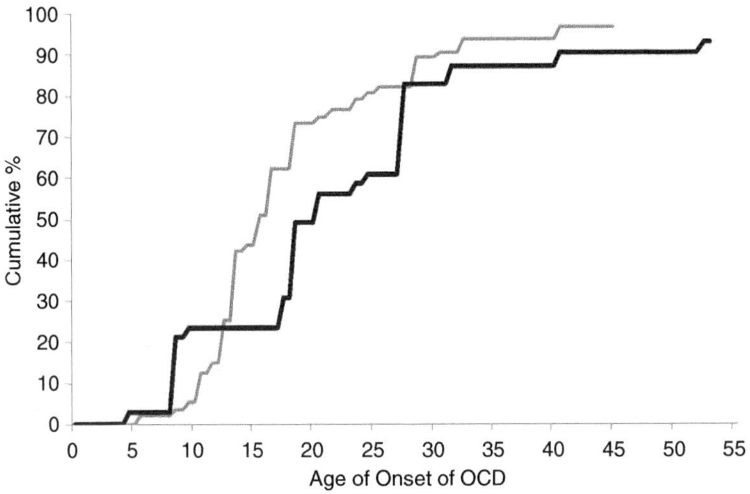

Figure 10.1 Age of onset of first obsession or compulsion among individuals with lifetime obsessive-compulsive disorder (OCD) in the National Comorbidity Survey Replication. The cumulative age-of-onset distributions differ significantly for males and females (Chi-square 8.1, $P = 0.004$). Gray line = females; black line = males. Reprinted with permission from Ruscio AM, Stein DJ, Chiu WT, Kessler R. The epidemiology of obsessive-compulsive disorder in the National Comorbidity Survey Replication. *Molecular Psychiatry* 2008; 15: 53–63.

Impairment and Treatment Seeking

A number of epidemiological studies have convincingly demonstrated that individuals affected by OCD are profoundly impaired in social and occupational functioning and that the emergence of OCD may reduce quality of life [12,16,30,31,32]. In the NCS-R, nearly two-thirds of the individuals with a 12-month diagnosis reported severe role impairments [12]. Severely affected individuals reported the greatest impairments, with the highest impairment ratings in the domains of relationships and social functioning. There is some evidence that individuals affected by OCD seem to be more impaired in daily life than not only individuals who are mentally healthy, but also individuals affected by other mental disorders [31].

Epidemiological studies also found evidence that subclinical forms of OCD are associated with poorer functioning in work or social activities [11,21,30]. The results of the GHS-MHS show that even obsessive or compulsive symptoms alone are considerably associated with impairments in daily life [16]. The findings reported by the Dunedin Multidisciplinary Health and Development Study also indicate that obsessions and compulsions may cause interference even in people who do not meet full diagnostic criteria for OCD, with higher distress in individuals with obsessions than in individuals with compulsions [15].

Addressing the question of treatment-seeking rates of individuals affected by OCD, epidemiological studies have revealed somewhat contradictory findings. While some studies indicate rather low treatment-seeking rates (e.g., Subramanian et al. [32] and Nestadt et al. [33]), others suggest higher treatment rates. For example, the NCS-R reported that half of the individuals with a 12-month diagnosis reported receiving treatment during the last 12 months [12]. In the GHS-MHS, 68% of individuals with 12-month OCD received at least a minimal intervention [16,34].

Torres et al. [31] analyzed services use by adults with OCD living in private households in Great Britain and showed that 40% of the individuals with OCD received treatment. This rate was matched by the population-based Zurich study, in which 40% of individuals with OCD reported seeking professional treatment [30]. Torres et al. [35] found that individuals with OCD were more likely than people with other mental disorders to receive treatment (40% vs. 23%), but within the OCD group, individuals with pure OCD were much less likely than those with comorbid other mental disorders (14% vs. 56%).

The findings by Torres et al. [31] are consistent with the results of other epidemiological studies that found evidence that comorbidity with other mental conditions seems to be a powerful predictor of help seeking among individuals with OCD [34,36]. Studies that evaluated delay in treatment seeking demonstrated a lag of 9–14 years from the first manifestation of OCD symptoms to the time the affected individuals sought treatment [32,37,38]. These delays are somewhat longer than those reported for mood disorders but comparable to delays reported for other anxiety disorders [39]. From the NCS-R, reported median years of delay were 9 years for generalized anxiety disorder (GAD), 10 years for panic disorder, 12 years for agoraphobia and post-traumatic stress disorder (PTSD), 16 years for social phobia, 20 years for specific phobia and 23 years for separation anxiety disorder. Treatment contact among patients with OCD seems to occur with about the same delay as those with GAD, panic disorder, agoraphobia and PTSD reported in the NCS-R. One might speculate that these anxiety disorders show shorter delays due to their highly associated impairments in daily life.

Comorbidity

Relationship Between OCD and Other Disorders

Epidemiological studies have consistently demonstrated the comorbidity of OCD and a wide range of mental disorders. Pure cases are the exception rather than the rule, with 84–90% of patients with OCD meeting criteria for at least one other mental disorder in 12-month [16] and lifetime [12,40] comorbidity estimates. Similar patterns for the most common comorbid disorders in OCD have emerged from epidemiological studies, with the highest rates for comorbid anxiety (67–76%) [12,16] and affective disorders (63–70%) [11,12,16] followed by impulse control disorders (56%) [12], substance use disorders (13.3–40.1%) [11,12,16,20] and eating disorders (1.7–6.5%) [11,16]. Findings from epidemiological studies on the associations between OCD and specific comorbid disorders are presented in Table 10.1.

Comorbidity with affective disorders: There is consistent evidence from longitudinal and cross-sectional epidemiological surveys for both 12-month [16] and lifetime [8,42,44,45] association between OCD and bipolar disorder. In the NCS-R, individuals with OCD in comparison with individuals without OCD had seven-fold higher odds of developing bipolar disorder over their lifetime [12]. Most studies examining lifetime [12,41,43,44,45] and 12-month [16,23,40] rates have shown an association between OCD and major depressive disorder. However, Fineberg et al. [42] assumed that in some studies cases of bipolar disorder may have been misclassified as major depression, resulting in false positive associations between OCD and major depression.

Comorbidity with other anxiety disorders: Many individuals with OCD have also been found to meet criteria for other anxiety disorders over the past 12 months [16] or over their lifetime [12,41]. Both 12-month [16,23,40] and lifetime [11,12,43] specific and social phobia have consistently been associated with OCD. For the associations between OCD and panic disorder, agoraphobia, and GAD, inconsistent results have been reported (Table 10.1). Surprisingly, the comorbidity of OCD and PTSD has not been well documented in epidemiological samples. Results based on the NCS-R suggest that lifetime OCD is significantly associated with lifetime PTSD [12].

Comorbidity with substance use disorders: Most epidemiological studies have reported a relationship between OCD and substance use disorders with 30–40% of individuals with OCD meeting criteria for a substance-related disorder [11,12,16]. There is, however, less consistency between studies in terms of the substance used. Whereas most studies did not find a link between OCD and illicit substances, Nestadt et al. [43] and Douglass et al. [40] found a link between OCD and marijuana use. These conflicting findings may be related to Cuzen et al.'s [49] heuristic, which argues that comorbidity with substance use disorders in OCD increases with increasing severity of OCD but only to a certain threshold. Beyond this threshold compulsivity may decrease the risk of incidence of substance use disorders. Thus, it may be that the severity of OCD in subjects between the samples investigated was variable.

Comorbidity with other mental disorders: Only a few community sample studies have examined the association between OCD and eating, impulse control and personality disorders. Given the low prevalence rates of both OCD and eating disorders, it is not surprising that a considerable number of community-based studies have not reported any comorbid cases of OCD and any eating disorder. Others, however, have reported positive associations between lifetime OCD and bulimia nervosa [20,48] and binge eating disorder [48] but not anorexia nervosa [40,48].

In contrast, in the NCS-R, lifetime OCD has been linked to all of the examined impulse-control disorders [12]. In the British National Survey of Psychiatric Morbidity 2000, Torres et al. [50] showed a considerable comorbidity of OCD and almost all cluster A, B and C personality disorders. A remarkable 74% of individuals who met criteria for OCD over the past month also met criteria for any personality disorder over the past month.

Temporal Pattern of Comorbid Disorders

Information on the temporal pattern of OCD and comorbid disorders based on community samples is

Table 10.1 Comorbidity of obsessive-compulsive disorder (OCD) and other mental disorders in epidemiological studies.

Other mental disorder	Association	No association
Any other anxiety disorder	Adam et al. [16]; Ruscio et al. [12]; Weissman et al. [41]	
Panic disorder	de Bruijn et al.[11]; Fineberg et al. [42]; Ruscio et al. [12]	Douglass et al. [40]; Nestadt et al. [43]
Agoraphobia	Adam et al. [16]; de Bruijn et al. [11]; Douglass et al. [40]; Ruscio et al. [12]	Fineberg et al. [42]; Nestadt et al. [43]
Specific phobia	Adam et al. [16]; de Bruijn et al. [11]; Douglass et al. [40]; Nestadt et al. [43]; Ruscio et al. [12]; Valleni-Basile et al. [23]	Fineberg et al. [42]
Social phobia	Adam et al. [16]; de Bruijn et al. [11]; Douglass et al. [40]; Fineberg et al. [42]; Nestadt et al. [43]; Ruscio et al.[12]	
Generalized anxiety disorder	Adam et al. [16]; de Bruijn et al. [11]; Fineberg et al. [42]	Douglass et al. [40]; Nestadt et al. [43]; Ruscio et al. [12]
Post-traumatic stress disorder	Ruscio et al. [12]	
Any affective disorder		
Major depression	Adam et al. [16]; Chen and Dilsaver [44]; de Graaf et al. [45]; Douglass et al. [40]; Nestadt et al. [43]; Ruscio et al. [12]; Valleni-Basile et al. [23]; Weissman et al. [41]	Fineberg et al. [42]
Any bipolar disorder	Adam et al. [16]; Chen and Dilsaver [44]; de Graaf et al. [45]; Fineberg et al. [42]; Ruscio et al. [12]	
Dysthymia	Adam et al. [16]; de Graaf et al. [45]; Douglass et al. [40]; Ruscio et al.[12]	
Any substance use disorder	Adam et al. [16]; de Bruijn et al. [11]; Ruscio et al. [12]	Angst et al. [20]
Nicotine dependence	Adam et al. [16]	Isensee et al. [46]
Alcohol abuse/ dependence	Adam et al. [16]; Ruscio et al. [12]; Douglass et al. [40]	Angst et al. [20]; Nestadt et al. [43]
Drug abuse/ dependence	Ruscio et al. [12]; Nestadt et al. [43] (marijuana); Douglass et al. [40] (marijuana)	Adam et al. [16]; Angst et al. [20] (any illicit); Nestadt et al. [43] (sedative, cocaine, stimulant)
Eating disorder	de Bruijn et al. [11]	Adam et al. [16]; Rapoport et al. [47] (no cases)
Anorexia nervosa		Hudson et al. [48] (no cases); Douglass et al. [40] (no cases)
Bulimia nervosa	Angst et al. [20]; Hudson et al. [48]	Douglass et al. [40] (no cases)
Binge eating disorder	Hudson et al. [48]	Angst et al. [20]
Any impulse control disorder	Ruscio et al. [12]	
Any personality disorder	Torres et al. [31]	
Any disorder	Adam et al. [16]; Ruscio et al. [12]	

scarce. Given the low prevalence of OCD, numbers of comorbid cases with specific mental disorders are often rather small [51,52]. Thus, for the temporal pattern of comorbid cases, we consider only studies with at least 10 comorbid cases.

Affective disorders: In the analyses of lifetime comorbidity of OCD and affective disorders, the proportion of OCD predating affective disorders is similar to the proportion of OCD following affective disorders [12]. More than 50% of the individuals meeting criteria for both OCD and major depression disorder reported a prior onset of OCD (57%) in the NSC-R [12]. A clear temporal pattern of OCD and bipolar disorder has not yet been established. In the Netherlands Mental Health Survey and Incidence Study, OCD frequently began in the same year as bipolar disorder (43% to 64%) or was reported as the initial disorder [45]. In the NSC-R, OCD frequently followed bipolar disorder (52%) [12].

Anxiety disorders: The onset of other anxiety disorders generally predates the onset of OCD [4,12,53]. In the NSC-R, for example, almost 80% of all anxiety disorders predated the onset of OCD. A disorder-specific pattern seems to exist for PTSD, with equal proportions of individuals reporting prior onset of OCD or PTSD [12]. Furthermore, the onset of OCD has been reported to predate the onset of panic disorder in 30% to 40% of comorbid individuals [4,12].

Substance use disorders: Substance use disorders frequently manifest prior to the onset of OCD (59%) [12]. Regarding the temporal pattern of specific substances, however, an earlier onset of OCD has been reported in a substantial proportion of comorbid cases of OCD and alcohol abuse or dependence (53%; 46%) [4,12] and other drug abuse or dependence (62%) [4].

Risk Factors

The identification of risk factors for mental disorders is one of the most important but also most challenging areas in epidemiological research. In this chapter, we use Kraemer et al.'s [54] concept that conceptualizes a risk factor as a characteristic that occurs before the outcome. Because of a reliance on retrospective recall, the proper identification of risk factors according to this concept is almost impossible in cross-sectional studies (with some exceptions, such as gender or independently documented early factors, e.g., prenatal complications).

For the investigation of most risk factors, longitudinal studies that start with a group of individuals who lack a positive history of the outcome of interest and who are exposed to the risk factor or not are needed. Only with this study design can potential risk factors be examined properly. Whenever temporal precedence between the factor and the outcome under study cannot be demonstrated, the factor should be labeled just a "correlate."

In this chapter, we aim to give an overview of risk factors that have been identified so far in epidemiological studies. We have therefore relied on population-based longitudinal studies that took into account the temporal precedence of risk factors and OCD. It should be noted that even in these studies the interpretation of results might be compromised by methodological problems, such as low number of incident individuals [55] or remaining uncertainties about the temporal order of risk factors and onset of OCD [40,56].

Sociodemographic Variables

The investigation of sociodemographic variables did not result in a coherent picture. Valleni-Basile et al. [55] found that a higher socioeconomic status was associated with higher odds of developing OCD. The odds ratio (OR) could not be calculated since all five incident individuals had a middle to high socioeconomic status. Crum and Anthony [51] found that unemployed women had the highest odds (OR 3.9) of developing OCD when compared with employed women (OR 2.3), unemployed men (OR 1.6) or employed men (reference group).

In the studies by Douglass et al. [40] and Nestadt et al. [43] however, socioeconomic status or household income was not associated with occurrence of OCD. Black race was associated with substantially higher odds (OR 23.38) of developing OCD compared with white race in the study by Valleni-Basile et al. [48]. No significant association between race and OCD was found in the study by Nestadt et al. [43], nor between grades and OCD or marital status and OCD.

Most epidemiological studies have found a preponderance of female incident individuals. The following pooled "best estimates" of 12-month and lifetime prevalence rates separately for men and women were provided by a systematic review [9]: 12-month prevalence rate, male 0.31% (95% CI 0.08–0.65%), female 0.5% (95% CI 0.31–0.76%); lifetime prevalence rate, male 1.0% (95% CI 0.67–1.60%), female 1.6% (95% CI 1.0–2.2%).

Fontenelle et al. [8] confirmed these findings in their review and concluded that the majority of epidemiological studies found an increased risk of adult women developing OCD compared with men. The tendency for more women than men to develop OCD was also found in more recent epidemiological studies; that is, higher odds of onset (OR 2.1) among females than males [12]. However, it should also be noted that some epidemiological studies failed to find gender differences [15,16,32].

Childhood Experiences

So far, not many childhood experiences have been identified as risk factors for OCD. In the Dunedin Multidisciplinary Health and Development Study, none of the childhood risk factors were increased in a group of individuals diagnosed with OCD at age 18 years compared to individuals with anxiety, depressive or conduct disorders, and also individuals without any mental disorder [40]. The investigated factors included perinatal problems (e.g., diabetes or hypertension of the mother, delivery other than spontaneous, low Apgar score at birth, preterm birth), behavior problems at home or at school between the ages of 5 and 11 years (e.g., nail biting, temper tantrums, stuttering, fearfulness), childhood temperament (at ages 3 and 5 years), speech problems at age 13 years (e.g., incoherent speech, parroting) and neurodevelopmental problems between the ages of 3 and 9 years and at age 13 years.

The 12-month prevalence of OCD was reassessed at ages 26 and 32 years, and at these time points two factors were associated with increased odds of OCD compared with anxious and healthy controls: social isolation in childhood (OR 1.4) and negative emotionality at age 18 years (OR 1.7) [56]. Additionally, in adolescents, undesirable life events within the last 12 months (OR 1.21) have been found to be associated with increased odds of OCD, and fewer desirable life events within the last 12 months (OR 0.78) and high familial cohesion (OR 0.90) with decreased odds of OCD [55].

Intelligence Quotient

Inconsistent findings emerged from prospective studies investigating intelligence quotient (IQ) as a predictor of OCD. There was no significant association between childhood IQ and OCD at age 18 years [40], 26 years [50] or 32 years [56]. Peterson et al. [52] found a positive association between IQ and OCD: the higher the IQ in late adolescence, the greater the increase in OCD symptoms in early adulthood.

Other Risk Factors or Correlates of Obsessive-Compulsive Disorder

A broad range of other potential risk factors for OCD have been investigated in studies not based on prospective, population-based designs (e.g., in clinical samples, case control or twin studies). Brandner et al. [57] identified factors involved in the reproductive cycle (e.g., pregnancy and postpartum period) and stressful or traumatic life events (e.g., loss, family disruption, illness or injury, physical or sexual abuse) as potential candidates for increasing the risk for OCD. Consistent with this conclusion, a meta-analysis confirmed that women are at greater risk of developing OCD during pregnancy and the postpartum period than women from the general population [58].

On the other hand, only limited evidence suggests that family size, parental age, season of birth or birth order, parental rearing practices (e.g., overprotection, parental rejection, parental care), infections, traumatic brain injury or vitamin deficiency are likely to be risk factors for OCD according to Brandner et al. [57]. The authors also emphasized that at the time of publication none of the discussed factors could be conclusively declared a risk factor for OCD; nor could any of these factors be definitely excluded as a potential risk factor, since the study designs and methodological problems of the reported studies did not allow such conclusions.

Mental Disorders as Risk Factors for Obsessive-Compulsive Disorder

Comorbid mental disorders are among the most frequently investigated potential risk factors for OCD.

Affective disorders: The relevance of depression as a potential risk factor has been examined in a few epidemiological studies. In a prospective study of adolescents, individuals with higher depressive symptoms were at higher risk of developing OCD in the following year (OR 1.08) [55]. Similarly, major depression increased the risk of OCD by 140% in the ECA [51]. In line with these results, Douglass et al.

[40] found that individuals with OCD at age 18 years were significantly more depressed than a healthy group at age 11 years (OR 3.2) and 15 years (OR 10.38) but not at age 13 years (OR 2.93). Particularly high risk estimates were found for OCD and a prior history of bipolar disorder [51].

Anxiety disorders: In the EDSP study, Goodwin et al. [59] showed that individuals with panic attacks at baseline had an increased risk of first onset of OCD compared with individuals without panic attacks at baseline (OR 9.5). However, after adjusting for differences in all comorbid disorders at baseline, the association between panic attack at baseline and the risk of incident OCD failed to reach significance.

Another study of the EDSP sample examined the impact of specific phobia on the risk of incident OCD over the 10-year follow-up [60]. Specific phobia was found to elevate the risk of developing subsequent OCD by 279%. Individuals affected by two subtypes of specific phobia were at a remarkably higher risk of developing OCD compared with individuals affected by only one subtype. In line with these results are the associations between the risk of OCD and prior history of phobic disorders and panic disorder that have been demonstrated in the ECA [51].

Substance use disorders: The longitudinal comorbidity of OCD and substance use disorder was investigated in the longitudinal Northwestern–UCLA Youth Emotion Project [61]. At baseline, alcohol use disorders but not substance use disorders in general increased the risk of subsequent onset of OCD in the four-year follow-up. Notably, OCD was the only anxiety disorder that was predicted by prior substance use disorder.

This association was supported by results from the ECA, for which alcohol use disorders were found to increase the risk of OCD by 120% [51]. Furthermore they demonstrated an increased risk of OCD for the use of marijuana only (190%) and the use of cocaine and marijuana (620%). Substance abuse at age 15 years predicted OCD at age 18 years in the Dunedin cohort study [40].

Psychosis: The two longitudinal epidemiological studies that have investigated the relationship between prior psychosis and the risk of OCD suggested that schizophrenic disorders [51], schizotypal signs and schizophrenia nuclear symptoms [62] may predict OCD and therefore may constitute another important risk factor for OCD.

Cross-Diagnostic Approaches and Their Implications for Classification and Diagnosis

Given that this book takes a transdiagnostic approach to OCD and related disorders, one might ask how epidemiological findings can inform the classification and diagnosis of OCD. One of the major epidemiological issues that we have discussed is the often empirically shown comorbidity of OCD with other mental disorders. Using unselected representative samples, studies have shown that OCD co-occurs in the majority of cases with anxiety, affective, substance use and eating disorders. When considering a transdiagnostic approach, one might use these observations specifically in the discussion of the conceptualization of OCD in relation to other mental disorders.

To date, the classification of mental disorders has generally been challenged by the complexity of these disorders, including clinical diversity and overlap of symptoms, diverse theoretical approaches, and the assumed complexity of underlying neurobiological and psychological mechanisms. This classification challenge also applies to comorbidity findings since boundaries between disorders are a matter of continuing debate. The conceptualization of a disorder in relation to phenomenologically similar psychopathologies influences scientific and clinical approaches, such as strategies for the detection of etiologically relevant mechanisms, diagnostic assessment and clinical interventions.

In the DSM-IV, OCD was categorized as an anxiety disorder. Although the DSM-IV argument for this categorization was not comorbidity with anxiety disorders (rather, it was the causation of marked anxiety by obsessions and/or the neutralization of the anxiety through compulsions), this categorization fits well with what epidemiological studies have observed: OCD often goes hand in hand with other anxiety disorders. It is still not totally clear how this observed comorbidity can be explained: whether anxiety disorder increases the risk for subsequent OCD, whether prior OCD increases the risk for subsequent anxiety disorders, whether both temporal risk associations exist, whether there are common risk factors, or whether there are shared vulnerability factors, such as common neurobiological or psychological vulnerabilities.

The DSM-5, released in 2013, included a new chapter on so-called obsessive-compulsive and related disorders (OCRDs) [63]. According to the American Psychiatric Association (APA), the disorders grouped in this new chapter (i.e., hoarding disorder, OCD, body dysmorphic disorder, trichotillomania and excoriation disorder) "have features in common such as obsessive preoccupation and repetitive behaviors" [64]. This new chapter was included "to reflect the increasing evidence of these disorders' relatedness to one another and distinction from other anxiety disorders, as well as to help clinicians better identify and treat patients suffering from those disorders ... The disorders included in this new chapter have enough similarities to group them together in the same diagnostic classification but enough important differences between them to exist as distinct disorders" [64].

Since "relatedness to one another and distinction from other anxiety disorders" [64] was the rationale for the APA in taking OCD out of the anxiety disorders and to group it with other disorders, one might ask from an epidemiological perspective whether comorbidity findings from unselected community samples offer empirical support for this new grouping of the DSM-5. For the old inclusion of OCD in the DSM-IV anxiety disorders group, as we have seen above, there is a fairly impressive number of comorbidity findings based on methodologically sound epidemiological studies that argue for this "old" conceptualization. However, as far as we know, no population-based large-scale epidemiological study has examined the comorbidity between OCD and the disorders included in the new DSM-5 OCRD group. Therefore, even though the APA has taken epidemiologically observed comorbidity as a transdiagnostic argument for the grouping of disorders, there is currently no robust epidemiological evidence to support this OCRD grouping.

Clinical Implications of Cross-Diagnostic Approaches for Treatment and Prevention

Epidemiological data about comorbidity rates are important to consider when performing a comprehensive assessment of mental disorders, since knowing about common comorbidities diminishes the risk of missing important diagnoses. Additionally, knowledge of comorbidity rates from epidemiological studies can help reduce the delay of treatment for comorbid disorders, since they will not only be detected in time but can also be treated concurrently or in quick succession.

Regarding clinical implications, several epidemiological studies have suggested that OCD may predict the first onset of subsequent other mental disorders, such as schizophrenia [65,66], anorexia nervosa [67–69], anxiety disorders [70] and affective disorders [65,70–72]. From these findings, one might conclude that early efforts to treat OCD can potentially result in transdiagnostic prevention of different forms of subsequent psychopathology. However, to date we can only speculate on this transdiagnostic effect of early treatment of OCD, as empirical evidence is still completely lacking.

From another perspective and as briefly discussed above, epidemiological comorbidity findings suggest that OCD and its comorbid disorders might share *transdiagnostic risk factors* (i.e., factors that play a role across multiple disorders). Prevention approaches that target such factors might prove efficient for reducing the overall incidence of common mental health disorders [73]. Using the risk factor conceptualization of Kraemer et al. [54], specifically causal risk factors are relevant targets for prevention efforts [74]. Within this concept, causal risk factors are factors that can be changed and, when manipulated, can change the risk of the outcome under consideration [54]. Thus, for preventative interventions to be based on solid evidence, only causal risk factors should be used. Considering the dearth of evidence regarding causal risk factors for OCD, the lack of prevention interventions for OCD is not surprising.

Transdiagnostic Risk Factors

In the following, we give an overview of a few selected potential risk factors for OCD and the evidence thereof for OCD and other mental disorders to evaluate whether they might be transdiagnostic risk factors. On the basis of a systematic review of potential environmental risk factors for OCD [75], we have chosen to focus on adverse life events, parental rearing practices, social isolation and reproductive cycle events. As already described in our risk factor section, we have relied primarily on population-based studies with a longitudinal design in which the precedence of a risk factor over the onset of the outcome disorder was established.

Adverse life events. There is evidence that traumatic events increase vulnerability to various mental health disorders. In a 2016 study [76], traumatic events were shown to increase the risk for the new onset of OCD. Some prospective population-based studies have examined the predictive role of traumatic events for subsequent affective disorders. Traumatic events at baseline were associated with the incidence of major depressive [77,78] and manic [79] episodes. There is evidence that traumatic events and childhood adversities also predict the subsequent onset of anxiety disorders such as specific phobia [79], PTSD [79] or panic disorder [80]. Traumatic events have further been shown to increase the risk of cannabis abuse and/or dependence [81] and nicotine dependence [82]. On the basis of these epidemiological findings, traumatic events do not seem to be a specific risk factor for OCD but increase the risk for a broad range of mental disorders. Thus, traumatic events may identify those at risk for a broad range of mental disorders and early prevention interventions might be put in place prior to there being a diagnosable disorder.

Parental rearing practices. Self-reported retrospective data suggest that a perceived overprotective rearing style and paternal rejection may be associated with OCD [76]. However, whether these rearing styles are risk factors or rather consequences of OCD is not clear, since we could not identify a longitudinal, population-based study that took into account the temporal order of parental rearing and OCD. Turning to other mental disorders, inconsistent findings have emerged from population-based studies investigating parental rearing practices as a risk factor for the subsequent onset of psychopathology. In the Netherlands Mental Health Survey and Incidence Study-2, a prospective study of adults aged between 16 and 64 years at baseline who were assessed three times over 3 years, recollection of parental rearing during the first 16 years of life was assessed on two main dimensions: lack of care and overprotection [75]. Lack of care was found to be associated with more incident mental disorders than overprotection. Paternal lack of care predicted the subsequent onset of major depressive disorder, dysthymia, social phobia, drug abuse and alcohol dependence, whereas maternal lack of care predicted the subsequent onset of panic disorder, agoraphobia and alcohol abuse. With regard to overprotection, only maternal overprotection increased the risk of major depressive disorder, whereas paternal overprotection was not longitudinally associated with any mental disorder. Overall, perceived parental lack of care seemed to be nonspecifically associated with the incidence of DSM-III-R disorders [5].

In another longitudinal study of Dutch adolescents, perceived parental rejection and emotional warmth at age 11 years were examined as risk factors for the subsequent first onset of anxiety and depressive disorders [83]. Emotional warmth did not predict the onset of affective or anxiety disorders. Parental rejection was associated with the onset of depressive but not anxiety disorders.

We can draw only preliminary conclusions, as these studies examined different domains of parental rearing, and findings need replication. Furthermore, OCD was not examined in the two aforementioned studies. Results of the reported studies suggest that lack of care may increase the risk of a broad range of mental disorders. Maternal overprotection increased only the risk for major depressive disorder. Parental rejection was associated with the subsequent onset of depressive but not anxiety disorder. Future studies that include a broad range of mental disorders are needed to investigate if parental rejection and overprotection are indeed specific risk factors for affective disorders. Furthermore, we need prospective population-based studies to evaluate if certain parental rearing practices also increase the risk of OCD. Given the existing evidence, however, it is unlikely that parental rearing is a specific risk factor for OCD.

Social isolation. As mentioned above, compared with anxious and healthy controls, subjects who experienced social isolation in childhood had an increased risk of OCD, which might suggest that social isolation is a risk factor specific to OCD. However, there is some indication that social isolation is also related to other mental disorders. For example, one prospective population-based study found that older adults (50 years or over) who had in-person social contact only every few months or less had a higher risk of developing clinically significant depressive symptoms two years later than older adults who had in-person social contact at least once or twice per month [84]. A cross-sectional population-based study including a representative sample of 34,653 American community members found associations between current social isolation and an increased risk of major depressive disorder, dysthymic disorder, social phobia and GAD [85]. Yet no association was found between social isolation and drug or alcohol dependence or abuse, which might mean that obsessive-compulsive, affective and anxiety disorders share social isolation as a risk factor. It has to be noted that the temporal order was not controlled in this study and that social isolation could also be a consequence of the mental disorder, rather than a preceding risk factor. In sum, population-based prospective studies investigating social isolation as a risk factor for mental disorders are scarce, and firm conclusions about whether social isolation is a specific risk factor for OCD seem premature.

Pregnancy and the postpartum period. Women are at greater risk of developing OCD during pregnancy and the postpartum period than women from the general population [58]. Martini et al. [86] found OCD incident cases during the postpartum period but not during pregnancy, which they interpreted as reflecting either hormonal changes or changes in responsibility after childbirth. Major depressive disorder has also been found to increase during the postpartum period [86]. Regarding the prevalence of anxiety disorders during pregnancy and the postpartum period, a recent meta-analysis [87] concluded that there is a lack of large epidemiological studies including appropriate comparison groups, and so it is not possible to draw conclusions about whether anxiety disorders are more common in pregnant or postpartum women than in women in the general population. Thus, there appears to be insufficient evidence from population-based studies to answer the question of whether pregnancy and the postpartum period are also risk factors for anxiety disorders. Since OCD after delivery is associated with considerable impairment and impacts negatively on mother–child interactions [58], a prevention program to target obsessive-compulsive symptoms during this vulnerable time was developed. It successfully reduced obsessive-compulsive symptoms during the postpartum period compared with a control condition [88].

Future Directions

Based on the aforementioned research findings and conclusions, future directions should address the following topics:

1. The evaluation of risk factors for OCD, as well as their causal role in the etiopathogenesis of OCD, and additionally in the etiopathogenesis of the newly included DSM-5 OCRD chapter [63]. Risk factors should address the whole range of biological, psychological and social risk factors, their interplay and causal status in the development of OCRDs. Likewise, it would be important to study whether such factors are involved in the transition from symptomatic to subthreshold to threshold forms of OCRDs.
2. So far, no population-based large-scale epidemiological study has examined the comorbidity between OCD and the disorders included in DSM-5 OCRD group. Such efforts however would need the development and validation of diagnostic interviews designed to assess all disorders subsumed under the umbrella of OCRDs.
3. Prevention programs to target obsessive-compulsive symptoms in vulnerable populations should be developed. The ideal prevention would address empirically confirmed vulnerability or risk factors that put individuals to a higher probability of OCD compared with individuals without the respective factor. Besides prevention, the detection and intervention of early subclinical forms of OCD would be important. Such interventions may be helpful in preventing trajectories from symptomatic into chronic forms of full-blown OCD.
4. New approaches such as machine learning or network analyses may be helpful to identify transdiagnostic subtypes across OCD and comorbid disorders. Such subtypes may offer new ideas for intervention targets.

Conclusion

Despite the use of reliable diagnostic assessment instruments, available prevalence estimates of OCD vary substantially in epidemiological studies. This variation can best be explained by differences in assessment instruments, country studied and response rates. Nevertheless, we can conclude from epidemiological studies that a substantial proportion of individuals in the general population are or have over their lifetime been affected by OCD, and that obsessions and compulsions are common in the adult population. Subclinical obsessions and compulsions should therefore be taken into account in research and intervention efforts. Epidemiological studies have additionally shown that OCD typically is associated with remarkable impairments in daily life.

Epidemiological findings further suggest that the risk for first onset of OCD is highest between late childhood and early to middle adulthood. Our chapter has also shown that individuals with OCD have elevated odds of experiencing other mental disorders, for example, affective, other anxiety or substance use disorders. As discussed above, there is considerable uncertainty regarding risk factors for OCD since the available literature is limited by both number of studies and methodological issues. Future research efforts that investigate risk factors for OCD, as well as their causal role in the etiopathogenesis of OCD, are clearly needed. The information gained in such studies would be highly relevant to the development of preventive strategies.

References

1. Lieb R. Concepts and methods of epidemiology. In: Wright JD, ed. *International Encyclopedia of the Social and Behavioral Sciences*. Volume 7. 2nd ed. Amsterdam: Elsevier; 2015:824–831.
2. Bijl RV, de Graaf R, Hiripi E, et al. The prevalence of treated and untreated mental disorders in five countries. *Health Affairs*. 2003;22(3):122–133.
3. Karno M, Golding JM, Sorenson SB, Burnam MA. The epidemiology of obsessive-compulsive disorder in five US communities. *Arch Gen Psychiatry*. 1988;45(12):1094–1099.
4. American Psychiatric Association. *Diagnostic and Statistical Manual of Mental Disorders*, 3rd ed. Washington, DC: APA; 1980.
5. American Psychiatric Association. *Diagnostic and Statistical Manual of Mental Disorders*, 3rd ed., revised. Washington, DC: APA; 1987.
6. American Psychiatric Association. *Diagnostic and Statistical Manual of Mental Disorders*, 4th ed. Washington, DC: APA; 1994.
7. World Health Organization. *International Statistical Classification of Diseases and Related Health Problems, 10th Revision*. Geneva: WHO; 1990.
8. Fontenelle LF, Mendlowicz MV, Versiani M. The descriptive epidemiology of obsessive-compulsive disorder. *Prog Neuropsychopharmacol Biol Psychiatry*. 2006;30(3):327–337.
9. Somers JM, Goldner EM, Waraich P, Hsu L. Prevalence and incidence studies of anxiety disorders: a systematic review of the literature. *Can J Psychiatry*. 2006;51(2):100–113.
10. Caraveo-Anduaga JJ, Bermudez EC. The epidemiology of obsessive-compulsive disorder in Mexico City. *Salud Mental*. 2004;27(2):1–6.
11. de Bruijn C, Beun S, de Graaf R, ten Have M, Denys D. Subthreshold symptoms and obsessive-compulsive disorder: evaluating the diagnostic threshold. *Psychol Med*. 2010;40(6):989–997.
12. Ruscio AM, Stein DJ, Chiu WT, Kessler RC. The epidemiology of obsessive-compulsive disorder in the National Comorbidity Survey Replication. *Mol Psychiatry*. 2010;15(1):53–63.
13. Kessler RC, Berglund P, Demler O, Jin R, Merikangas KR, Walters EE. Lifetime prevalence and age-of-onset distributions of DSM-IV disorders in the National Comorbidity Survey Replication. *Arch Gen Psychiatry*. 2005;62(6):593–602.
14. Crino R, Slade T, Andrews G. The changing prevalence and severity of obsessive-compulsive disorder criteria from DSM-III to DSM-IV. *Am J Psychiatry*. 2005;162(5):876–882.
15. Jacobi F, Hofler M, Siegert J, et al. Twelve-month prevalence, comorbidity and correlates of mental disorders in Germany: the Mental Health Module of the German Health Interview and Examination Survey for Adults (DEGS1-MH). *Int J Methods Psychiatr Res*. 2014;23(3):304–319.
16. Adam Y, Meinlschmidt G, Gloster AT, Lieb R. Obsessive-compulsive disorder in the community: 12-month prevalence, comorbidity and impairment. *Soc Psychiatry Psychiatr Epidemiol*. 2012;47(3):339–349.
17. Kessler RC, Chiu WT, Demler O, Merikangas KR, Walters EE. Prevalence, severity, and comorbidity of 12-month DSM-IV disorders in the National Comorbidity Survey Replication. *Arch Gen Psychiatry*. 2005;62(6):617–627.
18. Wittchen HU, Jacobi F, Rehm J, et al. The size and burden of mental disorders and other disorders of the brain in Europe 2010. *Eur Neuropsychopharmacol*. 2011;21(9):655–679.
19. Fullana MA, Vilagut G, Rojas-Farreras S, et al. Obsessive-compulsive symptom dimensions in the general population: results from an epidemiological study in six European countries. *J Affect Disord*. 2010;124(3):291–299.
20. Angst J, Gamma A, Endrass J, et al. Obsessive-compulsive severity spectrum in the community: prevalence, comorbidity, and course. *Eur Arch Psychiatry Clin Neurosci*. 2004;254(3):156–164.
21. Grabe HJ, Meyer C, Hapke U, et al. Prevalence, quality of life and psychosocial function in obsessive-compulsive disorder and subclinical obsessive-compulsive disorder in northern Germany. *Eur Arch Psychiatry Clin Neurosci*. 2000;250(5):262–268.
22. Stein MB, Forde DR, Anderson G, Walker JR. Obsessive-compulsive disorder in the community: an epidemiologic survey with clinical reappraisal. *Am J Psychiatry*. 1997;154(8):1120–1126.

23. Valleni-Basile LA, Garrison CZ, Jackson KL, et al. Frequency of obsessive-compulsive disorder in a community sample of young adolescents. *J Am Acad Child Adolesc Psychiatry.* 1994;33(6):782–791.
24. Weissman MM, Bland RC, Canino GJ, et al. The cross national epidemiology of obsessive compulsive disorder. The Cross National Collaborative Group. *J Clin Psychiatry.* 1994;55(Suppl):5–10.
25. Cilli AS, Telcioglu M, Askin R, Kaya N, Bodur S, Kucur R. Twelve-month prevalence of obsessive-compulsive disorder in Konya, Turkey. *Compr Psychiatry.* 2004;45(5):367–374.
26. Karno M, Golding JM, Sorenson SB, Burnam MA. The epidemiology of obsessive-compulsive disorder in 5 United-States communities. *Arch Gen Psychiatr.* 1988;45(12):1094–1099.
27. Kessler RC, Amminger GP, Aguilar-Gaxiola S, Alonso J, Lee S, Ustun TB. Age of onset of mental disorders: a review of recent literature. *Curr Opin Psychiatr.* 2007;20(4):359–364.
28. Mohammadi MR, Ghanizadeh A, Rahgozar M, et al. Prevalence of obsessive-compulsive disorder in Iran. *BMC Psychiatry.* 2004;4:2.
29. Burke KC, Burke JD, Regier DA, Rae DS. Age at onset of selected mental-disorders in 5 community populations. *Arch Gen Psychiatr.* 1990;47(6):511–518.
30. Fineberg NA, Hengartner MP, Bergbaum CE, et al. A prospective population-based cohort study of the prevalence, incidence and impact of obsessive-compulsive symptomatology. *Int J Psychiatry Clin Pract.* 2013;17(3):170–178.
31. Torres AR, Prince MJ, Bebbington PE, et al. Obsessive-compulsive disorder: prevalence, comorbidity, impact, and help-seeking in the British National Psychiatric Morbidity Survey of 2000. *Am J Psychiatry.* 2006;163(11):1978–1985.
32. Subramaniam M, Abdin E, Vaingankar JA, Chong SA. Obsessive–compulsive disorder: prevalence, correlates, help-seeking and quality of life in a multiracial Asian population. *Soc Psychiatry Psychiatr Epidemiol.* 2012;47(12):2035–2043.
33. Nestadt G, Samuels JF, Romanoski AJ, Folstein MF, McHugh PR. Obsessions and compulsions in the community. *Acta Psychiatr Scand.* 1994;89(4):219–224.
34. Jacobi F, Wittchen HU, Holting C, et al. Prevalence, co-morbidity and correlates of mental disorders in the general population: results from the German Health Interview and Examination Survey (GHS). *Psychol Med.* 2004;34(4):597–611.
35. Torres AR, Prince MJ, Bebbington PE, et al. Treatment seeking by individuals with obsessive-compulsive disorder from the British psychiatric morbidity survey of 2000. *Psychiatr Serv.* 2007;58(7):977–982.
36. Mayerovitch JI, du Fort GG, Kakuma R, Bland RC, Newman SC, Pinard G. Treatment seeking for obsessive-compulsive disorder: role of obsessive-compulsive disorder symptoms and comorbid psychiatric diagnoses. *Compr Psychiatry.* 2003;44(2):162–168.
37. Cullen B, Samuels JF, Pinto A, et al. Demographic and clinical characteristics associated with treatment status in family members with obsessive-compulsive disorder. *Depress Anxiety.* 2008;25(3):218–224.
38. Pinto A, Mancebo MC, Eisen JL, Pagano ME, Rasmussen SA. The Brown Longitudinal Obsessive Compulsive Study: clinical features and symptoms of the sample at intake. *J Clin Psychiatry.* 2006;67(5):703–711.
39. Wang PS, Berglund P, Olfson M, Pincus HA, Wells KB, Kessler RC. Failure and delay in initial treatment contact after first onset of mental disorders in the National Comorbidity Survey Replication. *Arch Gen Psychiatry.* 2005;62(6):603–613.
40. Douglass HM, Moffitt TE, Dar R, McGee R, Silva P. Obsessive-compulsive disorder in a birth cohort of 18-year-olds: prevalence and predictors. *J Am Acad Child Adolesc Psychiatry.* 1995;34(11):1424–1431.
41. Weissman MM, Bland RC, Canino GJ, et al. Cross-national epidemiology of obsessive-compulsive disorder. *CNS Spectrums.* 1998;3:6–9.
42. Fineberg NA, Hengartner MP, Bergbaum C, Gale T, Rossler W, Angst J. Lifetime comorbidity of obsessive-compulsive disorder and sub-threshold obsessive-compulsive symptomatology in the community: impact, prevalence, socio-demographic and clinical characteristics. *Int J Psychiatry Clin Pract.* 2013;17(3):188–196.
43. Nestadt G, Bienvenu OJ, Cai G, Samuels J, Eaton WW. Incidence of obsessive-compulsive disorder in adults. *J Nerv Ment Dis.* 1998;186(7):401–406.
44. Chen YW, Dilsaver SC. Comorbidity for obsessive-compulsive disorder in bipolar and unipolar disorders. *Psychiatry Res.* 1995;59(1–2):57–64.
45. de Graaf R, Bijl RV, Spijker J, Beekman AT, Vollebergh WA. Temporal sequencing of lifetime mood disorders in relation to comorbid anxiety and substance use disorders – findings from the Netherlands Mental Health Survey and Incidence Study. *Soc Psychiatry Psychiatr Epidemiol.* 2003;38(1):1–11.
46. Isensee B, Wittchen HU, Stein MB, Hofler M, Lieb R. Smoking increases the risk of panic: findings from a prospective community study. *Arch Gen Psychiatry.* 2003;60(7):692–700.
47. Rapoport JL, Inoff-Germain G, Weissman MM, et al. Childhood obsessive-compulsive disorder in the NIMH MECA study: parent versus child identification

of cases. Methods for the Epidemiology of Child and Adolescent Mental Disorders. *J Anxiety Disord.* 2000;14(6):535–548.

48. Hudson JI, Hiripi E, Pope HG Jr., Kessler RC. The prevalence and correlates of eating disorders in the National Comorbidity Survey Replication. *Biol Psychiatry.* 2007;61(3):348–358.
49. Cuzen NL, Stein DJ, Lochner C, Fineberg NA. Unconscious habit systems in compulsive and impulsive disorders. *Behav Brain Sci.* 2014;37(2):141.
50. Torres AR, Moran P, Bebbington P, et al. Obsessive-compulsive disorder and personality disorder: evidence from the British National Survey of Psychiatric Morbidity 2000. *Soc Psychiatry Psychiatr Epidemiol.* 2006;41(11):862–867.
51. Crum RM, Anthony JC. Cocaine use and other suspected risk factors for obsessive-compulsive disorder: a prospective study with data from the Epidemiologic Catchment Area surveys. *Drug Alcohol Depend.* 1993;31:281–295.
52. Peterson BS, Pine DS, Cohen P, Brook JS. Prospective, longitudinal study of tic, obsessive-compulsive, and attention-deficit/hyperactivity disorders in an epidemiological sample. *J Am Acad Child Adolesc Psychiatry.* 2001;40(6):685–695.
53. Grabe HJ, Meyer C, Hapke U, et al. Lifetime-comorbidity of obsessive-compulsive disorder and subclinical obsessive-compulsive disorder in Northern Germany. *Eur Arch Psychiatry Clin Neurosci.* 2001;251(3):130–135.
54. Kraemer HC, Kazdin AE, Offord DR, Kessler RC, Jensen PS, Kupfer DJ. Coming to terms with the terms of risk. *Arch Gen Psychiatry.* 1997;54(4):337–343.
55. Valleni-Basile LA, Garrison CZ, Waller JL, et al. Incidence of obsessive-compulsive disorder in a community sample of young adolescents. *J Am Acad Child Adolesc Psychiatry.* 1996;35(7):898–906.
56. Grisham JR, Fullana MA, Mataix-Cols D, Moffitt TE, Caspi A, Poulton R. Risk factors prospectively associated with adult obsessive-compulsive symptom dimensions and obsessive-compulsive disorder. *Psychol Med.* 2011;41(12):2495–2506.
57. Brandner G, Perez-Vigil A, Larsson H, Mataix-Cols D. Systematic review of environmental risk factors for obsessive-compulsive disorder: a proposed roadmap from association to causation. *Neurosci Biobehav Rev.* 2016;65:36–62.
58. Russell EJ, Fawcett JM, Mazmanian D. Risk of obsessive-compulsive disorder in pregnant and postpartum women: a meta-analysis. *J Clin Psychiatry.* 2013;74(4):377–385.
59. Goodwin RD, Lieb R, Hoefler M, et al. Panic attack as a risk factor for severe psychopathology. *Am J Psychiatry.* 2004;161:2207–2214.
60. Lieb R, Miche M, Gloster AT, Beesdo-Baum K, Meyer AH, Wittchen HU. Impact of specific phobia on the risk of onset of mental disorders: a 10-year prospective-longitudinal community study of adolescents and young adults. *Depress Anxiety.* 2016;33(7):667–675.
61. Wolitzky-Taylor K, Bobova L, Zinbarg RE, Mineka S, Craske MG. Longitudinal investigation of the impact of anxiety and mood disorders in adolescence on subsequent substance use disorder onset and vice versa. *Addict Behav.* 2012;37(8):982–985.
62. Rossler W, Hengartner MP, Ajdacic-Gross V, Haker H, Gamma A, Angst J. Sub-clinical psychosis symptoms in young adults are risk factors for subsequent common mental disorders. *Schizophr Res.* 2011;131(1–3):18–23.
63. American Psychiatric Association. *Diagnostic and Statistical Manual of Mental Disorders.* 5th ed. Washington, DC: APA; 2013.
64. American Psychiatric Association. *Obsessive Compulsive and Related Disorders.* DSM-5 Factsheet. Washington, DC: APA; 2013. Available from: www.psychiatry.org/psychiatrists/practice/dsm/educational-resources/dsm-5-fact-sheets (accessed July 8, 2018).
65. Cederlof M, Lichtenstein P, Larsson H, et al. Obsessive-compulsive disorder, psychosis, and bipolarity: a longitudinal cohort and multigenerational family study. *Schizophr Bull.* 2015;41(5):1076–1083.
66. Meier SM, Petersen L, Pedersen MG, et al. Obsessive-compulsive disorder as a risk factor for schizophrenia: a nationwide study. *JAMA Psychiatry.* 2014;71(11):1215–1221.
67. Buckner JD, Silgado J, Lewinsohn PM. Delineation of differential temporal relations between specific eating and anxiety disorders. *J Psychiatr Res.* 2010;44(12):781–787.
68. Cederlof M, Thornton LM, Baker J, et al. Etiological overlap between obsessive-compulsive disorder and anorexia nervosa: a longitudinal cohort, multigenerational family and twin study. *World Psychiatry.* 2015;14(3):333–338.
69. Meier SM, Bulik CM, Thornton LM, Mattheisen M, Mortensen PB, Petersen L. Diagnosed anxiety disorders and the risk of subsequent anorexia nervosa: a Danish population register study. *Eur Eat Disord Rev.* 2015;23(6):524–530.
70. Kessler RC, Ormel J, Petukhova M, et al. Development of lifetime comorbidity in the World Health

Organization world mental health surveys. *Arch Gen Psychiatry.* 2011;68(1):90–100.

71. Goodwin RD. Anxiety disorders and the onset of depression among adults in the community. *Psychol Med.* 2002;32(6):1121–1124.

72. Meier SM, Petersen L, Mattheisen M, Mors O, Mortensen PB, Laursen TM. Secondary depression in severe anxiety disorders: a population-based cohort study in Denmark. *Lancet Psychiatry.* 2015;2(6):515–523.

73. Brown TA, Barlow DH. A proposal for a dimensional classification system based on the shared features of the DSM-IV anxiety and mood disorders: implications for assessment and treatment. *Psychol Assess.* 2009;21(3):256–271.

74. Offord DR, Kraemer HC. Risk factors and prevention. *Evid Based Ment Health.* 2000;3(3):70–71.

75. Overbeek G, ten Have M, Vollebergh W, de Graaf R. Parental lack of care and overprotection. Longitudinal associations with DSM-III-R disorders. *Soc Psychiatry Psychiatr Epidemiol.* 2007;42(2):87–93.

76. Brander G, Perez-Vigil A, Larsson H, Mataix-Cols D. Systematic review of environmental risk factors for obsessive-compulsive disorder: a proposed roadmap from association to causation. *Neurosci Biobehav Rev.* 2016;65:36–62.

77. Zimmermann P, Bruckl T, Lieb R, et al. The interplay of familial depression liability and adverse events in predicting the first onset of depression during a 10-year follow-up. *Biol Psychiatry.* 2008;63(4):406–414.

78. Zimmermann P, Bruckl T, Nocon A, et al. Interaction of FKBP5 gene variants and adverse life events in predicting depression onset: results from a 10-year prospective community study. *Am J Psychiatry.* 2011;168(10):1107–1116.

79. Asselmann E, Wittchen HU, Lieb R, Perkonigg A, Beesdo-Baum K. Incident mental disorders in the aftermath of traumatic events: a prospective-longitudinal community study. *J Affect Disord.* 2017;227:82–89.

80. Goodwin RD, Fergusson DM, Horwood LJ. Childhood abuse and familial violence and the risk of panic attacks and panic disorder in young adulthood. *Psychol Med.* 2005;35(6):881–890.

81. von Sydow K, Lieb R, Pfister H, Hofler M, Wittchen HU. What predicts incident use of cannabis and progression to abuse and dependence? A 4-year prospective examination of risk factors in a community sample of adolescents and young adults. *Drug Alcohol Depend.* 2002;68(1):49–64.

82. Breslau N, Davis GC, Schultz LR. Posttraumatic stress disorder and the incidence of nicotine, alcohol, and other drug disorders in persons who have experienced trauma. *Arch Gen Psychiatry.* 2003;60(3):289–294.

83. Oldehinkel AJ, Hartman CA, Van Oort FV, Nederhof E. Emotion recognition specialization and context-dependent risk of anxiety and depression in adolescents. *Brain Behav.* 2015;5(2):e00299.

84. Teo AR, Choi H, Andrea SB, et al. Does mode of contact with different types of social relationships predict depression in older adults? Evidence from a nationally representative survey. *J Am Geriatr Soc.* 2015;63(10):2014–2022.

85. Chou KL, Liang K, Sareen J. The association between social isolation and DSM-IV mood, anxiety, and substance use disorders: wave 2 of the National Epidemiologic Survey on Alcohol and Related Conditions. *J Clin Psychiatry.* 2011;72(11):1468–1476.

86. Martini J, Petzoldt J, Einsle F, Beesdo-Baum K, Hofler M, Wittchen HU. Risk factors and course patterns of anxiety and depressive disorders during pregnancy and after delivery: a prospective-longitudinal study. *J Affect Disord.* 2015;175:385–395.

87. Goodman JH, Watson GR, Stubbs B. Anxiety disorders in postpartum women: a systematic review and meta-analysis. *J Affect Disord.* 2016;203:292–331.

88. Timpano KR, Abramowitz JS, Mahaffey BL, Mitchell MA, Schmidt NB. Efficacy of a prevention program for postpartum obsessive-compulsive symptoms. *J Psychiatr Res.* 2011;45(11):1511–1517.

Chapter 11

Symptoms, Diagnosis and Specifiers of Obsessive-Compulsive Disorder

Leonardo F. Fontenelle

Introduction

In the latest edition of *Goodwin and Guze's Psychiatric Diagnosis* [1], it is argued that, in the absence of a diagnosis, "medicine largely becomes a tower of Babel where no one understands what is going on". Indeed, the whole conceptual basis of medical and other clinical professions lies in the diagnostic process. The process allows clinicians to communicate with one another, it determines (predicts) outcomes (as the old aphorism says, "diagnosis is prognosis"), and is the ultimate target of our therapeutic efforts. However, in no other clinical areas has diagnosis been so much attacked as in psychiatry and clinical psychology. Yet, the fact that psychiatrists and psychologists keep diagnosing and treating obsessive-compulsive disorder (OCD) patients since the time of Jean-Étienne Dominique Esquirol is a tacit indication that this approach is still the most effective way of dealing with impairing levels of obsessions and/or compulsions. In this chapter, we provide an overview of diagnosis and classification of OCD.

The acts of diagnosing and classifying any mental disorder, including OCD, are not synonyms. Diagnosing is a cognitive procedure performed by a clinician or a researcher [2]. In contrast, classifying is a scientific heuristic procedure; that is, a method not guaranteed to be perfect, but sufficient for our immediate goals [2]. While the specific diagnostic criteria for a given mental disorder should be considered a proxy for ideal prototypes (as described below), its classification corresponds to a specific place in a nosological system; for example, in DSM-5 [3], body dysmorphic disorder is an obsessive-compulsive related disorder (OCRD). The clinician who is merely including a patient's case in a "nosographic table" is not diagnosing nor classifying, but just performing a bureaucratic-administrative procedure [4]. In fact, the error of comparing the act of diagnosing a psychiatric disorder to simple labeling has been stimulated by the bad habit of using diagnostic criteria to pigeonhole people, leaving aside the patient as a person [4].

Open Interviews

A diagnosis is a recognition of a totality under conditions of limited or incomplete information [4]. In daily clinical practice, it is usually based on what Schwartz and Wiggs termed typification [5]; that is, "a basic human cognitive feature" which clinicians automatically employ to structure and organize their own experiences during examination as "salient units or certain Gestalts" [6]. Typification is a skill developed through exposure to prototypes (or, according to Jaspers, "ideal types") [7], and categories that resemble, but do not belong to, them [6]. In psychiatry, as in other areas of medicine, the ability to typify a case is usually acquired during clinical training. Typification is thought to explain controversial historical concepts, such as the so-called *praecox feeling* described by Rümke as diagnostic of schizophrenia [5]. However, besides orienting and guiding the first steps in psychiatric diagnosis, typification is most useful when being constantly revised and called into question [6].

Robins and Guze [8] have proposed a list of validators (e.g., family history) [1] deemed relevant for the characterization of mental disorders. In open interviews performed in clinical settings, this sort of information is constantly compared and reviewed against our prototypical or ideal types. For instance, if an astute clinician meets a fearful patient and describing a family history of Tourette's disorder, he or she may automatically consider OCD. Alternatively, a depressed patient reporting the sudden onset of "negative repetitive thoughts" after a loss of a loved one may actually have an acute grief reaction. Given the widespread availability of diagnostic criteria, such as the *Diagnostic and Statistical*

Manual of Mental Disorders, fifth edition (DSM-5) [3], sometimes clinicians also see patients arguing to suffer from a specific mental disorder that proves to be different from the one first claimed, including OCD [9]. However, as open interviews are associated with low reliabilities, they are not considered to be scientifically rigorous.

Structured Interviews

Broadly speaking, structured interviews almost integrally reproduce criteria listed in well-known classification systems, such as DSM and the International Classification of Diseases (ICD), which have already been described in simple language by their developers. The rationale for this approach, which does not leave much space for clinical judgment, is to increase interrater and test–retest reliabilities. These interviews are particularly important in situations where well-trained clinicians are not available (e.g., epidemiological studies), although they may also be desirable in clinical studies as a way to assure that diagnosis follows current diagnostic criteria. However, structured interviews are generally time consuming and cumbersome; they may affect rapport with the patient negatively, and they often require extensive training [10]. In the context of OCD, structured interviews may be particularly difficult, as patients may provide an excessive amount of information or overly precise details for each question [11], although this problem may affect open interviews as well.

Although the problems related to the use of structured interviews in OCD samples may be minimized by discussions that inform that both patients and clinicians will need to keep focus during the interview [11], these interviews also decrease diagnostic validity by ignoring accessory diagnostic elements, such as the slowness, rigidity and prolixity of OCD [12]. Consider the way OCD symptoms, particularly obsessions, are assessed in a fully structured diagnostic instrument such as the Mini International Neuropsychiatric Interview; that is, "In the past month, have you been bothered by recurrent thoughts, impulses, or images that were unwanted, distasteful, inappropriate, intrusive, or distressing?" [13]. Clearly, patients may respond positively to these questions despite having other phenomena (such as depressive ruminations, schizophrenic delusions, post-traumatic stress disorder flashbacks and so on), which may only be disclosed after further open assessments. In structured interviews, the process of typification is eliminated or severely constrained at the outset.

In medicine, clinical phenomena can be conceptualized along three progressively increasing degrees of complexity: symptoms, syndromes and clinical (or nosological) entities. A symptom is the most elemental sign by which an underlying pathological process is evident (e.g., an obsession). A syndrome is a group of more or less coherent symptoms as they are usually correlated with one another (e.g., obsessions and compulsions). Finally, a nosological entity is a condition that describes the most important essential characteristics of the pathological process (e.g., OCD). In the case of psychiatric disorders, it includes specific courses and/or lack of clearly recognizable etiological factors. The diagnosis of OCD starts at the identification of obsessions and/or compulsions as symptoms and ends at the establishment of its specifiers. In this chapter, the evolution of obsessions, compulsions and OCD characterization through different diagnostic systems is described.

Obsessions

Although early German writers, such as Westphal, considered obsessions to be disorders of the course of thinking [14], most current definitions conceptualize it as a complex symptom involving several facets that cannot be captured within the limits of a single mental function. In fact, obsessions are thought to involve thought, imagery and volitional aspects. This pleomorphic nature has been officially recognized since the DSM-III, which defined obsessions as "recurrent, persistent ideas, thoughts, images, or impulses" [15]. It also remained essentially the same throughout most of the post-DSM-III [15–17] and ICD-10 history [18]. However, recent concerns about a potential confusion between impulses that have been experienced but not acted upon (an OCD symptom) and impulses that have been actually enacted (key to impulse control disorders) have led developers of the most recent DSM-5 to substitute the term "impulses" for a better expression [3].

Accordingly, it was felt that the term "urges" had a few advantages over "impulses", including a better coverage of the so-called "sensory" or "just-right phenomena" (e.g., uncomfortable sensations localized in a specific region of the body, desires for things to feel, look or sound just right, feelings of incompleteness, inner tensions or energies that build up and need to be released by certain behaviors) [19] and the fact that "urges" is seen as a more long-lasting and persistent phenomenon as compared with impulses (which are usually considered more paradoxical and short-lived). A similar path is likely to be followed by ICD-11, which will probably keep both terms (impulses/urges) [20], as they can have different meanings and be differentially emphasized in individuals from different cultures [21–23]. However, the term "urge" is not free from criticism, as it can also imply a gratifying aspect of obsessions that most would consider inadequate [20].

The DSM-5 has required these symptoms to be experienced, "at some time during the disturbance, as intrusive and unwanted" [3]. This prerequisite represents a change from the argument that obsessions need to be "senseless and repugnant" in DSM-III [15], "intrusive and senseless" in DSM-III-R [16] and "intrusive and inappropriate" in DSM-IV [24] and DSM-IV-TR [17]. In fact, all these terms represented attempts to operationalize the traditional concepts of ego-dystonicity [20]. Although the intruding quality of obsessions has been perceived as still valid and worth being kept in DSM-5 [3], it was considered that the term "inappropriate" was value laden and subject to different interpretations contingent on cultures, genders and ages [20]. Thus, "inappropriate" was substituted by "unwanted", which was resurrected from earlier DSM versions [25,26] and is also likely to be adopted by ICD-11 [21,22].[1] Also, the perception that ego-dystonicity can fluctuate along the course of the illness, a phenomenon that was recognized since the DSM-III-R [16] remained in DSM-5 [3]. However, no minimum duration of ego-dystonicity was mentioned in the later system [27].

The relationship between obsessions and anxiety/distress has changed over the course of DSM history. For instance, in DSM-I, anxiety had an apparent etiological role in OCD [25]. In DSM-II, anxiety and distress were said to be "often present" but only if patients were prevented from ritualizing or if they were concerned about being unable to control themselves [26]. Conversely, obsessions were argued to be a "source" [26] or "cause" [16] of distress in DSM-III and DSM-III-R, but anxiety was largely ignored as one of its key components.[2] In DSM-IV, "anxiety or distress" reappeared together as necessary outcomes of obsessions [17,28]. ICD-10 argued that obsessions were almost invariably distressing because of their repugnant content or senselessness [18]. More recently, though, DSM-5 admitted that obsessions cause "anxiety or distress" in "most" (but not all) individuals [3]. Instead, the DSM-5 text mentions that a range of affective responses can be noted when individuals are confronted with situations that trigger obsessions (and compulsions), including panic attacks, disgust and incompleteness [3]. It is likely that this view will be endorsed by ICD-11, as the current draft describes obsessions as "commonly associated" with anxiety [22].

According to early psychopathologists, "the feeling that one must resist" an obsession is an essential feature, which may or may not be followed by "the innumerable devices, rituals and repetitions of the obsessional" [28]. This feature was officially incorporated into DSM-III [15] and ICD-10 [18],[3] and remained as such ever since. It was kept in DSM-5 as the attempt to ignore, suppress or neutralize the obsession with some other thought or action (i.e., by performing a compulsion) and is likely to be present in ICD-11 as well [22]. Though not completely clear in these systems, it has been suggested that performing a compulsion is just one of different forms developed to "fight against" obsessions. For instance, researchers have found a variety of neutralizing strategies that are not "stereotyped" (DSM-III-R wording) nor "rigidly applied" (DSM-IV/DSM-5 wording), but have identical functional properties to compulsions, such as saying "stop" to oneself and self-questioning [30]. If one performs a semantic exercise and considers these behaviors to be compulsive based on their functional similarities with DSM compulsions, there might be

[1] The "unwanted" nature of obsessions was already stressed in ICD-10, which described them as "involuntary and repugnant".

[2] Although anxiety was not included as a key element of obsessions in the DSM-III, OCD was considered to be anxiety disorder from DSM-III until DSM-IV-TR.

[3] In ICD-10, among all OCD symptoms, there must be at least one thought or act that is still resisted without success, even though resistance to other symptoms may have disappeared (as in delusions) [17]. In other words, at least one obsession or compulsion must be present that is acknowledged as excessive or unreasonable [29]. Diagnostic criteria mention that, if very long standing, resistance to some obsessions or compulsions may be minimal [29].

greater support for the non-existence of individuals with pure obsessions.

Lastly, given the similarities between obsessions and cognitions core to the diagnosis of other mental disorders (see Chapter 1), recent DSM editions have been concerned with symptom delimitation. They have consistently attempted to disentangle obsessions from other phenomena. Firstly, only thought insertion, "obsessions of schizophrenia", and symptoms of comorbid axis I disorder such as eating disorders, substance use disorder or major depression were excluded [16]. Subsequently schizophrenia's thought insertion and generalized anxiety disorder (GAD) excessive worries about real-life problems [17,24] were added to the exclusion criteria. The ICD-10 also argued that the thoughts were not pleasurable (as in fantasies) and that individuals suffering from recurrent depressive disorder could develop "obsessional thoughts" during their episodes of depression [18]. The DSM-V Anxiety, OC Spectrum, Post-traumatic and Dissociative Disorders Work Group did not find a clear advantage to including information on differential diagnosis under the definition of obsessions [20]. Thus, DSM-5 changed its approach and, instead of trying to differentiate obsessions *per se* from other symptoms, required the "disturbance" (OCD) not to be "explained by" (or "understood as",[4] if one uses Jaspers' terms [7]) the symptoms of another disorder, including a list of 14 different diagnostic examples [3].

Compulsions

Unlike obsessions, which have been the focus of specific interest by philosophers and alienists since the nineteenth century, compulsions have received less attention and have been seen more as the visible byproduct of obsessions. In fact, although there are many descriptions of compulsive behaviors by many classical authors (e.g., Steinberg et al. [31]), it has been difficult to find early proper definitions of the phenomena, which have also been described as "obsessional acts" [32]. Before DSM-III, attempts to describe compulsive behaviors were understandably broad. For instance, DSM-I referred to "compulsion to repetitive actions" that "often" accompanied "recurring thoughts", without too much further explanation [25]. Later, the DSM-II added that anxiety and distress could be present if patients were prevented from completing their rituals [26]. Greater psychopathological rigor was seen in DSM-III [15], which provided a paragraph-long description of compulsions. However, it was only after DSM-III-R operationalization of four essential features previously listed on DSM-III that the modern view of compulsive behaviors actually emerged [15].

The DSM-III defined compulsions as "repetitive and seemingly purposeful behaviors that are performed according to certain rules or in a stereotyped fashion" [15]. The fact that compulsions not just looked purposeful, but were actually intentional and had a true goal (e.g., to prevent discomfort or some dreaded event or situation) was later recognized in DSM-III-R, along with the fact that it could also occur in response to an obsession [16]. Perhaps under the influence of the later manuals, the ICD-10 defined compulsive acts or rituals as stereotyped behaviors that are repeated again and again [18]. Later, DSM-IV expanded the concept of compulsions to include not only overt repetitive behaviors (e.g., hand washing, ordering, checking) but also covert mental acts (e.g., praying, counting, repeating words silently) that the person felt driven to perform in response to an obsession, or according to rules that must be applied rigidly [17,24]. Fortunately, DSM-5 has kept the later, and broader, definition of compulsions [3].

Although the term "stereotyped" was not included in DSM-IV criteria, it was kept in the accompanying text [17,24]. In contrast, in DSM-5, the stereotypical nature of OCD compulsions has been completely removed [3]. This is a welcome change, as stereotypical behaviors have been listed as symptoms of many different disorders that could be easily confused with OCD, including stereotypic movement disorders, autism spectrum disorders, stimulant intoxication and the behavioral variant of frontotemporal neurocognitive disorder, among others [3]. It is likely that the ICD-11 definition of compulsions will avoid references to stereotypies as well, while maintaining that it can occur as a response to an obsession, according to rigid rules, or to achieve a sense of "completeness" [22]. The later addition has been based on the need to cover compulsions that are not just fear related, but often performed to alleviate the so-called "sensory phenomena" [19], including a feeling of incompleteness [33].

[4] According to Jaspers, author of the hallmark book on descriptive psychopathology, it is through "understanding" that the examiner grasps how a mental phenomenon arises from another mental phenomenon in a meaningful way [7].

In DSM-III, a compulsion was "not an end in itself", but a behavior with a distal implication; that is, the production or the prevention of some future event or situation [15]. In contrast, DSM-III-R and the subsequent editions had slightly different wordings. First, they eliminated the statement requiring the compulsion not to be "an end in itself", as this sentence excluded many OCD behaviors that had short-term objectives, such as the alleviation of discomfort resulting from symmetry and arranging symptoms. Second, instead of including behaviors that could produce some event (e.g., superstitions), post-DSM-III editions attempted to include only compulsions that actually avoided unwanted scenarios. For instance, compulsions neutralized or prevented "discomfort" (i.e., in DSM-III-R [16]), prevented or reduced "distress" (i.e., in DSM-IV [17,24]), prevented or reduced "anxiety or distress" (i.e., in DSM-5 [23]), or prevented some dreaded event or situation (in DSM-III-R [16], DSM-IV [17,24] and the DSM-5 [3]).

Since the DSM-III [1,15,16,17,24], the criteria stating that compulsive behaviors or mental acts "are not connected in a realistic way with what they are designed to neutralize or prevent, or are clearly excessive" has remained mostly unchanged. The only exception to this tenet has been the addition, in DSM-5, of examples that are now provided in the text illustrating symptoms that are qualitatively disconnected from the feared event (e.g., "arranging items symmetrically to prevent harm to a loved one")[5] or are simply excessive (e.g., "showering for hours each day" [3]). Different diagnostic manuals have underlined the fact that the individual with OCD generally recognizes the "senselessness" (DSM-III) [15], excessiveness or unreasonableness (DSM-III-R and DSM-IV) [15,17,24] or ineffectuality (ICD-10) [17] of the compulsive behaviors, although they have also acknowledged that this may not be true for people whose obsessions have evolved into overvalued ideas [16], or for young children [15,17,24]. In DSM-5, children's potential inability to recognize the unsuitability of their behaviors has been substituted by inability to "articulate the aims of these behaviors or mental acts" [3].

There has been a requirement, both as part of the compulsions criteria [15] and as a comment in the text [16], that the person showing the OCD compulsion "desires to resist the compulsion". In DSM-IV, the attempts to resist compulsions (or obsessions) were linked to the recognition of these phenomena as excessive or unreasonable, a prerequisite that had to be present "at some point during the course of the disorder" (criterion B) [17,24]. A similar remark has been made in the ICD-10 diagnostic guidelines [18]. Until recently, different DSM editions have noted that, after repeated failures to resist the compulsions (or the obsessions) [15,17,24] the individual could give up, no longer experience a desire to resist these symptoms, and incorporate the compulsions into his or her daily routines. According to the ICD-10, this resistance could be minimal in very long standing cases [18]. Since insight (or the recognition of the "senselessness", "excessiveness", "unreasonableness" or "ineffectuality" of symptoms) is not a requirement for OCD diagnosis, DSM-5 is silent when it comes to the patient's attempt to resist compulsions [3].

Though only included as a criterion for compulsions in the DSM-III [15], the text of remaining DSM editions [1,16,17,24], as well as the ICD-10 [17], has always been concerned with not allowing the diagnosis of OCD compulsions if the behaviors were performed for pleasure or gratification. However, these diagnostic systems have continuously recognized that compulsive behaviors could lead to relief from "mounting tension" [15,16], "mounting anxiety or tension" [17,24] or "anxiety or distress" [3]. We speculate that the progressive disappearance of the term "tension" and the associated emergence of "anxiety and distress" can reflect greater attempts to disentangle OCD compulsions (more linked to relief from anxiety or distress) from cravings and patterns of compulsive drug use (more linked to relief of tension). Paradoxically, this move has been made in the context of an ever-increasing literature linking OCD and behavioral addictions (e.g., Ferreira et al. [35]). In ICD-10, compulsive acts or rituals do not result in the completion of inherently useful tasks [18].

Finally, despite being listed in initial editions of the DSM, the experience of "subjective compulsion" [28,36] has been completely eliminated after the DSM-IV [17,24]. This ambiguous concept has been initially discussed within traditional psychopathology texts (e.g., Kurt Schneider's *Clinical Psychopathology* [36]) as the most important signature of OCD, e.g.,

[5] Though not clearly mentioned in the criteria, nor in the text, this example is consistent with the concept of "magical thinking"; that is, beliefs that defy scientific or culturally accepted laws of causality [34].

"every compulsive experience has an ego character; it is always a 'subjective' compulsion and not one that comes from without, as in schizophrenic passivity experiences" (p. 103) [36]. It was first included as criterion for compulsion in DSM-III, although the DSM wording: "a sense of subjective compulsion coupled with a desire to resist the compulsion (at least initially)" [15] did not seem to reflect Schneider's intention to differentiate the phenomenon from schizophrenia symptoms. Later, the expression was restricted to the text of DSM-III-R [16] and finally excluded in DSM-IV [17,24]. The DSM-5 does not include any reference to "subjective compulsion" [2].

Diagnosis

Early Conceptualizations

Although poets and priests have recognized OCD symptoms since the medieval period, it was no earlier than 1838 that Esquirol first described "instinctive monomania", considered to be the first medical report of a case of OCD [37]. However, as reported above, the origins of the OCD "label" appear to date back to Krafft-Ebing, who in 1867 coined the term *Zwangvorstellung* to describe the "compelling forces" that subdued many depressed (and, curiously, not clearly OCD) patients [14]. According to Berrios, *Zwangvorstellung* was translated in the United Kingdom as "obsessive" and in the United States as "compulsive", thus suggesting that the well-established term "obsessive-compulsive" was in fact a compromise between two different translations [37]. Regardless of linguistic discussions, Kraepelin was among the first clinicians who suggested obsessive-compulsive phenomena to be an "independent clinical entity ... in which obsessive ideas play a special role" (*Zwangsvorstellungskrankheit*) [31]. However, the exact place of OCD in early classification systems was a little more controversial. Throughout the last part of the nineteenth and the beginning of the twentieth century, OCD has been successively classified as a "neurosis" (or a "disease of the emotions"), a psychosis (a delusional state), and, finally, as a member of the newly formed class of "neuroses" (the newer psychoanalytical concept) [38].

Diagnostic and Statistical Manuals

The origins of the *Diagnostic and Statistical Manual for Mental Disorders* date back to 1952, when the American Psychiatric Association issued its first edition [25]. This version of the DSM, which was based on the ICD-6 and largely influenced by Adolf Meyer's psychobiological view of mental illnesses, conceptualized OCD a "psychoneurotic disorder" and form of reaction of the individual to different psychological, social and biological factors [39]. According to DSM-I, this "obsessive-compulsive reaction" would be characterized by anxiety leading to "the persistence of unwanted ideas and repetitive impulses to perform acts that may be considered morbid by the patient" [25]. In DSM-II, the terms "psychoneurosis" and "reaction" were abandoned in favor of the simpler designation "obsessive-compulsive neurosis" [26]. However, DSM-II kept a definition of "obsessive-compulsive neurosis" that was quite similar to DSM-I's "obsessive-compulsive reaction", adding that anxiety could result if the patient did not perform his rituals or feared losing control [26].

DSM-III

The modern view of OCD began to be defined with the publication of the DSM-III in 1980 [15]. This version of DSM adopted an atheoretical approach to psychopathology. In other words, it eliminated any speculation regarding the etiology or pathophysiology of OCD, as it did for many other disorders. In fact, the DSM-III was concerned exclusively with the description of symptoms and reliability of the diagnosis. Accordingly, the term "obsessive-compulsive neurosis", which was considered ambiguous and heavily influenced by psychodynamic concepts,[6] was first questioned and officially substituted for by the broad designation "obsessive compulsive *disorder* (or obsessive compulsive neurosis)" [40]. Interestingly, DSM-III required the presence of obsessions *or* compulsions for a diagnosis of OCD [15], a wording that was only slightly changed in DSM-IV. It also contained simple and separate definitions of obsessions and compulsions; for example, it required obsessions to be ego-dystonic (without insight), and compulsions to be associated with a sense of "subjective compulsion".[7]

However, the DSM-III did not mention a minimum time per day occupied by OCD symptoms.

[6] According to DSM-III, neurosis was ambiguous because it had both descriptive and etiological meanings [14].
[7] This feature may reflect the influence of Kurt Schneider's work on DSM-III criteria for OCD [34].

It was also heavily hierarchical, as it excluded a diagnosis of OCD in individuals with Tourette's disorder, schizophrenia, major depression or organic mental disorders [15]. There was a certain rationale in the hierarchal approach to the diagnosis of psychiatric disorders in general. Few people would argue that diagnosing schizophrenia in patients with Alzheimer's disease or bipolar disorder in patients with schizophrenia would make much clinical sense nowadays. However, it is fortunate that rigid algorithms to diagnose OCD were abandoned in subsequent editions of the DSM, as these algorithms would not have allowed researchers to unveil the close genetic relationship between OCD and Tourette's disorder [41] or to discover that OCD is actually quite common among schizophrenia individuals [42] (while the opposite is certainly not true).

Like DSM-III, DSM-III-R required the presence of "obsessions or compulsions" for a diagnosis of OCD [16]. However, in DSM-III-R, there was an attempt to detail the core features of obsessions and compulsions in four and three separate sets of features, respectively [16]. Although the DSM-III-R did not mention the possibility that obsessions could be associated with poor insight, it required obsessions to be intrusive and senseless "at least initially" [17]. The DSM-III-R also tried to differentiate obsessions from symptoms that were core to other disorders (e.g., thought insertion), even though no such attempt has been made in relation to compulsions [16]. Further, although compulsions were described exclusively as behaviors (and not as thoughts), the DSM-III-R criteria for obsessions required the person to neutralize their obsessions with *some other thought* or action (my emphasis) [16]. Thus, the DSM-III-R seemed to be ambiguous about what would be later described in DSM-IV as mental compulsions [24].

Insight toward OCD symptoms was dealt somewhat idiosyncratically in DSM-III-R [16]. For instance, it allowed patients with OCD to show obsessions not considered intrusive or senseless at later stages of their illness (see above), but it unexpectedly required compulsions to be recognized by the person as excessive or unreasonable throughout the course of the disorder. As reported above, DSM-III-R also introduced the possibility of diagnosing OCD in the presence of other disorders, including Tourette's disorder, schizophrenia and major depression, a movement that allowed the growth of comorbidity research in OCD [16]. Finally, an attempt to draw a line between clinical and sub-threshold OCD was made, with the requirement that obsessions or compulsions had to cause marked distress, are time consuming (take more than an hour a day), or significantly interfere with the person's normal routine, occupational functioning or usual social activities or relationships with others [16].

DSM-IV

The DSM criteria for OCD have been tested in a field trial study that included 431 OCD patients from seven different US centers [43]. This study had three major results, which led to critical changes in DSM-III-R wording, and resulted in the DSM-IV criteria for OCD. First, the authors of this field trial tested whether the OCD subtypes listed in ICD-10 (obsessive, compulsive or mixed) actually existed. They found equivocal results that did not support the inclusion of these subtypes in DSM-IV (e.g., while patients with OCD frequently classified themselves into one of these three subtypes, the ratio between their obsessions and compulsions sub-scores in the Yale-Brown Obsessive-Compulsive Scale were distributed along a unimodal, and not trimodal, curve [43]). Second, the authors also found that 5% of patients with OCD reported never having insight into their symptoms, and 25% were mostly certain that their symptoms were reasonable [43]. Thus, DSM-IV criteria were changed to acknowledge the existence of individuals with OCD who had reduced insight into their symptoms and included the so-called "poor insight" specifier.

Finally, this field trial also found that most (79.5%) of their patients with OCD reported having both mental and behavioral compulsions [43]. These findings prompted DSM-IV developers to acknowledge the existence of "mental acts (e.g., praying, counting, repeating words silently)" that the person felt driven to perform in response to an obsession, or according to rules that must be applied rigidly (i.e., mental compulsions). The origins of the remaining DSM-IV criteria [17] for OCD can be traced back to DSM-III-R. For instance, DSM-IV used the same phraseology of DSM-III-R to disentangle OCD from subthreshold OCD. In addition, as in DSM-III-R, DSM-IV required that, if another axis I disorder was present (the DSM diagnosis was multiaxial by then), the content of the obsessions or compulsions should not be restricted to it. Fortunately, by maintaining the later strategy, DSM-IV-TR continued to allow the comorbid diagnosis to OCD to be made. Finally, in DSM-IV, OCD was required not to be due to the direct physiological effects of a substance or a general medical condition. The DSM-IV-TR criteria for OCD were identical to those of DSM-IV.

DSM-5

In DSM-5, the wording of criterion A has been changed from "Either obsessions or compulsions" to the clearer "Presence of obsessions, compulsions, or both". In other words, provided that individuals fulfill other criteria for OCD, a diagnosis of OCD can be given to anyone showing "pure" obsessions (without concomitant compulsions), "pure compulsions" (without concomitant obsessions) or both symptoms (the majority of cases). However, there remains some discussion as to the validity of such a method. Some studies have suggested that patients with OCD who display "pure" obsessions are likely to be rare, as individuals with OCD who do not show "overt" (motor) compulsions will often show "covert" (mental) compulsions [44]. In other words, according to many researchers and clinicians, whenever someone comes across an individual showing true "pure obsessions" (i.e., repetitive unwanted cognitions without mental concomitant ritual), a diagnosis other than OCD should be entertained, including, for instance, the preoccupations of GAD, or the ruminations of major depressive disorder.

To draw a clearer line between OCD and subclinical OCD symptoms, DSM-5 has also improved its wording. The former DSM-IV criterion C ("The obsessions or compulsions cause marked distress, are time consuming, take more than 1 hour a day, or significantly interfere with the person's normal routine, occupational, or academic, functioning, or usual social activities or relationships") was a source of potential misunderstanding. For instance, the author has seen inattentive clinicians arguing that a DSM-IV diagnosis of OCD requires marked distress, a minimum of one hour a day spent on symptoms *and* interference in different areas to be present. The DSM-5 criterion B, which substitutes DSM-IV's criterion C, is now much clearer by requiring obsessions or compulsions to be time consuming (e.g., to take more than one hour per day) *or* to cause clinically significant distress *or* impairment in social, occupational or other important areas of functioning. The cut-off of a minimum of one hour per day spent with symptoms is also now given as an example rather than as an arbitrary prerequisite for a diagnosis.

The DSM-V Anxiety, OC Spectrum, Posttraumatic and Dissociative Disorders Work Group has raised several interesting questions in relation to the DSM item that excludes a diagnosis of OCD whenever OCD symptoms are attributable to the physiological effects of a substance (e.g., a drug of abuse, a medication) or another ("general", in DSM-IV terms) medical condition [20]. For instance, while few clinicians would argue that an OCD diagnosis according to the current DSM-5 criteria should be excluded in the presence of strokes affecting the corticostriatothalamocortical system but probably maintained in the presence of Tourette's disorder, a clear guideline is lacking in relation to other biomedical conditions, including the so-called pediatric autoimmune neuropsychiatric disorders associated with streptococcal infections. Accordingly, DSM-5 could have made clearer statements; for example, either excluding a diagnosis of OCD in the presence of any medical cause or allowing a diagnosis of OCD in the presence of any medical cause. Unfortunately, DSM-5 has ignored these discussions and eventually none of these reflections has been included, neither in the criteria nor in the text.

ICD-10

Chapter 5, Mental and Behavioral Disorders, of ICD-10 was made available in different versions, including the clinical descriptions and diagnostic guidelines (also known as the Blue Book), which was intended for general clinical, educational and service use by psychiatrists and other mental health professionals [18]. Also included were the diagnostic criteria for research (also known as the Green Book), which was for research purposes and had to be used in conjunction with the Blue Book [29], and the Glossary, which was for use by coders or clerical workers [45]. These versions included overlapping definitions of OCD, although with some particularities. For instance, the clinical description and diagnostic guidelines were broad and narrative, while the diagnostic criteria for research was focused and bulleted.

For an ICD-10 diagnosis of OCD according to the diagnostic criteria for research, individuals had to display: (i) obsessive thoughts, compulsive acts or both, which had been present on most days for at least 2 weeks; (ii) obsessions and compulsions that (a) had not been imposed by an outside person or influence, (b) had been resisted (even though there could be symptoms that the patient no longer resisted), (c) had not been pleasurable and (d) had been repetitive;

(iii) obsessions or compulsions that had caused distress or interfered with the subject's social or individual functioning, usually by wasting time and (iv) obsessions or compulsions that had not been caused by other mental disorders, such as schizophrenia, related disorders or mood disorders [29]. In addition, the description and diagnostic guidelines posited that OCD could lack autonomic anxiety symptoms.

While ICD-10 made several consistent remarks about OCD, including its early age of onset [46], its variable course [47], and its frequent association with depression [47,48], a number of statements were not fully supported by the available data [18]. For instance, the ICD-10 claimed that OCD was equally common in men and women, when several epidemiological studies suggested a slight female preponderance [49]. It also argued that OCD individuals often show prominent anankastic features in the underlying personality, when in fact obsessive-compulsive personality disorder has been shown to be just one (and not necessarily the most common) personality disorder among a plethora of other personality disorders [50,51]. Finally, ICD-10 suggested that the course of OCD was likely to be chronic in the absence of significant depressive symptoms when, in general, the chronic course predominates, regardless of the presence of associated depression [52].

The ICD-10 has also been criticized for providing guidelines on differential diagnosis that "are not consistent with the current literature, nor, arguably, with good clinical practice" [21]. For instance, whenever OCD and depression coexisted, ICD-10 argued that: (i) preference should be given to diagnosing the condition whose symptoms developed first (which, generally, is OCD) and (ii) a diagnosis of OCD (which is usually a chronic condition) [52] should be given if obsessive thoughts arise or persist in the absence of a depression [18]. Thus, the adherence to ICD-10 guidelines could lead to serious underdiagnosis and undertreatment of depression in those with OCD [21]. In contrast, ICD-10 also recommended diagnosing depression when neither OCD not depression predominates, an approach that could also result in underdiagnosis of OCD. The fact that ICD-10 did not allow a diagnosis of OCD in the presence of schizophrenia or Tourette's disorder was also a severe limitation of this diagnostic system.

ICD-11

The ICD-11 is due to be published in 2018 [53] (ICD-11 for Mortality and Morbidity Statistics was published in June 2018 [22]). The Working Group on the Classification of Obsessive-Compulsive and Related Disorder published its recommendations in 2014 [21]. Although there is no complete guarantee that they will be accepted, it is likely that many suggestions of the working group will. We have already addressed many of the changes proposed by the ICD-11 on the sections on obsessions and compulsions, including the substitution of "impulse" to "impulse/urge" under the definition of obsessions, and both the abandonment of the term "stereotyped" and inclusion of mental acts under the definition of compulsions [21]. Two additional suggestions for inclusion in the text were the recognition that OCD individuals can experience a wide range of emotions when confronted with one of their OCD triggers (such as anxiety/panic, disgust or incompleteness) and that compulsions were performed "in relationship to" (versus "in response to") obsessions to reflect the fact that the former may precede the latter [21].

Other than the proposed changes in the definition of obsessions and compulsions, a number of suggestions have been made in terms of the diagnostic guidelines of OCD itself. These include the removal of the minimum duration requirement of two weeks and the inclusion, in the text, of a cautionary note recommending a careful evaluation of patients showing OCD symptoms for less than one month or children showing an acute and fulminant onset of OCD suggestive of a medical etiology [54]. The working group also suggested the inclusion of a list of mental disorders that are known to be comorbid with OCD in the ICD-11 text, as well as a more detailed description of conditions that should be differentiated from OCD, such as other obsessive-compulsive and related disorders, tic disorders, psychotic disorders, eating disorders, mood disorders and anxiety disorders [21].

Obsessive-Compulsive Disorder Specifiers

DSM

DSM-IV

As reported above, the inclusion of a poor insight specifier in DSM-IV was prompted by field trial findings showing that 5% of patients with OCD lacked insight into their symptoms and were mostly certain that their symptoms were reasonable in another 25% [43]. Thus, DSM-IV allowed patients to be specified with poor insight "if, for most of the time during the current episode, the person does not recognize that the obsessions and compulsions are excessive or unreasonable." Although history has witnessed a pendulum between the recognition and the denial of the existence of lack of insight in OCD [55], this specification seems important, as greater severity and worse outcome among those with poor insight may indicate an underlying biology closer to that of schizophrenia spectrum disorders [56]. There are a few problems with the insight approach to OCD in DSM-IV, though.

First, the poor insight specifier in DSM-IV is somewhat broad and heterogeneous, including OCD showing either delusions or overvalued ideas within the same category. Although there are researchers who believe that these symptoms lie within a single insight continuum, there are also authors who see delusions and overvalued ideas as concepts that are categorically different [57]. Second, the DSM-IV allows additional diagnoses of either delusional disorder or psychotic disorder not otherwise specified to patients with OCD who are delusional, thus creating the unusual scenario where a patient with a single disorder can have three possible diagnoses. Third, the DSM-IV requirement that insight had to be decreased for "most of the time during the current episode" is probably too subjective and most likely based on an imprecise assessment (either from the clinician or from the patient) [58] not to mention that OCD is not typically an episodic illness [20].

DSM-5

While a poor insight specifier was restricted to OCD and hypochondriasis in DSM-IV, such specifier has been added to all DSM-5 OCRDs with an evident cognitive component, including OCD, body dysmorphic disorder and hoarding disorder [3]. It has been argued that the use of an insight specifier across these OCRDs highlights to clinicians how the assessment and therapeutic strategies used in these patients are shared but also different from those employed in other groups of disorders, including schizophrenia spectrum disorders [59]. However, for unknown reasons, the DSM-5 also dropped a poor-insight specifier from illness anxiety disorder, which partially overlaps with DSM-IV hypochondriasis and is now characterized as being associated with preserved insight. Of note, the DSM-5 also added an additional tic-related specifier that was not present in earlier versions of the DSM [3].

In fact, most, but not all, problems associated with the poor insight specifier in DSM-IV OCD have been addressed in DSM-5. For instance, there is now the possibility of specifying the insight of patients with OCD as being good or fair ("The individual thinks OCD beliefs are definitely or probably not true or that they may or may not be true"), poor ("The individual thinks OCD beliefs are probably true") or absent/delusional ("The individual is completely convinced that OCD beliefs are true"), thus offering clinicians a wider range of more homogeneous groups. Additional diagnoses of delusional disorder or psychotic disorder not otherwise specified for patients with OCD who are delusional are no longer allowed. Finally, the DSM-5 has reworded the specifiers and eliminated ambiguous expressions, such as "most of the time", "episode", "excessive" and "unreasonable". However, such specifiers should not be considered categorical subtypes of OCD, as there is evidence that poor insight fluctuates according to exposure to different threats and/or in different periods in a patient's life.

In DSM-5, the diagnosis of a tic-related OCD is based on a lifetime (current or past) history of a tic disorder, which is reported to occur in up to 30% of OCD cases [3]. The inclusion of a tic-related specifier in DSM-5 was supported by a number of distinctive features (as reviewed in Leckman et al. [20]), including a predominance of males; an earlier onset and earlier peak of severity of OCD followed by increased likelihood of remission; greater frequency of sensory phenomena (e.g., muscle–skeletal sensations, "just-right" perceptions), symmetry/ordering symptoms and forbidden thoughts; increased rates of disruptive, impulsive and developmental disorders; worse response to serotonin reuptake inhibitors (SRIs), and increased response to neuroleptic augmentation. There is also compelling genetic evidence of a tic-related OCD, which has been associated with higher rates of OCD and tics among first-degree family members. Curiously, the augmentation studies used to support a tic-related specifier are based on current rather than lifetime presence of tics.

ICD

ICD-10

Despite acknowledging the common coexistence of obsessions and compulsions, the ICD-10 clinical descriptions and diagnostic guidelines suggest that specifying the symptoms which predominate in a patient with OCD may be useful, as obsessions and compulsions, according to the ICD-10, respond to different treatments [18]. Although it is doubtful whether this tenet would hold true according to present day data, it was believed at the time that ICD-10 was issued that obsessive thoughts were more closely associated with depression and compulsive acts were more readily remediated by behavioral therapies. Therefore, in ICD-10 patients with OCD could be specified into those showing predominantly obsessional thoughts or ruminations (particularly those with aggressive, sexual/religious or pseudophilosophical content), predominantly compulsive acts (in which washing, checking and ordering symptoms dominate), mixed obsessional thoughts and compulsive acts, and the rather unclear "other obsessive-compulsive disorders" and "obsessive-compulsive disorder, unspecified" [18].

ICD-11

The ICD-11 working group recommended the removal of the ICD-10 specifiers, as they were not validated in DSM-IV field trials [43] and may be difficult to establish. For instance, in many cases, deciding whether a symptom (obsession or compulsion) dominates the clinical picture can be quite arbitrary, as ICD-10 did not mention a specific guideline for making this differentiation. The group has also assessed whether to include DSM-5's insight and tic-related specifiers [1,21], as well as a few other specifiers (i.e., age at onset, symptom dimensions, history of infection, the underlying motivations, course and severity) [21]. The inclusion of an insight specifier was eventually recommended, as it was thought to avoid patients being misdiagnosed with delusional disorders and mistreated with monotherapy with antipsychotics. In contrast, the addition of a tic-related OCD specifier was thought to be redundant, as the group had already recommended tic disorders and Tourette syndrome to be listed in the OCRDs chapter.

Cross-Diagnostic Approaches and Their Implications for Classification and Diagnosis

Although a resurgence of the interest in the concept of "obsessive-compulsive spectrum" was seen in the past 25 years, the traditional psychopathological literature had already emphasized the links between OCD and other non-OCD conditions, such as body dysmorphic disorder [60] and tics, for more than a century [61]. The recognition that OCD shares many characteristics (the so-called "11 validators")[8] with a heterogeneous group of mental disorders (some newly described and some originating from other DSM-IV chapters), while also differing substantially from panic, phobic and generalized anxiety disorders, had a major impact in the organization of DSM-5 [59,62]. However, the fact that OCRDs immediately follow the anxiety disorders chapter still reflects the important role for fear and anxiety in some OCRDs (e.g., OCD) and the close relationship between some of the disorders listed in these chapters (e.g., body dysmorphic disorder and social anxiety disorder).

The OCRDs chapter comprises complex, cognitively based, high-order disorders including not only OCD itself, classified as an anxiety disorder in DSM-IV, but also other conditions discussed more in depth in other chapters of this book, such as body dysmorphic disorders, classified as a somatoform disorder in DSM-IV; and hoarding disorder, new to DSM-5. However, DSM-5 OCRDs also include less complex, motorically based and low-order disorders that are reminiscent of tics and stereotypies, such as trichotillomania (hair pulling disorder), originally an impulse control not elsewhere specified in DSM-IV; and excoriation (skin picking) disorder, new to DSM-5 [59]. Although a couple of other disorders were not classified as OCRDs in DSM-5, ICD-11 is likely to include them as so; namely, olfactory reference disorder, health (or illness, in DSM terms) anxiety disorder (hypochondriasis) and Tourette's disorder and personality disorder with anankastic features as cross-referenced disorders that could legitimately be placed in more than one section of the classification [61].

There are a few problems with the rationale supporting the creation of the OCRDs group. For instance, data from different validators may eventually conflict, and it is currently unclear whether a few validators should have greater weight than the others [59]. The OCRD specifiers may also have broader implications for diagnosis and classifications

[8] The relatedness of disorders to one another was based on an expanded version of the validators proposed by Robins and Guze [8], including shared symptom similarity, high comorbidity between disorders, course of illness, familiality, genetic and environmental risk factors, neutral substrates, biomarkers, temperament, emotional/cognitive processing profile, and response to treatment.

for other psychiatric disorders. Although insight has been included as a specifier for high-order OCRDs in DSM-5, and is also recommended for inclusion in the criteria for the same group of disorders in ICD-11, it may have potential implications that transcend the diagnostic limits of the later conditions, being potentially relevant for the characterization of phenotypes of eating [63] and social anxiety disorders [64]. Finally, it is unclear whether the presence of tics may be valuable in other disorders, of which autism spectrum disorders and other developmental disorders would be natural candidates [65]. Alternatively, autistic features may also differentiate Tourette's disorder.

Clinical Implications of Cross-Diagnostic Approaches for Treatment and Prevention

There are a few practical implications of a cross-diagnostic approach to OCD. First, patients with OCD need to be assessed for conditions known to "orbit around" or be frequently comorbid with OCD. Although they obviously include the official OCRDs, other mental disorders that can be even more frequently found among those with OCD, such as different depressive, bipolar and anxiety disorders, should not be dismissed. Secondly, as OCD and OCRDs tend to affect different individuals in the same family, another clinical implication of a cross-diagnostic approach to OCD is the increased importance of assessing family history of OCRDs among patients with OCD and those without. A positive family history for an OCRD can be particularly valuable in cases presenting diagnostic challenges.

For sharing with OCD intrusive thoughts and/or repetitive behaviors as their core psychopathological features, patients with OCD and OCRDs can have their severity assessed in similar ways, including how much time the individual spends with symptoms, how much interference their symptoms cause, what is the degree of distress/anxiety generated by their intrusive thoughts or the prevention of repetitive behaviors, how much the patient resists and/or controls their symptoms, and to what extent they avoid specific situations because of their symptoms. This can be done by using specific versions of the Yale-Brown Obsessive-Compulsive Scale or the Florida Obsessive-Compulsive Inventory adapted for the OCRD of interest. It should be mentioned, though, that OCRDs are not simply subtypes of OCD, as they do have qualitative differences compared with the latter category.

Another clinical implication of a cross-diagnostic approach to OCD is the fact that all related high-order, cognitively based OCRDs can be assessed in terms of insight into their core beliefs. The prompt identification of cases of OCRDs that exhibit poor insight can lead to lower misdiagnosis, as these patients are frequently labeled as having schizophrenia spectrums and other psychotic disorders (e.g., delusional disorder, somatic type, in the case of poor insight BDD); and consequently, to lower prescription rates of monotherapy with antipsychotics. Similarly, tic-related OCD and other low-order, motorically based OCRDs (including trichotillomania and excoriation disorders), have to be differentiated from stereotypic movement disorders (which are more purposeless and rhythmical) and "pure" (non-OCD related) tic disorders (which are sudden, rapid and recurrent).

Finally, the reunion of OCRDs under the same rubric also had positive implications for treatment. For instance, it is now widely recognized that the first-line drug treatments for both OCD and body dysmorphic disorder are SRIs, although these conditions seem to differ in terms of response to augmentation strategies (i.e., neuroleptics). However, the creation of the OCRDs group has also resulted in a few additional misconceptions and unwanted outcomes. For example, it has been assumed that SRIs are the standard pharmacological treatment for all OCRDs, although the evidence supporting their use in hoarding disorder and low-order OCRDs is not unequivocal. Similarly, while exposure and response prevention is the first-line treatment for OCD, other OCRDs have to incorporate specific components to their treatment, such as motivational interviewing (for low-insight OCRDs) and habit reversal (for low-order OCRDs).

Future Directions

One of the greatest challenges that psychiatry has faced throughout its history is the absence of valid biomarkers of DSM and ICD-10 "discretely defined" mental disorders. A biomarker has been defined as a "characteristic that is objectively measured and evaluated as an indicator of normal biological processes, pathogenic processes, or pharmacologic responses to a therapeutic intervention" [66]. Although there has been at least one proposal to incorporate a biomarker in OCRDs criteria (i.e., the evidence of fronto-striatal brain circuitry dysfunction, e.g., caudate hyperactivity) [67] and also subtle findings suggesting that differences in brain activation patterns may predict responses to specific types of anti-OCD treatments [68], the evidence is probably not mature enough for OCD biomarkers to be incorporated in clinical practice.

Lately, to clarify the pathogenic processes underlying mental disorders and develop treatments that are more specifically targeted at dysfunctional biological parameters, the attention has shifted toward the Research Domains Criteria (RDoC), an initiative by the US National Institute of Mental Health that promises to result in more personalized/precise treatments. Thus, rather than trying to decipher the underlying biology of an arbitrarily-defined OCD and propose treatments focusing on symptoms, the RDoC would use what is presently known about the molecular, cellular, circuit, physiological, and cognitive basis of biologically valid brain systems to either expand or narrow the boundaries of OCD (and/or other neurodevelopmental disorders).

For instance, deletions or duplications at 16p13.11 have been implicated in a wide range of disorders, including OCD, Tourette's disorder, autism spectrum disorders, intellectual disability and seizures [69,70]. Thus, future studies could investigate the consequences of 16p13.11 copy number variants for brain systems and how treatments could be developed to remediate phenotypes related to this locus. Hypothetically, such an approach could be made both on a syndromal (e.g., OCD) and a brain system level (say, for instance, problems in response to sustained threat or habit formation), a strategy that is reminiscent of the multiaxial approach used by the DSM system until its fourth edition (for a greater discussion on the prospects of the RDoC strategy in relation to OCRDs, see Chapter 1).

Conclusions

For a diagnosis of OCD, mental health professionals do not need to have a *"fameuse oreille"* [2]. Instead, they should perform a sufficient number of open interviews, which help them creating a "prototype" or gestalt of OCD cases. This may be facilitated by attendance to OCRDs clinics. The recognition of global patterns and identification of information that may be missing on particular cases allow clinicians to search for diagnostic validators of different kinds. For instance, the revelation of compulsive behavior by a patient with OCD during an open interview may lead a clinician to search for the corresponding obsessions. However, this strategy may also generate a less reliable diagnosis, as clinicians can differ on their prototypes and personal opinions of a particular case, and can change their own opinion over time.

Open assessments can be complemented, especially in early years of training, by the performance of structured or semi-structured interviews that guide the examiner through the most recent diagnostic criteria for OCD. Structured interviews are thought to increase reliability of diagnosis. They are based on existing criteria (e.g., DSM or ICD), which should be data (research) driven, but also informed by clinical experience. An ideal scenario is one where data and "prototypes" converge toward a common diagnosis. This is why, over the years, diagnostic systems have evolved and been shaped and ultimately improved, to reproduce a hypothetical truth. For instance, it is now recognized that poor insight, mental compulsions and emotions other than anxiety may be integral parts of some OCD cases.

References

1. North C, Yutzy S. *Goodwin and Guze's Psychiatric Diagnosis*, 6th ed. Oxford University Press; 2010.
2. Leme Lopes J. *O diagnóstico psiquiátrico*. Rio de Janeiro-RJ: Editora Cultura Médica; 1980.
3. American Psychiatric Association. *Diagnostic and Statistical Manual of Mental Disorders*. 5th ed. Washington, DC: APA; 2013.
4. de Miranda-Sá Júnior LS. *Compêndio de psicopatologia e semiologia psiquiátrica*. ArtMed; 2000.
5. Schwartz MA, Wiggins OP. Typifications: the first step for clinical diagnosis in psychiatry. *J Nerv Ment Dis*. 1987;175(2):65–77.
6. Jansson L, Nordgaard J. The psychiatric interview: theoretical aspects. In: Jansson L, Nordgaard J, eds. *The Psychiatric Interview for Differential Diagnosis*. Switzerland: Springer International Publishing; 2016:17–26.
7. Jaspers K. *General Psychopathology*. University of Chicago Press; 1963.
8. Robins E, Guze SB. Establishment of diagnostic validity in psychiatric illness: its application to schizophrenia. *Am J Psychiatry*. 1970;126(7):983–987.
9. Fontenelle LF, Lins-Martins NM, Melca IA, et al. Exaggerating, mislabeling or simulating

obsessive-compulsive symptoms: case reports of patients claiming to have obsessive-compulsive disorder. *Compr Psychiatry*. 2014;55(5):1188–1194.

10. Aboraya A, France C, Young J, Curci K, Lepage J. The validity of psychiatric diagnosis revisited: the clinician's guide to improve the validity of psychiatric diagnosis. *Psychiatry (Edgmont)*. 2005;2(9):48–55.
11. Dorfan NM, Woody SR. Assessing OCD symptoms and severity. In: Steketee G, ed. *The Oxford Handbook of Obsessive Compulsive and Spectrum Disorders*. Oxford University Press; 2011:253–274.
12. Berrios GE. Trastorno obsesivo-compulsivo y enfermedad neurológica: estado actual de la cuestión. In: Ruiloba JV, Berrios GE, eds. *Estados obsesivos*. 3a. edición ed. Barcelona: Masson; 2006:487–519.
13. Sheehan DV, Lecrubier Y, Sheehan KH, et al. The Mini-International Neuropsychiatric Interview (M.I.N.I.): the development and validation of a structured diagnostic psychiatric interview for DSM-IV and ICD-10. *J Clin Psychiatry*. 1998;59(Suppl 20):22–33.
14. de Haan S, Rietveld E, Denys D. *On the nature of obsessions and compulsions*. Vol 29. Basel: Karger; 2013.
15. American Psychiatric Association. *Diagnostic and Statistical Manual of Mental Disorders (DSM-III)*. 3rd ed. Washington, DC: APA; 1980.
16. American Psychiatric Association. *Diagnostic and Statistical Manual of Mental Disorders (DSM-III-R)*. 3rd revised ed. Washington, DC: APA; 1987.
17. American Psychiatric Association. *Diagnostic and Statistical Manual of Mental Disorders: DSM-IV-TR*. Washington, DC: APA; 2000.
18. World Health Organization. *The ICD-10 Classification of Mental and Behavioural Disorders: Clinical Descriptions and Diagnostic Guidelines*. Geneva: WHO; 1992.
19. Ferrao YA, Shavitt RG, Prado H, et al. Sensory phenomena associated with repetitive behaviors in obsessive-compulsive disorder: an exploratory study of 1001 patients. *Psychiatry Res*. 2012;197(3):253–258.
20. Leckman JF, Denys D, Simpson HB, et al. Obsessive–compulsive disorder: a review of the diagnostic criteria and possible subtypes and dimensional specifiers for DSM-V. *Depress Anxiety*. 2010;27(6):507–527.
21. Simpson HB, Reddy YCJ. Obsessive-compulsive disorder for ICD-11: proposed changes to the diagnostic guidelines and specifiers. *Revista Brasileira de Psiquiatria*. 2014;36:3–13.
22. World Health Organization. International Classification of Diseases-11 for Mortality and Morbidity Statistics (ICD-11 MMS) 2018 version. Available from: https://icd.who.int/browse11/l-m/en (accessed July 9, 2018).
23. Marras A, Fineberg N, Pallanti S. Obsessive compulsive and related disorders: comparing DSM-5 and ICD-11. *CNS Spectr*. 2016;21(4):324–333.
24. American Psychiatric Association. *Diagnostic and Statistical Manual of Mental Disorders: DSM-IV*. Washington, DC: APA; 1994.
25. American Psychiatric Association. *Diagnostic and Statistical Manual: Mental Disorders* Washington, DC: APA; 1952.
26. American Psychiatric Assoociation. *Diagnostic and Statistical Manual of Mental Disorders (DSM-II)*. 2nd. ed. Washington, DC: APA; 1968.
27. Fontenelle LF. New neuropsychological data might help build a model of poor insight in obsessive-compulsive disorder: an editorial comment to Kashyap H, Kumar K, Kandavel T, Janardhan Reddy YC. "Neuropsychological correlates of insight in obsessive-compulsive disorder" (1). *Acta Psychiatr Scand*. 2012;126(2):83–84.
28. Lewis A. Problems of obsessional illness: section of psychiatry. *Proc R Soc Med*. 1936;29(4):325–336.
29. WHO. *The ICD-10 Classification of Mental and Behavioural Disorders: Diagnostic Criteria for Research*. Geneva: World Health Organization; 1993.
30. Ladouceur R, Freeston MH, Rheaume J, et al. Strategies used with intrusive thoughts: a comparison of OCD patients with anxious and community controls. *J Abnorm Psychol*. 2000;109(2):179–187.
31. Steinberg H, Carius D, Fontenelle LF. Kraepelin's views on obsessive neurosis: a comparison with DSM-5 criteria for obsessive-compulsive disorder. *Rev Brasil Psiquiatr*. 2017;39:355–364.
32. Freud S, Strachey J, Freud A. *Complete Psychological Works of Sigmund Freud*. London: Vintage; 2001.
33. Pietrefesa AS, Coles ME. Moving beyond an exclusive focus on harm avoidance in obsessive compulsive disorder: considering the role of incompleteness. *Behav Ther*. 2008;39(3):224–231.
34. Einstein DA, Menzies RG. Magical thinking in obsessive-compulsive disorder, panic disorder and the general community. *Behav Cogn Psychother*. 2006;34(3):351–357.
35. Ferreira GM, Yücel M, Dawson A, Lorenzetti V, Fontenelle LF. Investigating the role of anticipatory reward and habit strength in obsessive-compulsive disorder. *CNS Spectr*. 2017;22(3):295–304.
36. Schneider K. *Clinical Psychopathology*. New York: Grune and Stratton; 1959.
37. Berrios GE. *The History of Mental Symptoms: Descriptive Psychopathology Since the Nineteenth Century*. Cambridge University Press; 1996.

38. Berrios GE. Obsessive-compulsive disorder: its conceptual history in France during the 19th century. *Compr Psychiatry*. 1989;30(4):283–295.

39. APA. DSM History. 2017. Available from: www.psychiatry.org/psychiatrists/practice/dsm/history-of-the-dsm (accessed March 17, 2017).

40. First M, Caban DK, Lewis-Fernández R. Development of the nosology of anxiety disorders. In: Simpson HB, Neria Y, Lewis-Fernández R, Schneier F, eds. *Anxiety Disorders: Theory, Research and Clinical Perspectives*. Cambridge University Press; 2010:20–39.

41. Grados MA. The genetics of obsessive-compulsive disorder and Tourette syndrome: an epidemiological and pathway-based approach for gene discovery. *J Am Acad Child Adolesc Psychiatry*. 2010;49(8):810–819.

42. Lysaker PH, Whitney KA. Obsessive-compulsive symptoms in schizophrenia: prevalence, correlates and treatment. *Expert Rev Neurother*. 2009;9(1):99–107.

43. Foa EB, Kozak MJ, Goodman WK, Hollander E, Jenike MA, Rasmussen SA. DSM-IV field trial: obsessive-compulsive disorder. *Am J Psychiatry*. 1995;152(1):90–96.

44. Williams MT, Farris SG, Turkheimer E, et al. Myth of the pure obsessional type in obsessive–compulsive disorder. *Depress Anxiety*. 2011;28(6):495–500.

45. World Health Organization. *Pocket Guide to ICD-10 Classification of Mental and Behavioural Disorders: With Glossary and Diagnostic Criteria for Research*. Edinburgh: Churchill Livingstone; 1994.

46. Fontenelle LF, Mendlowicz MV, Marques C, Versiani M. Early- and late-onset obsessive-compulsive disorder in adult patients: an exploratory clinical and therapeutic study. *J Psychiatr Res*. 2003;37(2):127–133.

47. Kichuk SA, Torres AR, Fontenelle LF, et al. Symptom dimensions are associated with age of onset and clinical course of obsessive-compulsive disorder. *Prog Neuropsychopharmacol Biol Psychiatry*. 2013;44:233–239.

48. Quarantini LC, Torres AR, Sampaio AS, et al. Comorbid major depression in obsessive-compulsive disorder patients. *Compr Psychiatry*. 2011;52(4):386–393.

49. Fontenelle LF, Hasler G. The analytical epidemiology of obsessive-compulsive disorder: risk factors and correlates. *Prog Neuropsychopharmacol Biol Psychiatry*. 2008;32(1):1–15.

50. Torres AR, Moran P, Bebbington P, et al. Obsessive-compulsive disorder and personality disorder: evidence from the British National Survey of Psychiatric Morbidity 2000. *Soc Psychiatry Psychiatr Epidemiol*. 2006;41(11):862–867.

51. Melca IA, Yücel M, Mendlowicz MV, de Oliveira-Souza R, Fontenelle LF. The correlates of obsessive-compulsive, schizotypal, and borderline personality disorders in obsessive-compulsive disorder. *J Anxiety Disord*. 2015;33:15–24.

52. Bloch MH, Green C, Kichuk SA, et al. Long-term outcome in adults with obsessive-compulsive disorder. *Depress Anxiety*. 2013;30(8):716–722.

53. World Health Organization. ICD-11 is here! Available from: www.who.int/classifications/icd/en (accessed July 9, 2018).

54. Singer HS, Gilbert DL, Wolf DS, Mink JW, Kurlan R. Moving from PANDAS to CANS. *J Pediatr*. 2012;160(5):725–731.

55. Spitzer M, Sigmund D. The phenomenology of obsessive-compulsive disorder. *Int Rev Psychiatry*. 1997;9(1):7–14.

56. Poyurovsky M. *Schizo-Obsessive Disorder*. Cambridge University Press; 2013.

57. Veale D. Over-valued ideas: a conceptual analysis. *Behav Res Ther*. 2002;40(4):383–400.

58. Fontenelle LF. New neuropsychological data might help build a model of poor insight in obsessive–compulsive disorder. *Acta Psychiatr Scand*. 2012;126(2):83–84.

59. Phillips KA, Stein DJ. Introduction and major changes for the obsessive-compulsive and related disorders in DSM-5. In: Phillips KA, Stein DJ, eds. *Handbook on Obsessive-Compulsive and Related Disorders*. Washington, DC: American Psychiatric Publishing; 2015:1–24.

60. Steinberg H, Carius D, Fontenelle LF. Kraepelin's views on obsessive neurosis: a comparison with DSM-5 criteria for obsessive-compulsive disorder. *Rev Bras Psiquiatr*. 2017;39:355–364.

61. Pitman RK. Pierre Janet on obsessive-compulsive disorder (1903). Review and commentary. *Arch Gen Psychiatry*. 1987;44(3):226–232.

62. Stein DJ, Kogan CS, Atmaca M, et al. The classification of obsessive–compulsive and related disorders in the ICD-11. *J Affect Disord*. 2016;190:663–674.

63. Konstantakopoulos G, Tchanturia K, Surguladze SA, David AS. Insight in eating disorders: clinical and cognitive correlates. *Psychol Med*. 2011;41(9):1951–1961.

64. Vigne P, de Menezes GB, Harrison BJ, Fontenelle LF. A study of poor insight in social anxiety disorder. *Psychiatry Res*. 2014;219(3):556–561.

65. Clarke RA, Lee S, Eapen V. Pathogenetic model for Tourette syndrome delineates overlap with related

neurodevelopmental disorders including Autism. *Transl Psychiatry*. 2012;2:e158.

66. Biomarkers Definitions Working Group. Biomarkers and surrogate endpoints: preferred definitions and conceptual framework. *Clin Pharmacol Ther*. 2001;69(3):89–95.
67. Hollander E, Braun A, Simeon D. Should OCD leave the anxiety disorders in DSM-V? The case for obsessive compulsive-related disorders. *Depress Anxiety*. 2008;25(4):317–329.
68. Frydman I, de Salles Andrade JB, Vigne P, Fontenelle LF. Can neuroimaging provide reliable biomarkers for obsessive-compulsive disorder? A narrative review. *Curr Psychiatry Rep*. 2016;18(10):90.
69. McGrath LM, Yu D, Marshall C, et al. Copy number variation in obsessive-compulsive disorder and Tourette syndrome: a cross-disorder study. *J Am Acad Child Adolesc Psychiatry*. 2014;53(8):910–919.
70. Gazzellone MJ, Zarrei M, Burton CL, et al. Uncovering obsessive-compulsive disorder risk genes in a pediatric cohort by high-resolution analysis of copy number variation. *J Neurodev Disord*. 2016;8(1):36.

Chapter 12

The Natural History of Obsessive-Compulsive Disorder across the Lifespan

Eesha Sharma and Y. C. Janardhan Reddy

Introduction

The course of psychiatric disorders begins with a phase of susceptibility, characterized by biological and environmental risk factors, followed by a stage of subclinical/prodromal symptoms, and then a stage of clinical manifestations [1]. Therapeutic interventions may abort further illness progression and lead to recovery; or the untreated disorder may proceed to lifelong disability with individual and environmental factors influencing fluctuations in severity [1]. Adequate understanding about the course of a disorder has diagnostic, prognostic, interventional and research implications. In this chapter, we critically review scientific literature on the course and outcome of obsessive-compulsive disorder (OCD) and related disorders (OCRDs). OCD, with a community prevalence between 0.5% and 3% [2,3,4], ranks among the top 10 causes of disability [5]. The disorder typically follows a chronic course with incomplete remissions [6], with help seeking delayed for several years [7]. This chapter aims to be an informative resource on the course and outcome of OCD and related disorders.

Measurement of Course and Outcome in Obsessive-Compulsive Disorder

For OCD, the 10-item Yale-Brown Obsessive-Compulsive Scale (Y-BOCS) with a maximum score of 40 is the gold-standard instrument for defining treatment outcomes [8,9]. Remission is defined as a reduction of the total Y-BOCS score to less than 16 or less than 12. Studies using signal detection analyses observed that a Y-BOCS score of 14 or lower best predicts remission, whereas a score of 12 or lower predicts "wellness" on quality of life measures [10]. According to the 2016 Delphi survey of experts, remission is defined as a Y-BOCS score of 12 or lower (Table 12.1) [11].

The Longitudinal Interval Follow-up Evaluation (LIFE) assesses illness course [12]. A semi-structured tool, LIFE can be used at variable time intervals (weekly, biweekly, six-monthly) to record outcome at a cross-sectional time point, and also course, incident life events, treatment and functioning. LIFE uses psychiatric status ratings (PSRs), which takes into account Y-BOCS scores to measure outcome. PSR1/PSR2 corresponds to "full remission" (Y-BOCS score less than 8), and PSR3 corresponds to partial remission (Y-BOCS score 8–15) [13].

Course and Outcome of Obsessive-Compulsive Disorder in Pre-Serotonin-Reuptake Inhibitor/Cognitive Behavioral Therapy Studies

The natural course of OCD is best depicted by studies published before the introduction of serotonin reuptake inhibitors (SRIs) and cognitive behavior therapy (CBT). In one review of 13 such studies, OCD had a favorable outcome with spontaneous remissions/recovery in almost one-third of patients [14]. Patients who were hospitalized had a chronic course with only one-third of them improving symptomatically, whereas outpatients had a rather good prognosis, with almost 60–80% "improved" 1–5 years after diagnosis. In the landmark 40-year follow-up of 141 patients, a majority (83%) improved and about half (48%) recovered with no clinically relevant symptoms for the preceding 5 years [15]. Early age at onset, presence of both obsessions and compulsions, low baseline social functioning, chronic course and magical obsessions predicted poor prognosis. The study findings appear optimistic, but one-fifth of the patients relapsed after remission for more than two decades. Thus, early recovery correlated with good prognosis but did not exclude the possibility of a later relapse.

Table 12.1 Consensus definitions and operationalization of treatment response, partial response, remission, recovery and relapse for obsessive-compulsive disorder (reproduced with permission from the lead author of the Delphi survey [11]).

	Conceptual Definition	Operationalization
Treatment response	A clinically meaningful reduction in symptoms (time, distress and interference associated with obsessions, compulsions and avoidance) relative to baseline severity in an individual who meets diagnostic criteria for OCD	A ≥ 35% reduction in (C) Y-BOCS scores plus CGI-I rating of 1 (very much improved) or 2 (much improved), lasting for at least 1 week
Partial response		A ≥ 25% but < 35% reduction in (C) Y-BOCS scores plus CGI-I rating of at least 3 (minimally improved), lasting for at least 1 week
Remission	The patient no longer meets syndromal criteria for the disorder and has no more than minimal symptoms. Residual obsessions, compulsions and avoidance may be present but are not time consuming and do not interfere with the person's everyday life	*If a structured diagnostic interview is feasible*, the person no longer meets diagnostic criteria for OCD for at least one week *If a structured diagnostic interview is not feasible*, a score of ≤ 12 on the (C) Y-BOCS plus CGI-S rating of 1 (normal, not at all ill) or 2 (borderline mentally ill), lasting for at least 1 week
Recovery	The patient no longer meets syndromal criteria for the disorder and has had no more than minimal symptoms. Residual obsessions, compulsions and avoidance may be present and slightly fluctuate in severity over time but, overall, they are not time consuming and do not interfere with the person's everyday life and therefore require no further treatment. The clinician may begin to consider discontinuation of treatment or, if the treatment continues, the aim is to prevent relapse	*If a structured diagnostic interview is feasible*, the person no longer meets diagnostic criteria for OCD for at least 1 year *If a structured diagnostic interview is not feasible*, a score of ≤ 12 on the (C) Y-BOCS plus CGI-S rating of 1 (normal, not at all ill' or 2 (borderline mentally ill), lasting for at least 1 year
Relapse	After response or remission or recovery was achieved, the patient experiences a return of symptoms. For patients who were in remission or recovered, obsessions, compulsions and avoidance are again sufficiently time consuming, distressing and impairing for the individual to meet diagnostic criteria for OCD	*For responders who did not necessarily remit/recover*: The person no longer meets the definition of ≥ 35% reduction on (C) Y-BOCS scores (relative to pre-treatment) plus CGI-I rating of 6 (much worse) or higher for at least 1 month *For remitters/recovered*: OCD criteria are met again, according to a structured interview (if feasible). Alternatively, the person no longer meets the definition of remission/recovery (i.e., the person again scores 13 or above on the (C) Y-BOCS) plus CGI-I rating of 6 (much worse) or higher for at least 1 month or needs to be withdrawn prematurely from the trial before 1 month has elapsed due to a severe worsening of OCD symptoms. Discontinuation of the trial due to reasons other than a worsening in OCD symptoms (e.g., suicide risk) is not considered a relapse

CGI-I, Clinical Global Impression Improvement; CGI-S, Clinical Global Impression Severity; (C) Y-BOCS, (Children's) Yale-Brown Obsessive Compulsive Scale; OCD, obsessive-compulsive disorder.

The ability to generalize from findings from these studies is limited due to methodological shortcomings such as lack of standardized diagnostic criteria, interview techniques and rating scales; inclusion of cases with obsessive-compulsive symptoms in the context of psychotic/mood disorders or non-OCD phobic disorders; unclear definitions of outcome; heterogeneous samples comprising outpatients, inpatients and patients treated psychosurgically; retrospective designs and varying durations of follow-up [16,17].

Course and Outcome of Obsessive-Compulsive Disorder in Recent Studies

Onset

Large clinical [16,18,19] and community samples [20,21] have reported mean age at onset of around 20 years, with peaks at 9–11 years and 20–23 years [22,23]. A juvenile (less than 18 years) onset is seen in 30–50% patients [18], while onset after the fourth decade occurs in less than 10% of cases [24,25]. Juvenile onset OCD is more familial [26,27], usually seen in males [19,25], and is associated with high rates of comorbid tic and attention deficit hyperactivity disorders [28]. A positive family history could contribute to anticipation in age at onset [29]. Adult onset OCD has equal gender distribution, and has high rate of comorbid mood, anxiety and substance use disorders [28]. Late onset OCD (i.e., after 30–40 years) has a female predominance [24,25].

Stressful life events have been associated with onset of OCD in 37–60% cases [30,31]. OCD starting within one year of a stressful life event is associated with an abrupt onset, overrepresentation in older women, history of obstetric complications, lower rates of family history of OCD and comorbidity with mood disorders [30,31]. Interestingly, gray-matter volume differences are seen between patients who have and have not experienced a stressful life event [32].

Course

OCD has an insidious onset and treatment is often delayed for years [33]. Duration of untreated illness, an important prognostic factor in psychotic disorders, does not seem to influence treatment outcome in OCD [33,34], but those with shorter duration of untreated illness have a later age at onset (over 20 years of age) and higher rates of mood/anxiety disorders and stressful life events [33]. Typically, OCD follows a chronic course (symptoms persistently present) spanning several decades, with waxing and waning severity [6,16]. However, an 11–13-year naturalistic follow-up of 75 patients from India who were largely treatment-naïve, and help-seeking, found a chronic course in only 24% of patients; 65% had "subclinical OCD" or "no OCD". Notably, 37% of patients were in "true remission" (no illness even when off treatment) for 11 years (median) [35]. Another study from the same center found a chronic course in less than 30% of patients [36].

Episodic OCD is associated with female gender [37,38], higher comorbidity with, and a higher family loading of, mood disorders [39,40], a later age at onset [37], autoimmune neuropsychiatric disorders [41], lesser compulsive symptoms [39] and possibly a better outcome [37]. Episodic course is less common in adult patients [35,42], whereas in children and adolescents it may be seen in 20–40% of patients [38]. In adults who have OCD comorbid with bipolar disorders, an episodic course may be seen in 75% of patients[42]; symptoms worsen with depression and improve with mania/hypomania [42]. OCD with bipolar disorder may be part of a bipolar diagnosis, rather than an independent entity.

Outcome

Naturalistic studies on patients treated with SRIs/CBT, followed up for at least one year are tabulated in Table 12.2 [13,17,21,35,36,43,44,45,46,47,48,49,50,51,52,53,54,55,56,57,58,59,60,61,62,63,64]. These studies differ in sample characteristics, outcome criteria and duration of follow-up. It is also evident from the table that remission rates in long-term follow-up studies vary widely, from 12% [17] to 76% [35].

We meta-analyzed 17 long-term studies on adult (18 years and over) patients with OCD treated with SRIs/CBT, followed-up for 1 year or more [16]. Primary outcome measure was rate of remission (i.e., Y-BOCS score < 16 at follow-up) [65]. The pooled sample size was 1265. Follow-up duration ranged from 1 to 15 years, average around 5 years. Pooled mean duration of illness was 14 years and pooled mean baseline Y-BOCS score was 24. We could not control for treatment since it varied among studies. However, 60–90% of patients were reportedly on treatment. The pooled rate of remission was 53%. Interestingly, studies from our center in India had a higher rate of remission (71%) than from predominantly Western countries (48%). Better outcome from our center could be related to sample characteristics (self-referred, drug-naïve, outpatient, shorter illness duration, low comorbidity rates and moderate illness severity) and, perhaps, as yet unexplored cultural factors. The meta-analysis was optimistic in that approximately 50% of patients achieved remission. However, there were few data on quality of life and functioning.

Most long-term outcome studies, including those in the meta-analysis, focused on a treatment-seeking population. Fineberg et al. have reported outcomes over 30 years in a community sample, recruited at age 19–20 years [66]. Serial interviews showed that 63.5% of those with OCD and 81.5% of those with sub-threshold obsessive-compulsive syndrome attained complete remission. Remission in this study was defined as complete absence of obsessive-compulsive symptoms over three consecutive years. Mean age at remission, for OCD and sub-threshold obsessive-compulsive syndrome, lay in the late-30s and mid-30s, respectively.

Predictors of Outcome in OCD

In our meta-analysis, meta-regression revealed four predictors of outcome – age at onset, gender, duration of illness and baseline illness severity [16]. However, predictors of outcome for OCD are generally inconsistent [16]. Table 12.3 summarizes some of the predictors of outcome in OCD. Of all the predictors studied, early onset [16], longer duration of illness [13,16,51], greater baseline symptom severity [13,16,51,67], poor insight [68], certain symptoms (especially hoarding and tics) [69,70,71], family accommodation [63] and the presence of certain personality disorders [72] such as schizotypal [73] and obsessive-compulsive personality disorder [74], seem to be the most consistent in predicting poor outcome. Similarly, lower baseline severity, good initial treatment response [56,64], full remission of symptoms and long-term treatment with SRIs [75,76,77] predicted good outcome.

Course and Outcome of Obsessive-Compulsive Disorder in Children

The prevalence of OCD in children and adolescents (1–3%) is comparable to that in adults [78,79]. Adults with OCD usually report an onset in late adolescence or early adulthood. This suggests that in a sizeable proportion, childhood onset OCD does not persist into adulthood. Data from follow-up studies in children also suggest that the outcome of childhood OCD may not be all that pessimistic. A meta-analysis of 16 long-term follow-up studies of pediatric-onset OCD found that 60% of the sample had at least a partial remission from illness [80]. Inpatient care, earlier age at onset and longer illness duration at baseline were associated with persistent illness at follow-up.

The largest follow-up study on childhood-onset OCD ($n = 142$) found that 60% of the sample remitted at five years, even though only 50% of the sample was on any treatment [81]. Duration of illness predicted illness persistence. Those with comorbid tic disorder had lower rates of persistence. Interestingly, this study found that other anxiety disorders were present at follow-up in approximately 40% of individuals. A study that compared 60 adolescents and 221 adults over three years of follow-up found that rate of "at least partial remission" increased in the youth from 9% at six months to 53% at three years, whereas in the adult group this change was only from 11% to 34% [82]. A shorter latency to initial treatment and lesser baseline functional impairment predicted better outcome in the youth.

Course and Outcome of Obsessive-Compulsive Disorder in the Elderly

There is a paucity of literature on course and outcome in the elderly. Onset of OCD after the sixth decade is rare, usually occurring in the context of neurological illnesses [83]. Symptoms usually remit with treatment of the primary illness [84].

Course and Outcome of Obsessive-Compulsive Related Disorders

Body Dysmorphic Disorder

In a retrospective follow-up study of 95 patients with BDD, 17% attained full remission and 38% attained partial remission by the end of four years [85]. Although a majority of treated patients improved at some time during the follow-up, improvement was usually partial with frequent relapses. Longer duration of treatment predicted remission from illness while higher baseline severity, comorbid depression and social anxiety predicted poor outcome. In a four-year prospective follow-up of 183 patients, with 84% of the sample on treatment, over 80% reported a *continuous* course, with less than one month of remission [86,87]. Remission rates increased from 9% at one year to 20% at four years. While more than 50% of the individuals reported at least a partial remission of illness, probability of relapse was over 60%. In an eight-year follow-up of 22 patients, only 13% remitted at one year; at eight years, 75% of patients reported full recovery at some time during the course with a subsequent 14% probability of relapse [88]. Baseline severity and a longer duration of illness predicted poorer outcome [87,88]. Importantly, gender, age at onset, "delusionality" of the BDD beliefs and comorbidities did not affect long-term outcome [86]. From the available data, we conclude that BDD begins in adolescence, and follows a continuous course with remissions and frequent relapses.

Hoarding Disorder

The age at *onset* of hoarding is similar to OCD [70,89,90], but the two differ in the age at *presentation*. Typical age at presentation in hoarders is around

Table 12.2 Recent long-term naturalistic follow-up studies in obsessive-compulsive disorder.

Study	Patients (n)	Sample characteristics	Follow-up duration (years)	Design	Age (years) mean ± SD	Age at onset (years) mean ± SD
Cottraux 1993 [43]	33	Treatment seeking	1.5	P	~35	
Orloff 1994 [45]	85	Treatment seeking	2	R	38.3 ± 10.5	17.2 ± 8.9
Mundo 1995 [44]	105	Treatment seeking	1	P	34.3 ± 12.6	20.7 ± 10
Eisen 1999 [17]	66	Treatment seeking	2	P		
Zitterl 2000 [46]	70	Treatment seeking Comorbid depression in 63.5%	1.5	P	34.9 ± 13.1	
Alonso 2001 [47]	60	Treatment seeking 36.7% treatment resistant	2.5	P	30.2 ± 10	17.5 ± 7.6
Hembree 2003 [49]	62	Treatment seeking	1–1.5	P	35.1 ± 10.5	-
Rufer 2005 [50]	30	Treatment seeking	7	R	32.4 ± 9.2	24 ± 9.3
Biondi 2005 [48]	32	Treatment seeking	2	P	32	
Reddy 2005 [35]	75	Largely self-referred (84%), drug-naïve (72%), outpatients (80%)	12	R	30.1 ± 9.5	24.5 ± 9.5
van Oppen 2005 [53]	102	Treatment seeking;	5	P	36.2 ± 10.7	

Duration of illness (years) mean ± SD	Baseline Y-BOCS mean ± SD	Treatment	Outcome	Notes
13		SRIs ± ERP	All followed up patients improved	No difference among SRI, ERP and placebo
	23.7 ± 6.7	SRIs ± augmentation ± BT	Y-BOCS score reduction > 75% in 33% 50–75% in 31% 25–49% in 24% < 24% in 9%	Effect size for improvement > 2
13.3 ± 10.7	24.2 ± 8.2	SRIs	Y-BOCS score reduction > 75% in 18% 50–75% in 25.7% 25–49%in 21.9% < 24% in 30.4%	
		SRI in 77% BT in 18%	Full remission in 12% Partial remission in 47%	48% relapsed after achieving remission
	23.8 ± 5.3	SRI + CBT	> 25% Y-BOCS score reduction in 43% Y-BOCS < 16 in 31%	Comorbid depression did not influence outcome
11.9 ± 10.1	24.7±6.6	SRIs ± CBT High doses in resistant cases	63.3% responders (Y-BOCS < 16 OR score reduced ≥ 35%)	Non-responders had more sexual/religious obsessions
13.6 ± 11.0		39% SRIs; 61% ERP ± SRIs	50% (SRIs only) – 70% (ERP ± SRIs) response rates	Response rates higher in the ERP groups even after medication discontinuation
8.3 ± 7.3	27.6 ± 4.3	CBT ± SRI	60% responded (Y-BOCS reduction ≥ 35%) 43% remitted (Y-BOCS < 16)	37% patients re-hospitalized during follow-up had higher depression scores, and were more likely to be unmarried. 30% patients did not take treatment during follow-up: depression scores higher in those who continued medication
>5	21.7	73% SRIs 27% SRIs + CBT	62.5% remitted	Rate of relapse in SRI alone group double that of combined treatment group. Time to relapse around 2 years in SRI alone group, vs 11 years in integrated treatment group
3		SRIs + CBT	76% No OCD or subclinical OCD 37% in "true remission" for 11 years	At follow-up 71% not on treatment for ~8 years. Good outcome correlated with functional recovery
12.8 ± 10.3	25.3 ± 7	SRIs/CBT/combination	73% recovered (Y-BOCS ≤ 12)	Treatment dropouts also showed a significant change in symptom status, but less than treatment completers

(*continued*)

Table 12.2 *(cont.)*

Study	Patients (n)	Sample characteristics	Follow-up duration (years)	Design	Age (years) mean ± SD	Age at onset (years) mean ± SD
Catapano 2006 [51]	55	73.4% treated earlier; < 20% adequately treated	3	P	31.5 ± 10.3	22.5 ± 8.9
Math 2007 [36]	77	50% 'mixed' and 50% 'pure obsessional' OCD	5	R	36.3 ± 11.04	22.9 ± 9.66
Olsen 2008 [52]	25	Treatment seeking outpatients at a private clinic 52% treated earlier	3.5	R	33	24 ± 10.3
Whittal 2008 [60] (Sample 1)	41		2	P	36.1 ± 11.4	23.4 ± 13.9
Whittal 2008 [60] (Sample 2)	45		2	P	35.4 ± 9.82	22.5 ± 9.9
Reddy 2010 [59]	36	Treatment resistant sample (≥ 2 SRI trials)	4.5	R	29.77 ± 8.27	16.58 ± 5.85
Braga 2010 [56]	42	Comorbidities in 80% 40.5% on long term treatment	1	P	36.8 ± 13.2	14.8 ± 6.9
Cabedo 2010 [57]	36		1	P	34.16 ± 8.61	
Anholt 2011 [55]	121	Comorbidities in 44.6% 67.8% treated earlier Pure obsessional OCD excluded from study	5.5	R	35.1 ± 10.7	
Anand 2011 [54]	26	Medication 'non-responders' (treatment ≥ 1year, inadequate response to at least 2 adequate SRI trials, Y-BOCS ≥ 20); Comorbidities in 71%	1	P	29.87 ± 8.16	19.48 ± 6.13

Duration of illness (years) mean ± SD	Baseline Y-BOCS mean ± SD	Treatment	Outcome	Notes
8.9 ± 6.5	27.1 ± 6.5	SRIs	Probability of remission increased from 42% at 1 year to 65% at 3 years 'Full remission' increased from 10% after 1 year to 38% at 3years	Of those who did not respond to first SRI (~70%), 31.6% responded to 2nd and 10.5% to ≥ 3 trials Of those who achieved at least partial remission 38% relapsed at 1 year and 60% at 3 years Symptom severity predicted poor outcome
		Largely SRIs; < 20% on CBT	70% remitted 26% in 'true remission'	Similar course and outcome in mixed and pure obsessional OCD
10.6 ± 10.9	21.7 ± 7.5	CBT ± SRIs	Y-BOCS score reduction: ≥ 70% in 50% 31–69% in 28%	Symptom reduction correlated with functional recovery
13.1 ± 11.8			61% maintained recovery (Y-BOCS < 12)	Study comparing maintenance of treatment gains after individual vs. group CBT; Only those who responded to initial treatment were followed up; 55–60% were on SRIs at follow-up; change in medication or medication status were not related to outcome; relapse rates 8.1%; Thus, 40–60% of those who responded to treatment sustained improvement over ~2 years
13 ± 8.9		CBT ± SRIs	40% maintained recovery (Y-BOCS < 12)	
8.74 ± 6.03	27.36 ± 6.73	SRI/CBT	39% at least partially remitted	Long duration of illness, poor quality of life at baseline, not having received CBT and age at onset were associated with poor outcome
21.5 ± 11.6	25.6 ± 5.29	CBT ± SRIs	76% had at least partial remission at 1 year (Y-BOCS reduction ≥ 35% + CGI = 2) 38% showed 'full remission' (Y-BOCS ≥ 8 + CGI < 2)	Study on maintenance of treatment gains after group CBT; 35.5% relapsed in follow-up; relapse rates were higher in those with <54% reduction in Y-BOCS score after treatment; baseline severity, age at onset and comorbidity did not influence relapse rates
9.4 ± 10.04	25.36 ± 5.67	CBT	67% remission (Y-BOCS ≥ 12)	
	24.94 ± 6.95	CT/BT/SRI or combination		Long-term outcome not affected by baseline severity of OCD or depression
> 10	32.09 ± 4.17	SRI + CBT	61% responders 48% remitters (Y-BOCS < 16)	Open label study – generalizability limited; but emphasizes utility of combination treatment even in non-responders; quality of homework compliance predicted remission

(continued)

Table 12.2 *(cont.)*

Study	Patients (n)	Sample characteristics	Follow-up duration (years)	Design	Age (years) mean ± SD	Age at onset (years) mean ± SD
Marcks 2011 [58]	42	Treatment seeking Comorbid anxiety disorders in 78%	15	P	35.21 ± 11.9	17.42 ± 10.44
Jakubovski 2013 [64]	75	Drug-naïve Comorbidities in 87.5%	2	P	33.6 ± 10.6	12.8 ± 8.2
Bloch 2013 [61]	83		11	R	42 ± 9.9	23.4 ± 7.9
Eisen 2013 [13]	213	Treatment seeking	5	P	39.8 ± 12.8	17.9 ± 9.5
Fineberg 2013 [66]	30	Community sample	30	P	19–20	18
Cherian 2014 [62]	106	Treatment seeking Juvenile (< 18) onset in 46%; 41% drug-naïve Comorbidities in 64%	4	P	28.05 ± 9.06	21.09 ± 7.58

Duration of illness (years) mean ± SD	Baseline Y-BOCS mean ± SD	Treatment	Outcome	Notes
17.89 ± 11.84		SRIs/CBT/both	Remission (PSR1 for ≥ 8 weeks) – 16% at year 1 to 42% at year 15	Recurrence (PSR3 for ≥ 4 weeks) in those with full remission 7% at 1 year to 25% later on. Not being married, receiving SRIs at intake (correlated with severity) and comorbid depression predicted poor outcome
20.9 ± 10.6	26.3 ± 5.4	SRIs/CBT/both	50.1% responders (Y-BOCS reduction ≥ 35%) 21.3% remitters (Y-BOCS < 8)	Response at 12 weeks predicted response at 2 years; From the baseline sample 42.6% responders at 2 years. Comorbid disorders, baseline depression severity, duration of illness >30 years, family history of anxiety or tics associated with poor outcome; Later age at onset associated with better outcome
15.9 ± 11.9		SRIs/CBT/both	20% remitters (Y-BOCS < 8) 31% – subclinical OCD (Y-BOCS 8–15)	Initial response to SRIs predicted remission at follow-up
21.9 ± 13.6	23.4 ± 5.7	SRIs/CBT/ both	39% had at least partial remission	Lower baseline severity, shorter duration of illness, 'over-responsibility' predicted remission. Hoarding associated with poor outcome 59% of remitters relapsed; partial remitters and comorbid OCPD more likely to relapse
		One-third *professionally treated*	63.5%	Studied both OCD and "OCS"; i.e., subthreshold cases. 81.5% remission rate in subthreshold cases. Remission defined as *complete absence of symptoms for 3 years.*
6.89 ± 6.70	23.25 ± 7.07	SRIs	53% full remission (Y-BOCS < 8) 28% partial remission (Y-BOCS 8–15)	Cumulative Probability of *at least partial remission* increased from 70% at 1 year to 93% at 5 years Cumulative probability of full remission increased from 53% at 1 year to 65% at 5 years Probability of relapse in those who at least achieved partial remission increased from 13% at 1 year to 36% at 5 years Drug-naïve status at baseline and percentage of time on treatment predicted *at least partial remission;* percentage of time on treatment predicted full remission Doubts/checking symptoms and achieving full remission associated with lesser likelihood of relapse Most patients who remitted did so in the first two years

(continued)

Table 12.2 *(cont.)*

Study	Patients (n)	Sample characteristics	Follow-up duration (years)	Design	Age (years) mean ± SD	Age at onset (years) mean ± SD
Cherian 2014 [63]	94	39% drug-naive at baseline; 52% with juvenile onset (< 18) Comorbidities in 48%	1	P	27.6 ± 8.5	19.8 ± 7

BT, behavioral therapy; CBT, cognitive behavioral therapy; CT, cognitive therapy; ERP, exposure and response prevention; OCD, obsessive-compulsive disorder; OCPD, obsessive-compulsive personality disorder; OCS, obsessive-compulsive symptoms; OR, odds ratio; PSR, psychiatric status rating SD, standard deviation; SRIs, serotonin reuptake inhibitors; Y-BOCS, Yale-Brown Obsessive Compulsive Scale.

Table 12.3 Predictors of outcome in obsessive-compulsive disorder.

Type	Predictors of Good Outcome	Predictors of Poor Outcome
Sociodemographic	1. Being married [50,58]	1. Pediatric (around adolescence) onset of illness [16] 2. Male gender [16,17]
Illness characteristics	1. Over-responsibility as primary symptom [13] 2. Doubts/checking symptoms [62]	1. Longer duration [13,16,51] 2. Greater baseline severity [13,16,51,67] 3. Mixed subtype of OCD [35] 4. Lack of insight [68] 5. Sexual/religious obsessions [47,69] 6. Washing compulsions [69] 7. Hoarding [70,89,91] 8. Continuous course (vs. episodic) [37]
Treatment	1. Robust initial treatment response [56,64] 2. 'Full remission' [61,62] 3. Continued treatment with SRIs [75,76]	1. Discontinuation of SRI [77]
Comorbid disorders		1. Depression [58,64] 2. Schizotypal disorder [73] 3. Any lifetime axis I comorbidity [35,64] 4. Chronic tic disorder [71] 5. Borderline/avoidant/paranoid/OCPD [72,74]
Other factors	1. Combination treatment with SRIs and CBT [48]	1. Family accommodation & Involvement behaviors [63]

OCD, obsessive-compulsive disorder; OCPD, obsessive-compulsive personality disorder; SRI, serotonin reuptake inhibitor.

Duration of illness (years) mean ± SD	Baseline Y-BOCS mean ± SD	Treatment	Outcome	Notes
7.9 ± 7	27.7 ± 5.8	SRIs ± CBT	58% in remission (Y-BOCS < 16)	Probability of remission increased from 23% at 3 months to 58% at 12 months 11% of those who achieved remission relapsed Mean duration to achieve remission ~7 months Non-remitters had higher family accommodation, lesser sexual obsessions, greater illness severity and functional impairment at baseline. Lower family accommodation, sexual obsessions and percentage time on treatment predicted time to remission. Long duration of illness, comorbidities were negatively associated with time to remission

40 years [91], whereas those with OCD typically seek help in their 20s and 30s. The presence of hoarding, generally associated with poor insight and comorbidities, is related with poorer response to treatment [92]. In the Brazilian clinical cohort of 1000 patients with OCD, those with hoarding had a "worsening with later plateau" or a "constant" course, whereas those with other symptom dimensions had higher rates of "episodic" and "waxing–waning" course [70]. Reports from follow-up of hoarders corroborate a chronic unremitting course in 70–80% of patients [89,91]. In a study of hoarding with or without OCD, CBT was effective in more than 60% of patients and the gains were maintained at 3–12 months [93]. There is a need to study the clinical features, course, treatment–response and outcome of hoarding disorder as defined in DSM-5.

Trichotillomania and Skin-Picking Disorder

Trichotillomania and skin-picking disorder have similar clinical profiles [94]. Trichotillomania has three peaks in age at onset of symptoms – early childhood, adolescence and adulthood [95,96]. Early childhood onset, developmentally related to normative tactile exploration by children, is a benign self-remitting habit similar to thumb sucking [95,97,98]. The most typical age at onset of trichotillomania is late childhood or early adolescence [94,99]. The disorder usually follows a chronic, relapsing course spanning decades; a large proportion of patients do not seek help [100,101]. Prevalence of clinically significant skin picking ranges from 1% to 5% [94]. Skin picking is frequently comorbid with disorders like BDD and trichotillomania; it could start in childhood, adolescence or later and follows a chronic course with fluctuations [102].

A Transdiagnostic Approach in Obsessive-Compulsive Disorder and Obsessive-Compulsive and Related Disorders

OCD and OCRDs have distinctive but overlapping clinical presentations. It is evident that several aspects of these illnesses may have a transdiagnostic valence with potential impact on classification, clinical management and research.

Age at Onset and Etiopathological Basis of Illness

OCD and OCRDs typically start at a young age. Studies have shown that childhood onset OCD has a somewhat benign course with a high likelihood of remission before adulthood. Childhood-onset OCD is also more commonly associated with attention deficit hyperactivity disorder and tic disorders. These phenomena suggest that childhood-onset OCRDs could have a developmental etiology. However, since they occur at a critical life stage, they could influence long-term developmental outcomes. Adolescent or adult onset is commonly found in treatment-seeking populations, suggesting that onset at this age is more likely to lead to persistent illness. An onset after 30–40 years of age may be influenced by pre-existing psychopathology, such as mood disorders, or neuropathology, as is the case with OCD in the elderly population, and environmental factors such as stressful life events. One might ask – is there a shift in the etiopathological basis from a primary pathology that is more genetic and developmental in childhood to a secondary pathology that is more environmental and neurological in late adulthood? Neuroimaging studies show differential age trajectories in the growth of individual brain regions that could influence gene–brain–environment interactions in the pathogenesis of mental disorders [103]. These transdiagnostic observations have implications for neurobiological enquiry and treatment decisions.

'Course of Illness' as a Specifier

Current classificatory systems have specifiers alongside diagnostic criteria. The ICD-11 guidelines [104,105] and the DSM-5 [6] have insight specifiers but no course specifiers. The proposed modifications to diagnostic guidelines for OCD in ICD-11 discuss the pros and cons of different illness specifiers that have been researched in terms of their nosological and clinical utility [105]. *Course of illness* was considered a potential specifier for OCD but was not recommended for inclusion because of factors that may have contributed to varying courses reported across different studies. These factors include heterogeneity in samples studied, varying definitions of course and outcome, associated comorbidity, nature of treatment received and length of follow-up. It was thought that there was lack of clear data to support clinical utility of a course specifier. However, we think there is a case for using a uniform course specifier for all disorders now classified under OCRD because of their somewhat similar course over the long run. This has been established with some clarity in OCD, BDD and trichotillomania [16,88,100] while the data on other categories are limited.

The disorders seem to run a varying course, some people remitting fully and some partially, while others run an episodic or a chronic course with remissions and relapses, much the same as in other psychiatric illnesses such as schizophrenia. It is now well recognized that the course specifier for schizophrenia in DSM-IV and DSM-5 has enormous clinical utility. For example, treatment strategy for a first episode of schizophrenia that remits fully is different from that for schizophrenia that is either chronic or has multiple relapses [106]. Similarly, the course specifier for OCRDs may have important implications for both clinical and research purposes. OCRD that remits completely following treatment may not require long-term treatment with medications. In the Indian data, a significant proportion of patients were asymptomatic for many years without any form of long-term maintenance treatment, implying that indefinite long-term treatment may not be required for all [35,107]. OCD that runs an episodic course when comorbid with bipolar disorder is perhaps primarily a mood disorder that needs to be treated primarily with mood stabilizers and not SSRIs [42]. Although the data on OCRDs other than OCD are limited, there is a reason to believe that a course specifier may also be useful for the other categories.

A transdiagnostic approach toward the course of an illness may also be useful for identifying a distinct and shared neural basis for these disorders that in turn may influence treatment choices. Categorical classificatory systems serve the purpose of enhancing reliability in diagnosis [108] and help to generate evidence-based treatments, but have not been very successful in aiding our understanding of the relationship between psychopathology and underlying neurobiological mechanisms [109]. Today, there is an attempt to understand the neurobiological processes of clinical phenomenology cutting across diagnostic categories within the OCRDs and other similar categories such as behavioral addictions and eating disorders [110]. While these efforts are primarily focused on understanding the neurobiological processes behind constructs such as compulsivity–impulsivity, indecision, obsessionality–delusionality and cognitive-motor aspects of phenomenology that cut across diagnostic categories, there is perhaps a need to explore beyond phenomenology and examine whether different courses have something shared and distinct. Such an approach would be in accordance with that recently proposed by the Research Domain

Criteria [111] and the Roadmap for Mental Health Research in Europe [112].

A Case for Early Intervention

There is indirect evidence from naturalistic studies of OCD that those with a shorter duration of illness have a better outcome if treated early [16]. Therefore, it is possible to speculate that initiating treatment early in the course of illness may modify the course by preventing relapses. The OCRDs that remit completely may also be neurobiologically distinct from the disorders that do not remit, and these mechanisms could be similar across the OCRDs that share many phenotypic characteristics.

Summary

A review of natural history of OCD reveals that, in most patients, illness starts in adolescence and persists into adulthood. Childhood-onset OCD, although not unusual, has a substantial rate of remission by adulthood. OCD in adults tends to run a chronic course with fluctuations in symptom severity. Modern treatments (SRIs and CBT) are efficacious in improving short-term outcomes. While a handful of studies demonstrate their long-term effects, these are yet to be clearly enunciated.

It is interesting to note that long-term outcomes of OCD were not all that pessimistic, even prior to the advent of effective treatments. There is variability in the course and outcome of illnesses reported in naturalistic long-term follow-up studies, possibly due to methodological differences and varying duration of follow-up and treatment. Although no consistent predictors of long-term course and outcome are identified, it appears that those with a less severe, short-duration illness may have a favorable outcome.

Those who respond early, achieve remission and continue to receive long-term treatment also seem to do well in the long run. What is unclear from the data is the differential effects of individual treatments, or their combinations, on the course of illness. With new inroads into biological psychiatry, the future may lead us to harder markers for predicting outcome. Our meta-analysis of long-term studies has indicated that outcome of OCD could be better in India, a finding that needs to be replicated in larger and diverse samples from India.

OCRDs are no less common in clinical practice, but surprisingly the data on the naturalistic course and outcome of these disorders are scarce. With the publication of DSM-5 and inclusion of these disorders as disorders related to OCD, we could hope for a spurt in literature in the next decade or so. However, from what we know, it appears that all OCRDs run a chronic course similar to OCD.

In conclusion, there is a need for large well-conducted multicenter studies on course and outcome of OCD and OCRDs, with uniformity in assessment and follow-up methods across cohorts.

References

1. Strauss JS, Hafez H, Lieberman P, Harding CM. The course of psychiatric disorder, III: longitudinal principles. *Am J Psychiatry.* 1985;142:289–296.
2. Fontenelle LF, Mendlowicz MV, Versiani M. The descriptive epidemiology of obsessive-compulsive disorder. *Prog Neuropsychopharmacol Biol Psychiatry.* 2006;30:327–337.
3. Gururaj G, Varghese M, Benegal V, et al. *National Mental Health Survey of India, 2015–16: Summary Report.* Bengaluru: National Institute of Mental Health and Neurosciences; 2016.
4. Jaisoorya TS, Reddy YCJ, Nair BS, et al. Prevalence and correlates of obsessive-compulsive disorder and subthreshold obsessive-compulsive disorder among college students in Kerala, India. *Indian J Psychiatry.* 2017;59:56–62.
5. Eaton WW, Martins SS, Nestadt G, et al. The burden of mental disorders. *Epidemiol Rev.* 2008;30:1–14.
6. American Psychiatric Association. *Diagnostic and Statistical Manual of Mental Disorders*, 5th ed. Washington, DC: APA; 2013.
7. Dell'Osso B, Benatti B, Oldani L, Spagnolin G, Altamura AC. Differences in duration of untreated illness, duration, and severity of illness among clinical phenotypes of obsessive-compulsive disorder. *CNS Spectr.* 2015;20:474–478.
8. Goodman WK, Price LH, Rasmussen SA, et al. The Yale-Brown Obsessive Compulsive Scale. I. Development, use, and reliability. *Arch Gen Psychiatry.* 1989;46:1006–1011.
9. Goodman WK, Price LH, Rasmussen SA, et al. The Yale-Brown Obsessive Compulsive Scale. II. Validity. *Arch Gen Psychiatry.* 1989;46:1012–1016.
10. Farris SG, McLean CP, Van Meter PE, Simpson HB, Foa EB. Treatment response, symptom remission, and wellness in obsessive-compulsive disorder. *J Clin Psychiatry.* 2013;74:685–690.
11. Mataix-Cols D, Fernandez de la Cruz L, Nordsletten AE, et al. Towards an international expert consensus

for defining treatment response, remission, recovery and relapse in obsessive-compulsive disorder. *World Psychiatry.* 2016;15:80–81.

12. Keller MB, Lavori PW, Friedman B, et al. The Longitudinal Interval Follow-up Evaluation. A comprehensive method for assessing outcome in prospective longitudinal studies. *Arch Gen Psychiatry.* 1987;44:540–548.
13. Eisen JL, Sibrava NJ, Boisseau CL, et al. Five-year course of obsessive-compulsive disorder: predictors of remission and relapse. *J Clin Psychiatry.* 2013;74:233–239.
14. Goodwin DW, Guze SB, Robins E. Follow-up studies in obsessional neurosis. *Arch Gen Psychiatry.* 1969;20:182–187.
15. Skoog G, Skoog I. A 40-year follow-up of patients with obsessive-compulsive disorder. *Arch Gen Psychiatry.* 1999;56:121–127.
16. Sharma E, Thennarasu K, Reddy YC. Long-term outcome of obsessive-compulsive disorder in adults: a meta-analysis. *J Clin Psychiatry.* 2014;75:1019–1027.
17. Eisen JL, Goodman WK, Keller MB, et al. Patterns of remission and relapse in obsessive-compulsive disorder: a 2-year prospective study. *J Clin Psychiatry.* 1999;60:346–351.
18. Dell'Osso B, Benatti B, Buoli M, et al. The influence of age at onset and duration of illness on long-term outcome in patients with obsessive-compulsive disorder: a report from the International College of Obsessive Compulsive Spectrum Disorders (ICOCS). *Eur Neuropsychopharmacol.* 2013;23:865–871.
19. Dell'Osso B, Benatti B, Hollander E, et al. Childhood, adolescent and adult age at onset and related clinical correlates in obsessive-compulsive disorder: a report from the International College of Obsessive-Compulsive Spectrum Disorders (ICOCS). *Int J Psychiatry Clin Pract.* 2016;20:210–217.
20. Burke KC, Burke JD, Jr, Regier DA, Rae DS. Age at onset of selected mental disorders in five community populations. *Arch Gen Psychiatry.* 1990;47:511–518.
21. Angst J, Gamma A, Endrass J, et al. Obsessive-compulsive severity spectrum in the community: prevalence, comorbidity, and course. *Eur Arch Psychiatry Clin Neurosci.* 2004;254:156–164.
22. Delorme R, Golmard JL, Chabane N, et al. Admixture analysis of age at onset in obsessive-compulsive disorder. *Psychol Med.* 2005;35:237–243.
23. De Luca V, Gershenzon V, Burroughs E, Javaid N, Richter MA. Age at onset in Canadian OCD patients: mixture analysis and systematic comparison with other studies. *J Affect Disord.* 2011;133:300–304.
24. Frydman I, do Brasil PE, Torres AR, et al. Late-onset obsessive-compulsive disorder: risk factors and correlates. *J Psychiatr Res.* 2014;49:68–74.
25. Sharma E, Shyam Sundar A, Thennarasu K, Reddy YCJ. Is late-onset OCD a distinct phenotype? Findings from a comparative analysis of age-at-onset groups. *CNS Spectrums.* 2015;20:508–514.
26. Chabane N, Delorme R, Millet B, et al. Early-onset obsessive-compulsive disorder: a subgroup with a specific clinical and familial pattern? *J Child Psychol Psychiatry.* 2005;46:881–887.
27. Arumugham SS, Cherian AV, Baruah U, et al. Comparison of clinical characteristics of familial and sporadic obsessive-compulsive disorder. *Compr Psychiatry.* 2014;55:1520–1525.
28. de Mathis MA, Diniz JB, Hounie AG, et al. Trajectory in obsessive-compulsive disorder comorbidities. *Eur Neuropsychopharmacol.* 2013;23:594–601.
29. Cavallini MC, Albertazzi M, Bianchi L, Bellodi L. Anticipation of age at onset of obsessive-compulsive spectrum disorders in patients with obsessive-compulsive disorder. *Psychiatry Res.* 2002;111:1–9.
30. Real E, Labad J, Alonso P, et al. Stressful life events at onset of obsessive-compulsive disorder are associated with a distinct clinical pattern. *Depress Anxiety.* 2011;28:367–376.
31. Rosso G, Albert U, Asinari GF, Bogetto F, Maina G. Stressful life events and obsessive-compulsive disorder: clinical features and symptom dimensions. *Psychiatry Res.* 2012;197:259–264.
32. Real E, Subira M, Alonso P, et al. Brain structural correlates of obsessive-compulsive disorder with and without preceding stressful life events. *World J Biol Psychiatry.* 2016;17:366–377.
33. Poyraz CA, Turan S, Saglam NG, et al. Factors associated with the duration of untreated illness among patients with obsessive compulsive disorder. *Compr Psychiatry.* 2015;58:88–93.
34. Dell'Osso B, Buoli M, Hollander E, Altamura AC. Duration of untreated illness as a predictor of treatment response and remission in obsessive-compulsive disorder. *World J Biol Psychiatry.* 2010;11:59–65.
35. Reddy YC, D'Souza SM, Shetti C, et al. An 11- to 13-year follow-up of 75 subjects with obsessive-compulsive disorder. *J Clin Psychiatry.* 2005;66:744–749.
36. Math SB, Thoduguli J, Janardhan Reddy YC, et al. A 5-year course of predominantly obsessive vs. mixed subtypes of obsessive-compulsive disorder. *Indian J Psychiatry.* 2007;49:250–255.
37. Ravizza L, Maina G, Bogetto F. Episodic and chronic obsessive-compulsive disorder. *Depress Anxiety.* 1997;6:154–158.

38. Thomsen PH. Obsessive-compulsive disorder in children and adolescents: predictors in childhood for long-term phenomenological course. *Acta Psychiatr Scand.* 1995;92:255–259.

39. Tukel R, Oflaz SB, Ozyildirim I, et al. Comparison of clinical characteristics in episodic and chronic obsessive-compulsive disorder. *Depress Anxiety.* 2007;24:251–255.

40. Zutshi A, Kamath P, Reddy YC. Bipolar and nonbipolar obsessive-compulsive disorder: a clinical exploration. *Compr Psychiatry.* 2007;48:245–251.

41. Leonard HL, Swedo SE. Paediatric autoimmune neuropsychiatric disorders associated with streptococcal infection (PANDAS). *Int J Neuropsychopharmacol.* 2001;4:191–198.

42. Amerio A, Odone A, Liapis CC, Ghaemi SN. Diagnostic validity of comorbid bipolar disorder and obsessive-compulsive disorder: a systematic review. *Acta Psychiatr Scand.* 2014;129:343–358.

43. Cottraux J, Mollard E, Bouvard M, Marks I. Exposure therapy, fluvoxamine, or combination treatment in obsessive-compulsive disorder: one-year followup. *Psychiatry Res.* 1993;49:63–75.

44. Mundo E, Erzegovesi S, Bellodi L. Follow-up of obsessive-compulsive patients treated with proserotonergic agents. *J Clin Psychopharmacol.* 1995;15:288–289.

45. Orloff LM, Battle MA, Baer L, et al. Long-term follow-up of 85 patients with obsessive-compulsive disorder. *Am J Psychiatry.* 1994;151:441–442.

46. Zitterl W, Demal U, Aigner M, et al. Naturalistic course of obsessive compulsive disorder and comorbid depression. Longitudinal results of a prospective follow-up study of 74 actively treated patients. *Psychopathology.* 2000;33:75–80.

47. Alonso P, Menchon JM, Pifarre J, et al. Long-term follow-up and predictors of clinical outcome in obsessive-compulsive patients treated with serotonin reuptake inhibitors and behavioral therapy. *J Clin Psychiatry.* 2001;62:535–540.

48. Biondi M, Picardi A. Increased maintenance of obsessive-compulsive disorder remission after integrated serotonergic treatment and cognitive psychotherapy compared with medication alone. *Psychother Psychosom.* 2005;74:123–128.

49. Hembree EA, Riggs DS, Kozak MJ, Franklin ME, Foa EB. Long-term efficacy of exposure and ritual prevention therapy and serotonergic medications for obsessive-compulsive disorder. *CNS Spectr.* 2003;8:363–371, 381.

50. Rufer M, Hand I, Alsleben H, et al. Long-term course and outcome of obsessive-compulsive patients after cognitive-behavioral therapy in combination with either fluvoxamine or placebo: a 7-year follow-up of a randomized double-blind trial. *Eur Arch Psychiatry Clin Neurosci.* 2005;255:121–128.

51. Catapano F, Perris F, Masella M, et al. Obsessive-compulsive disorder: a 3-year prospective follow-up study of patients treated with serotonin reuptake inhibitors OCD follow-up study. *J Psychiatr Res.* 2006;40:502–510.

52. Olsen T, Mais AH, Bilet T, Martinsen EW. Treatment of obsessive-compulsive disorder: personal follow-up of a 10-year material from an outpatient county clinic. *Nord J Psychiatry.* 2008;62:39–45.

53. van Oppen P, van Balkom AJ, de Haan E, van Dyck R. Cognitive therapy and exposure in vivo alone and in combination with fluvoxamine in obsessive-compulsive disorder: a 5-year follow-up. *J Clin Psychiatry.* 2005;66:1415–1422.

54. Anand N, Sudhir PM, Math SB, Thennarasu K, Janardhan Reddy YC. Cognitive behavior therapy in medication non-responders with obsessive-compulsive disorder: a prospective 1-year follow-up study. *J Anxiety Disord.* 2011;25:939–945.

55. Anholt GE, Aderka IM, van Balkom AJ, et al. The impact of depression on the treatment of obsessive-compulsive disorder: results from a 5-year follow-up. *J Affect Disord.* 2011;135:201–207.

56. Braga DT, Manfro GG, Niederauer K, Cordioli AV. Full remission and relapse of obsessive-compulsive symptoms after cognitive-behavioral group therapy: a two-year follow-up. *Rev Bras Psiquiatr.* 2010;32:164–168.

57. Cabedo E, Belloch A, Carrio C, et al. Group versus individual cognitive treatment for obsessive-compulsive disorder: changes in severity at post-treatment and one-year follow-up. *Behav Cogn Psychother.* 2010;38:227–232.

58. Marcks BA, Weisberg RB, Dyck I, Keller MB. Longitudinal course of obsessive-compulsive disorder in patients with anxiety disorders: a 15-year prospective follow-up study. *Compr Psychiatry.* 2011;52:670–677.

59. Reddy YC, Alur AM, Manjunath S, Kandavel T, Math SB. Long-term follow-up study of patients with serotonin reuptake inhibitor-nonresponsive obsessive-compulsive disorder. *J Clin Psychopharmacol.* 2010;30:267–272.

60. Whittal ML, Robichaud M, Thordarson DS, McLean PD. Group and individual treatment of obsessive-compulsive disorder using cognitive therapy and exposure plus response prevention: a 2-year follow-up of two randomized trials. *J Consult Clin Psychol.* 2008;76:1003–1014.

61. Bloch MH, Green C, Kichuk SA, et al. Long-term outcome in adults with obsessive-compulsive disorder. *Depress Anxiety.* 2013;30:716–722.

62. Cherian AV, Math SB, Kandavel T, Reddy YC. A 5-year prospective follow-up study of patients with obsessive-compulsive disorder treated with serotonin reuptake inhibitors. *J Affect Disord.* 2014;152–154:387–394.

63. Cherian AV, Pandian D, Bada Math S, Kandavel T, Janardhan Reddy YC. Family accommodation of obsessional symptoms and naturalistic outcome of obsessive-compulsive disorder. *Psychiatry Res.* 2014;215:372–378.

64. Jakubovski E, Diniz JB, Valerio C, et al. Clinical predictors of long-term outcome in obsessive-compulsive disorder. *Depress Anxiety.* 2013;30:763–772.

65. Pallanti S, Hollander E, Bienstock C, et al. Treatment non response in OCD: methodological issues and operational definitions. *Int J Neuropsychopharmacol.* 2002;5:181–191.

66. Fineberg NA, Hengartner MP, Bergbaum C, et al. Remission of obsessive-compulsive disorders and syndromes; evidence from a prospective community cohort study over 30 years. *Int J Psychiatry Clin Pract.* 2013;17:179–187.

67. Steketee G, Eisen J, Dyck I, Warshaw M, Rasmussen S. Predictors of course in obsessive-compulsive disorder. *Psychiatry Res.* 1999;89:229–238.

68. Ravi Kishore V, Samar R, Janardhan Reddy YC, Chandrasekhar CR, Thennarasu K. Clinical characteristics and treatment response in poor and good insight obsessive-compulsive disorder. *Eur Psychiatry.* 2004;19:202–208.

69. Shetti CN, Reddy YC, Kandavel T, et al. Clinical predictors of drug nonresponse in obsessive-compulsive disorder. *J Clin Psychiatry.* 2005;66:1517–1523.

70. Kichuk SA, Torres AR, Fontenelle LF, et al. Symptom dimensions are associated with age of onset and clinical course of obsessive-compulsive disorder. *Prog Neuropsychopharmacol Biol Psychiatry.* 2013;44:233–239.

71. McDougle CJ, Epperson CN, Pelton GH, Wasylink S, Price LH. A double-blind, placebo-controlled study of risperidone addition in serotonin reuptake inhibitor-refractory obsessive-compulsive disorder. *Arch Gen Psychiatry.* 2000;57:794–801.

72. Baer L, Jenike MA. Personality disorders in obsessive compulsive disorder. *Psychiatr Clin North Am.* 1992;15:803–812.

73. Huang LC, Hwang TJ, Huang GH, Hwu HG. Outcome of severe obsessive-compulsive disorder with schizotypal features: a pilot study. *J Formos Med Assoc.* 2011;110:85–92.

74. Cavedini P, Erzegovesi S, Ronchi P, Bellodi L. Predictive value of obsessive-compulsive personality disorder in antiobsessional pharmacological treatment. *Eur Neuropsychopharmacol.* 1997;7:45–49.

75. Koran LM, Hackett E, Rubin A, Wolkow R, Robinson D. Efficacy of sertraline in the long-term treatment of obsessive-compulsive disorder. *Am J Psychiatry.* 2002;159:88–95.

76. Romano S, Goodman W, Tamura R, Gonzales J. Long-term treatment of obsessive-compulsive disorder after an acute response: a comparison of fluoxetine versus placebo. *J Clin Psychopharmacol.* 2001;21:46–52.

77. Grant JE, Mancebo MC, Weinhandl E, et al. Longitudinal course of pharmacotherapy in obsessive-compulsive disorder. *Int Clin Psychopharmacol.* 2013;28:200–205.

78. Valleni-Basile LA, Garrison CZ, Jackson KL, et al. Frequency of obsessive-compulsive disorder in a community sample of young adolescents. *J Am Acad Child Adolesc Psychiatry.* 1994;33:782–791.

79. Narrow WE, Rae DS, Robins LN, Regier DA. Revised prevalence estimates of mental disorders in the United States: using a clinical significance criterion to reconcile 2 surveys' estimates. *Arch Gen Psychiatry.* 2002;59:115–123.

80. Stewart SE, Geller DA, Jenike M, et al. Long-term outcome of pediatric obsessive-compulsive disorder: a meta-analysis and qualitative review of the literature. *Acta Psychiatr Scand.* 2004;110:4–13.

81. Micali N, Heyman I, Perez M, et al. Long-term outcomes of obsessive-compulsive disorder: follow-up of 142 children and adolescents. *Br J Psychiatry.* 2010;197:128–134.

82. Mancebo MC, Boisseau CL, Garnaat SL, et al. Long-term course of pediatric obsessive-compulsive disorder: 3 years of prospective follow-up. *Compr Psychiatry.* 2014;55:1498–1504.

83. Jenike MA. Geriatric obsessive-compulsive disorder. *J Geriatr Psychiatry Neurol.* 1991;4:34–39.

84. Philpot MP, Banerjee S. Obsessive-compulsive disorder in the elderly. *Behav Neurol.* 1998;11:117–121.

85. Phillips KA, Grant JE, Siniscalchi JM, Stout R, Price LH. A retrospective follow-up study of body dysmorphic disorder. *Compr Psychiatry.* 2005;46:315–321.

86. Phillips KA, Pagano ME, Menard W, Fay C, Stout RL. Predictors of remission from body dysmorphic disorder: a prospective study. *J Nerv Ment Dis.* 2005;193:564–567.

87. Phillips KA, Menard W, Quinn E, Didie ER, Stout RL. A 4-year prospective observational follow-up study of course and predictors of course in body dysmorphic disorder. *Psychol Med.* 2013;43:1109–1117.

88. Bjornsson AS, Dyck I, Moitra E, et al. The clinical course of body dysmorphic disorder in the Harvard/Brown Anxiety Research Project (HARP). *J Nerv Ment Dis.* 2011;199:55–57.

89. Tolin DF, Meunier SA, Frost RO, Steketee G. Course of compulsive hoarding and its relationship to life events. *Depress Anxiety.* 2010;27:829–838.

90. Ayers CR, Saxena S, Golshan S, Wetherell JL. Age at onset and clinical features of late life compulsive hoarding. *Int J Geriatr Psychiatry.* 2010;25:142–149.

91. Grisham JR, Frost RO, Steketee G, Kim HJ, Hood S. Age of onset of compulsive hoarding. *J Anxiety Disord.* 2006;20:675–686.

92. Bloch MH, Bartley CA, Zipperer L, et al. Meta-analysis: hoarding symptoms associated with poor treatment outcome in obsessive-compulsive disorder. *Mol Psychiatry.* 2014;19:1025–1030.

93. Muroff J, Steketee G, Frost RO, Tolin DF. Cognitive behavior therapy for hoarding disorder: follow-up findings and predictors of outcome. *Depress Anxiety* 2014;31:964–971.

94. Grant JE, Stein DJ. Body-focused repetitive behavior disorders in ICD-11. *Rev Bras Psiquiatr.* 2014;36(Suppl 1):59–64.

95. Sah DE, Koo J, Price VH. Trichotillomania. *Dermatol Ther.* 2008;21:13–21.

96. Cohen LJ, Stein DJ, Simeon D, et al. Clinical profile, comorbidity, and treatment history in 123 hair pullers: a survey study. *J Clin Psychiatry.* 1995;56:319–326.

97. Bloch MH. Trichotillomania across the life span. *J Am Acad Child Adolesc Psychiatry.* 2009;48:879–883.

98. Bruce TO, Barwick LW, Wright HH. Diagnosis and management of trichotillomania in children and adolescents. *Paediatr Drugs.* 2005;7:365–376.

99. Flessner CA, Lochner C, Stein DJ, et al. Age of onset of trichotillomania symptoms: investigating clinical correlates. *J Nerv Ment Dis.* 2010;198:896–900.

100. Christenson GA, Mackenzie TB, Mitchell JE. Characteristics of 60 adult chronic hair pullers. *Am J Psychiatry.* 1991;148:365–370.

101. Odlaug BL, Kim SW, Grant JE. Quality of life and clinical severity in pathological skin picking and trichotillomania. *J Anxiety Disord.* 2010;24:823–829.

102. Grant JE, Odlaug BL, Chamberlain SR, et al. Skin picking disorder. *Am J Psychiatry.* 2012;169:1143–1149.

103. Lenroot RK, Giedd JN. The changing impact of genes and environment on brain development during childhood and adolescence: initial findings from a neuroimaging study of pediatric twins. *Dev Psychopathol.* 2008;20:1161–1175.

104. Stein DJ, Kogan CS, Atmaca M, et al. The classification of Obsessive-Compulsive and Related Disorders in the ICD-11. *J Affect Disord.* 2016;190:663–674.

105. Simpson HB, Reddy YC. Obsessive-compulsive disorder for ICD-11: proposed changes to the diagnostic guidelines and specifiers. *Rev Bras Psiquiatr.* 2014;36(Suppl 1):3–13.

106. Kreyenbuhl J, Buchanan RW, Dickerson FB, Dixon LB, Schizophrenia Patient Outcomes Research Team. The Schizophrenia Patient Outcomes Research Team (PORT): updated treatment recommendations 2009. *Schizophr Bull.* 2010;36:94–103.

107. Reddy YC, Srinath S, Prakash HM, et al. A follow-up study of juvenile obsessive-compulsive disorder from India. *Acta Psychiatr Scand.* 2003;107:457–464.

108. Regier DA, Narrow WE, Clarke DE, et al. DSM-5 field trials in the United States and Canada, Part II: test-retest reliability of selected categorical diagnoses. *Am J Psychiatry.* 2013;170:59–70.

109. Sanislow CA, Pine DS, Quinn KJ, et al. Developing constructs for psychopathology research: research domain criteria. *J Abnorm Psychol.* 2010;119:631–639.

110. Gillan CM, Fineberg NA, Robbins TW. A trans-diagnostic perspective on obsessive-compulsive disorder. *Psychol Med.* 2017;47:1528–1548.

111. Insel TR. The NIMH Research Domain Criteria (RDoC) Project: precision medicine for psychiatry. *Am J Psychiatry.* 2014;171:395–397.

112. Haro JM, Ayuso-Mateos JL, Bitter I, et al. ROAMER: roadmap for mental health research in Europe. *Int J Methods Psychiatr Res.* 2014;23(Suppl 1):1–14.

Chapter 13

Sub-Diagnostic Obsessive-Compulsive Symptoms

Albina R. Torres and Leonardo F. Fontenelle

The boundary between mental disorder and normality is inherently unclear and wherever the artificial line is drawn, some people who need treatment will be missed and some who should avoid treatment will be diagnosed.

(Allen Frances, Psychology Today, *2010)*

Introduction

Psychopathological symptoms in general present a broad spectrum of severity, ranging from very mild to extremely severe, not only among individuals, but also in the same person, along the course of illness. Several studies, particularly community-based studies, show that clinical thresholds always involve some degree of arbitrariness, since even individuals who do not meet diagnostic criteria for a given psychiatric disorder may present persistent symptoms that lead to considerable psychosocial impairment, including disability, suicidality and healthcare use [1]. While individuals presenting minimal or very severe symptomatology are easily recognized, those in the intermediate levels of severity are more challenging to deal with.

The implications of this problem are not negligible, since some individuals may have been denied proper treatment and others receive unnecessary and even noxious interventions. Nevertheless, there is a relative lack of data on this important area of "sub-diagnostic" psychiatric symptoms [1], including the symptoms of obsessive-compulsive disorder (OCD). Sub-diagnostic OCD has been defined by the presence of obsessions and/or compulsions not severe enough to meet standardized diagnostic criteria. For example, to meet OCD diagnostic criteria according to the *Diagnostic and Statistical Manual of Mental Disorders*, 5th edition (DSM-5) [2], the obsessions and/or compulsions must be time consuming (e.g. at least one hour a day) or cause significant distress or interfere with the person's daily life. However, these later criteria are not very precise and involve a considerable degree of subjective judgment [3].

Perhaps the first problem faced in this field is related to terminology. We have found at least 15 different terms to describe our main focus of interest in this chapter, including simply obsessions and compulsions [4,5,6], obsessive-compulsive symptoms [7,8,9] and obsessive-compulsive syndromes [10,11,12,13,14]; sub-clinical OCD [15,16], sub-clinical obsessions and compulsions [17] and sub-clinical obsessive-compulsive symptoms [18]; unwanted intrusive thoughts [19], unwanted mental intrusions [20] and intrusive thoughts [21]; sub-threshold symptoms [22], sub-threshold OCD [23,24], sub-threshold symptomatology [12,13,14]; sub-syndromal OCD [25], protracted symptom phase [26] and compulsive-like behaviors [27].

Thus, the difficulty in interpreting the findings of these studies seems obvious, not only because these terms are interchangeably used to describe similar phenomena, but also because the same terms may refer to a different clinical picture depending on the study. For instance, in the Zurich follow-up study, the authors have used the Structured Psychopathological Interview and Rating of the Social Consequences for Epidemiology criteria to describe at least three different conditions that only partly fulfill criteria for OCD, i.e., (1) obsessive-compulsive "syndrome" [obsessions or compulsions causing either (a) some distress, *or* (b) interfering with social or professional function], (2) obsessions and (3) compulsions [10,11,12,13,14]. In this chapter, we have decided to keep the terminology employed in the original studies while using the broader term "sub-diagnostic obsessive-compulsive symptoms" (OCS) to refer to any of these phenomena. The reader might want to refer to the original studies to check specificities of each definition.

Although being core symptoms of OCD, obsessions and compulsions frequently occur in individuals presenting other neuropsychiatric disorders (see Chapter 32) and also in non-clinical populations worldwide. Therefore, obsessions and compulsions extend much beyond the traditional nosological boundaries of OCD [28]. An important study with 777 university students of 13 countries across six continents found that 93.6% experienced at least one unwanted intrusive thought in the previous three months, which were qualitatively similar to the obsessive thoughts of OCD sufferers, involving on average 2.77 content areas [21]. Since unwanted intrusive thoughts, images or impulses are normative phenomena almost universally experienced by ordinary people without mental disorders, several researchers have investigated possible risk factors associated with the transformation of intrusive thoughts into clinical obsessions [19,29,30].

Sub-diagnostic Obsessive-Compulsive Symptoms and the Cognitive Models of Obsessive-Compulsive Disorder

Cognitive models of OCD propose that the main aspects involved in the origins of clinically significant OCS are the misinterpretation of unwanted intrusive thoughts as unacceptable and the maladaptive attempts made by the individual to control them [21]. This faulty appraisal of intrusions leads to higher levels of anxiety and to avoidance and/or to (overt or covert) compulsive behaviors aimed at ignoring, neutralizing or suppressing them. However, as the individual focuses the attention in the unwanted intrusive thoughts, they become more and more upsetting, long lasting and harder to dismiss, and a detrimental feedback develops [19,21,29,30].

According to Salkovskis [29], unwanted intrusive thoughts should be regarded as cognitive stimuli that generate negative automatic thoughts (cognitive responses) typically linked to dysfunctional beliefs concerning personal responsibility for harm to self or others if the person does not take preventive measures. These exaggerated responsibility appraisals trigger negative emotional responses (e.g. anxiety) that lead to engagement in compulsive rituals, which in turn negatively reinforce the dysfunctional beliefs. The metacognitive model of OCD proposes that the unwanted intrusive thoughts are misinterpreted because of metacognitive beliefs, with a central causal role of thought fusion beliefs; that is, beliefs about the power and significance or meaning of one's thoughts/feelings (e.g. danger), and the consequent worry and need for control [7,31].

Therefore, contemporary cognitive behavioral theories of OCD (and related psychotherapeutic protocols) generally state that the intrusions are not problematic of themselves, but they may become more frequent and lead to emotional distress, fear, guilt, avoidance and compulsive behaviors, depending on the way the individuals react to, interpret, appraise and/or try to control them [21]. These theories presuppose a dimensional approach (i.e., continuity between unwanted intrusive thoughts experienced by mentally healthy individuals and the repetitive, persistent and distressing obsessions experienced by OCD patients [4,19]). Several factors may be involved in this aggravation process, including not only dysfunctional beliefs, but factors related to personality characteristics, self-view discrepancies, culture and context [19].

Interestingly, obsessions and compulsions may be particularly frequent and even expected phenomena in certain periods of life, including childhood (e.g., nighttime rituals [27]), pregnancy and postpartum period (e.g. repetitive intrusive thoughts about the health of the fetus or checking rituals on the wellbeing of new-born babies [32]). From an evolutionary perspective, OCS can be considered adaptive in certain circumstances, since some behavioral patterns (e.g. checking, washing, ordering or hoarding compulsions) could have been beneficial early in evolution, conferring survival advantages [33]. Interestingly, some normal behaviors observed in new parents, especially of a first child (e.g. anxious thoughts associated with threat detection and harm avoidant behaviors) have a close resemblance to OCS and share overlapping neural circuits [32]. In fact, compulsive-like behaviors have also been observed in other species, and several animal models have been proposed for symptoms of OCD and related disorders (see Chapter 7).

Recent Research Findings

The Neuropsychology of Sub-diagnostic Obsessive-Compulsive Symptoms

There is also increasing evidence that sub-diagnostic OCS are associated with distinctive neuropsychological features. For instance, compared with healthy controls, patients presenting sub-clinical OCD displayed more deficits in executive functioning, with higher rates of total error, perseverative errors and perseverative responses [34]. Likewise, a moderate deficiency in response inhibition in a go/no-go task was found in a sub-clinical OCD sample, compared with a control sample with low OCS [15]. Lastly, using a sample of 201 14-year-old Bengali students, Malakar and Basu [18] found that sub-clinical OCS were associated with poorer cognitive processes and lower achievement, indicating the need for detection of OCS and early interventions for these adolescents.

The Impact of Sub-diagnostic Obsessive-Compulsive Symptoms on Quality of Life and Help-Seeking Behaviors

As already discussed, OCS present a dimensional rather than a categorical nature [15,19] varying in a continuum of severity from very mild to extremely severe, distressing and incapacitating manifestations [35]. Nevertheless, obsessions and compulsions may lead to considerable burden even among those without a full-blown OCD diagnosis. For instance, the high prevalence of "sub-syndromal" OCD in the National Comorbidity Survey Replication (only 2.3% and 1.2% of the 2073 participants met full *Diagnostic and Statistical Manual of Mental Disorders*, fourth edition (DSM-IV) criteria for lifetime and 12-month OCD, but up to 28.2% experienced lifetime obsessions or compulsions), led the authors to emphasize the potential high public health burden of "sub-syndromal" OCD, whose clinical significance warrants more attention and research [25]. Interestingly, checking and hoarding compulsions were the most frequent in this community sample, but more uncommon types of symptoms were associated with higher risk of OCD [35].

Goracci et al. [24] explored quality of life in 202 Italian subjects free of any axis I or II diagnoses, and found a significant correlation between a scale that explores threshold and sub-threshold OCS (Questionnaire for Obsessive-Compulsive Spectrum) and the following quality of life domains: physical health, subjective feelings, work, school, social relationships and general activities. In other words, subjects with sub-threshold OCD presented poorer quality of life compared with those without obsessions or compulsions. Similarly, Blom et al. [36] examined the occurrence of obsessions in the general population of the Netherlands and described lifetime and one-year prevalence of 5.3% and 1.7%, respectively. Among individuals with a psychiatric disorder, these rates were 10.3% and 6.8%. Patients with obsessions presented worse quality of life in all domains, even when controlling for the presence of co-occurring mental disorders.

Among 591 adults from the general population [12,13,14], OCS clearly presented as a continuum of severity, ranging from mild symptoms with moderate distress to severe symptoms with high distress. Importantly, even participants with lesser symptoms were more distressed than the control group with no obsessions or compulsions. Compared with OCD, sub-threshold OCD was associated with less psychosocial impairment (e.g. suicidality was only associated with OCD), but compared with controls, this group also presented more workplace and marital problems. Moreover, treatment-seeking behaviors increased exponentially according to OCS severity.

Fullana et al. [5] conducted an important community-based prospective study in New Zealand, which showed that obsessions and/or compulsions were present in 13–17% of the adults with no mental disorder and in 31–49% of those with mental disorders. Overall, 21–25% of individuals from the general population presented obsessions and/or compulsions, whereas only 2–3% presented OCD, according to DSM-IV criteria. Compared with compulsions, obsessions caused more interference and led to more help-seeking behaviors, particularly for individuals presenting shameful/taboo thoughts or thoughts of hurting, killing or accidentally harming others. One-quarter of those reporting obsessions experienced them for more than one hour/day and 15% were upset or bothered by them.

In a large study conducted with 7076 Dutch individuals from the community [22], 4.9% presented sub-threshold symptoms and only 0.9% full-blown *Diagnostic and Statistical Manual of Mental Disorders*, third edition, revised (DSM-III-R) OCD. Importantly, those with OCD and sub-threshold OCD had similar levels of health, functionality, psychological vulnerability and psychiatric comorbidity, all worse compared with patients without obsessions or compulsions. These findings indicate that considerable disability and emotional suffering are related to having obsessions and compulsions, even in sub-clinical levels.

Comorbidity of Sub-diagnostic Obsessive-Compulsive Symptoms

Perhaps the first study to describe the frequency of comorbid disorders, and associated symptoms among individuals from the general population showing sub-diagnostic OCS was performed by Degonda et al.

in Switzerland [10]. Owing to the very low prevalence of *Diagnostic and Statistical Manual of Mental Disorders*, third edition (DSM-III) OCD, the authors applied a lower diagnostic threshold and found, at age 30 years, a prevalence of 5.5% of OCS. Interestingly, sub-clinical OCD was associated with depressive disorders, social phobia and agoraphobia. In another community-based study with 4075 adults in Germany, somatoform pain disorder was only associated with OCD but high rates of comorbid depressive disorders were found both in OCD and in sub-clinical OCD subjects [16].

In Germany, among 4181 adults from the community [23], the one-year prevalence of OCD, sub-threshold OCD (i.e. individuals fulfilling some but not all core DSM-IV criteria) and OCS were 0.7%, 4.5% and 8.3%, respectively. Importantly, all these three outcomes were associated with increased odds of substance use, mood, anxiety, somatoform and psychotic disorders. Moreover, compared with participants without OCS, those with any level of OCS presented higher impairment and health-care use. Therefore, this study suggests that, besides relevant psychiatric comorbidity and functional impairment, individuals with sub-clinical OCD present increased health-care utilization.

In a 30-year prospective study conducted in Zurich, Switzerland, with 591 subjects from the general population [12,13,14], 5.1% presented OCD diagnosis, 14.7% sub-diagnostic or sub-threshold OCD ('OC syndrome', conceptualized as at least one symptom plus *either* distress *or* interference) and 12.5%, just obsessions or compulsions. Also, 60% of the 30 participants who presented OCD at some point presented either OCS or "obsessive-compulsive syndrome" at least in one time point during the study period, indicating the wax and waning course of OCD. Interestingly, panic disorder was associated with all OCD-related manifestations, while bipolar disorder, social phobia and generalized anxiety disorder were associated with OCD and "OC syndrome".

In a prospective cohort study with 461 women screened for OCS at two weeks postpartum [6], 11.2% presented OCD and 37.5% sub-clinical OCD. Compared with women without obsessions or compulsions, those with sub-clinical symptoms presented increased rates of depression and state trait anxiety. Alvarenga et al. [37] investigated OCS in a large sample of schoolchildren aged 6–12 years (n = 9937) in Brazil, their siblings, mothers and fathers, obtaining prevalence estimates of 14.7%, 15.6%, 34.6% and 12.1%, respectively. Of note, OCS were more prevalent among older children and were associated with other psychiatric symptoms and with behavioral/school impairment.

In another study by the same group of researchers [38], 2512 of these children were divided in three groups: 77 with OCD, 488 with OCS and 1947 unaffected controls. Although the OCD group presented higher scores in some psychopathological measures and higher rates of separation anxiety, generalized anxiety and major depressive disorders, the OCS group had similar levels of overall functional impairment, including school problems and delinquent behaviors. Therefore, these results suggest the existence of a psychopathological continuum between OCS and OCD in this age group.

Jaisoorya and coworkers investigated the prevalence of sub-diagnostic and fully diagnosable self-reported OCS among 5784 students (age range of 18–25 years) hailing from 58 colleges within a specific Indian district [39]. Compared with individuals without OCD, "sub-threshold" OCD cases (8.5% of the sample) exhibited greater rates of lifetime alcohol use, psychological distress, suicidal thoughts and attempts, sexual abuse and higher attention deficit hyperactivity symptom scores. Importantly, the only difference between sub-threshold and full-blown OCD (3.3% of the sample) was higher psychological distress scores among the latter group.

Using data from the 1998 German Mental Health Survey, which included 4181 adults representative of the general population, Witthauer et al. [40] compared three groups of individuals (no OCS, OCS without any core DSM-IV criteria and sub-threshold OCD or OCD) in relation to physical diseases. Compared with patients without obsessions or compulsions, the latter group – patients with either some or all core DSM-IV criteria – were more likely to have respiratory diseases and migraine headaches. However, persons presenting just obsessions and compulsions had higher prevalence rates of migraine headaches, allergies and thyroid disorders than those without these symptoms.

Prevalence of Sub-diagnostic Obsessive-Compulsive Symptoms in Children and Adolescents

Among 2323 Brazilian adolescent students [41], the one-month prevalence of OCS was 18.3%, significantly higher among girls than boys (24.8% vs.

14.4%), whereas the OCD point prevalence was 3.3%, also higher among females (4.9% vs. 1.4%). A similar rate of OCS (19%) had been previously reported among 3283 adolescents in the United States [42], but a higher rate (26.2%) was described among adolescent and young adult students in Egypt [8], and lower rates (11–12%) in adolescents from Iran [9] and Italy [11].

Follow-Up Studies of Sub-diagnostic Obsessive-Compulsive Symptoms

Several studies of OCD onset and course have shown that patients usually suffer from sub-clinical symptoms for many years before the diagnostic threshold of duration and interference is achieved (see Chapter 12). In spite of the problematic issue of retrospective recall, most adults with OCD remember having minor or sub-threshold symptoms in childhood. However, many studies have considered age at onset of OCD to be the age at which symptoms become severe enough to meet full diagnostic criteria for the disorder [3]. Over two-thirds of the 199 patients with OCD investigated by Coles et al. [26] reported an insidious onset of symptoms, with a slow progression from sub-clinical to clinical manifestations, taking on average five years until OCD criteria of duration and interference was met. This long sub-clinical phase was observed in early and late onset cases, but was particularly protracted among the latter.

Similar findings are also reported in epidemiological samples. For instance, in a Brazilian epidemiological study with 2323 school adolescents [41], the mean age of onset of OCS was 9.7 years and of OCD was 13.8 years, indicating that sub-clinical symptoms persist for a fairly long time until full-blown OCD starts. In a multicenter clinical sample of 1001 patients in Brazil [43], the mean age of OCS onset was 12.6 years, whereas the mean age of interference (i.e., OCD onset) was 21.8 years. Importantly, the first treatment for OCD occurred on average at 29.4 years of age (i.e., more than seven years after the disorder onset).

In a prospective study with participants from the community in Switzerland [12,13,14], OCD was also frequently preceded by sub-diagnostic OCS. In 82% of these cases, less severe symptoms predated the onset of the disorder but only a minority of cases presenting any level of sub-clinical symptoms developed full-blown OCD. More specifically, only 6 of 107 participants with just obsessions or compulsions and 9 of 98 of those presenting an "obsessive-compulsive syndrome" (defined as above) converted into a full diagnosis of OCD (i.e., at least one symptom, *plus* significant distress or anxiety when trying to stop, *plus* impairment in work and social life). Nevertheless, some interventions have been proposed for individuals presenting sub-clinical OCS to prevent them from developing full-blown OCD. For example, a cognitive behavioral workshop was offered for youngsters aged 18–22 years with sub-clinical obsessions and compulsions, which resulted in fewer symptoms and less thought-act fusion after five months [17].

Also, longitudinal studies demonstrate that several patients who do respond to treatments continue to present sub-clinical obsessions and/or compulsions. For example, in a 40-year follow-up study [44], 28% of the patients who recovered still presented sub-clinical symptoms, while 20% presented a complete recovery. Similarly, in a five-year prospective study with 213 adults with DSM-IV OCD, only 16.9% presented full remission and 22.1%, partial remission [45]. Importantly, the latter group was more likely to relapse compared with the former (70% vs. 45%). The authors conclude that full remission should be a target in treatment to minimize the risk of relapse.

Familial-Genetic Aspects of Sub-diagnostic Obsessive-Compulsive Symptoms

Like genetic environmental twin studies, several adult and child family studies have included in the analyses first-degree relatives presenting not only OCD but also OCD "features" or sub-diagnostic OCD [46]. The general conclusion of studies with child or adolescent probands is that both OCD and sub-diagnostic OCD are genetically linked, given the significantly higher rates of sub-diagnostic OCD among relatives of patients with OCD, compared with controls or with general population rates, and *vice versa*. With a few exceptions, family studies with adult probands also found a higher familial aggregation of diagnostic and sub-diagnostic OCD [46], including a study with treatment-seeking patients and individuals from the community who had never been treated [47]. In a prospective controlled family study with the 7–18-year-old offspring of adults with OCD (i.e., "high-risk" subjects) [48], intermediate levels of psychopathology were present in children with sub-clinical symptoms, compared with those with OCD and those without any symptoms.

Cross-Diagnostic Approaches and Their Implications for Classification and Diagnosis

We have seen that sub-diagnostic OCS can occur across different mental disorders, including substance use, mood, anxiety, somatoform and psychotic disorders. Traditional approaches to diagnosis could conceptualize sub-diagnostic OCS as a manifestation of these conditions. As a consequence, it seems interesting to investigate the utility of the addition of an "obsessive-compulsive symptoms" specifier to the above-mentioned disorders. For instance, a differentiated etiology (e.g., atypical antipsychotics use), as well as a specific impact on the basic phenotype [49], may underscore some clinical usefulness of this conceptualization of OCS in schizophrenia [50]. There is also some evidence suggesting that serotonin reuptake inhibitors may effectively treat OCS in the context of psychotic disorders [51]. However, it is unclear whether the same holds true for other conditions associated with OCS.

In fact, earlier studies have indicated that the relationships between sub-diagnostic OCD and other co-occurring diagnoses can be quite complex and should not be trivialized. For instance, Gittleson has divided depressed patients into "gainers", "keepers", "losers" and "nevers", depending on whether they develop new, keep or lose old, or had never developed "obsessional neurosis symptoms". Thus, the longitudinal course of sub-diagnostic OCS in relation to comorbid disorder should also be taken into account, as the latter may overshadow the former. Finally, a truly cross-diagnostic approach to sub-diagnostic OCD may prompt the investigation of common environmental and/or biological risk factors with other conditions, which could ultimately result in improved treatments and even prevention of OCD itself (see below for a discussion).

Another important cross-diagnostic aspect of sub-diagnostic OCD that has classification and diagnostic implications is the optimal diagnostic cut-off of OCD (i.e. the point where the clinician should draw the line dividing OCD from non-OCD, including sub-diagnostic OCD). Currently, the DSM approach to OCD has emphasized time consumption (e.g., at least one hour per day), distress and/or impairment as the ultimate features differentiating these states. However, the World Health Organization has adopted a different stance. The International Classification of Functioning, Disability, and Health (ICF) posits that functional status and disability should not be part of the definitions and criteria for the diagnostic entities classified by the International Classification of Diseases (ICD) systems, including mental disorders [52]. This approach mirrors the definition of clinical entities in other areas of medicine (e.g., no functional status and disability is required, for instance, for a diagnosis of asthma). According to this model, constructs such as impairment, disability and handicap are the consequences rather than part of the disorders themselves.

Although disentangling the concept of "disorder" from impaired functional status/disability may prove to be a difficult task [52], the ICF approach to psychiatric diagnoses would also avoid circular definitions of mental disorders. For instance, it might not be considered very informative to find increased disability rates in OCD if the disorder itself embeds some level of impairment in its definition. Thus, the ICF would provide more reliable information on the impact of poor mental health in general, and OCD in particular. Finally, the consideration that the cut-off between full-blown and sub-diagnostic OCD is somewhat arbitrary and is likely to be affected by many factors unrelated to OCD itself (e.g., cultural influences)[1] has consequences for the research on the pathophysiology of OCD as well. The recognition that many non-affected individuals may in fact suffer from an OCD may be helpful for the elucidation of the genetic-environmental basis of the condition.

Clinical Implications of Cross-Diagnostic Approaches for Treatment and Prevention

During the last 30 years, many advances have been noted in the clinical management of OCD, including the demonstration of the efficacy of exposure and response prevention, high doses of serotonin reuptake inhibitors, deep brain stimulation and neurosurgery. However, the use of these strategies in patients

[1] For instance, it is unknown whether Western individuals with sub-diagnostic OCD would be more likely to be diagnosed with OCD in a non-Western environment (due to increased distress) rather than in a Western environment.

with milder or sub-diagnostic conditions is unwarranted and/or unrealistic, as these strategies are not widely available (e.g., exposure and response prevention), do have adverse effects (e.g., serotonin reuptake inhibitors), are excessively costly (e.g., deep brain stimulation) and/or result in persistent handicaps (e.g., neurosurgery) [53]. The use of Internet delivered cognitive behavioral treatments seems to be a viable and appropriate treatment for these patients, yet we are not aware of any study testing its efficacy in sub-diagnostic cases. Similarly, therapeutic strategies targeting lifestyles, such as meditation-based therapies and interventions focusing on eliminating sedentarism, seem to be promising approaches [53].

It is important to clarify what sort of advice clinicians should give to individuals with sub-diagnostic OCS. Theoretically, the treatment of these symptoms could avoid the later development of full-blown OCD. Yet, there are very few studies on the topic, and the area has several gaps and methodological challenges. For instance, although retrospective studies indicate that patients with OCD typically report an insidious onset of (sub-diagnostic) symptoms [26], there are also prospective studies suggesting that individuals showing sub-diagnostic OCS ascertained in the community and followed for several years do not convert to full-blown OCD very often [12,13,14]. These data are consistent with the view that sub-diagnostic OCS can be extremely frequent [5] and yet the conversion rates to OCD quite rare. Thus, it seems that we can reassure patients that their sub-diagnostic OCS will not necessarily evolve into OCD in most cases.

Future Directions

Yet, if only a few patients with sub-diagnostic OCS seem to convert to full-blown OCD, efforts should be made to target those subjects that are more likely to convert to illness. For example, other "at-risk" phenotypes in psychiatry have included a number of features in their characterization in addition to sub-diagnostic (or "attenuated") symptoms, such as a recent decrease in functioning plus a pre-existing schizotypal personality disorder or a first-degree relative with a history of psychosis [54]. This strategy has led to the identification of an "enriched" phenotype that shows conversion to psychosis at the end of 12 months in up to 30% of cases (though these rates have decreased in recent years, perhaps as a result of effective prevention) [54]. It is presently unclear whether a similar approach could be adopted in relation to OCD and we can only speculate about which additional features, besides sub-diagnostic OCS, would be pertinent to consider, but a positive family history of OCD or related disorders would be a natural candidate.

As the ultimate implications of research into sub-diagnostic forms of psychopathology include prevention of more severe cases, future research should pay particular attention to the identification of OCS among specifically vulnerable age groups [55]. The onset of OCD often occurs earlier than of other psychiatric disorders (e.g., schizophrenia), thus suggesting that the prevention of full-blown OCD should target younger populations than those considered in traditional mental health units for patients "at risk" for psychosis [54]. For instance, a few early studies on the epidemiology of OCD have shown that up to 80% of cases have their onset of symptoms during childhood and the adolescent years [56]. Thus, sub-diagnostic OCS in this population may be more unstable and subject to further deterioration than at later ages. However, an additional challenge would be the differentiation (if possible) between sub-diagnostic OCS in childhood and normal behaviors in this developmental phase, such as night-time rituals [27]. Although individuals with sub-diagnostic OCS have shown decreased quality of life in different domains, another particular challenge for future studies is how to engage these subjects in treatment, as they are obviously less impaired.

Finally, since most patients with OCD report an insidious onset of symptoms (e.g., over an average of five years in one study [26]), the exact point of conversion of sub-diagnostic OCD into fully diagnosable OCD may be blurred, thus hindering a clear differentiation between converted and non-converted cases. Important life events and their impact on OCS should not be forgotten. Therefore, the identification of an at-risk phenotype for OCD may need to include data collection done through multiple assessments over a prolonged period of time, rather than just a single snapshot of individuals with sub-diagnostic symptoms taken in one particular day of their lives [57]. As our ability to manage increased amounts of data improves, this collection could be accomplished by means of mobile devices or online assessments. Thus, technological advances could allow an early identification of changes in symptom patterns that could predict future

OCD cases, as well as the clarification of the exact role of potential risk factors (e.g., stressful life events) in the conversion to full-blown OCD.

Conclusions

Obsessive-compulsive manifestations are better conceptualized as a non-specific, diverse and dimensional construct. These manifestations are not pathognomonic of OCD, but rather almost ubiquitous both in clinical and non-clinical populations. They range from very mild to extremely severe symptoms and, as the severity increases the levels of emotional distress, interference and psychosocial impact also increase. In other words, the construct is not a black and white phenomenon, but certainly is better represented by several shades of gray that vary in severity (and in content) from person to person and also within each individual during the natural course of illness, or according to treatment response.

Sub-threshold psychiatric symptoms in general are still understudied and a matter of debate. According to Allen Frances [58], "normality is an endangered species", as the current diagnostic system is already overinclusive and captures too many people who might be better off with no diagnosis and no treatment. Nevertheless, it is important to note that individuals presenting sub-diagnostic OCD can be considerably upset by their obsessions and compulsions, which may negatively impact several life domains and increase the use of healthcare resources. A high personal, family and public health burden is possibly associated with sub-diagnostic OCD, due to its prevalence and significance. Therefore, more research is certainly necessary to better determine which interventions (if any) can be beneficial to a large number of individuals in this situation.

References

1. Stein DJ. Subthreshold and residual symptoms in depression and anxiety disorders: where next? *Medicographia.* 2014;36(4):452–457.
2. APA. *Diagnostic and Statistical Manual of Mental Disorders.* 5th ed. Washington, DC: APA; 2013.
3. Rasmussen SA, Eisen JL. The course and clinical features of obsessive-compulsive disorder. In: Davis KL, Charney DC, Coyle JT, Nemeroff C, eds. *Neuropsychopharmacology: The Fifth Generation of Progress.* Philadelphia, PA: Lippincott, Williams, & Wilkins; 2002:1593–1608.
4. Abramowitz JS, Fabricant LE, Taylor S, Deacon BJ, McKay D, Storch EA. The relevance of analogue studies for understanding obsessions and compulsions. *Clin Psychol Rev.* 2014;34(3):206–217.
5. Fullana MA, Mataix-Cols D, Caspi A, et al. Obsessions and compulsions in the community: prevalence, interference, help-seeking, developmental stability, and co-occurring psychiatric conditions. *Am J Psychiatry.* 2009;166(3):329–336.
6. Miller ES, Hoxha D, Wisner KL, Gossett DR. Obsessions and compulsions in postpartum women without obsessive compulsive disorder. *J Womens Health (Larchmt).* 2015;24(10):825–830.
7. Myers SG, Wells A. Obsessive-compulsive symptoms: the contribution of metacognitions and responsibility. *J Anxiety Disord.* 2005;19(7):806–817.
8. Okasha A, Ragheb K, Attia AH, Seif el Dawla A, Okasha T, Ismail R. Prevalence of obsessive compulsive symptoms (OCS) in a sample of Egyptian adolescents. *Encephale.* 2001;27(1):8–14.
9. Shams G, Foroughi E, Esmaili Y, Amini H, Ebrahimkhani N. Prevalence rates of obsessive-compulsive symptoms and psychiatric comorbidity among adolescents in Iran. *Acta Med Iran.* 2011;49(10):680–687.
10. Degonda M, Wyss M, Angst J. The Zurich Study. XVIII. Obsessive-compulsive disorders and syndromes in the general population. *Eur Arch Psychiatry Clin Neurosci.* 1993;243(1):16–22.
11. Maina G, Albert U, Bogetto F, Ravizza L. Obsessive-compulsive syndromes in older adolescents. *Acta Psychiatr Scand.* 1999;100(6):447–450.
12. Fineberg NA, Hengartner MP, Bergbaum C, Gale T, Rossler W, Angst J. Lifetime comorbidity of obsessive-compulsive disorder and sub-threshold obsessive-compulsive symptomatology in the community: impact, prevalence, socio-demographic and clinical characteristics. *Int J Psychiatry Clin Pract.* 2013;17(3):188–196.
13. Fineberg NA, Hengartner MP, Bergbaum C, Gale T, Rossler W, Angst J. Remission of obsessive-compulsive disorders and syndromes; evidence from a prospective community cohort study over 30 years. *Int J Psychiatry Clin Pract.* 2013;17(3):179–187.
14. Fineberg NA, Hengartner MP, Bergbaum CE, et al. A prospective population-based cohort study of the prevalence, incidence and impact of obsessive-compulsive symptomatology. *Int J Psychiatry Clin Pract.* 2013;17(3):170–178.
15. Abramovitch A, Shaham N, Levin L, Bar-Hen M, Schweiger A. Response inhibition in a subclinical obsessive-compulsive sample. *J Behav Ther Exp Psychiatry.* 2015;46:66–71.

16. Grabe HJ, Meyer C, Hapke U, et al. Lifetime-comorbidity of obsessive-compulsive disorder and subclinical obsessive-compulsive disorder in Northern Germany. *Eur Arch Psychiatry Clin Neurosci.* 2001;251(3):130–135.
17. Zucker BG, Craske MG, Blackmore MA, Nitz A. A cognitive behavioral workshop for subclinical obsessions and compulsions. *Behav Res Ther.* 2006;44(2):289–304.
18. Malakar P, Basu J. Subclinical obsessive-compulsive symptoms, cognitive processes, school achievement, and intelligence-achievement relationship in adolescents. *Int J School Educ Psychol.* 2017;5(2):115–125.
19. Clark DA, Inozu M. Unwanted intrusive thoughts: cultural, contextual, covariational, and characterological determinants of diversity. *J Obsess Compuls Relat Disord.* 2014;3(2):195–204.
20. Pascual-Vera B, Roncero-Sanchis M, Belloch Fuster A. Are unwanted mental intrusions a transdiagnostic variable? *Psicothema.* 2017;29(2):166–171.
21. Radomsky AS, Alcolado GM, Abramowitz JS, et al. Part 1 – You can run but you can't hide: intrusive thoughts on six continents. *J Obsess Compuls Relat Disord.* 2014;3(3):269–279.
22. de Bruijn C, Beun S, de Graaf R, ten Have M, Denys D. Subthreshold symptoms and obsessive–compulsive disorder: evaluating the diagnostic threshold. *Psychol Med.* 2009;40(6):989–997.
23. Adam Y, Meinlschmidt G, Gloster AT, Lieb R. Obsessive-compulsive disorder in the community: 12-month prevalence, comorbidity and impairment. *Soc Psychiatry Psychiatr Epidemiol.* 2012;47(3):339–349.
24. Goracci A, Martinucci M, Kaperoni A, et al. Quality of life and subthreshold obsessive-compulsive disorder. *Acta Neuropsychiatr.* 2007;19(6):357–361.
25. Ruscio AM, Stein DJ, Chiu WT, Kessler RC. The epidemiology of obsessive-compulsive disorder in the National Comorbidity Survey Replication. *Mol Psychiatry.* 2010;15(1):53–63.
26. Coles ME, Johnson EM, Schubert JR. Retrospective reports of the development of obsessive compulsive disorder: extending knowledge of the protracted symptom phase. *Behav Cogn Psychother.* 2011;39(5):579–589.
27. Evans DW, Leckman JF, Carter A, et al. Ritual, habit, and perfectionism: the prevalence and development of compulsive-like behavior in normal young children. *Child Dev.* 1997;68(1):58–68.
28. Fullana MA, Vilagut G, Rojas-Farreras S, et al. Obsessive-compulsive symptom dimensions in the general population: results from an epidemiological study in six European countries. *J Affect Disord.* 2010;124(3):291–299.
29. Salkovskis PM. Obsessional-compulsive problems: a cognitive-behavioural analysis. *Behav Res Ther.* 1985;23(5):571–583.
30. Calkins AW, Berman NC, Wilhelm S. Recent advances in research on cognition and emotion in OCD: a review. *Curr Psychiatry Rep.* 2013;15(5):357.
31. Myers SG, Wells A. An experimental manipulation of metacognition: a test of the metacognitive model of obsessive-compulsive symptoms. *Behav Res Ther.* 2013;51(4–5):177–184.
32. Leckman JF, Herman AE. Maternal behavior and developmental psychopathology. *Biol Psychiatry.* 2002;51(1):27–43.
33. Leckman JF, Mayes LC. Understanding developmental psychopathology: how useful are evolutionary accounts? *J Am Acad Child Adolesc Psychiatry.* 1998;37(10):1011–1021.
34. Kim M-S, Jang K-M, Kim B-N. The neuropsychological profile of a subclinical obsessive-compulsive sample. *J Int Neuropsychol Soc.* 2009;15(2):286–290.
35. Apter A, Fallon TJ, Jr, King RA, et al. Obsessive-compulsive characteristics: from symptoms to syndrome. *J Am Acad Child Adolesc Psychiatry.* 35(7):907–912.
36. Blom RM, Hagestein-de Bruijn C, de Graaf R, ten Have M, Denys DA. Obsessions in normality and psychopathology. *Depress Anxiety.* 2011;28(10):870–875.
37. Alvarenga PG, Cesar RC, Leckman JF, et al. Obsessive-compulsive symptom dimensions in a population-based, cross-sectional sample of school-aged children. *J Psychiatr Res.* 2015;62:108–114.
38. Alvarenga PG, do Rosario MC, Cesar RC, et al. Obsessive-compulsive symptoms are associated with psychiatric comorbidities, behavioral and clinical problems: a population-based study of Brazilian school children. *Eur Child Adolesc Psychiatry.* 2016;25(2):175–182.
39. Jaisoorya T, Janardhan Reddy Y, Nair B, et al. Prevalence and correlates of obsessive-compulsive disorder and subthreshold obsessive-compulsive disorder among college students in Kerala, India. *Indian J Psychiatry.* 2017;59(1):56–62.
40. Witthauer C, Gloster AT, Meyer AH, Lieb R. Physical diseases among persons with obsessive compulsive symptoms and disorder: a general population study. *Soc Psychiatry Psychiatr Epidemiol.* 2014;49(12):2013–2022.
41. Vivan Ade S, Rodrigues L, Wendt G, Bicca MG, Braga DT, Cordioli AV. Obsessive-compulsive symptoms and obsessive-compulsive disorder in adolescents: a population-based study. *Rev Bras Psiquiatr.* 2014;36(2):111–118.

42. Valleni-Basile LA, Garrison CZ, Waller JL, et al. Incidence of obsessive-compulsive disorder in a community sample of young adolescents. *J Am Acad Child Adolesc Psychiatry.* 1996;35(7):898–906.

43. Torres AR, Fontenelle LF, Ferrao YA, et al. Clinical features of obsessive-compulsive disorder with hoarding symptoms: a multicenter study. *J Psychiatr Res.* 2012;46(6):724–732.

44. Skoog G, Skoog I. A 40-year follow-up of patients with obsessive-compulsive disorder. *Arch Gen Psychiatry.* 1999;56(2):121–127.

45. Eisen JL, Sibrava NJ, Boisseau CL, et al. Five-year course of obsessive-compulsive disorder: predictors of remission and relapse. *J Clin Psychiatry.* 2013;74(3):233–239.

46. Pauls DL. The genetics of obsessive-compulsive disorder: a review. *Dialogues Clin Neurosci.* 2010;12(2):149–163.

47. Grabe HJ, Ruhrmann S, Ettelt S, et al. Alexithymia in obsessive-compulsive disorder – results from a family study. *Psychother Psychosom.* 2006;75(5):312–318.

48. Black DW, Gaffney GR. Subclinical obsessive-compulsive disorder in children and adolescents: additional results from a "high-risk" study. *CNS Spectr.* 2008;13(9 Suppl 14):54–61.

49. Zink M. Comorbid obsessive-compulsive symptoms in schizophrenia: insight into pathomechanisms facilitates treatment. *Adv Med.* 2014;2014:18.

50. Lysaker PH, Whitney KA. Obsessive-compulsive symptoms in schizophrenia: prevalence, correlates and treatment. *Expert Rev Neurother.* 2009;9(1):99–107.

51. Stryjer R, Dambinsky Y, Timinsky I, et al. Escitalopram in the treatment of patients with schizophrenia and obsessive-compulsive disorder: an open-label, prospective study. *Int Clin Psychopharmacol.* 2013;28(2):96–98.

52. International Advisory Group for the Revision of ICDM, Behavioural D. A conceptual framework for the revision of the ICD-10 classification of mental and behavioural disorders. *World Psychiatry.* 2011;10(2):86–92.

53. Fontenelle LF, Zeni-Graiff M, Yucel M. Is there a role for lifestyle interventions in obsessive-compulsive and related disorders? *Curr Med Chem.* 2018 Jan 4. doi: 10.2174/0929867325666180104150854.

54. Yung AR, Nelson B. Young people at ultra high risk for psychosis: research from the PACE clinic. *Rev Bras Psiquiatr.* 2011;33(Suppl 2):s143–s160.

55. Fontenelle LF, Hasler G. The analytical epidemiology of obsessive-compulsive disorder: risk factors and correlates. *Prog Neuropsychopharmacol Biol Psychiatry.* 2008;32(1):1–15.

56. Grados MA, Labuda MC, Riddle MA, Walkup JT. Obsessive-compulsive disorder in children and adolescents. *Int Rev Psychiatry.* 1997;9(1):83–98.

57. Nelson B, McGorry PD, Wichers M, Wigman JTW, Hartmann JA. Moving from static to dynamic models of the onset of mental disorder: a review. *JAMA Psychiatry.* 2017;74(5):528–534.

58. Frances A. Psychiatric fads and overdiagnosis: normality is an endangered species. *Pyschol Today.* 2010 June 2. Available from: www.psychologytoday.com/blog/dsm5-in-distress/201006/psychiatric-fads-and-overdiagnosis (accessed July 9, 2018).

Chapter 14

Assessment Instruments for Obsessive-Compulsive Disorder

Andrew G. Guzick, Adam M. Reid and Eric A. Storch

Introduction

Despite changes in the classification of obsessive-compulsive disorder (OCD) in the *Diagnostic and Statistical Manual of Mental Disorders*, fifth edition (DSM-5) [1], the diagnostic criteria for OCD have remained relatively similar since the third edition (DSM-III) in 1980. The clinical hallmarks of the disorder are: obsessions, or repetitive, intrusive, distressing thoughts; and compulsions, or excessive and/or ritualistic behaviors that are done to neutralize obsessions or prevent feared outcomes. To meet criteria for the disorder, an individual must experience obsessions and/or compulsions that occupy at least one hour per day or cause clinically significant distress or functional impairment (American Psychiatric Association) [1].

Several semi-structured diagnostic interviews have been shown to reliably assess OCD, including the Anxiety Disorders Interview Schedule for DSM-IV [2] and the Structured Clinical Interview for DSM-IV Axis I Disorders [3] for adults with OCD, and the Schedule for Affective Disorders and Schizophrenia for School-age Children-Present and Lifetime Version [4] and the Child and Parent versions of the Anxiety Disorders Interview Schedule [5] for children and adolescents. Updates to these interviews are only beginning to be published to reflect DSM-5 criteria and thus are not widely validated, although they are expected to produce reliable OCD diagnoses, as the criteria are similar to those found in in DSM-IV.

Recent Research Findings

Interviewer-Rated Scales

The most widely used measures of OCD severity are the Yale-Brown Obsessive-Compulsive Scale (Y-BOCS) [6] and the children's version of the Y-BOCS (CY-BOCS) [7], which are both semi-structured interviews. The Y-BOCS and CY-BOCS have two sections: a symptom checklist that assesses whether patients are currently experiencing an array of obsessions and compulsions (in the past week) and if they ever have, and a severity section in which patients are asked about how symptoms have affected them in the past week. After completing the checklist, respondents are prompted to consider the three or four most severe obsessions, the three or four most severe compulsions, as well as any avoidance behavior that may accompany them (e.g., not using public restrooms to avoid obsessions related to contamination, not tidying a room to avoid initiating perfectionistic ordering rituals).

The severity scale consists of ten items: five that inquire about the impact of obsessions and five that assess compulsions in the following domains: (i) time taken by symptoms; (ii) functional impairment; (iii) distress they cause; (iv) resistance against them and (v) perceived control over them; generating total scores from 0 to 40. The following severity cutoffs have been recommended based on the most recent psychometric evaluations of the measures: CY-BOCS: slight illness: 0–4; mild: 5–13; moderate: 14–24; moderate-severe: 25–30; severe: 31–40 [8]; Y-BOCS: mild: 0–13; moderate: 14–25; moderate-severe: 26–34; severe: 35–40 [9].

The adult and childhood versions of the Y-BOCS are largely similar, with some minimal differences in developmentally appropriate language used and content of the symptom checklists. When using the CY-BOCS, parental input in the interview is recommended, particularly when the child does not recognize the excessiveness of symptoms. The CY-BOCS administration instructions recommend that a clinician interviews a parent and child independently at first and then collaboratively, though in many cases a collaborative interview alone suffices [9].

The Y-BOCS and CY-BOCS both have strong psychometric properties, including high internal consistency, interrater reliability and test-retest reliability [8,9,10]. A 35% reduction in Y-BOCS or CY-BOCS across treatment, and a post-treatment score of 12 or lower are the most widely-accepted definitions of treatment response and remission, respectively [11]. Signal detection analyses suggest that a reduction of 25% and 45–50% on the CY-BOCS and 30% and 40–50% reductions on the Y-BOCS correspond with treatment response and remission, respectively [12,13].

The Y-BOCS second edition (Y-BOCS-II) was developed to address some of the limitations of the original Y-BOCS [14]. Specifically, four alterations were proposed: (i) including two items that assess avoidance due to obsessions and compulsions; (ii) a wider Likert range (0–5) to increase sensitivity of the measure in severe cases; (iii) elimination of the "resistance" items, as patients are often instructed to actively face and/or accept obsessive thoughts during treatment (a recommendation that could paradoxically increase Y-BOCS scores) and (iv) changes to wording in the symptom checklist to better capture "not just right" experiences as well as symptoms that are based in specific fears [14].

While the Y-BOCS is the most widely used clinician-rated measure of OCD severity, other clinician-rated assessment measures have merit. Most notably, the National Institute of Mental Health Global Obsessive-Compulsive Scale (NIMH-GOCS) is a single-item measure [15] and the Dimensional Yale-Brown Obsessive Compulsive Scale (DY-BOCS) evaluates the severity of symptoms across six OCD symptom "dimensions" [16]. The NIMH-GOCS is a single-item rating that ranges from 0–15, with 0 representing no illness and 15 representing the most severe form of the disorder, which has been widely used as an overall assessment of OCD severity [15]. The DY-BOCS is a more extensive assessment that was developed to assess OCD severity in six symptom dimensions: aggression, moral/sexual/religious scrupulosity, symmetry, contamination, hoarding and "miscellaneous" (e.g., superstitions, special colors/numbers, brief assessment of related phenomena like body-image disturbance and body-focused repetitive behaviors) [16]. The DY-BOCS includes symptom checklists that incorporate both obsessions and compulsions in each of these categories followed by five items assessing the severity, avoidance, distress, frequency and impairment due to symptoms, and also includes a section that assesses overall symptoms. The DY-BOCS is validated for use with children and adults [16].

Self-Report Measures

Since obsessions can easily be confused with other cognitive phenomena like ruminations and worries, interviewer-rated measures of OCD are generally considered first-line. Regardless, many self-report questionnaires have been used to assess OCD and demonstrate sound psychometric properties. The American Psychiatric Association guidelines recommend two questionnaires: the Obsessive-Compulsive Inventory Revised (OCI-R) [17] and the Florida Obsessive-Compulsive Scale (FOCI) [18,19]. The OCI-R is an 18-item scale that assesses the distress associated with 18 common obsessive-compulsive symptoms, corresponding with six dimensions: washing, obsessing, hoarding, ordering, checking and neutralizing [19,20]. The FOCI follows the format of the Y-BOCS-II by first inquiring about 10 common obsessions and 10 common compulsions as part of a symptom checklist, and then includes a 5-item severity scale [20]. An empirically derived score of 21 on the OCI-R indicates significant likelihood of an OCD diagnosis [19].

The Child Version of the Obsessive Compulsive Inventory (OCI-CV) was validated in children ages 7–17 years, with a symptom checklist that parallels the 6-dimension structure of the adult version of the measure [21]. The OCI-CV assesses distress caused by 21 common obsessive-compulsive symptoms using a smaller Likert scale than in the adult measure (range 0–2) [22]. The Children's FOCI (C-FOCI) was modified to include developmentally appropriate language but follows the format of the FOCI, including a checklist of 17 common obsessions and compulsions experienced in childhood as rated on a "present" or "not present" scale, followed by 5 items assessing severity [23]. Both show strong internal consistency, convergent validity with interview-rated measures of OCD severity and sensitivity to treatment [22,24].

Self-report measures have been developed to capture the different dimensions of obsessive-compulsive symptoms. The Dimensional Obsessive-Compulsive Scale is a self-report measure that prompts respondents to rate the time taken, distress, avoidance, impairment and control caused by obsessions or compulsions in the following dimensions by providing a description of each with examples: contamination, responsibility (e.g., for harm or aggression), and unacceptable thoughts, and symmetry [22]. The DY-BOCS also includes a self-report version [18]. Both measures provide psychometrically sound ways of assessing different types of obsessive-compulsive symptoms [16,25].

Cross-Diagnostic Approaches and Their Implications for Classification and Diagnosis

What did change in DSM-5 was an increased recognition that many psychiatric syndromes are characterized by distressing, repetitive thoughts and/or behaviors, generating the new "obsessive-compulsive related disorders" (OCRD) category [24]. Distressing, irrational thoughts and repetitive behaviors occur in many mental health conditions beyond OCD. Thus, even if patients do not meet strict diagnostic criteria for OCD, they may still experience obsessions or compulsions and related clinical phenomena. The remainder of this chapter provides information about the boundaries of obsessions and compulsions compared with other types of repetitive thoughts and behaviors, and also provides suggestions of features to assess in those with obsessions and compulsions, including insight into the excessiveness of symptoms, family accommodation, maladaptive beliefs, functional motivators of symptoms and temperamental sensitivities.

Rumination and Worry Compared with Obsessions

Repetitive thoughts about distressing topics is a process that occurs across emotional disorders [25]. Most prominently, "repetitive negative thinking" appears to occur as "worries" in anxiety disorders, "rumination" in affective disorders like major depressive disorder, and obsessions in OCD and other related disorders like body dysmorphic disorder (BDD) [25,26].

Researchers have pointed to differences between the content and qualitative experience of worries/ruminations and obsessions, often suggesting that ruminations and worries are largely similar processes that differ in their temporal focus (i.e., the past in rumination and the future in worry) [25,27]. Worries are excessive preoccupations about everyday problems that are relevant to a person's quality of life, while ruminations are past-based, negative thoughts about real-life events and their potential consequences [25,27]. Compared with both worries and ruminations, obsessions tend to be: (i) less rational; (ii) experienced as intrusive and unwanted rather than self-initiated and (iii) prompt stronger urges to act on a compulsive urge (though it is worth noting that worries/ruminations can motivate some compulsive behaviors like reassurance-seeking and checking) [26,28,29,30]. Obsessions are now recognized in several DSM-5 disorders, most prominently in BDD, although future research may evaluate the obsessionality of thinking processes in other disorders like hoarding, and putative OCRDs like body-focused repetitive behavior disorders.

Insight

Although it was once thought that most people with OCD have complete recognition of the irrationality of their symptoms, it has since been recognized that insight exists in a continuous dimension in OCD, with some people completely acknowledging the senselessness of the thoughts and behaviors, others describing complete conviction in their intrusive thoughts and need to complete compulsions, and many others falling in between [31]. If the patient also has symptoms of a thought disorder (e.g., flat or inappropriate affect, hallucinations, paranoia), a comorbid diagnosis should also be considered. Generally speaking, even patients with low insight into the irrationality of their obsessions are able to articulate some doubt that they may not be true. When patients are completely convinced of the validity of their intrusive thoughts or delusions have themes (e.g., delusions of grandeur, of reference), they are more likely to be considered as delusions rather than obsessions.

The Brown Assessment of Beliefs Scale (BABS) is a semi-structured interview that provides a detailed assessment of a patient's recognition of the irrationality of psychiatric symptoms and has been validated for use among adults with OCD [32]. After prompting a patient for a specific belief they hold (e.g., "I will get AIDS unless I spend three hours per day washing a particular way"), the BABS interviewer asks seven questions that assess insight into the irrationality of the belief across different domains (e.g., conviction, perceptions of others' views, whether they could acknowledge another perspective). The BABS has been used to assess insight in those with OCD, BDD and other psychiatric conditions [32,33].

Ego-Dystonic Obsessions and Compulsions Compared with Ego-Syntonic Repetitive Thoughts and Interests

Repetitive thoughts and behaviors can be conceptualized on a continuous dimension of ego-dystonic compared with ego-syntonic processes. On the one end of the spectrum exist ego-dystonic obsessions and compulsions, which cause distress and are unwanted, and on the other end exist ego-syntonic thoughts and interests, such as pedophilic or homicidal ideations, hyperfocused interests and behaviors often described in those with autism spectrum disorder (ASD), and a need for perfectionism that is experienced as desired rather than burdensome. These distinctions are described below.

Unlike in homicidal individuals or people with pedophilic urges, obsessions about these topics produce intensive discomfort and often drive them to avoid any situations that may be perceived as dangerous (e.g., holding a knife around others, making eye contact with children). Similarly, people with OCD may have obsessive doubts about their own sexual orientation. While many people with non-heterosexual sexual orientations fear the consequences of their orientation (e.g., due to cultural biases), people with obsessive sexual orientation fears are concerned about whether they are romantically or sexually attracted toward a different sex even when they truly are not [34].

Another psychiatric disorder that is characterized by excessive and repetitive behaviors is ASD, though again research supports a delineation between repetitive thoughts and behaviors in each disorder (although they often co-occur) [35,36]. In ASD, individuals take interest in very particular activities and engage in them repetitively, contrasting with compulsions, which are driven by obsession-induced anxiety or discomfort. For instance, an individual with ASD may love a particular book and read it repetitively because they are interested in re-experiencing the story, while someone with OCD may re-read lines within a book until it feels "just right". Sensory sensitivities that are common in individuals with ASD may also appear to be driven by just right obsessions, but again the distinction between ego-syntonic experiences patients enjoy and ego-dystonic thoughts patients wish to stop is relevant. In these cases, an assessment of the function of the avoidance or behaviors may elucidate the appropriate diagnosis [37]. For instance, some people with OCD may need to readjust their clothing or tie their shoes repetitively to attain a just right sensation but wish they could stop, while those with ASD may not tolerate wearing certain clothing because it causes intense sensory discomfort, but may perceive this simply as a preference that they may not wish to change.

With regard to perfectionism, obsessive-compulsive personality disorder (OCPD) is characterized by excessive preoccupation with order and detail, perfection, and an inability to show flexibility, to the extent that these traits interfere with task completion and relationships [1]. Again, although these phenomena are prevalent in those with OCD, primary distinctions between these processes involve ego-dystonic needs for certainty/perfection in OCD and ego-syntonic perfectionism in OCPD [38,39]. For instance, a person with OCD is more likely to recognize the excessiveness of ordering compulsions and would seek treatment to experience relief from this need. A person with OCPD, however, is more likely to see excessive ordering as truly necessary to stay organized and may impose this need on family members, which could in turn lead to conflict and their recommendation for their family member to seek treatment [39].

Compulsions Compared With Tics or Impulse Control Behaviors

Though impulses, tics and compulsions all reflect an inability to inhibit a behavior, compulsions are driven by a desire to avoid harm or minimize distress, impulses are done to elicit some positive emotional experience, and tics are sudden movements or sounds done to satisfy a sensory urge like blinking, shaking or sniffing [40,41]. Common impulses include excessive shopping, stealing, skin picking and hair pulling, and common tics include blinking, sniffing, jerking and shrugging [42,43]. In contrast, common compulsions include cleaning, checking, ordering, counting and reassurance seeking. That said, some people with OCD experience compulsions as more impulsive than others (i.e., they perceive them as more rational and do not feel as strong a need to resist or control them), which has been related to more severe symptoms, a longer duration of illness and poorer treatment outcome [44,45]. Similarly, behaviors typically considered to be "impulse control" problems or tics may serve a compulsive function, like repetitive skin picking done to groom perceived skin flaws, or a shaking tic done to get rid of a "bad" thought. Thus, a particular symptom never determines whether repetitive behaviors are impulsive or compulsive. Rather, impulses and compulsions occur across diagnoses, and assessing the function of each (i.e., to elicit relief/pleasure or to alleviate distress) is the only way to determine where on the impulsive–compulsive continuum a behavior lies.

Cognitive Distortions

The Obsessive Beliefs Questionnaire (OBQ) was developed by an international group of OCD experts to capture common cognitive distortions among those with OCD [46]. Factor analyses of the OBQ suggested a three-factor structure of obsessive beliefs that included 44 items, generating the OBQ-44 [47]. These factors assess cognitions in the following domains: increased sense of responsibility for harm/estimation of the probability of threat, perfectionism/intolerance of uncertainty and a sense of the importance/control of thoughts [47]. Further validation of the OBQ-44 showed that perfectionism/intolerance of uncertainty and responsibility/threat estimation are transdiagnostic vulnerabilities that also correlate with depression and anxiety [46,48,49], while the importance of/need to control thoughts appears to be more directly related to OCD [49]. These domains are also beginning to be demonstrated in putative OCRDs, such as BDD and hoarding disorder, which have been shown to be related to the perfectionism domain [50,51].

Incompleteness Compared With Harm Avoidance

Coles' and Summerfeldt's bifactor model of OCD complements the work of the Obsessive Compulsive Cognitions Working Group, classifying two major motivators of obsessive-compulsive symptoms: (i) a sensory sense of "just not right" or incompleteness and (ii) a desire to avoid harm [52,53]. These two motivators are proposed to cut across overt symptoms dimensions like contamination, symmetry and aggressive/taboo thoughts; some people with OCD may check things repeatedly to attain a sense of completeness, while other may do so to prevent some feared outcome [54]. Both are likely present in many cases as the two constructs are significantly correlated; for instance, someone may wash their hands until it feels just right to avoid contracting a serious disease [54,55].

Incompleteness appears to more specifically motivate obsessive-compulsive symptoms compared with harm avoidance, which correlates similarly with other forms of emotional distress like depression and anxiety [55,56]. An interviewer-rated rating scale (the Obsessive-Compulsive Core Dimensions Interview) and a self-rated questionnaire (the Obsessive-Compulsive Core Dimensions Questionnaire) assess this bi-dimensional model of symptom motivators [57]. Incompleteness compared with harm avoidance has primarily been studied in OCD, though preliminary research suggests that incompleteness may also be a motivator of OCRD phenomena like body-image checking [58] and may be more prevalent in those with tic-related OCD [59].

Disgust and Anxiety Sensitivity

Two psychological vulnerabilities that have been proposed to be relevant to the development and maintenance of OCD and related disorders are sensitivity to experiences of disgust and anxiety [57,60]. Specifically, people with OCD may believe that the affective experience of anxiety following intrusive thoughts is unacceptable [60]. Anxiety sensitivity has been shown to be as prevalent in OCD as in anxiety disorders, except for panic disorder [61], and may also be linked to hoarding behaviors [62]. The Anxiety Sensitivity Index 3 (ASI-3) is an 18-item, psychometrically sound measure of anxiety sensitivity that was validated with a large number of clinical and nonclinical respondents across several countries [63]. The ASI-3 captures the most consistently replicated three-factor structure of anxiety sensitivity, including items that concern how anxiety will affect a person across social (i.e., looking anxious), physical (i.e., unpleasant physiological symptoms) and cognitive (i.e., losing control of thoughts) domains [63]. The ASI-3 is internally consistent and converges with theoretically similar subscales from previous anxiety sensitivity measures [63].

Disgust sensitivity refers to the extent of reactivity people experience in the face of disgusting stimuli, which has been most prominently characterized in three domains: core (i.e., consuming the stimulus would be associated with danger like garbage, rotting food), animal reminder (i.e., stimuli that remind people of mortality like injury or death) and contamination (i.e., contact with others who may be ill or dangerous) [64]. Disgust sensitivity has been prominently linked to disorders characterized by intuitively "disgusting" stimuli like contamination-based OCD and blood-injury injections or spider phobias [65], but have also been linked to anxiety disorder symptomology more generally even after controlling for negative affect [66]. The Disgust Propensity and Sensitivity Scale Revised (DPSS-R) is a 16-item questionnaire that assesses both disgust propensity, of the frequency of disgust experiences, and disgust sensitivity, or the affective impact of experiencing disgust [67,68]. The DPSS-R is internally consistent, shows a reliable two-factor structure, and has been validated for use among people with nonclinical respondents, as well as people with OCD and anxiety disorders [67,68].

Family Accommodation of Symptoms

Excessive accommodation of symptoms (e.g., participating in rituals, changing plans to avoid obsession triggers) can negatively reinforce symptoms, as do compulsions or avoidance [69]. A recent meta-analysis of 41 studies showed a large, significant correlation between family accommodation and OCD severity [70]. Though family accommodation was a process that was first formerly characterized in OCD, emerging research (particularly conducted with parents of children) indicates that family accommodation is a transdiagnostic process that is just as prevalent in anxiety disorders as it is in OCD [71], and has been shown to be common in related syndromes like chronic tic disorders [72]. The most common forms of family accommodation are listed on the Family Accommodation Scale for Obsessive-Compulsive Disorder, which has Interview Administered (FAS-IR) [73], Self-Report (FAS-SR; i.e., completed by caregivers) [74] and Patient Report (FAS-PR) [75] versions. All versions begin with an inquiry into different types of obsessions and compulsions that a family member may have, and are followed by an assessment of the extent to which family members are engaging in different types of accommodating behaviors (e.g., reassurance, waiting for ritual completion, participating in compulsions, helping avoid trigger situations). Although the FAS-IR is recommended by its developers, the FAS-SR and FAS-PR versions are psychometrically valid and are acceptable alternatives for untrained raters without sufficient time to administer the FAS-IR [79,80].

Clinical Implications of Cross-Diagnostic Approaches for Treatment and Prevention

Treatment Implications for Low Insight and Ego-Syntonic Obsessions or Compulsions

Poor insight has also been related to worse treatment outcome in most [76,77,78], but not all [79,80], studies that have assessed this issue. Even in people with poorer recognition of the excessiveness of their symptoms, however, insight has been shown to increase after OCD treatment [79]. Although OCD with poor insight has been proposed to be related to psychotic disorders, serotonin reuptake inhibitors have been shown to be effective even in cases of OCD with poor insight and with BDD, which often suggests poorer insight relative to typical patients with OCD [79,81]. In these cases, particular emphasis on motivational enhancement may be necessary to help patients focus on how their symptoms have interfered with their personal goals and values, rather than on providing evidence for and against the irrationality of symptoms. Similarly, for those with ego-syntonic symptoms of perfectionism (i.e., those with OCPD), motivational interviewing may help patients discover how imposing their rigidity on others may interfere with their goals. Using contingency management in younger people with ego-syntonic symptoms may also be an appropriate strategy.

Treatment Implications of Compulsions Compared With Tics and Impulse Control Behaviors

Accurate assessment of compulsions compared with impulse control behaviors and tics is necessary for treatment planning, as each indicates slightly different behavioral approaches. Although interventions for each symptom are similar in that patients find new ways to act to inhibit an undesired behavior, distinctions should be noted. The key behavioral tool for compulsions is exposure and response prevention, which involves patients facing obsession-provoking situations without participating in compulsions, while the core behavioral approach for impulse control behaviors like skin picking, hair pulling and tics, is habit reversal training, which involves patients using competing responses that are physically incompatible with the target behavior [82]. Further, comorbid tics have been shown to impede psychopharmacological treatment outcome in those with OCD, though cognitive-behavioral therapy outcomes do not appear to be affected by comorbid tics [83].

Family Accommodation of Symptoms

Family accommodation has been found to predict treatment outcome in multiple studies [76,84], although it is important to note that successful treatment generally corresponds with reductions in family accommodation [84]. Accordingly, a recent meta-analysis showed that increased emphasis on family accommodation during family-based cognitive behavioral therapy results in improved treatment outcomes [85], suggesting that clinicians should always make an effort to involve family members in treatment, particularly with very accommodating relatives.

Anxiety and Disgust Sensitivity

There is emerging evidence that psychoeducation about anxiety sensitivity and interoceptive exposure, or exposure to physiological sensations of anxiety, can result in meaningful reductions in anxiety sensitivity [86]. Relatively less has been done to investigate treatments specific to disgust sensitivity, though disgust reactions have been shown to decrease following cognitive behavioral therapy for anxiety disorders [87], although they may decline at a slower rate than fear [88].

Future Directions

As the OCRDs attract more research support and the transdiagnostic approach to psychopathology gains more momentum, diagnostic assessment, and treatment planning will only become more refined for people with clinically significant obsessions and compulsions. Specific diagnoses will be less likely to be used in this new framework, and, instead, many of the processes reviewed in this chapter may be assessed across diagnostic populations, which will only grow our understanding of these constructs.

Some dimensions may cut across people with OCD and anxiety disorders, like intolerance of uncertainty, threat avoidance, subjective and physiological arousal in the face of symptom triggers. Other dimensions may be relevant to the study of people presenting with other symptoms like tics or body-focused repetitive behavior disorders, such as sensory incompleteness experiences or neural circuits involving the basal ganglia. It will be interesting to see how processes that have been primarily linked to OCD, like the belief in the importance of thoughts, catastrophic interpretations of intrusions and incompleteness are related to other symptoms, and whether these processes correspond with consistent outcomes across diagnostic populations (e.g., treatment response, symptom severity, age of onset, neural circuit mechanisms). Likewise, bringing concepts typically studied in other disorders into OCD and other diagnoses may also prove useful. For example, body-focused repetitive behaviors are often described as either "focused" or "automatic," in that some people report realizing when they are engaging in these habits and others may not be aware of them at all [89]. In our clinical experience, we notice patients who do not realize they are engaging in more subtle compulsions or avoidance behaviors like reassurance seeking, mental compulsions or avoiding eye contact. Conceptualizing compulsions and avoidance on a similar automatic–focused continuum may be useful in the assessment of OCRDs and anxiety disorders.

To adequately study these processes across diagnoses, rating scales and other assessments must be developed that are relatively agnostic to specific symptom presentations. Many investigators have already recognized the importance of designing cross-diagnostic assessments, such as the BABS. Rather than assessing insight for a specific disorder, the BABS prompts respondents to consider a core belief associated with a symptom, whether it be a depressive cognition, an obsessive belief or a paranoid delusion, before going on to inquire about perceptions of this belief. Developing tools like the BABS that assess other clinically significant concepts like impulsivity, compulsivity or intrusiveness across symptom presentations, will give researchers and clinicians more reliable ways to assess these constructs across diagnoses.

Using self-report measures that use consistent formats may be another way to more consistently compare across symptom presentations. LeBeau and colleagues from the DSM-5 working group on obsessive-compulsive related disorders provided one example of this in their validation of four brief assessments of OCRDs that include questions based on the FOCI (i.e., time, distress, control, avoidance and interference caused by the four other DSM-5 OCRDs) [90]. Measures like these that use consistent methods to assess repetitive thoughts and behaviors across specific symptoms may bring more parsimony to our understanding of putative obsessive-compulsive syndromes.

As research into continuous dimensions that affect people with a variety of psychiatric symptoms grows, it may give clinicians more guidance as to how to conduct flexible, clinically applicable assessment. For instance, treatment protocols for hoarding disorder and BDD call for more of an emphasis on cognitive interventions and motivational enhancement compared with many treatment manuals for OCD; clinical investigators have reported making this decision due to lower insight reported in these populations [90,91]. For individuals with OCD with low insight, however, these motivational enhancement strategies are likely equally important. Likewise, treatment that primarily emphasizes exposure and response prevention may be more efficient for people with BDD or hoarding problems with better insight.

As this research translates to clinical practice, clinicians may evaluate continuous constructs and formulate them into the treatment planning in addition to following treatment manuals for specific disorders. Indeed, many clinicians already sense the need to assess these characteristics continuously, as treatment manuals for specific diagnoses are often criticized as being too rigid, leading to an emergence of more "transdiagnostic" psychosocial treatments (e.g., the Unified Protocol) [92]. Tailoring our assessments to use a similar framework, which assesses clinically relevant constructs across diagnoses, will ensure that our psychiatric assessment corresponds with these more flexible treatment approaches.

References

1. American Psychiatric Association. *Diagnostic and Statistical Manual of Mental Disorders (DSM-5)*. Washington, DC: APA; 2013.
2. Brown TA, Barlow DH, DiNardo PA. *Anxiety Disorders Interview Schedule for DSM-IV, Adult Version: Client Interview Schedule*. New York, NY: Graywind Publications; 1994.
3. First MB, Spitzer RL, Gibbon M, Williams JB. *Structured Clinical Interview for DSM-IV Axis I Disorders*. New York, NY: New York State Psychiatric Institute; 1995.
4. Kaufman J, Birmaher B, Brent D, et al. Schedule for affective disorders and schizophrenia for school-age children-present and lifetime version (K-SADS-PL): initial reliability and validity data. *J Am Acad Child Adolesc Psychiatry*. 1997;36(7):980–988.
5. Silverman WK, Albano AM, Barlow DH. *Manual for the ADIS-IV-C/P*. New York, NY: Psychological Corporation; 1996.
6. Goodman WK, Price LH, Rasmussen SA, et al. The Yale-Brown Obsessive Compulsive Scale: II. Validity. *Arch Gen Psychiatry*. 1989;46(11):1012–1016.
7. Scahill L, Riddle MA, McSwiggin-Hardin M, et al. Children's Yale-Brown Obsessive Compulsive Scale: reliability and validity. *J Am Acad Child Adolesc Psychiatry*. 1997;36(6):844–852.
8. Lewin AB, Piacentini J, De Nadai AS, et al. Defining clinical severity in pediatric obsessive-compulsive disorder. *Psychol Assess*. 2014;26(2):679.
9. Storch EA, De Nadai AS, do Rosário MC, et al. Defining clinical severity in adults with obsessive–compulsive disorder. *Compr Psychiatry*. 2015;63:30–35.
10. Storch EA, Murphy TK, Geffken GR, et al. Psychometric evaluation of the Children's Yale–Brown Obsessive-Compulsive Scale. *Psychiatry Res*. 2004;129(1):91–98.
11. Mataix-Cols D, de la Cruz LF, Nordsletten AE, Lenhard F, Isomura K, Simpson HB. Towards an international expert consensus for defining treatment response, remission, recovery and relapse in obsessive-compulsive disorder. *World Psychiatry*. 2016;15(1):80–81.
12. Storch EA, Lewin AB, De Nadai AS, Murphy TK. Defining treatment response and remission in obsessive-compulsive disorder: a signal detection analysis of the Children's Yale-Brown Obsessive Compulsive Scale. *J Am Acad Child Adolesc Psychiatry*. 2010;49(7):708–717.
13. Tolin DF, Abramowitz JS, Diefenbach GJ. Defining response in clinical trials for obsessive-compulsive disorder: a signal detection analysis of the Yale-Brown obsessive compulsive scale. *J Clin Psychiatry*. 2005;66(12):1549–1557.
14. Storch EA, Rasmussen SA, Price LH, Larson MJ, Murphy TK, Goodman WK. Development and psychometric evaluation of the Yale–Brown Obsessive-Compulsive Scale – Second Edition. *Psychol Assess*. 2010;22(2):223.
15. Insel TR, Murphy DL, Cohen RM, Alterman I, Kilts C, Linnoila M. Obsessive-compulsive disorder: a double-blind trial of clomipramine and clorgyline. *Arch Gen Psychiatry*. 1983;40(6):605–612.
16. Rosario-Campos MC, Miguel EC, Quatrano S, et al. The Dimensional Yale–Brown Obsessive–Compulsive

Scale (DY-BOCS): an instrument for assessing obsessive–compulsive symptom dimensions. *Mol Psychiatry*. 2006;11(5):495–504.

17. Foa EB, Huppert JD, Leiberg S, et al. The Obsessive-Compulsive Inventory: development and validation of a short version. *Psychol Assess*. 2002;14(4):485.
18. Storch EA, Bagner D, Merlo LJ, et al. Florida obsessive-compulsive inventory: development, reliability, and validity. *J Clin Psychol*. 2007;63(9):851–859.
19. Koran LM, Simpson HB. *Guideline Watch (March 2013): Practice Guideline for the Treatment of Patients with Obsessive-Compulsive Disorder*. Arlington, VA: American Psychiatric Association; 2013.
20. Huppert JD, Walther MR, Hajcak G, et al. The OCI-R: validation of the subscales in a clinical sample. *J Anxiety Disord*. 2007;21(3):394–406.
21. Foa EB, Coles M, Huppert JD, Pasupuleti RV, Franklin ME, March J. Development and validation of a child version of the obsessive compulsive inventory. *Behav Ther*. 2010;41(1):121–132.
22. Abramowitz JS, Deacon BJ, Olatunji BO, et al. Assessment of obsessive-compulsive symptom dimensions: development and evaluation of the Dimensional Obsessive-Compulsive Scale. *Psychol Assess*. 2010;22(1):180.
23. Storch EA, Khanna M, Merlo LJ, et al. Children's Florida obsessive compulsive inventory: psychometric properties and feasibility of a self-report measure of obsessive–compulsive symptoms in youth. *Child Psychiatry Hum Dev*. 2009;40(3):467–483.
23. Abramowitz JS, Deacon BJ, Olatunji BO, et al. Assessment of obsessive-compulsive symptom dimensions: development and evaluation of the Dimensional Obsessive-Compulsive Scale. *Psychol Assess*. 2010;22(1):180.
24. Phillips KA, Stein DJ, Rauch SL, et al. Should an obsessive–compulsive spectrum grouping of disorders be included in DSM-V? *Depress Anxiety*. 2010;27(6):528–555.
25. Ehring T, Watkins ER. Repetitive negative thinking as a transdiagnostic process. *Int J Cogn Ther*. 2008;1(3):192–205.
26. Wahl K, Schönfeld S, Hissbach J, et al. Differences and similarities between obsessive and ruminative thoughts in obsessive-compulsive and depressed patients: a comparative study. *J Behav Ther Exp Psychiatry*. 2011;42(4):454–461.
27. McEvoy PM, Mahoney AE, Moulds ML. Are worry, rumination, and post-event processing one and the same? Development of the Repetitive Thinking Questionnaire. *J Anxiety Disord*. 2010;24(5):509–519.
28. Turner SM, Beidel DC, Stanley MA. Are obsessional thoughts and worry different cognitive phenomena? *Clin Psychol Rev*. 1992;12(2):257–270.
29. Schut AJ, Castonguay LG, Borkovec TD. Compulsive checking behaviors in generalized anxiety disorder. *J Clin Psychol*. 2001;57(6):705–715.
30. Beesdo-Baum K, Jenjahn E, Höfler M, Lueken U, Becker ES, Hoyer J. Avoidance, safety behavior, and reassurance seeking in generalized anxiety disorder. *Depress Anxiety*. 2012;29(11):948–957.
31. Foa EB, Kozak MJ. DSM-IV field trial: obsessive-compulsive disorder. *Am J Psychiatry*. 1995;152(1):90–96.
32. Eisen JL, Phillips KA, Baer L, Beer DA, Atala KD, Rasmussen SA. The Brown assessment of beliefs scale: reliability and validity. *Am J Psychiatry*. 1998;155(1):102–108.
33. Eisen JL, Phillips KA, Coles ME, Rasmussen SA. Insight in obsessive compulsive disorder and body dysmorphic disorder. *Compr Psychiatry*. 2004;45(1):10–15.
34. Williams MT, Farris SG. Sexual orientation obsessions in obsessive–compulsive disorder: prevalence and correlates. *Psychiatry Res*. 2011;187(1):156–159.
35. Ruzzano L, Borsboom D, Geurts HM. Repetitive behaviors in autism and obsessive–compulsive disorder: new perspectives from a network analysis. *J Autism Dev Disord*. 2015;45(1):192–202.
36. Zandt F, Prior M, Kyrios M. Repetitive behaviour in children with high functioning autism and obsessive compulsive disorder. *J Autism Dev Disord*. 2007;37(2):251–259.
37. Ben-Sasson A, Hen L, Fluss R, Cermak SA, Engel-Yeger B, Gal E. A meta-analysis of sensory modulation symptoms in individuals with autism spectrum disorders. *J Autism Dev Disord*. 2009;39(1):1–1.
38. Eisen JL, Coles ME, Shea MT, et al. Clarifying the convergence between obsessive compulsive personality disorder criteria and obsessive compulsive disorder. *J Pers Disord*. 2006;20(3):294–305.
39. Mancebo MC, Eisen JL, Grant JE, Rasmussen SA. Obsessive compulsive personality disorder and obsessive compulsive disorder: clinical characteristics, diagnostic difficulties, and treatment. *Ann Clin Psychiatry*. 2005;17(4):197–204.
40. Hollander E, Benzaquen SD. The obsessive-compulsive spectrum disorders. *Int Rev Psychiatry*. 1997;9(1):99–110.
41. Shprecher D, Kurlan R. The management of tics. *Mov Disord*. 2009;24(1):15
42. Dell'Osso B, Altamura AC, Allen A, Marazziti D, Hollander E. Epidemiologic and clinical updates on impulse control disorders: a critical review. *Eur Arch Psychiatry Clin Neurosci*. 2006;256(8):464–475.

43. Leckman JF, Riddle MA, Hardin MT, et al. The Yale Global Tic Severity Scale: initial testing of a clinician-rated scale of tic severity. *J Am Acad Child AdolescPsychiatry*. 1989;28(4):566–573.

44. Fontenelle LF, Oostermeijer S, Harrison BJ, Pantelis C, Yücel M. Obsessive-compulsive disorder, impulse control disorders and drug addiction. *Drugs*. 2011;71(7):827–840.

45. Kashyap H, Fontenelle LF, Miguel EC, et al. "Impulsive compulsivity" in obsessive-compulsive disorder: a phenotypic marker of patients with poor clinical outcome. *J Psychiatr Res*. 2012;46(9):1146–1152.

46. Obsessive Compulsive Cognitions Working Group. Development and initial validation of the obsessive beliefs questionnaire and the interpretation of intrusions inventory. *Behav Res Ther*. 2001;39(8):987–1006.

47. Obsessive Compulsive Cognitions Working Group. Psychometric validation of the obsessive belief questionnaire and interpretation of intrusions inventory – Part 2: factor analyses and testing of a brief version. *Behav Res Ther*. 2005;43(11):1527–1542.

48. Gentes EL, Ruscio AM. A meta-analysis of the relation of intolerance of uncertainty to symptoms of generalized anxiety disorder, major depressive disorder, and obsessive–compulsive disorder. *Clin Psychol Rev*. 2011 Aug 31;31(6):923–933.

49. Tolin DF, Worhunsky P, Maltby N. Are "obsessive" beliefs specific to OCD?: a comparison across anxiety disorders. *Behav Res Ther*. 2006;44(4):469–480.

50. Abramowitz JS, Lackey GR, Wheaton MG. Obsessive–compulsive symptoms: the contribution of obsessional beliefs and experiential avoidance. *J Anxiety Disord*. 2009;23(2):160–166.

51. Blakey SM, Abramowitz JS, Mahaffey BL. Do obsessive beliefs predict body image disturbance? *J Obsess-Compuls Rel*. 2016;11:96–100.

52. Coles ME, Heimberg RG, Frost RO, Steketee G. Not just right experiences and obsessive–compulsive features: experimental and self-monitoring perspectives. *Behav Res Ther*. 2005;43(2):153–167.

53. Summerfeldt LJ. Understanding and treating incompleteness in obsessive-compulsive disorder. *J Clin Psychol*. 2004;60(11):1155–1168.

54. Summerfeldt LJ, Kloosterman PH, Antony MM, Swinson RP. Examining an obsessive-compulsive core dimensions model: structural validity of harm avoidance and incompleteness. *J Obsess-Compuls Rel*. 2014;3(2):83–94.

55. Taylor S, McKay D, Crowe KB, et al. The sense of incompleteness as a motivator of obsessive-compulsive symptoms: an empirical analysis of concepts and correlates. *Behav Ther*. 2014;45(2):254–262.

56. Pietrefesa AS, Coles ME. Moving beyond an exclusive focus on harm avoidance in obsessive-compulsive disorder: behavioral validation for the separability of harm avoidance and incompleteness. *Behav Ther*. 2009;40(3):251–259.

57. Olatunji BO, Ebesutani C, David B, Fan Q, McGrath PB. Disgust proneness and obsessive–compulsive symptoms in a clinical sample: structural differentiation from negative affect. *J Anxiety Disord*. 2011;25(7):932–938.

58. Summers BJ, Matheny NL, Cougle JR. "Not just right" experiences and incompleteness in body dysmorphic disorder. *Psychiatry Res*. 2017;247:200–207.

59. da Silva Prado H, do Rosario MC, Lee J, Hounie AG, Shavitt RG, Miguel EC. Sensory phenomena in obsessive-compulsive disorder and tic disorders: a review of the literature. *CNS Spectr*. 2008;13(5):425–432.

60. Robinson LJ, Freeston MH. Emotion and internal experience in obsessive compulsive disorder: reviewing the role of alexithymia, anxiety sensitivity and distress tolerance. *Clin Psychol Rev*. 2014;34(3):256–271.

61. Olatunji BO, Wolitzky-Taylor KB. Anxiety sensitivity and the anxiety disorders: a meta-analytic review and synthesis. *Psychol Bull*. 2009;135(6):974–999.

62. Timpano KR, Buckner JD, Richey JA, Murphy DL, Schmidt NB. Exploration of anxiety sensitivity and distress tolerance as vulnerability factors for hoarding behaviors. *Depress Anxiety*. 2009;26(4):343–353.

63. Taylor S, Zvolensky MJ, Cox BJ, et al. Robust dimensions of anxiety sensitivity: development and initial validation of the Anxiety Sensitivity Index-3. *Psychol Assess*. 2007;19(2):176.

64. Olatunji BO, Broman-Fulks JJ. A taxometric study of the latent structure of disgust sensitivity: converging evidence for dimensionality. *Psychol Assess*. 2007;19(4):437.

65. Olatunji BO, Cisler J, McKay D, Phillips ML. Is disgust associated with psychopathology? Emerging research in the anxiety disorders. *Psychiatry Res*. 2010;175(1–2):1–10.

66. Olatunji BO, Armstrong T, Elwood L. Is disgust proneness associated with anxiety and related disorders? A qualitative review and meta-analysis of group comparison and correlational studies. *Perspect Psychol Sc*. 2017;12(4):613–648.

67. Van Overveld WJM, de Jong PD, Peters ML, Cavanagh K, Davey GCL. Disgust propensity and disgust sensitivity: separate constructs that are differentially related to specific fears. *Pers Individ Dif*. 2006;41(7):1241–1252.

68. Olatunji BO, Cisler JM, Deacon BJ, Connolly K, Lohr JM. The disgust propensity and sensitivity

scale-revised: psychometric properties and specificity in relation to anxiety disorder symptoms. *J Anxiety Disord.* 2007;21(7):918–930.

69. Lebowitz ER, Panza KE, Su J, Bloch MH. Family accommodation in obsessive–compulsive disorder. *Expert Rev Neurother.* 2012;12(2):229–238.

70. Wu MS, McGuire JF, Martino C, Phares V, Selles RR, Storch EA. A meta-analysis of family accommodation and OCD symptom severity. *Clin Psychol Rev.* 2016;45:34–44.

71. Lebowitz ER, Scharfstein LA, Jones J. Comparing family accommodation in pediatric obsessive-compulsive disorder, anxiety disorders, and nonanxious children. *Depress Anxiety.* 2014;31(12):1018–1025.

72. Storch EA, Johnco C, McGuire JF, et al. An initial study of family accommodation in children and adolescents with chronic tic disorders. *Eur Child Adolesc Psychiatry.* 2017;26(1):99–109.

73. Calvocoressi L, Mazure CM, Kasl SV, et al. Family accommodation of obsessive-compulsive symptoms: instrument development and assessment of family behavior. *J Nerv Ment Dis.* 1999;187(10):636–642.

74. Pinto A, Van Noppen B, Calvocoressi L. Development and preliminary psychometric evaluation of a self-rated version of the Family Accommodation Scale for Obsessive-Compulsive Disorder. *J Obsess-Compuls Rel.* 2013;2(4):457–465.

75. Wu MS, Pinto A, Horng B, et al. Psychometric properties of the Family Accommodation Scale for Obsessive–Compulsive Disorder–Patient Version. *Psychol Assess.* 2016;28(3):251.

76. Garcia AM, Sapyta JJ, Moore PS, et al. Predictors and moderators of treatment outcome in the Pediatric Obsessive Compulsive Treatment Study (POTS I). *J Am Acad Child Adolesc Psychiatry.* 2010;49(10):1024–1033.

77. Kishore VR, Samar R, Reddy YJ, Chandrasekhar CR, Thennarasu K. Clinical characteristics and treatment response in poor and good insight obsessive–compulsive disorder. *Eur Psychiatry.* 2004;19(4):202–208.

78. Himle JA, Van Etten ML, Janeck AS, Fischer DJ. Insight as a predictor of treatment outcome in behavioral group treatment for obsessive–compulsive disorder. *Cognit Ther Res.* 2006;30(5):661–666.

79. Eisen JL, Rasmussen SA, Phillips KA, et al. Insight and treatment outcome in obsessive-compulsive disorder. *Compr Psychiatry.* 2001;42(6):494–497.

80. Alonso P, Menchón JM, Segalàs C, et al. Clinical implications of insight assessment in obsessive-compulsive disorder. *Compr Psychiatry.* 2008;49(3):305–312.

81. Phillips KA, Hollander E. Treating body dysmorphic disorder with medication: evidence, misconceptions, and a suggested approach. *Body Image.* 2008;5(1):13–27.

82. Himle MB, Woods DW, Piacentini JC, Walkup JT. Brief review of habit reversal training for Tourette syndrome. *J Child Neurol.* 2006;21(8):719–725.

83. March JS, Franklin ME, Leonard H, et al. Tics moderate treatment outcome with sertraline but not cognitive-behavior therapy in pediatric obsessive-compulsive disorder. *Biol Psychiatry.* 2007;61(3):344–347.

84. Merlo LJ, Lehmkuhl HD, Geffken GR, Storch EA. Decreased family accommodation associated with improved therapy outcome in pediatric obsessive–compulsive disorder. *J Consult Clin Psychol.* 2009;77(2):355.

85. Thompson-Hollands J, Edson A, Tompson MC, Comer JS. Family involvement in the psychological treatment of obsessive–compulsive disorder: a meta-analysis. *J Fam Psychol.* 2014;28(3):287–298.

86. Schmidt NB, Capron DW, Raines AM, Allan NP. Randomized clinical trial evaluating the efficacy of a brief intervention targeting anxiety sensitivity cognitive concerns. *J Consult Clin Psychol.* 2014;82(6):1023–1033.

87. Taboas W, Ojserkis R, McKay D. Change in disgust reactions following cognitive-behavioral therapy for childhood anxiety disorders. *Int J Clin Health Psychol.* 2015;15(1):1–7.

88. Mason EC, Richardson R. Treating disgust in anxiety disorders. *Clin Psychol.* 2012;19(2):180–194.

89. Flessner CA, Woods DW, Franklin ME, Cashin SE, Keuthen NJ, Board TL. The Milwaukee inventory for subtypes of trichotillomania-adult version (MIST-A): development of an instrument for the assessment of "focused" and "automatic" hair pulling. *J Psychopathol Behav Assess.* 2008;30(1):20–30.

90. Wilhelm S, Phillips KA, Steketee G. *Cognitive-Behavioral Therapy for Body Dysmorphic Disorder: A Treatment Manual.* New York, NY: Guilford Press; 2014.

91. Tolin DF, Worden BL, Wootton BM, Gilliam CM. *CBT for Hoarding Disorder: A Group Therapy Program Therapist's Guide.* Hoboken, NJ: John Wiley & Sons; 2017.

92. Barlow DH, Farchione TJ, Fairholme CP, et al. *Unified Protocol for Transdiagnostic Treatment of Emotional Disorders: Therapist Guide.* Oxford: Oxford University Press; 2010.

Chapter 15

Pharmacological Treatments for Obsessive-Compulsive and Related Disorders: A Transdiagnostic Perspective

Ricky A. Sachdev, Risha Ruparelia, Jemma E. Reid, Davis Mpavenda, Eduardo Cinosi and Naomi A. Fineberg

Case Study

Mr. X is a 40-year-old man with a longstanding history of distressing obsessions of a murderous and sexual nature. Associated compulsions include the need to examine all his thoughts, motivated either by the desire to eradicate any that do not "feel right", or by the desire to prevent him acting aggressively. Mr. X also experiences repeated, distressing impulsive urges that predate the onset of the obsessive-compulsive symptomatology, including the urge to hit his wife, break his car windscreen and grind his teeth, which at times he cannot resist, and which appear to have become habitual. They are characterized by a prodromal period of tension with a feeling of release at the time of the act. Mr. X also described the habit of picking his skin around his nails to the point that they bleed.

Mr. X meets diagnostic criteria for obsessive-compulsive disorder, "other habit and impulse disorder" and skin-picking disorder. He gave a childhood history of inattentiveness, which together with his impulse control problems was suggestive of attention deficit hyperactivity disorder, but he did not fulfill all the criteria for this diagnosis. There were traits, but again insufficient evidence to sustain a diagnosis of obsessive-compulsive personality disorder or autism spectrum disorder.

This complex pattern of symptoms and syndromes, characterized by a shift over time from impulsive to compulsive behavior, is commonly seen in the psychiatry clinic, is inadequately captured by the current psychiatric taxonomy and can be difficult to treat. Mr. X's symptoms have so far proved resistant to conventional OCD treatments, including multiple trials of cognitive behavioral therapy (CBT) with exposure and response prevention, as well as treatment with clomipramine, several selective serotonin reuptake inhibitors and adjunctive first- and second-generation antipsychotics. He has also failed to respond to adjunctive treatment with methylphenidate targeting poor attention and impulse control and anti-epileptics (lamotrigine, carbamazepine, pregabalin) targeting emotional lability and anxiety. Further treatment options under consideration include exposure and response prevention augmented with habit reversal strategies, venlafaxine, N-acetylcysteine and naltrexone, based on experimental findings in studies of obsessive-compulsive and related disorders.

Introduction

Drug development in psychiatry is traditionally based on categorical diagnostic models that define psychiatric disorders according to symptoms and syndromes. Faced with the growing concern that existing treatments are inadequate and the shortage of new compounds entering phase II trials, the European Union Roadmap for Mental Health Research in Europe [1] and the US National Institute of Mental Health, Research Domain Criteria [2] have called for new ways of classifying psychopathology to better support treatment development. The proposed models are to be based on dimensions of observable behavior with established biological validity, irrespective of diagnosis, and represent an attempt to minimize the considerable biological heterogeneity that exists within the current taxonomy, which is thought to be hampering identification of the underpinning mechanisms that may serve as therapeutic targets.

In response to these concerns, the *Diagnostic and Statistical Manual of Mental Disorders*, 5th edition (DSM-5) placed greater weight than hitherto on clustering psychiatric disorders according to neurobiological factors, in the expectation that this would also enhance treatment discovery. Based largely on its distinctive treatment profile, obsessive-compulsive disorder (OCD) was placed at the head of a new obsessive-compulsive and related disorder (OCRD) grouping. Other OCRDs were included on the basis of shared aspects of phenomenology, including the performance of distressing and functionally disabling compulsive behaviors, as well as a tendency to co-exist both within the same individual and within family groups, implying the existence of shared etiological mechanisms [3]. However, relatively little is known about shared and disorder-specific neurobiological abnormalities that might mediate traits and symptoms seen across the OCRD grouping and that could act as substrates for transdiagnostic treatments [4].

The DSM-5 OCRD cluster, comprising OCD, body dysmorphic disorder (BDD), hoarding disorder, hair-pulling disorder and skin-picking disorder, represents some of the most costly, functionally disabling and treatment-resistant brain disorders [5,6]. By gathering together diagnoses previously listed in the DSM-IV under anxiety disorders, somatoform disorders, and impulse control disorders not elsewhere classified into a coherent OCRD grouping, the DSM-5 classification is generally expected to advance the scientific study of these disorders, as well as to improve their clinical recognition and management. It is fully expected that the forthcoming International Classification of Diseases 11th revision will adopt a similar approach and may even include additional new diagnoses among the OCRD grouping, such as olfactory reference syndrome (or disorder) [7].

Of these disorders, OCD is by far the most well understood. The disorder is characterized by the selective response to the strongly serotonergic tricyclic clomipramine and the more highly selective serotonin reuptake inhibitors (SSRIs) delivered at high doses, combined with the lack of response to anxiolytic agents of other classes (see below), as well as brain imaging findings implicating the involvement of corticostriatal neural circuitry outside the recognized fear pathways. However, approximately 40% of those receiving evidence-based therapies fail to respond and there is no way of predicting a priori, with any degree of certainty, the extent to which treatment-related benefits or adverse effects will emerge.

Whereas other OCRDs have so far been subjected to little systematic research and their treatment remains largely empirical, it is becoming increasingly clear that across the OCRDs grouping there are areas of overlap but also key differences in the treatment response, presumably reflecting differences in the underlying illness mechanisms. Moreover, there is a great deal of unexplained heterogeneity within each disorder, to the extent that the same treatment cannot be assumed to benefit all members of the diagnostic group. A diverse range of drugs belonging to different classes have been found to be potentially effective in the OCRDs (see below), and have also been investigated in treatment-resistant OCD, with mixed results. Furthermore, treatments usually used for other diagnoses such as psychotic or addictive disorders may also have a role in treating OCRDs. However, the shortage of effective treatments, in the face of an overall decline in the pace of psychiatric treatment discovery, represents a key and pressing challenge [8].

In the case of OCD, most treatment trials have investigated the relatively "pure" disorder, in which patients with major psychiatric comorbidity were excluded in an attempt to reduce potential sources of confound. In clinical practice, however, OCD is frequently associated with significant multiple psychiatric comorbidity. Common comorbid diagnoses include mood, anxiety and psychotic disorders, as well as other OCRDs and personality disorders [9]. Phenotypic signs of an altered neurodevelopmental trajectory are also commonly observed in patients with OCRDs, such as traits or symptoms of tic disorder, autism spectrum disorder (ASD) and attention deficit hyperactivity disorder (ADHD) [10,11]. These comorbid traits and diagnoses appear to cluster in the same patient or within their family members, hinting that shared, heritable neurobehavioral mechanisms contribute to the expression of a broad spectrum of compulsive behavior.

For example, a recent study in patients with tic disorders identified two independent, heritable, symptom-based factors (one involving the urge to attain symmetry, the other involving behavioral disinhibition) as possible transdiagnostic phenotypes of compulsive behavior [12]. These complex syndromes do not easily fit into the existing diagnostic classification, are challenging to manage, and often fail to respond to conventional treatments. The above vignette, in which highly treatment-resistant OCD is associated with multiple mixed impulsive and compulsive symptomatology, exemplifies just such a case. The presence of this co-existing symptomatology hints that the discovery of treatments that target transdiagnostic symptom dimension constructs commonly associated with OCDs, such as compulsivity and impulsivity, obsessionality and delusionality, cognitive (obsession) and motoric (stereotypies, habits and tics), harm avoidance and incompleteness, would be of great value for the field. Unfortunately, however, there is a shortage of published trial data relating to "comorbid" – or "complex" OCRD and a lack of a standardized battery of instruments to define and measure the symptom dimensions. Therefore, the clinical management of cases such as these remains largely empirical.

In this chapter, we review the shared and disorder-specific clinical psychopharmacology of OCD and the disorders related to it, from a transdiagnostic perspective. We focus on OCD, as the exemplar disorder for which the majority of the data pertains. We therefore start by defining the "typical" characteristics of the OCD treatment response. We draw comparisons with the emerging trial data relating to the other OCRDs, and, where relevant, with other psychiatric disorders thought to share a relationship with OCRDs, such as Tourette's disorder, ASD and addictive disorders. Improved understanding of the areas of overlap and differences in treatment response among these disorders may help to clarify what is currently known about treating compulsivity and the boundaries of OCD and related disorders, unveil areas worthy of future research and aid the development of new assessment tools and treatment targets. We additionally explore the extent to which the presence of specific compulsive symptoms or cognitive behavioral traits might impact upon OCRD treatment outcomes, as a step in the path toward developing treatment algorithms based on transdiagnostic phenomena.

Pharmacotherapy of Obsessive-Compulsive Disorders

Individuals with OCRDs are usually unforthcoming about their symptoms; for example, through a sense of shame or lack of knowledge that they represent recognized mental disorders. As a result, the OCRDs are poorly recognized and there is usually a lag of several years between the onset of symptoms and initiation of effective treatment. The duration of untreated illness, which in the case of OCD still reaches on average 15 years, represents one of the principal factors determining clinical and health outcomes [13], emphasizing the importance of early diagnosis and institution of effective treatment [14].

Selective Response to Clomipramine and the Selective Serotonin Reuptake Inhibitors

The efficacy of the tricyclic agent clomipramine, and the SSRIs fluoxetine, paroxetine, fluvoxamine, citalopram and escitalopram, has been conclusively demonstrated in a series of well-powered multicenter placebo-referenced randomized controlled trials (RCT) in adults and children with OCD (reviewed in Fineberg and Gale [15]; Fineberg et al. [16]; Stein et al. [17]), and a series of meta-analyses (see below). While response to medication does not necessarily imply symptom remission, it was usually associated with significant improvement in quality of life [18,19,20].

Soomro et al. [21] included 17 adulthood OCD studies, with a total of 3097 recruits, and demonstrated that SSRIs were twice as likely as placebo to effect a clinical response, while McGuire et al. [22] found a moderate effect size for treatment efficacy (g = 0.50), treatment response (relative risk, RR, 1.80) and remission (RR 2.06) in a meta-analysis of SSRI and clomipramine trials involving 789 young people with OCD. A 2016 systematic review and network meta-analysis of randomized controlled treatment trials in adults with OCD reaffirmed that clomipramine and all the SSRIs had superior efficacy against drug placebo [23]. These drugs act as powerful inhibitors of the synaptic reuptake of serotonin (5-hydroxytryptamine, 5-HT). In contrast, drugs lacking robust SRI effects (e.g. imipramine [24,25], clorgyline [26], phenelzine [27], amitriptyline [28], nortriptyline [29], lithium [30]), and non-antidepressant anxiolytics such as the azapirone buspirone [31], and the benzodiazepine alprazolam [32] turned out to be ineffective in RCTs (Table 15.1). Clonazepam, a benzodiazepine with possible serotonergic effects, may be of some benefit in OCD [33] but the results from two placebo-controlled trials were not positive [34,35].

The majority of the validating treatment studies excluded major psychiatric comorbidity, so as to be sure that the treatment was specifically working on OCD. Yet OCD is naturally highly comorbid with other psychiatric disorders such as anxiety, depression, OCRDs, bipolar disorder and neurodevelopmental disorders [36]. We therefore know relatively little about the impact of these comorbidities on the OCD treatment response.

Table 15.1 The pharmacological specificity of obsessive-compulsive disorder.

Effective	Ineffective
Potent SRIs:	Tricyclic antidepressants (except for clomipramine)
Clomipramine	Monoamine oxidase inhibitors
Fluvoxamine	Lithium
Fluoxetine	Benzodiazepines
Sertraline	Buspirone
Paroxetine	Agomelatine
Citalopram	
Escitalopram	

OCD with Comorbid Depression

Some of the early RCTs of clomipramine failed to exclude patients with depression and found that the drug was nevertheless effective (reviewed in Fineberg and Gale [15]). Hoehn-Saric et al. [37] allowed depression as a comorbidity and compared sertraline with desipramine. OCD responded equally well to sertraline (but not desipramine) whether or not depressive comorbidity was present. Interestingly, however, the depressive symptoms responded exclusively to sertraline, implying that an SSRI is needed to treat depression in the context of comorbid OCD and implying that the depressive symptomatology was integral or secondary to the OCD.

OCD with Comorbid Tic Disorder

Drugs used as antipsychotics are effective in the treatment of Tourette's disorder, presumably acting via dopamine receptor antagonist effects. They have also been found to be effective as adjunctive treatments with SRIs in OCD with tics [38], though a preferential effect for adjunctive antipsychotic in OCD with tic has yet to be robustly confirmed.

OCD with Comorbid Attention Deficit Hyperactivity Disorder

Highly discordant prevalence rates are reported for ADHD–OCD comorbidity. The extent to which attentional problems stemming from OCD symptoms are erroneously diagnosed as ADHD remains unclear [39]. Stimulants represent the first line of treatment for ADHD, but may lead to an exacerbation of anxiety or obsessive-compulsive symptoms [39]. However, case reports of children with OCD and ADHD hint that augmentation of SRI and CBT with either methylphenidate (a norepinephrine-dopamine reuptake inhibitor stimulant) or guanfacine (a noradrenergic alpha-2-a receptor agonist) might be of benefit for both conditions [40,41].

Incremental Response to Treatment with Serotonin Reuptake Inhibitors

The consensus from most OCD treatment trials is that the SRI response in OCD accrues slowly and gradually over weeks and months [15]. As the majority of studies included only a small number of subjects, the establishment of a significant drug–placebo difference was usually delayed by several weeks. However, two large multi-center double-blind RCTs were able to reveal a clinically significant difference between clomipramine and placebo in patients with OCD who were not depressed as early as the first week of administration [42,43]. A recent meta-analysis by Issaria et al. [44], involving 3276 patients, demonstrated placebo-referenced efficacy of SSRIs appearing as early as two weeks after treatment started. Furthermore, the largest treatment effect seemed to occur within this two-week period.

In a pragmatic naturalistic 12-week SRI trial [45], early improvement was the best predictor of treatment response. Only just over half the subjects who showed early improvement went on to achieve a full clinical response within the study period. However, other long-term follow-up data suggest that the percentage of OCD responders to SSRI increases for at least six months after treatment has started [19]. Additional gains continue to be made for at least two years, as long as treatment is continued [46]. Pulse loading, with either oral or intravenous clomipramine, may possibly advance the onset of response, but is not recognized to produce overall long-term benefit [47]. The extent to which these characteristics extend to other OCRDs, or are affected by comorbidity, is not well known.

Dose–Response Relationship

The finding from several fixed-dose studies that higher doses of SSRIs show greater efficacy in OCD (reviewed in Fineberg and Gale [15]) was confirmed in a meta-analysis [48]. A 2016 meta-analysis [44] demonstrated that higher doses of SSRIs were associated with greater improvement of OCD symptoms and that the onset of benefit occurs within three to six weeks of instituting high-dose treatment. Higher doses were however linked to poorer tolerability with an increased number of patient dropouts due to adverse effects. Therefore, most treatment guidelines [49,50,51] suggest gradual up-titration of SSRI to maximum licensed doses, factoring in sufficient time to evaluate treatment response. In contrast, there is no reliable dose-finding study data to inform the use of adjunctive antipsychotic in OCD, or the effects of dosage in other OCRDs.

Blunted Placebo Response

Placebo response rates in OCD are consistently lower than those seen in affective and anxiety disorders [52]. Rates are even lower in SSRI-resistant OCD. A systematic review of antipsychotic augmentation of SSRI [38] revealed a mean placebo response of 11%, and rates as low as 0% were reported in trials that augmented SRI with either lithium [30] or buspirone [31,53].

A random effects meta-analysis of 56 trials which directly compared antidepressant and placebo response rates between OCD, generalized anxiety disorder, panic disorder, post-traumatic stress disorder and social anxiety disorder revealed that OCD was associated with significantly lower pre–post effect sizes for placebo and antidepressant therapy although the drug–placebo effect sizes were not significantly different across the diagnoses [54].

It has been hypothesized that the placebo response may be closely tied to the reward neurocircuitry, involving projections linking the tegmental or prefrontal dopaminergic neurons and the dorsal and ventral striatum, and the activation of dopamine and endogenous opioid peptides in the nucleus accumbens [55,56,57]. As failures in the cortical control of frontostriatal neural circuits are thought to underpin the pathophysiology of OCD (reviewed in Figee et al. [58]; Fineberg et al. [59]; Stein et al. [17]) altered function of the reward based system may possibly explain the low placebo response rates seen in this condition. The extent to which a blunted placebo response extends transdiagnostically to other OCRDs or disorders of compulsive behavior remains to be explored.

Mechanism of Effect of Serotonin Reuptake Inhibitors in Obsessive-Compulsive Disorder

The weight of evidence suggests that the 5-HT system plays an important role in OCD, though the exact mechanism of effect of SRIs remains poorly understood [60]. El Mansari and Blier [61] reviewed the effects on 5-HT release and the adaptive changes in pre- and postsynaptic 5-HT receptor sensitivity induced by SRI treatment in rodent brain structures thought to be involved in OCD, including analogs of the orbitofrontal cortex. The time course of increased 5-HT release and terminal 5-HT_{1D} auto-receptor desensitization aligned with the course of the therapeutic response to SRI in OCD.

In addition, consistent with the dose-dependent therapeutic effect of SRIs, a greater dose of SRI induced greater reuptake inhibition, which played an essential role in this phenomenon. The authors hypothesized that the effect of enhanced 5-HT release in the orbitofrontal cortex is mediated by the activation of postsynaptic 5-HT_2-like receptors and underlies the therapeutic action of SRI in OCD. The potentially beneficial effect of hallucinogens with 5-HT_2 agonist properties (e.g., psilocybin [62]) in obtaining a therapeutic response may provide some support for this theory.

Long-Term Outcomes

A prospective study in a community cohort of individuals with a spectrum of OCDs and syndromes found that over the course of 30 years, a majority of the participants entered sustained remission, though for many this took several years to achieve [14]. The presence of comorbid anxiety and affective disorders, and the need to seek psychiatric treatment, were associated with significantly reduced remission rates [36].

In contrast, OCD in the clinical setting usually pursues a chronic relapse–remitting course and full or sustained remission is infrequently achieved [63]. In a naturalistic five-year follow-up study of 213 patients with OCD, only 39% entered either partial (22.1%) or full (16.9%) remission, and 59% of those who remitted subsequently relapsed [64]. Primary hoarding disorder responded particularly poorly in this study. Participants who had only achieved partial remission were more likely to relapse compared with those who had achieved full remission (70% vs. 45%). Moreover, patients with obsessive-compulsive personality disorder traits (perfectionism, cognitive and behavioral rigidity and hoarding) were more than twice as likely to relapse.

For those patients who have responded to an SSRI or clomipramine, maintenance treatment (as opposed to discontinuation) sustains the symptomatic response [65] and contributes positively to measures of quality of life and psychosocial functioning [18]. In contrast, cessation of drug therapy is frequently, but not in all cases, associated with relapse, regardless of the duration of treatment (reviewed by the American Psychiatric Association [51]; Fineberg et al. [66]). Regular clinic appointments have been shown to enhance adherence [67] and are recommended as a means of reducing relapse in the international standards of care for OCD published in 2016 [68].

Predicting Treatment-Related Outcomes

Approximately 40% of patients with OCD fail to respond, despite a prolonged course of evidence-based treatment (reviewed in Fineberg et al. [16]). The literature on response predictors is sparse and inconsistent (reviewed in Fineberg et al. [16]). In sum, there are no reliable, clinical or demographic response predictors that can be used on an individual basis, although a growing consensus suggests that a long period of untreated illness predicts a poorer response to pharmacological and psychological treatment in both childhood [69] and adult cohorts [13,64], suggesting that early identification and treatment of symptoms may favorably alter the clinical course of the disorder. Another long-term study of treatment non-responders reported that a poor outcome was predicted by shorter duration of follow-up and not receiving CBT during the interval period [70].

Other clinical factors may play a role in outcome prediction. In some studies of children, lesser symptom severity and OCD-related functional impairment and greater insight were associated with better outcomes [71,72], whereas comorbid illnesses such as ADHD, tic disorder and oppositional defiant disorder [73] predicted poorer outcomes. Similarly, studies in adults have found the presence of concomitant personality disorders [74–76] to be associated with poor treatment outcomes. Erzegovesi et al. [77] found that non-responders to SSRIs were more likely to have poorer insight and somatic obsessions. In another study, adult patients with OCD with comorbid chronic tic were less likely than patients without tic to respond to SSRI monotherapy [78].

Obsessive-Compulsive Symptom Dimensions

Factor analysis has resulted in the identification of OCD symptom "dimensions" thought to delineate more biologically homogeneous subgroups. The "symmetry" dimension has been found to be associated with poor response to SRIs [79] and with comorbid tic disorder [10,72], which may itself be independently associated with poor treatment response in most studies [80], although not according to de Vries et al. [10], Bloch et al. [81], Conelea et al. [82] and Hojgaard et al. [83].

In addition, the presence of hoarding obsessions and compulsions predicted a poorer response to SRIs [84,85]. In the cohort study by Eisen et al. [64], fewer than 10% of individuals with primary hoarding achieved remission in five years, whereas individuals whose primary obsession included over-responsibility for harm were more than twice as likely to remit and half as likely to relapse. Similar Landeros-Weisenberger et al. [86] found that 60% of patients with OCD with the "harm/checking" dimension were "much or very much improved" in response to SRI treatment.

Increased Serotonin Reuptake Inhibitor Dose

Individuals who have failed to respond to SRIs without experiencing major adverse effects may also benefit from treatment with SSRIs at dosages that exceed the licensed recommendations [51,87]. Ninan and colleagues [88] randomized sertraline non-responders to daily dosages of 200 mg or 400 mg and found that the higher dose was well tolerated and produced better outcomes. In the case of clomipramine, the maximum recommended dose of 250 mg daily is not usually exceeded, given its propensity to cause serious dose-related adverse effects (e.g., seizures). Caution is also required if the licensed dose of citalopram or escitalopram is exceeded, owing to the potential for adverse effects on cardiac conduction [89].

Antipsychotics

There is limited evidence to suggest that antipsychotics as monotherapy can be effective in the treatment of OCD and most studies to date have been negative [90]. However aripiprazole monotherapy, which has been investigated in two open-label studies, was found to be moderately effective among patients who were not treatment refractory (n = 8) [91] and children with SSRI and CBT treatment resistance (n = 16) [92].

First- and second-generation antipsychotics appear to be effective as augmentation agents. These agents have almost exclusively been tested in SRI-resistant OCD [93]; however, a RCT found that adjunctive quetiapine was also effective in non-SRI-resistant OCD [94]. Overall, the effect size is modest, with only around one-third of patients responding to such treatments. Meta-analysis [38] found that augmentation with antipsychotic produced a greater effect in patients with OCD and comorbid tic disorder. In contrast, a pooled analysis of exclusively quetiapine studies [95] suggested that a history of fewer previously failed SRI trials and higher baseline OCD symptom severity, as well as counting/ordering and arranging compulsions, was associated with a favorable outcome.

A subsequent meta-analysis by Dold et al. [96] incorporating 394 patients found that risperidone was the most effective antipsychotic, whereas the results for aripiprazole and haloperidol were inconsistent. No evidence was found for the effectiveness of quetiapine or olanzapine in comparison with placebo. The most recent meta-analysis, from 2014, which was limited to second-generation antipsychotics and included 14 studies and 493 patients [97], showed aripiprazole and risperidone to be effective in the short term, whereas olanzapine and quetiapine were not. A meta-regression analysis [98] suggested that D_2 and D_3 receptor affinity correlated with the efficacy of antipsychotic drugs in OCD, implying that these compounds exert their effects via dopaminergic mechanisms.

Experimental Compounds

While serotonergic medications are effective in alleviating symptoms of OCD, it does not necessarily imply that serotonergic dysfunction is the primary pathological process in OCD. For example, SRIs may modify serotonergic function to compensate for underlying pathology in another system. Furthermore, owing to the considerable biological heterogeneity that exists within the OCD population, and the failure of so many patients to respond to SRIs, it is likely that interrelating and/or disparate neurochemical systems underpin the disorder. A number of alternative compounds are under investigation as potential new therapeutic agents. These include treatments which also appear potentially effective in the treatment of OCRDs (Table 15.2).

Drugs Modulating Glutamate Neurotransmission

Dysfunction of the corticostriatothalamocortical (CTSC) neurocircuitry has been implicated in the pathogenesis of OCD [17]. Glutamate is the major excitatory neurotransmitter within these circuits with the majority of axon terminals within the striatum being glutamatergic; mounting evidence from a number of sources seem to suggest that glutamatergic signaling within the CTSC neurocircuitry may be disrupted in OCD [119]. Results from magnetic resonance spectroscopy suggest an inverse relationship between glutamatergic concentrations in the anterior cingulate and striatum in OCD [120,121,123], as well as a difference between glutamate levels in the caudate nucleus before and after treatment [124]. Increased concentrations of glutamate in cerebrospinal fluid were also found in drug-naïve adult individuals with OCD (relative to matched controls), thereby suggesting failures in maintaining an overall glutamate balance in the brain [119]. There has thus been considerable interest in the role of glutamatergic compounds as treatments in OCD and its related disorders.

Memantine

Memantine, a non-competitive antagonist at glutamatergic N-methyl-D-aspartate (NMDA) receptors has a relatively desirable tolerability profile and is considered to have limited drug–drug interactions [125]. Positive effects seen in three small open-label studies which used memantine either as a single agent or as adjunct to SRI [126,127,128] were replicated in two small randomized placebo-referenced trials [104,105]. While memantine has consistently shown positive therapeutic effects as an adjunct to conventional SRI treatments, there are no clear indications which patients with OCD may show a clinical response. No studies have been conducted on the role of memantine for the OCRDs.

Ketamine

Like memantine, ketamine is a non-competitive antagonist of the NMDA receptor, but its affinity for the receptor is higher, leading to a number of different clinical effects. Recent interest in ketamine stems from its rapid effects in the treatment of depression [129,130]. The results from the initial small-sized studies on the efficacy of ketamine in OCD are conflicting. A randomized double-blind placebo-controlled trial in 15 patients who were drug-free found that those who received ketamine reported immediate improvements in their obsessional thoughts and 50% of these individuals demonstrated a clinical response after one week of the infusion [102].

Table 15.2 Placebo-controlled, randomized, double-blind clinical trials of effective experimental compounds as monotherapy or augmentation of the existing psychotropic regimen in obsessive-compulsive disorder (adapted from Marinova et al. [99]).

	Compound	Study	Patients (*n*)	Duration and Dose	Outcome
Monotherapy	D-amphetamine	Insel et al. [100]	12	Single dose: 30 mg	D-amphetamine > placebo
		Joffe et al. [101]	11	Single dose: 30 mg D-amphetamine Single dose: 40 mg methylphenidate	D-amphetamine > placebo Methylphenidate = placebo
	Ketamine	Rodriguez et al. [102]	15 (2 with mild or moderate comorbid depression)	Ketamine and saline iv infused at least 1 week apart in random order; dose 0.5 mg/kg	Ketamine > placebo at 7 days
	Mirtazapine	Koran et al. [103]	30	12 weeks of open-label treatment followed by 8 weeks double-blind discontinuation; final dose 60 mg/day	Mirtazapine > placebo
Augmentation	Memantine	Ghaleiha et al. [104]	42	8 weeks + fluvoxamine; final dose 20 mg/day	Memantine > placebo
		Haghighi et al. [105]	40	12 weeks + SRI; dose 5–10 mg/day	Memantine > placebo
	Riluzole	Grant et al. [106]	60 (pediatric; 17 with comorbid ASD)	12 weeks + SRI; final dose: 100 mg/day	Riluzole= placebo
		Pittenger et al. [107]	38	12 weeks + SRI followed by 2 weeks lead-on placebo; final dose 100 mg/day	Riluzole = placebo
		Emamzadehfard et al. [108]	50	10 weeks +fluvoxamine; final dose: 100 mg/day	Riluzole > placebo
	Lamotrigine	Bruno et al. [109]	40 (adult; 33 in final sample)	16 weeks + SRI; final dose 100 mg/day	Lamotrigine > placebo
		Khalkhali et al. [110]	53 (treatment resistant)	12 weeks + SRI; final dose 100 mg/day	Lamotrigine > placebo
	N-acetyl cysteine	Afshar et al. [111]	48 (treatment resistant)	12 weeks + SRI; dose up to 2.4 g/day	N-acetyl cysteine > placebo
		Sarris et al. [112]	44	16 weeks + existing treatment OR monotherapy	N-acetyl cysteine = placebo
		Paydary et al. [113]	44	10 weeks +fluvoxamine; dose 2 g/day	N-acetyl cysteine > placebo
		Costa et al. [114]	40	16 weeks +SRI; dose 3 g/day	N-acetyl cysteine = placebo
	Morphine	Koran et al. [115]	23 (treatment resistant)	2 weeks + existing therapy; 1st week dose 30 mg/day 2nd week dose: 15–45mg/day	Morphine > placebo
	Ondansetron	Heidari et al. [116]	46	8 weeks + fluvoxamine; dose 8 mg/day	Ondansetron > placebo
		Soltani et al. [117]	42	8 weeks + fluoxetine; dose 4 mg/day	Ondansetron > placebo
	Granisetron	Askari et al. [118]	42	8 weeks + fluvoxamine; dose 2 mg/day	Granisetron > placebo

SRI, serotonin reuptake inhibitor.

However, an open-label trial which administered a single dose of ketamine infusion to 10 individuals with treatment-resistant OCD and comorbid depression, showed significant antidepressant effects but only marginal anti-OCD effects, with less than 12% reduction in Yale-Brown Obsessive-Compulsive Scale (Y-BOCS) [131] scores three days after treatment [132]. Again, no studies appear to have been conducted on the role of ketamine for OCRDs.

Riluzole

Riluzole is a multifunctional glutamate modulator [133], which initially showed promise as an adjunct to conventional OCD treatments in open-label studies [134,135,136]. Interestingly, two of the five responders in the study by Coric et al. [134] showed predominantly hoarding phenotypes. A more recent double-blinded placebo-controlled trial in 50 adult patients with OCD reported that adjunctive riluzole produced greater reductions of the compulsion Y-BOCS subscale and total Y-BOCS [108]. However, a placebo-controlled trial in children with treatment-resistant OCD did not reveal any clinically significant effect [106], nor did another randomized placebo-controlled trial conducted in treatment-refractory adult OCD patients [107].

No controlled studies have so far investigated the role of riluzole in other OCRDs. A case study of a 52-year-old patient with DSM-IV OCD, anorexia nervosa and skin-picking behaviors, showed demonstrable improvements in Y-BOCS, Skin Picking Impact Scale scores, and observed feeding behaviors while on riluzole, suggesting a possible role in the treatment of compulsive and repetitive behaviors [137].

Anticonvulsants

Lamotrigine acts as a glutamate modulator by reducing glutamate outflow through voltage gated sodium channels [138]. Positive results were obtained in two small RCTs of adjunctive lamotrigine in OCD [109,110]. Topiramate moderates glutamate release from axon terminals via its interaction with voltage gated calcium channels [138]. A small RCT investigating topiramate as an adjunctive treatment in OCD demonstrated a positive effect but only in reducing compulsions [139]. A second RCT failed to demonstrate any therapeutic effect [140] and was associated with a number of adverse effects. It should be noted that case reports of OCD provocation associated with these anticonvulsants have also been described in the literature [141,142,143,144].

N-Acetyl Cysteine

N-acetyl cysteine (NAC) has both antioxidant and glutamate-modulating properties [138]. In a 12-week double-blind controlled trial of 48 adult patients with SRI-resistant OCD, adjunctive NAC produced a significant improvement in Y-BOCS scores and overall treatment response [111]. Another 10-week randomized placebo-controlled trial demonstrated a greater reduction of obsession subscale and total Y-BOCS scores in fluvoxamine treated adults with OCD [113]. However, a third trial conducted on 44 adult patients with SRI-treated OCD demonstrated no difference in Y-BOCS scores between adjunctive NAC and placebo [112].

Drugs Acting on the Opioid System

Opioid Antagonists

Long-acting opioid antagonists such as naltrexone are used in the treatment of addiction [145]. Naltrexone has been shown to be effective in the short-term treatment for relapse prevention in alcoholism [146]; a proposed mechanism for this action includes reduction of the opioid contribution to rewarding effects of alcohol in the mesolimbic dopamine pathway [147]. Commonalities between the substance use disorders, impulse control disorders and OCD imply that this brain system may have a role in some forms of compulsivity.

Naltrexone has also been found to improve symptoms of impulse control disorders [148], pathological gambling [149], kleptomania [150,151] and compulsive sexual behavior [150]. However, evidence supporting the efficacy of opioid antagonists in OCD is not strong. Improvements in both obsessive-compulsive symptoms and motor tics were observed in two patients with OCD and comorbid Tourette's disorder who were drug-free and treated with naloxone [152].

A randomized double-blind placebo-referenced trial found no significant improvement of obsessive-compulsive or anxiety symptoms when naloxone was administered [153]. Three of 13 patients also experienced exacerbation of their obsessive-compulsive and anxiety symptoms. A similar adverse effect was historically described in case reports of naloxone and OCD [154]. A further double-blind placebo-controlled study which investigated SRI augmentation with naltrexone demonstrated no significant effect on Y-BOCS scores for naltrexone and overall increases in affective and anxiety psychopathology when compared with placebo [155].

Opioid Agonists

Opiate agonists have also been investigated in the treatment of OCRDs. An open-label trial of seven patients who were drug-free with treatment-refractory OCD suggested therapeutic benefit from tramadol, a weak agonist of the μ opioid receptor and an inhibitor of serotonin and noradrenaline transporters [156]. Three individuals in the study experienced a large improvement in Y-BOCS scores in the first week; this rapid effect may allude to the possibility that the effect of tramadol is unlike that of SRIs and perhaps related to its action on the opioid system [156]. A short (two-week) double-blind trial of oral morphine also caused transient symptom relief in patients with SRI-resistant OCD [115].

Serotonin Receptor Agonists/Antagonists

Preliminary studies suggest that compounds which target the serotonergic system in a manner different to that of the SRIs may be of use in treatment-resistant OCD. Mirtazapine, a noradrenergic and specific serotonergic antidepressant (enhances or antagonizes serotonin neurotransmission at the 5-HT_1 receptor and the 5-HT_2 receptor, respectively) reduced rates of OCD relapse in a placebo-controlled discontinuation study of 15 open-label mirtazapine responders [103]. Anecdotal reports suggest that psychedelic agents may also relieve OCD. In a modified double-blind study, psilocybin, a potent 5-HT_{1A} and 5-$HT_{2A/2C}$ agonist, was safely used in nine patients with OCD and was associated with acute reductions in core OCD symptoms in several patients [62].

5-HT_3 Antagonists

The 5-HT_3 antagonists are thought to possess anxiolytic properties in selected animal models of anxiety and may therefore be of use in the treatment of OCD [157]. In a pilot study of eight patients with OCD treated with ondansetron monotherapy, three individuals showed a clinical response [157]. A single-blind study [158] and two RCTs [116,117] suggested a beneficial effect of ondansetron as an adjunct to SRI. However, no effect was seen on obsessive-compulsive symptoms in a three-week randomized double-blind placebo-controlled study of 30 patients with Tourette's disorder [159], or in a 12-week double-blind randomized controlled OCD trial [160]. Granisetron, another 5-HT_3 antagonist, was shown to be superior as an add-on agent to fluvoxamine when compared with a placebo adjunct in a randomized double-blind trial of 42 patients with OCD [118]. However, its ability to penetrate the blood–brain barrier is questionable.

Stimulants

Stimulants may have a role in the treatment of OCD and may prove beneficial in cases with comorbid ADHD. A single dose of dexamphetamine was shown to produce short-term therapeutic effects in patients with OCD [100], and a single-dose challenge of dexamphetamine but not methylphenidate had a significant effect on obsessive-compulsive symptoms relative to placebo in a small randomized double-blinded controlled trial [101]. Another RCT, comparing augmentation with dexamphetamine against augmentation with caffeine in patients with treatment-resistant OCD resulted in rapid and sustained improvements in obsessive-compulsive symptoms for both treatment arms [161]. Adjunctive dexamphetamine was no more effective than caffeine; which could suggest that response in both treatment groups represented a placebo effect. Conversely, as both compounds may result in dopamine release at the prefrontal cortex, a pharmacologically induced therapeutic effect may have arisen in both treatment arms.

Clinical Implications of Cross-Diagnostic Approaches for Treatment and Prevention

Table 15.3 summarizes the evidence-based treatment of the OCRDs as a group. Apart from some studies of OCD and BDD, the pharmacotherapies were almost exclusively tested in small unreplicated trials.

Body Dysmorphic Disorder

BDD has been studied less intensively than OCD but the available results from a small number of open-label case series [162,163,164,165] and RCTs suggest that the disorder responds to SSRIs in acute phase and relapse prevention studies [166,167,168]. One randomized double-blind crossover trial demonstrated the superior efficacy of clomipramine over the noradrenergic tricyclic desipramine, hinting at the existence of a similar selective response to SRIs

Table 15.3 Evidence-based treatments for the OCRDs (the efficacy of medications in bold type is supported by multiple randomized controlled trials).

Disorder	Responds to SRI	Course of Response	Positive Dose–Response Relationship on SSRI	Responds to Adjunctive Antipsychotic	Responds to Glutamatergic Drugs	Responds to Other Drugs
OCD	**SSRI, clomipramine**	Gradual, sustained	Yes	Yes	Memantine, ketamine, lamotrigine, N-acetyl cysteine	Dexamphetamine, morphine, mirtazapine
BDD	**SSRI,** clomipramine	Gradual, sustained	Yes	Limited evidence		
Hoarding disorder	SSRI, clomipramine	Uncertain	Uncertain	Limited evidence for adjunctive quetiapine		Methylphenidate, venlafaxine
Hair-pulling disorder	Clomipramine, possibly SSRI	Rapid, not sustained	Effect with lower doses	Olanzapine	N-acetyl cysteine	
Skin-picking disorder	Fluoxetine, fluvoxamine	Rapid, sustained	Effect with lower doses	Uncertain	N-acetyl cysteine, lamotrigine (subset only)	

BDD, body dysmorphic disorder; OCD, obsessive-compulsive disorder; SRI, serotonin reuptake inhibitor; SSRI, selective SRI.

[169]. A placebo response of just 18% was recorded in the placebo-referenced RCT for fluoxetine, which is also similar to the rate observed in OCD [166], suggesting overlapping changes in reward pathways.

Expert consensus also suggests that, like OCD, higher doses of SRI are more efficacious in BDD and that the clinical response to treatments is gradual [170,171], although no dose-finding studies have so far been performed. In addition, a chart review study which investigated SRI continuation compared with discontinuation in BDD suggested that clinical response endured as long as treatment was continued [172]. A more recent double-blind placebo-controlled trial convincingly demonstrated that maintenance of escitalopram for six months following acute response resulted in further improvement and delayed time to relapse, compared with discontinuing the SSRI and switching to placebo [167].

In the case of inadequate response to SRI monotherapy, there is very limited evidence as to which compounds may be of benefit. A small (and possibly underpowered) RCT found that augmentation of fluoxetine with the first-generation antipsychotic pimozide was ineffective [173]. In contrast, a retrospective naturalistic case note study found that patients with BDD offered an adjunctive antipsychotic were less likely to disengage prematurely from services compared with those offered an SSRI and CBT only, but there was no significant intergroup difference in the clinical response rate [168]. Aripiprazole produced a positive outcome in a single case report [174]. Well-powered randomized controlled studies are warranted, to determine clinical outcomes with adjunctive antipsychotic in BDD.

Hoarding Disorder

Studies investigating pharmacological treatments for compulsive hoarding are limited and hoarding has mainly been studied in the context of comorbid OCD. Morein-Zamir and colleagues [175] examined cognitive performance and found both commonalities and differences between OCD with hoarding and hoarding disorder, with robust evidence of executive impairment and impulsivity in both groups compared with healthy controls. A meta-analysis by Bloch et al. [84] revealed that patients with OCD who had hoarding symptoms were approximately 50% less likely than those without hoarding to respond to SSRIs. However the analysis excluded patients with hoarding who did not have other OCD symptoms.

Other retrospective studies suggest there may be value in SSRI treatment for compulsive hoarding [176] One open-label study of 79 participants which quantitatively measured response to paroxetine in patients with the compulsive hoarding syndrome regardless of whether they had OCD symptoms demonstrated that compulsive hoarders responded equally as well to SRI as patients with non-hoarding OCD [177]. Whereas the evidence supporting a role for venlafaxine in OCD is not strong [178,179], another open-label study of 24 patients with DSM-5 hoarding disorder treated with venlafaxine for 12 weeks suggested that SNRIs may be effective for patients with compulsive hoarding [180].

An open-label trial of nine participants with treatment-resistant OCD and predominant hoarding which augmented SRI with quetiapine provided insufficient evidence to support a role for antipsychotics as add-on agents [181]. Monotherapy with methylphenidate was investigated in a small, open-label case series (n = 4) [182] but the modest reductions in hoarding symptoms were outweighed by adverse effects including insomnia and palpitations, which resulted in treatment discontinuation in all participants.

Hair-Pulling Disorder

Unlike OCD and BDD, the data supporting the efficacy of SRIs in hair-pulling disorder are not strong. One double-blind crossover study showed that clomipramine was more effective than desipramine in the treatment of hair pulling [183]. A follow-up study of responders from this trial suggested that pharmacotherapy with SRIs may be of long-term benefit to some patients with hair-pulling disorder [184]. Hair pulling was also significantly reduced in three open-label studies of fluoxetine, citalopram and escitalopram [185,186,187], but two RCTs of fluoxetine [188,189] and one of sertraline [190] did not demonstrate evidence of a treatment effect [191]. Unlike OCD, but similar to impulse control disorders, SSRIs appeared to have a rapid onset of effect, which was not sustained over time [192]. Moreover, clomipramine could not be differentiated from placebo in a small RCT conducted by Ninan et al. [193].

A single RCT of olanzapine [194] produced evidence that antipsychotics could be effective. Small open-label trials also suggested that aripiprazole [195] and adjunctive pimozide [196] may be of some benefit, but larger randomized double-blind placebo-controlled studies are required to confirm this. While significant benefits were seen in 11 of 14 children in a small open-label study [197], naltrexone was not shown to be effective in a double-blind placebo-controlled study in 51 patients [198]. In the latter study, however, individuals with a family history of addiction showed a greater numerical decrease in the urges to pull, but this did not reach statistical significance [198].

Grant et al. [199] reported a double-blind randomized trial that demonstrated NAC to be superior to placebo in adults with hair-pulling disorder. The clinical effect took several weeks to develop, but no major adverse effects were recorded, which suggested good tolerability. However a more recent randomized, double-blind, placebo-controlled add-on trial of NAC in 35 pediatric patients with hair-pulling disorder failed to show benefit relative to placebo [200]. Explanations for this result might include differences in pathologies for pediatric and adult hair-pulling disorder [201].

Skin-Picking Disorder

A double-blind, placebo-controlled trial found that fluoxetine was beneficial in skin-picking disorder [202]. Another study in which all responders to initial treatment with open-label fluoxetine were subsequently randomized double-blind to either fluoxetine or placebo demonstrated that those assigned to active treatment showed sustained response, whereas the reverse was true of those who were assigned to placebo [203]. Open-label studies with fluvoxamine [204] and escitalopram [205] provide additional weak evidence supporting the use of SSRIs. In the above trials, the clinical response was more rapid than that seen in BDD and OCD and high doses were not required. In contrast, another randomized double-blinded placebo-controlled trial in 45 participants with skin-picking found that citalopram was no more effective than placebo [206].

NAC has also been investigated in skin-picking disorder. A randomized placebo-referenced trial of 12 weeks' duration involving 66 adults with skin-picking disorder demonstrated significant clinical improvements in patients treated with NAC. At the study's end point, 15 of the 32 participants (47%) receiving NAC were much or very much improved compared with 4 of the 21 participants (19%) receiving placebo [207]. NAC was also shown to be beneficial in an open-label study of skin picking in patients with Prader-Willi syndrome, a neurodevelopmental disorder caused by a chromosomal abnormality that is in part characterized by compulsive skin-picking [208].

Only two studies have investigated the effects of lamotrigine on skin picking; one open-label trial demonstrated a positive effect [209]. In another RCT by Grant et al. [210], no significant overall differences were noted between lamotrigine and placebo on the primary or secondary end points. However, those who responded to lamotrigine exhibited impaired cognitive flexibility (extradimensional shifting) at baseline compared with lamotrigine non-responders. These findings suggest that, although safe and well tolerated, lamotrigine treatment may not be efficacious in patients with skin-picking disorder as a whole. However, lamotrigine may be valuable in a subset of patients who exhibit relatively impaired cognitive flexibility. Opioid antagonists have not been well studied in skin-picking disorder. A single case report found significant benefits with naltrexone and fluoxetine on skin-picking behaviors in a child with Prader-Willi syndrome [211].

Summary and Clinical Implications

OCD and its related disorders, like almost all other psychiatric disorders, respond in a heterogeneous way to treatment. Inexplicably, some patients do well on a given treatment and many do poorly. Moreover, there appears to be a role for almost all, if not all, available psychotropic agents, including those acting on serotonergic, dopaminergic, glutamatergic, opioid and noradrenergic systems.

Notwithstanding the limitations of the study data, some compulsive disorders (e.g. OCD, BDD) exhibit a strikingly similar treatment response to SRIs, suggesting that the underpinning neural mechanisms may overlap significantly with those relating to anxiety and affective disorders. In contrast, others (hair-pulling and skin-picking disorders), together with SRI-resistant forms of OCD, appear to respond better to combination treatment with drugs acting on dopamine, glutamate, opioid and noradrenergic systems (i.e., potentially more like impulse control disorders or even behavioral addictions), consistent with a compulsive-impulsive diathesis model [59]. Yet another group of patients with prominent motor symptoms (tics, habits) may respond preferentially to adjunctive dopamine antagonists, known to modulate the corticostriatal motor circuitry involved in Tourette's disorder and animal models of excessive habit behavior. All this suggests that a dimensional approach to treatment is warranted.

To move forward to a more fully dimensional approach to the psychopharmacology of the OCRDs, treatments need to be studied with respect to a broader range of symptom dimensions than hitherto, such as compulsivity and impulsivity, obsessionality, delusionality, cognitive (obsession) and motoric (stereotypies, habits, tics), harm avoidance and incompleteness. One aim would be to determine the impact of the presence of these transdiagnostic dimensions on the treatment response, as a method to predict clinical outcomes. Another aim would be to determine the effect of treatment on these symptom domains, to unravel the underpinning mechanisms of effect and identify new targets for treatment development that may be applied to an extended group of compulsive disorders. To do this, we urgently need validated clinical instruments to reliably measure these dimensions across diverse patient groups, and possibly even across clinical and non-clinical populations.

In the interim, in managing OCRDs, clinicians should look out for the presence of other prominent symptom dimensions (e.g., attentional, impulsive, motoric – tics), and if present, consider using relevant augmentation strategies (as described in the sections above), in preference to SSRI or clomipramine monotherapy.

Cross Diagnostic Treatment Approaches and Their Implications for Classification and Diagnosis

A proposed obsessive-compulsive spectrum infers that OCD and its putatively related disorders are closely linked to one another through shared domains, including symptomatology, course of illness, comorbidity, familial loading, neurocircuitry, as well as treatment response. The pharmacological treatment response may be of particular value for parsing psychiatric disorders, and defining the boundaries of diagnostic family groups, depending as it does on the underpinning neuropsychological and biological mechanisms.

A cross-diagnostic approach to pharmacological treatment is supported by the trial data presented in this chapter. We demonstrate overlaps and differences in treatment responses between the different diagnoses within the DSM-5 OCRD grouping. SSRIs may have a role in treating each disorder, but there is growing evidence suggesting a graduated shift toward a more prominent role for treatments usually aimed at addiction and impulse control and a lesser role for SSRIs, as the diagnosis shifts from OCD through BDD to hair-pulling and skin-picking disorders – disorders which are also characterized by deficient impulse control and addictive symptomatology.

As the treatment trial data for hoarding disorder, hair pulling and skin picking accrue, it is possible that more convincing similarities will be found with disorders classified elsewhere in the DSM, such as the behavioral addictions (e.g. pathological gambling), impulse control disorders (e.g. kleptomania, intermittent explosive disorder) or even neurodevelopmental disorders (e.g. autism spectrum disorder, ADHD), challenging the current classification of these disorders within the OCRDs grouping. Alternatively, by taking a broad "compulsive impulsive" approach to the psychopharmacology of the OCRDs, the emerging evidence may instead be interpreted to support the inclusion of some of these other disorders into an expanded OCRDs grouping, together with disorders such as Tourette's disorder, hypochondriasis and obsessive-compulsive personality disorder.

Future Directions: A Transdiagnostic Approach for the Pharmacological Treatment of Obsessive-Compulsive and Related Disorders

Inconsistencies in the pharmacological treatment trial data described in this chapter implicate biological heterogeneity within the OCRD population. The future of pharmacotherapy for these disorders may lie in a better understanding of this heterogeneity [212]. Research into potential OCRD biomarkers, such as genes or neurocognitive changes, may provide new scope for optimizing treatment for individual patients on a more personalized basis.

Most existing studies investigating predictors of response are, however, limited by the heterogeneous nature of the study populations. The large number of potential predictors have not been evaluated with consistency across studies, to the extent that, at present, we do not have reliable predictive markers to determine which patients will respond to which treatment. The role of pharmacogenetics appears to be particularly underrepresented.

Considering that so many patients are resistant to SRI treatment, assessing predictors of response to alternative forms of treatment such as adjunctive antipsychotic, glutamatergic agents, opioid receptor agents and stimulants represents a research priority. Unfortunately, even fewer rigorous studies of such agents have been reported and most of the studies are simply too small to determine which participants respond to the treatment and which participants do not [212].

Randomized controlled treatment trials of adequate size and power to enable the detection of predictive outcome markers are needed to drive forward the clinical management of these disorders on an individualized basis. Based on the current data, a transdiagnostic approach to biomarker discovery, which seeks to define dimensions of obsessive-compulsive symptomatology at the level of the individual, could provide the means for capturing this heterogeneity and lead to the delivery of personalized treatment plans.

Table 15.4 lists some of the most commonly used rating scales for the individual OCRDs. Many represent adaptations of the Y-BOCS. For the most part they are reliable and sensitive to change. However, it is difficult to equate the magnitude of improvements across the different scales. In the case of patients presenting with complex compulsive and impulsive symptomatology (such as in the case study at the beginning of this chapter), a more dimensional approach to measuring symptom severity is needed.

The Dimensional Yale-Brown Obsessive-Compulsive scale was designed to measure the presence and severity of symptoms of OCD within six distinct dimensions that combine thematically related obsessions and compulsions. It includes sections on contamination, hoarding, symmetry, sex/religion, aggression and miscellaneous symptoms, and includes both self-report and interviewer-administered portions. In a validation study, severity scores for individual symptom dimensions were largely independent of one another, only modestly correlated with the global ratings, and were also differentially related to ratings of depression, anxiety and tic severity [223].

Another set of brief self-rated scales, designed by the DSM-5 sub-working group on obsessive-compulsive spectrum disorders to mirror current DSM-5 criteria for BDD, hoarding disorder, hair-pulling disorder and skin-picking disorder [224], represents a further potential advance. Preliminary examination of the psychometric properties on a large non-clinical sample revealed strong internal

Table 15.4 Commonly used rating scales in obsessive-compulsive and related disorders.

Disorder	Self-rated	Observer-rated
OCD	OCI-R, DOCS	Y-BOCS
BDD	–	BDD-Y-BOCS
Hoarding disorder	SI-R, DOCS	HRS-I, UHSS
Hair-pulling disorder	HPS, DOCS	PITS, NIMH-Trichotillomania Scale, Y-BOCS TM
Skin-picking disorder	SPS, DOCS	NE-Y-BOCS

BDD-Y-BOCS, Body Dysmorphic Disorder Modification of the Yale-Brown Obsessive-Compulsive Scale [213]; DOCS, Dimensional Obsessive-Compulsive Scale [214]; HPS, Massachusetts General Hospital Hair Pulling Scale [215]; HRS-I, Hoarding Rating Scale-Interview [216]; NE-Y-BOCS, Yale-Brown Obsessive-Compulsive Scale Modified for Neurotic Excoriation [204]; NIMH, National Institute of Mental Health [183]; OCI-R, Obsessive-compulsive Inventory Revised [217]; PITS, Psychiatric Institute Trichotillomania Scale [218]; SI-R: Saving Inventory-Revised [219]; SPS, Skin-picking scale [220]; UHSS, UCLA Hoarding Severity Scale [177]; Y-BOCS, Yale-Brown Obsessive-Compulsive Scale [131]; Y-BOCS-TM, Yale-Brown Obsessive-Compulsive Scale for Trichotillomania [221,222].

consistency, convergent validity, and showed significantly higher scoring on scales for participants who screened positive for the core symptoms relative to those who did not.

Arguably, the further development of dimensional assessment techniques, to capture a broad spectrum of clinically relevant compulsivity, including obsessions, compulsions, avoidance, impulse control, tic and habitual behaviors, would provide much needed instruments for investigating multiple transdiagnostic aspects of compulsive symptom severity that could be applied systematically across natural history, neuroimaging, treatment response and genetic studies.

Specifically, a more dimensional approach to measurement could be expected to increase the homogeneity of research samples and would provide opportunities to identify obsessive-compulsive symptom domains that more or less strongly correlate with the underlying pathology or predict response to particular treatments. This would advance our understanding of compulsivity and modernize our approach toward personalized prescribing. This approach may be of particular value for individuals with co-occurring conditions such as ADHD, ASD and Tourette's disorder, including those with symptoms not meeting the threshold required to make a categorical diagnosis. The possible utility of this approach is exemplified by considering the case vignette described at the start of the chapter.

References

1. Haro JM, Ayuso-Mateos JL, Bitter I, et al. ROAMER: roadmap for mental health research in Europe. *Int J Methods Psychiatr Res.* 2014;23(S1):1–14.
2. Insel T, Cuthbert B, Garvey M, et al. Research domain criteria (RDoC): toward a new classification framework for research on mental disorders. *Am J Psychiatry.* 2010;167(7):748–751.
3. Hollander E, Braun A, Simeon D. Should OCD leave the anxiety disorders in DSM-V? The case for obsessive compulsive-related disorders. *Depress Anxiety.* 2008;25(4):317–329.
4. Stein DJ, Kogan CS, Atmaca M, et al. The classification of obsessive-compulsive and related disorders in the ICD-11. *J Affect Disord.* 2016;190:663–674.
5. Fineberg NA, Menchon JM, Zohar J, Veltman DJ. Compulsivity: a new trans-diagnostic research domain for the Roadmap for Mental Health Research in Europe (ROAMER) and Research Domain Criteria (RDoC) initiatives. *Eur Neuropsychopharmacol.* 2016;26(5):797–799.
6. Hollander E, Doernberg E, Shavitt R, et al. The cost and impact of compulsivity: a research perspective. *Eur Neuropsychopharmacol.* 2016;26(5):800–809.
7. Marras A, Fineberg N, Pallanti S. Obsessive compulsive and related disorders: comparing DSM-5 and ICD-11. *CNS Spectr.* 2016;21(4):324–333.
8. Fineberg NA, Baldwin DS, Menchon JM, et al. Manifesto for a European research network into obsessive-compulsive and related disorders. *Eur Neuropsychopharmacol.* 2013;23(7):561–568.
9. Lochner C, Fineberg NA, Zohar J, et al. Comorbidity in obsessive-compulsive disorder (OCD): a report from the International College of Obsessive-Compulsive Spectrum Disorders (ICOCS). *Compr Psychiatry.* 2014;55(7):1513–1519.
10. De Vries FE, Cath DC, Hoogendoorn AW, et al. Tic-related versus tic-free obsessive-compulsive disorder: clinical picture and 2-year natural course. *J Clin Psychiatry.* 2016;77(10):e1240–e1247.

11. Kaur S, Wikramanayake M, Kolli S, et al. Autistic spectrum disorder in adults with obsessive compulsive disorder: results from a UK survey. *Eur Neuropsychopharmacol.* 2016;26(5):886–887.
12. Darrow SM, Hirschtritt ME, Davis LK, et al. Identification of two heritable cross-disorder endophenotypes for Tourette syndrome. *Am J Psychiatry.* 2016;174(4):387–396.
13. Dell'Osso B, Benatti B, Buoli M, et al. The influence of age at onset and duration of illness on long-term outcome in patients with obsessive-compulsive disorder: a report from the International College of Obsessive Compulsive Spectrum Disorders (ICOCS). *Eur Neuropsychopharmacol.* 2013;23(8):865–871.
14. Fineberg NA, Hengartner MP, Bergbaum C, Gale T, Rössler W, Angst J. Remission of obsessive-compulsive disorders and syndromes; evidence from a prospective community cohort study over thirty years. *Int J Psychiatry Clin Pract.* 2013;17(3):179–187.
15. Fineberg NA, Gale TM. Evidence-based pharmacotherapy of obsessive compulsive disorder. *Int J Neuropsychopharmacol.* 2005;8(1):107–129.
16. Fineberg NA, Brown A, Reghunandanan S, Pampaloni I. Evidence-based pharmacotherapy of obsessive-compulsive disorder. *Int J Neuropsychopharmacol.* 2012;15(8):1173–1191.
17. Stein DJ, Fineberg N, Reghunandanan S. *Obsessive-Compulsive and Related Disorders,* 2nd ed. Oxford University Press; 2015.
18. Hollander E, Stein DJ, Fineberg NA, Marteau F, Legault M. Quality of life outcomes in patients with obsessive-compulsive disorder: relationship to treatment response and symptom relapse. *J Clin Psychiatry.* 2010;71(6):784–792.
19. Stein DJ, Andersen EW, Tonnoir B, Fineberg N. Escitalopram in obsessive–compulsive disorder: a randomized, placebo-controlled, paroxetine-referenced, fixed-dose, 24-week study. *Curr Med Res Opin.* 2007;23(4):701–711.
20. Tenney NH, Denys DA, van Megen HJ, Glas G, Westenberg HG. Effect of a pharmacological intervention on quality of life in patients with obsessive–compulsive disorder. *Int Clin Psychopharmacol.* 2003;18(1):29–33.
21. Soomro GM, Altman D, Rajagopal S, Oakley-Browne M. Selective serotonin re-uptake inhibitors (SSRIs) versus placebo for obsessive compulsive disorder (OCD). *Cochrane Database Syst Rev.* 2008;1:CD001765.
22. McGuire JF, Piacentini J, Lewin AB, Brennan EA, Murphy TK, Storch EA. A meta-analysis of cognitive behavior therapy and medication for child obsessive-compulsive disorder: moderators of treatment efficacy, response, and remission. *Depress Anxiety.* 2015;32(8):580–593.
23. Skapinakis P, Caldwell DM, Hollingworth W, et al. Pharmacological and psychotherapeutic interventions for management of obsessive-compulsive disorder in adults: a systematic review and network meta-analysis. *Lancet Psychiatry.* 2016;3(8):730–739.
24. Foa EB, Steketee G, Kozak MJ, Dugger D. Effects of imipramine on depression and obsessive-compulsive symptoms. *Psychiatry Res.* 1987;21(2):123–136.
25. Volavka J, Neziroglu F, Yaryura-Tobias JA. Clomipramine and imipramine in obsessive-compulsive disorder. *Psychiatry Res.* 1985;14(1):85–93.
26. Insel TR, Murphy DL, Cohen RM, Alterman I, Kilts C, Linnoila M. Obsessive-compulsive disorder. A double-blind trial of clomipramine and clorgyline. *Arch Gen Psychiatry.* 1983;40(6):605–612.
27. Jenike MA, Baer L, Minichiello WE, Rauch SL, Buttolph ML. Placebo-controlled trial of fluoxetine and phenelzine for obsessive-compulsive disorder. *Am J Psychiatry.* 1997;154(9):1261–1264.
28. Ananth J, Pecknold JC, Van Den Steen N, Engelsmann F. Double-blind comparative study of clomipramine and amitriptyline in obsessive neurosis. *Prog Neuropsychopharmacol.* 1981;5(3):257–262.
29. Thoren P, Asberg M, Cronholm B, Jornestedt L, Traskman L. Clomipramine treatment of obsessive-compulsive disorder. I. A controlled clinical trial. *Arch Gen Psychiatry.* 1980;37(11):1281–1285.
30. McDougle CJ, Price LH, Goodman WK, Charney DS, Heninger GR. A controlled trial of lithium augmentation in fluvoxamine-refractory obsessive-compulsive disorder: lack of efficacy. *J Clin Psychopharmacol.* 1991;11(3):175–184.
31. Pigott TA, L'Heureux F, Hill JL, Bihari K, Bernstein SE, Murphy DL. A double-blind study of adjuvant buspirone hydrochloride in clomipramine-treated patients with obsessive-compulsive disorder. *J Clin Psychopharmacol.* 1992;12(1):11–18.
32. Stein DJ, Hollander E, Mullen LS, DeCaria CM, Liebowitz MR. Comparison of clomipramine, alprazolam and placebo in the treatment of obsessive-compulsive disorder. *Hum Psychopharmacol Clin.* 1992;7(6):389–395.
33. Hewlett WA, Vinogradov S, Agras WS. Clomipramine, clonazepam, and clonidine treatment of obsessive-compulsive disorder. *J Clin Psychopharmacol.* 1992;12(6):420–430.
34. Hollander E, Kaplan A, Stahl SM. A double-blind, placebo-controlled trial of clonazepam in obsessive-compulsive disorder. *World J Biol Psychiatry.* 2003;4(1):30–34.

35. Crockett BA, Churchill E, Davidson JR. A double-blind combination study of clonazepam with sertraline in obsessive-compulsive disorder. *Ann Clin Psychiatry.* 2004;16(3):127–132.

36. Fineberg NA, Hengartner MP, Bergbaum C, Gale T, Rössler W, Angst J. Lifetime comorbidity of obsessive-compulsive disorder and sub-threshold obsessive-compulsive symptomatology in the community: impact, prevalence, socio-demographic and clinical characteristics. *Int J Psychiatry Clin Pract.* 2013;17(3):188–196.

37. Hoehn-Saric R, Ninan P, Black DW, et al. Multicenter double-blind comparison of sertraline and desipramine for concurrent obsessive-compulsive and major depressive disorders. *Arch Gen Psychiatry.* 2000;57(1):76–82.

38. Bloch MH, Landeros-Weisenberger A, Kelmendi B, Coric V, Bracken MB, Leckman JF. A systematic review: antipsychotic augmentation with treatment refractory obsessive-compulsive disorder. *Mol Psychiatry.* 2006;11(7):622–632.

39. Abramovitch A, Dar R, Mittelman A, Schweiger A. Don't judge a book by its cover: ADHD-like symptoms in obsessive compulsive disorder. *J Obsessive-Compuls Relat Disord.* 2013;2(1):53–61.

40. King J, Dowling N, Leow F. Methylphenidate in the treatment of an adolescent female with obsessive-compulsive disorder and attention deficit hyperactivity disorder: a case report. *Australas Psychiatry.* 2016;25(2):178–180.

41. Taormina SP, Galloway MP, Rosenberg DR. Treatment efficacy of combined sertraline and guanfacine in comorbid obsessive–compulsive disorder and attention deficit/hyperactivity disorder: two case studies. *J Dev Behav Pediatr.* 2016;37(6):491–495.

42. The Clomipramine Collaborative Study Group. Clomipramine in the treatment of patients with obsessive-compulsive disorder. *Arch Gen Psychiatry.* 1991;48(8):730–738.

43. De Veaugh-Geiss J, Landau P, Katz R. Treatment of obsessive compulsive disorder with clomipramine. *Psychiatr Ann.* 1989; 19(2):97–99.

44. Issaria Y, Jakubovski E, Bartley CA, Pittenger C, Bloch MH. Early onset of response with selective serotonin reuptake inhibitors in obsessive-compulsive disorder: a meta-analysis. *J Clin Psychiatry.* 2016;77(5):e605–e611.

45. Da Conceição Costa DL, Shavitt RG, Cesar RC, et al. Can early improvement be an indicator of treatment response in obsessive-compulsive disorder? Implications for early-treatment decision-making. *J Psychiatr Res.* 2013;47(11):1700–1707.

46. Rasmussen S, Hackett E, Duboff E, et al. A 2-year study of sertraline in the treatment of obsessive-compulsive disorder. *Int Clin Psychopharmacol.* 1997;12(6):309–316.

47. Koran LM, Sallee FR, Pallanti S. Rapid benefit of intravenous pulse loading of clomipramine in obsessive-compulsive disorder. *Am J Psychiatry.* 1997;154(3):396–401.

48. Bloch MH, McGuire J, Landeros-Weisenberger A, Leckman JF, Pittenger C. Meta-analysis of the dose–response relationship of SSRI in obsessive-compulsive disorder. *Mol Psychiatry.* 2010;15(8):850–855.

49. Baldwin DS, Anderson IM, Nutt DJ, et al. Evidence-based guidelines for the pharmacological treatment of anxiety disorders: recommendations from the British Association for Psychopharmacology. *J Psychopharmacol.* 2005;19(6):567–596.

50. Baldwin DS, Anderson IM, Nutt DJ, et al. Evidence-based pharmacological treatment of anxiety disorders, post-traumatic stress disorder and obsessive-compulsive disorder: a revision of the 2005 guidelines from the British Association for Psychopharmacology. *J Psychopharmacol.* 2014;28(5):403–439.

51. American Psychiatric Association. *Practice Guideline for the Treatment of Patients with Obsessive-Compulsive Disorder.* Arlington, VA: American Psychiatric Association; 2007.

52. Andrews G. Placebo response in depression: bane of research, boon to therapy. *Br J Psychiatry.* 2001;178(3):192–194.

53. Grady TA, Pigott TA, L'Heureux F, Hill JL, Bernstein SE, Murphy DL. Double-blind study of adjuvant buspirone for fluoxetine-treated patients with obsessive-compulsive disorder. *Am J Psychiatry.* 1993;150(5):819–821.

54. Sugarman MA, Kirsch I, Huppert JD. Obsessive-compulsive disorder has a reduced placebo (and antidepressant) response compared to other anxiety disorders: a meta-analysis. *J Affect Disord.* 2017;218:217–226.

55. De la Fuente-Fernández R, Ruth TJ, Sossi V, Schulzer M, Calne DB, Stoessl AJ. Expectation and dopamine release: mechanism of the placebo effect in Parkinson's disease. *Science.* 2001;293(5532):1164–1166.

56. Enck P, Benedetti F, Schedlowski M. New insights into the placebo and nocebo responses. *Neuron.* 2008;59(2):195–206.

57. Scott DJ, Stohler CS, Egnatuk CM, Wang H, Koeppe RA, Zubieta JK. Placebo and nocebo effects are defined by opposite opioid and dopaminergic responses. *Arch Gen Psychiatry.* 2008;65(2):220–231.

58. Figee M, de Koning P, Klaassen S, et al. Deep brain stimulation induces striatal dopamine release in obsessive-compulsive disorder. *Biol Psychiatry.* 2014;75(8):647–652.

59. Fineberg NA, Chamberlain SR, Goudriaan AE, et al. New developments in human neurocognition: clinical, genetic, and brain imaging correlates of impulsivity and compulsivity. *CNS Spectr.* 2014;19(1):69–89.

60. Baumgarten HG, Grozdanovic Z. Role of serotonin in obsessive-compulsive disorder. *Br J Psychiatry Suppl.* 1998;(35):13–20.

61. El Mansari M, Blier P. Mechanisms of action of current and potential pharmacotherapies of obsessive-compulsive disorder. *Prog Neuro-psychopharmacol Biol Psychiatry.* 2006;30(3):362–373.

62. Moreno FA, Wiegand CB, Taitano EK, Delgado PL. Safety, tolerability, and efficacy of psilocybin in 9 patients with obsessive-compulsive disorder. *J Clin Psychiatry.* 2006;67(11):1735–1740.

63. Skoog G, Skoog I. A 40-year follow-up of patients with obsessive-compulsive disorder. *Arch Gen Psychiatry.* 1999;56(2):121–127.

64. Eisen JL, Sibrava NJ, Boisseau CL, et al. Five-year course of obsessive-compulsive disorder: predictors of remission and relapse. *J Clin Psychiatry.* 2013;74(3):233–239.

65. Fineberg NA, Pampaloni I, Pallanti S, Ipser J, Stein DJ. Sustained response versus relapse: the pharmacotherapeutic goal for obsessive–compulsive disorder. *Int Clin Psychopharmacol.* 2007;22(6):313–322.

66. Fineberg NA, Reghunandanan S, Brown A, Pampaloni I. Pharmacotherapy of obsessive-compulsive disorder: evidence-based treatment and beyond. *Aust N Z J Psychiatry.* 2013;47(2):121–141.

67. Santana L, Versiani M, Mendlowicz MV, Fontenelle LF. Predictors of adherence among patients with obsessive-compulsive disorder undergoing naturalistic pharmacotherapy. *J Clin Psychopharmacol.* 2010;30(1):86–88.

68. Menchón JM, van Ameringen M, Dell'Osso B, et al. Standards of care for obsessive-compulsive disorder centres. *Int J Psychiatry Clin Pract.* 2016;20(3):204–208.

69. Micali N, Heyman I, Perez M, et al. Long-term outcomes of obsessive-compulsive disorder: follow-up of 142 children and adolescents. *Br J Psychiatry.* 2010;197(2):128–134.

70. Reddy YC, Alur AM, Manjunath S, Kandavel T, Math SB. Long-term follow-up study of patients with serotonin reuptake inhibitor-nonresponsive obsessive-compulsive disorder. *J Clin Psychopharmacol.* 2010;30(3):267–272.

71. Garcia AM, Sapyta JJ, Moore PS, et al. Predictors and moderators of treatment outcome in the Pediatric Obsessive Compulsive Treatment Study (POTS I). *J Am Acad Child Adolesc Psychiatry.* 2010;49(10):1024–1033.

72. Storch EA, Milsom VA, Merlo LJ, et al. Insight in pediatric obsessive-compulsive disorder: associations with clinical presentation. *Psychiatry Res.* 2008;160(2):212–220.

73. Storch EA, Merlo LJ, Larson MJ, et al. Impact of comorbidity on cognitive-behavioral therapy response in pediatric obsessive-compulsive disorder. *J Am Acad Child Adolesc Psychiatry.* 2008;47(5):583–592.

74. Baer L, Jenike MA. Personality disorders in obsessive compulsive disorder. *Psychiatr Clin North Am.* 1992;15(4):803–812.

75. Baer L, Jenike MA, Black DW, Treece C, Rosenfeld R, Greist J. Effect of axis II diagnoses on treatment outcome with clomipramine in 55 patients with obsessive-compulsive disorder. *Arch Gen Psychiatry.* 1992;49(11):862–866.

76. Jenike MA, Baer L, Minichiello WE, Schwartz CE, Carey RJ Jr. Concomitant obsessive-compulsive disorder and schizotypal personality disorder. *Am J Psychiatry.* 1986;143(4):530–532.

77. Erzegovesi S, Cavallini MC, Cavedini P, Diaferia G, Locatelli M, Bellodi L. Clinical predictors of drug response in obsessive-compulsive disorder. *J Clin Psychopharmacol.* 2001;21(5):488–492.

78. McDougle CJ, Goodman WK, Leckman JF, Barr LC, Heninger GR, Price LH. The efficacy of fluvoxamine in obsessive-compulsive disorder: effects of comorbid chronic tic disorder. *J Clin Psychopharmacol.* 1993;13(5):354–358.

79. Hazari N, Narayanaswamy JC, Arumugham SS. Predictors of response to serotonin reuptake inhibitors in obsessive-compulsive disorder. *Expert Rev Neurother.* 2016;16(10):1175–1191.

80. Leckman JF, Rauch SL, Mataix-Cols D. Symptom dimensions in obsessive-compulsive disorder: implications for the DSM-V. *CNS Spectr.* 2007;12(5):376–387, 400.

81. Bloch MH, Craiglow BG, Landeros-Weisenberger A, et al. Predictors of early adult outcomes in pediatric-onset obsessive-compulsive disorder. *Pediatrics.* 2009; 124(4):1085–1093.

82. Conelea CA, Walther MR, Freeman JB, et al. Tic-related obsessive-compulsive disorder (OCD): phenomenology and treatment outcome in the Pediatric OCD Treatment Study II. *J Am Acad Child Adolesc Psychiatry.* 2014;53(12):1308–1316.

83. Højgaard DR, Skarphedinsson G, Nissen JB, Hybel KA, Ivarsson T, Thomsen PH. Pediatric obsessive-compulsive disorder with tic symptoms: clinical presentation and treatment outcome. *Eur Child Adolesc Psychiatry.* 2017; 26(6):681–689.

84. Bloch MH, Bartley CA, Zipperer L, et al. Meta-analysis: hoarding symptoms associated with poor

treatment outcome in obsessive-compulsive disorder. *Mol Psychiatry*. 2014;19(9):1025–1030.

85. Mataix-Cols D, Rauch SL, Manzo PA, Jenike MA, Baer L. Use of factor-analyzed symptom dimensions to predict outcome with serotonin reuptake inhibitors and placebo in the treatment of obsessive-compulsive disorder. *Am J Psychiatry*. 1999;156(9):1409–1416.

86. Landeros-Weisenberger A, Bloch MH, Kelmendi B, et al. Dimensional predictors of response to SRI pharmacotherapy in obsessive-compulsive disorder. *J Affect Disord*. 2010;121(1–2):175–179.

87. Koran LM, Simpson HB. *Guideline Watch (March 2013): Practice Guideline for the Treatment of Patients with Obsessive-Compulsive Disorder*. Arlington, VA: American Psychiatric Association; 2013.

88. Ninan PT, Koran LM, Kiev A, et al. High-dose sertraline strategy for nonresponders to acute treatment for obsessive-compulsive disorder: a multicenter double-blind trial. *J Clin Psychiatry*. 2006;67(1):15–22.

89. Fineberg NA, Reghunandanan S, Simpson HB, et al. Obsessive-compulsive disorder (OCD): practical strategies for pharmacological and somatic treatment in adults. *Psychiatry Res*. 2015;227(1):114–125.

90. Khalsa SS, Schiffman JE, Bystritsky A. Treatment-resistant OCD: options beyond first-line medications. *Curr Psychiatr*. 2011;10(11):45.

91. Connor KM, Payne VM, Gadde KM, Zhang W, Davidson JR. The use of aripiprazole in obsessive-compulsive disorder: preliminary observations in 8 patients. *J Clin Psychiatry*. 2005; 66(1):49–51.

92. Ercan ES, Ardic UA, Ercan E, Yuce D, Durak S. A promising preliminary study of aripiprazole for treatment-resistant childhood obsessive-compulsive disorder. *J Child Adolesc Psychopharmacol*. 2015;25(7):580–584.

93. Skapinakis P, Papatheodorou T, Mavreas V. Antipsychotic augmentation of serotonergic antidepressants in treatment-resistant obsessive-compulsive disorder: a meta-analysis of the randomized controlled trials. *Eur Neuropsychopharmacol*. 2007;17(2):79–93.

94. Vulink NC, Denys D, Fluitman SB, Meinardi JC, Westenberg HG. Quetiapine augments the effect of citalopram in non-refractory obsessive-compulsive disorder: a randomized, double-blind, placebo-controlled study of 76 patients. *J Clin Psychiatry*. 2009;70(7):1001.

95. Carey PD, Lochner C, Kidd M, Van Ameringen M, Stein DJ, Denys D. Quetiapine augmentation of serotonin reuptake inhibitors in treatment-refractory obsessive–compulsive disorder: is response to treatment predictable? *Int Clin Psychopharmacol*. 2012;27(6):321–325. Available at doi:10.1097/YIC.0b013e3283576881 (accessed April 19, 2017).

96. Dold M, Aigner M, Lanzenberger R, Kasper S. Antipsychotic augmentation of serotonin reuptake inhibitors in treatment-resistant obsessive-compulsive disorder: a meta-analysis of double-blind, randomized, placebo-controlled trials. *Int J Neuropsychopharmacol*. 2013;16(3):557–574.

97. Veale D, Miles S, Smallcombe N, Ghezai H, Goldacre B, Hodsoll J. Atypical antipsychotic augmentation in SSRI treatment refractory obsessive-compulsive disorder: a systematic review and meta-analysis. *BMC Psychiatry*. 2014;14(1):317.

98. Ducasse D, Boyer L, Michel P, et al. D2 and D3 dopamine receptor affinity predicts effectiveness of antipsychotic drugs in obsessive-compulsive disorders: a metaregression analysis. *Psychopharmacology*. 2014;231(18):3765–3770.

99. Marinova Z, Chuang DM, Fineberg N. Glutamate-modulating drugs as a potential therapeutic strategy in obsessive-compulsive disorder. *Curr Neuropharmacol*. 2017;15(7):977–995.

100. Insel TR, Hamilton JA, Guttmacher LB, Murphy DL. D-amphetamine in obsessive-compulsive disorder. *Psychopharmacology*. 1983;80(3):231–235.

101. Joffe RT, Swinson RP, Levitt AJ. Acute psychostimulant challenge in primary obsessive-compulsive disorder. *J Clin Psychopharmacol*. 1991;11(4):237–241.

102. Rodriguez CI, Kegeles LS, Levinson A, et al. Randomized controlled crossover trial of ketamine in obsessive-compulsive disorder: proof-of-concept. *Neuropsychopharmacology*. 2013;38(12):2475–2483.

103. Koran LM, Gamel NN, Choung HW, Smith EH, Aboujaoude EN. Mirtazapine for obsessive-compulsive disorder: an open trial followed by double-blind discontinuation. *J Clin Psychiatry*. 2005;66(4):515–520.

104. Ghaleiha A, Entezari N, Modabbernia A, et al. Memantine add-on in moderate to severe obsessive-compulsive disorder: randomized double-blind placebo-controlled study. *J Psychiatr Res*. 2013;47(2):175–180.

105. Haghighi M, Jahangard L, Mohammad-Beigi H, et al. In a double-blind, randomized and placebo-controlled trial, adjuvant memantine improved symptoms in inpatients suffering from refractory obsessive-compulsive disorders (OCD). *Psychopharmacology*. 2013;228(4):633–640.

106. Grant PJ, Joseph LA, Farmer CA, et al. 12-week, placebo-controlled trial of add-on riluzole in the treatment of childhood-onset obsessive–compulsive disorder. *Neuropsychopharmacology*. 2014;39(6):1453–1459.

107. Pittenger C, Bloch MH, Wasylink S, et al. Riluzole augmentation in treatment-refractory obsessive-compulsive disorder: a pilot randomized placebo-controlled trial. *J Clin Psychiatry*. 2015;76(8):1075–1084.

108. Emamzadehfard S, Kamaloo A, Paydary K, et al. Riluzole in augmentation of fluvoxamine for moderate to severe obsessive-compulsive disorder: randomized, double-blind, placebo-controlled study. *Psychiatry Clin Neurosci*. 2016;70(8):332–341.

109. Bruno A, Micò U, Pandolfo G, et al. Lamotrigine augmentation of serotonin reuptake inhibitors in treatment-resistant obsessive-compulsive disorder: a double-blind, placebo-controlled study. *J Psychopharmacol*. 2012;26(11):1456–1462.

110. Khalkhali M, Aram S, Zarrabi H, Kafie M, Heidarzadeh A. Lamotrigine augmentation versus placebo in serotonin reuptake inhibitors-resistant obsessive-compulsive disorder: a randomized controlled trial. *Iran J Psychiatry*. 2016;11(2):104–114.

111. Afshar H, Roohafza H, Mohammad-Beigi H, et al. N-acetylcysteine add-on treatment in refractory obsessive-compulsive disorder: a randomized, double-blind, placebo-controlled trial. *J Clin Psychopharmacol*. 2012;32(6):797–803.

112. Sarris J, Oliver G, Camfield DA, et al. N-acetyl cysteine (NAC) in the treatment of obsessive-compulsive disorder: a 16-week, double-blind, randomised, placebo-controlled study. *CNS Drugs*. 2015;29(9):801–809.

113. Paydary K, Akamaloo A, Ahmadipour A, Pishgar F, Emamzadehfard S, Akhondzadeh S. N-acetylcysteine augmentation therapy for moderate-to-severe obsessive-compulsive disorder: randomized, double-blind, placebo-controlled trial. *J Clin Pharm Ther*. 2016; 41(2):214–219.

114. Costa DLC, Diniz JB, Requena G, et al. Randomized, double-blind, placebo-controlled trial of n-acetylcysteine augmentation for treatment-resistant obsessive-compulsive disorder. *J Clin Psychiatry*. 2017;78(7):e766–e773.

115. Koran LM, Aboujaoude E, Bullock KD, Franz B, Gamel N, Elliott M. Double-blind treatment with oral morphine in treatment-resistant obsessive-compulsive disorder. *J Clin Psychiatry*. 2005;66(3):353–359.

116. Heidari M, Zarei M, Hosseini SM, et al. Ondansetron or placebo in the augmentation of fluvoxamine response over 8 weeks in obsessive–compulsive disorder. *Int Clin Psychopharmacol*. 2014;29(6):344–350.

117. Soltani F, Sayyah M, Feizy F, Malayeri A, Siahpoosh A, Motlagh I. A double-blind, placebo-controlled pilot study of ondansetron for patients with obsessive-compulsive disorder. *Hum Psychopharmacol Clin*. 2010;25(6):509–513.

118. Askari N, Moin M, Sanati M, et al. Granisetron adjunct to fluvoxamine for moderate to severe obsessive-compulsive disorder: a randomised, double-blind, placebo-controlled trial. *CNS Drugs*. 2012;26(10):883–892.

119. Wu K, Hanna GL, Rosenberg DR, Arnold PD. The role of glutamate signaling in the pathogenesis and treatment of obsessive–compulsive disorder. *Pharmacol Biochem Behav*. 2012;100(4):726–735.

120. Ting JT, Feng G. Glutamatergic synaptic dysfunction and obsessive-compulsive disorder. *Curr Chem Genomics*. 2008;2:62–75.

121. Pittenger C, Bloch MH, Williams K. Glutamate abnormalities in obsessive compulsive disorder: neurobiology, pathophysiology, and treatment. *Pharmacol Ther*. 2011;132(3):314–332.

122. Pauls DL, Abramovitch A, Rauch SL, Geller DA. Obsessive-compulsive disorder: an integrative genetic and neurobiological perspective. *Nat Rev Neurosci*. 2014;15(6):410–424.

123. Rosenberg DR, Mirza Y, Russell A, Tang J, Smith JM, Banerjee SP, Bhandari R, Rose M, Ivey J, Boyd C, Moore GJ. Reduced anterior cingulate glutamatergic concentrations in childhood OCD and major depression versus healthy controls. *J Am Acad Child Adolesc Psychiatry*. 2004;43(9):1146–53.

124. Rosenberg DR, MacMaster FP, Keshavan MS, Fitzgerald KD, Stewart CM, Moore GJ. Decrease in caudate glutamatergic concentrations in pediatric obsessive-compulsive disorder patients taking paroxetine. *J Am Acad Child Adolesc Psychiatry*. 2000; 39(9):1096–1103.

125. Kavirajan, H. Memantine: a comprehensive review of safety and efficacy. *Expert Opin Drug Saf*. 2009;8(1):89–109.

126. Aboujaoude E, Barry JJ, Gamel N. Memantine augmentation in treatment-resistant obsessive-compulsive disorder: an open-label trial. *J Clin Psychopharmacol*. 2009;29(1):51–55.

127. Bakhla AK, Verma V, Soren S, Sarkhel S, Chaudhury S. An open-label trial of memantine in treatment-resistant obsessive-compulsive disorder. *Ind Psychiatry J*. 2013;22(2):149–152.

128. Feusner JD, Kerwin L, Saxena S, Bystritsky A. Differential efficacy of memantine for obsessive-compulsive disorder vs. generalized anxiety disorder: an open-label trial. *Psychopharmacol Bull*. 2009;42(1):81–93.

129. Niciu MJ, Henter ID, Luckenbaugh DA, Zarate CA Jr, Charney DS. Glutamate receptor antagonists as fast-acting therapeutic alternatives for the treatment of depression: ketamine and other compounds. *Annu Rev Pharmacol Toxicol.* 2014;54:119–139.

130. Price RB, Nock MK, Charney DS, Mathew SJ. Effects of intravenous ketamine on explicit and implicit measures of suicidality in treatment-resistant depression. *Biol Psychiatry.* 2009;66(5):522–526.

131. Goodman WK, Price LH, Rasmussen SA, et al. The Yale-Brown Obsessive Compulsive Scale. I. Development, use, and reliability. *Arch Gen Psychiatry.* 1989;46(11):1006–1011.

132. Bloch MH, Wasylink S, Landeros-Weisenberger A, et al. Effects of ketamine in treatment-refractory obsessive-compulsive disorder. *Biol Psychiatry.* 2012;72(11):964–970.

133. Pittenger C, Coric V, Banasr M, Bloch M, Krystal JH, Sanacora G. Riluzole in the treatment of mood and anxiety disorders. *CNS Drugs.* 2008;22(9):761–786.

134. Coric V, Taskiran S, Pittenger C, et al. Riluzole augmentation in treatment-resistant obsessive–compulsive disorder: an open-label trial. *Biol Psychiatry.* 2005; 58(5):424–428.

135. Grant P, Lougee L, Hirschtritt M, Swedo SE. An open-label trial of riluzole, a glutamate antagonist, in children with treatment-resistant obsessive-compulsive disorder. *J Child Adolesc Psychopharmacol.* 2007;17(6):761–767.

136. Pittenger C, Kelmendi B, Wasylink S, Bloch MH, Coric V. Riluzole augmentation in treatment-refractory obsessive-compulsive disorder: a series of 13 cases, with long-term follow-up. *J Clin Psychopharmacol.* 2008;28(3):363–367. Available from: doi:10.1097/JCP.0b013e3181727548 (accessed April 19, 2017).

137. Sasso DA, Kalanithi PS, Trueblood KV, et al. Beneficial effects of the glutamate-modulating agent riluzole on disordered eating and pathological skin-picking behaviors. *J Clin Psychopharmacol.* 2006;26(6):685–687.

138. Pittenger C. Glutamatergic agents for OCD and related disorders. *Curr Treat Options Psychiatry.* 2015;2(3):271–283.

139. Berlin HA, Koran LM, Jenike MA, et al. Double-blind, placebo-controlled trial of topiramate augmentation in treatment-resistant obsessive-compulsive disorder. *J Clin Psychiatry.* 2011;72(5):716–721.

140. Afshar H, Akuchekian S, Mahaky B, Zarean E. Topiramate augmentation in refractory obsessive-compulsive disorder: a randomized, double-blind, placebo-controlled trial. *J Res Med Sci.* 2014;19(10):976–981. Available from: www.ncbi.nlm.nih.gov/pmc/articles/PMC4274576/ (accessed April 19, 2017).

141. Kemp DE, Gilmer WS, Fleck J, Dago PL. An association of intrusive, repetitive phrases with lamotrigine treatment in bipolar II disorder. *CNS Spectr.* 2007;12(2):106–111.

142. Kuloglu M, Caykoylu A, Ekinci O, Yilmaz E. Lamotrigine-induced obsessional symptoms in a patient with bipolar II disorder: a case report. *J Psychopharmacol.* 2009;23(8):1001–1003.

143. Ozkara C, Ozmen M, Erdogan A, Yalug, I. Topiramate related obsessive-compulsive disorder. *Eur Psychiatry.* 2005;20(1):78–79.

144. Thuile J, Even C, Guelfi JD. Topiramate may induce obsessive-compulsive disorder. *Psychiatry Clin Neurosci.* 2006;60(3):394.

145. Kreek MJ. Methadone-related opioid agonist pharmacotherapy for heroin addiction. History, recent molecular and neurochemical research and future in mainstream medicine. *Ann N Y Acad Sci.* 2000;909:186–216.

146. Srisurapanont M, Jarusuraisin N. Naltrexone for the treatment of alcoholism: a meta-analysis of randomized controlled trials. *Int J Neuropsychopharmacol.* 2005;8(2):267–280.

147. Lee YK, Park SW, Kim YK, et al. Effects of naltrexone on the ethanol-induced changes in the rat central dopaminergic system. *Alcohol Alcohol.* 2005;40(4):297–301.

148. Kim SW. Opioid antagonists in the treatment of impulse-control disorders. *J Clin Psychiatry.* 1998;59(4):159–164.

149. Kim SW, Grant JE, Adson DE, Shin YC. Double-blind naltrexone and placebo comparison study in the treatment of pathological gambling. *Biol Psychiatry.* 2001;49(11):914–921.

150. Grant JE, Kim SW. A case of kleptomania and compulsive sexual behavior treated with naltrexone. *Ann Clin Psychiatry.* 2001;13(4):229–231.

151. Grant JE, Kim SW. An open-label study of naltrexone in the treatment of kleptomania. *J Clin Psychiatry.* 2002;63(4):349–356.

152. Sandyk R. Naloxone abolishes obsessive-compulsive behavior in Tourette's syndrome. *Int J Neurosci.* 1987;35(1–2):93–94.

153. Keuler DJ, Altemus M, Michelson D, Greenberg B, Murphy DL. Behavioral effects of naloxone infusion in obsessive-compulsive disorder. *Biol Psychiatry.* 1996;40(2):154–156.

154. Insel TR, Pickar D. Naloxone administration in obsessive compulsive disorder: report of two cases. *Am J Psychiatry.* 1983;140(9):1219–1220.

155. Amiaz R, Fostick L, Gershon A, Zohar J. Naltrexone augmentation in OCD: a double-blind placebo-controlled cross-over study. *Eur Neuropsychopharmacol.* 2008;18(6):455–461.

156. Shapira NA, Keck PE Jr, Goldsmith TD, McConville BJ, Eis M, McElroy SL. Open-label pilot study of tramadol hydrochloride in treatment-refractory obsessive-compulsive disorder. *Depress Anxiety.* 1997;6(4):170–173.

157. Hewlett WA, Schmid SP, Salomon RM. Pilot trial of ondansetron in the treatment of 8 patients with obsessive-compulsive disorder. *J Clin Psychiatry.* 2003;64(9):1025–1030.

158. Pallanti S, Bernardi S, Antonini S, Singh N, Hollander E. Ondansetron augmentation in patients with obsessive-compulsive disorder who are inadequate responders to serotonin reuptake inhibitors: improvement with treatment and worsening following discontinuation. *Eur Neuropsychopharmacol.* 2014;24(3):375–380.

159. Toren P, Weizman A, Ratner S, Cohen D, Laor N. Ondansetron treatment in Tourette's disorder: a 3-week, randomized, double-blind, placebo-controlled study. *J Clin Psychiatry.* 2005;66(4):499–503.

160. Transcept Pharmaceuticals. Efficacy and safety study of low-dose ondansetron for adjunctive therapy in adult patients with obsessive-compulsive disorder. NCT01275248; 2011. Available from: https://clinicaltrials.gov/ct2/show/NCT01275248 (accessed July 13, 2018).

161. Koran LM, Aboujaoude E, Gamel NN. Double-blind study of dextroamphetamine versus caffeine augmentation for treatment-resistant obsessive-compulsive disorder. *J Clin Psychiatry.* 2009;70(11):1530–1535.

162. Perugi G, Giannotti D, Di Vaio S, Frare F, Saettoni M, Cassano GB. Fluvoxamine in the treatment of body dysmorphic disorder (dysmorphophobia). *Int Clin Psychopharmacol.* 1996;11(4):247–254.

163. Phillips KA. An open-label study of escitalopram in body dysmorphic disorder. *Int Clin Psychopharmacol.* 2006;21(3):177–179.

164. Phillips KA, Dwight MM, McElroy SL. Efficacy and safety of fluvoxamine in body dysmorphic disorder. *J Clin Psychiatry.* 1998;59(4):165–171.

165. Phillips KA, Najjar F. An open-label study of citalopram in body dysmorphic disorder. *J Clin Psychiatry.* 2003;64(6):715–720.

166. Phillips KA, Albertini RS, Rasmussen SA. A randomized placebo-controlled trial of fluoxetine in body dysmorphic disorder. *Arch Gen Psychiatry.* 2002;59(4):381–388.

167. Phillips KA, Keshaviah A, Dougherty DD, Stout RL, Menard W, Wilhelm S. Pharmacotherapy relapse prevention in body dysmorphic disorder: a double-blind, placebo-controlled trial. *Am J Psychiatry.* 2016;173(9):887–895.

168. Rashid H, Khan AA, Fineberg NA. Adjunctive antipsychotic in the treatment of body dysmorphic disorder – a retrospective naturalistic case note study. *Int J Psychiatry Clin Practice.* 2015;19(2):84–89.

169. Hollander E, Allen A, Kwon J, et al. Clomipramine vs desipramine crossover trial in body dysmorphic disorder: selective efficacy of a serotonin reuptake inhibitor in imagined ugliness. *Arch Gen Psychiatry.* 1999;56(11):1033–1039.

170. Ipser JC, Sander C, Stein DJ. Pharmacotherapy and psychotherapy for body dysmorphic disorder. *Cochrane Database Syst Rev.* 2009;1:CD005473.

171. National Institute for Health and Care Excellence. *Obsessive-Compulsive Disorder: Core Interventions in the Treatment of Obsessive-Compulsive Disorder and Body Dysmorphic Disorder.* Clinical Guideline CG31. London: NICE; 2006.

172. Phillips KA, Albertini RS, Siniscalchi JM, Khan A, Robinson M. Effectiveness of pharmacotherapy for body dysmorphic disorder: a chart-review study. *J Clin Psychiatry.* 2001;62(9):721–727.

173. Phillips KA. Placebo-controlled study of pimozide augmentation of fluoxetine in body dysmorphic disorder. *Am J Psychiatry.* 2005;162(2):377–379.

174. Uzun Ö, Özdemir B. Aripriprazole as an augmentation agent in treatment-resistant body dysmorphic disorder. *Clin Drug Investig.* 2010;30(10):707–710.

175. Morein-Zamir S, Papmeyer M, Pertusa A, et al. The profile of executive function in OCD hoarders and hoarding disorder. *Psychiatry Res.* 2014;215(3):659–667.

176. Saxena S. Pharmocotherapy of compulsive hoarding. *J Clin Psychol.* 2011;67(5):477–484.

177. Saxena S, Brody AL, Maidment KM, Baxter LR Jr. Paroxetine treatment of compulsive hoarding. *J Psychiatr Res.* 2007;41(6):481–487.

178. Denys D, van Megen HJ, van der Wee N, Westenberg HG. A double-blind switch study of paroxetine and venlafaxine in obsessive-compulsive disorder. *J Clin Psychiatry.* 2004;65(1):37–43.

179. Denys D, Van Nieuwerburgh F, Deforce D, Westenberg HG. Prediction of response to paroxetine and venlafaxine by serotonin-related genes in obsessive-compulsive disorder in a randomized, double-blind trial. *J Clin Psychiatry.* 2007;68(5):747–753.

180. Saxena S, Sumner J. Venlafaxine extended-release treatment of hoarding disorder. *Int Clin Psychopharmacol.* 2014;29(5):266–273.

181. Bogan AM, Koran LM, Chuong HW, Vapnik T, Bystritsky A. Quetiapine augmentation in obsessive-compulsive disorder resistant to serotonin reuptake inhibitors: an open-label study. *J Clin Psychiatry.* 2005;66(1):73–79.

182. Rodriguez CI, Bender J Jr, Morrison S, Mehendru R, Tolin D, Simpson HB. Does extended release methylphenidate help adults with hoarding disorder?: a case series. *J Clin Psychopharmacol.* 2013;33(3):444–447.

183. Swedo SE, Leonard HL, Rapoport JL, Lenane MC, Goldberger EL, Cheslow DL. A double-blind comparison of clomipramine and desipramine in the treatment of trichotillomania (hair pulling). *N Engl J Med.* 1989;321(8):497–501.

184. Swedo SE, Lenane MC, Leonard HL. Long-term treatment of trichotillomania (hair pulling). *N Engl J Med.* 1993;329(2):141–142.

185. Gadde KM, Ryan Wagner H 2nd, Connor KM, Foust MS. Escitalopram treatment of trichotillomania. *Int Clin Psychopharmacol.* 2007;22(1):39–42.

186. Koran LM, Ringold A, Hewlett W. Fluoxetine for trichotillomania: an open clinical trial. *Psychopharmacol Bull.* 1992;28(2):145–149.

187. Stein DJ, Bouwer C, Maud CM. Use of the selective serotonin reuptake inhibitor citalopram in treatment of trichotillomania. *Eur Arch Psychiatry Clin Neurosci.* 1997;247(4):234–236.

188. Christenson GA, Mackenzie TB, Mitchell JE, Callies AL. A placebo-controlled, double-blind crossover study of fluoxetine in trichotillomania. *Am J Psychiatry.* 1991;148(11):1566–1571.

189. Streichenwein SM, Thornby JI. A long-term, double-blind, placebo-controlled crossover trial. *Am J Psychiatry.* 1995;152(8):1192–1196.

190. Dougherty DD, Loh R, Jenike MA, Keuthen NJ. Single modality versus dual modality treatment for trichotillomania: sertraline, behavioral therapy, or both? *J Clin Psychiatry.* 2006;67(7):1086–1092.

191. Rothbart R, Amos T, Siegfried N, et al. Pharmacotherapy for trichotillomania. *Cochrane Database Syst Rev.* 2013;11:CD007662.

192. Pollard CA, Ibe IO, Krojanker DN, Kitchen AD, Bronson SS, Flynn TM. Clomipramine treatment of trichotillomania: a follow-up report on four cases. *J Clin Psychiatry.* 1991;52(3):128–130.

193. Ninan, PT, Rothbaum BO, Marsteller FA, Knight BT, Eccard MB. A placebo-controlled trial of cognitive-behavioral therapy and clomipramine in trichotillomania. *J Clin Psychiatry.* 2000;61(1):47–50.

194. Van Ameringen M, Mancini C, Patterson B, Bennett M, Oakman J. A randomized, double-blind, placebo-controlled trial of olanzapine in the treatment of trichotillomania. *J Clin Psychiatry.* 2010;71(10):1336–1343.

195. White MP, Koran LM. Open-label trial of aripiprazole in the treatment of trichotillomania. *J Clin Psychopharmacol.* 2011;31(4):503–506.

196. Stein DJ, Hollander E. Low-dose pimozide augmentation of serotonin reuptake blockers in the treatment of trichotillomania. *J Clin Psychiatry.* 1992;53(4):123–126.

197. De Sousa A. An open-label pilot study of naltrexone in childhood-onset trichotillomania. *J Child Adolesc Psychopharmacol.* 2008;18(1):30–33.

198. Grant JE, Odlaug BL, Schreiber LR, Kim SW. The opiate antagonist, naltrexone, in the treatment of trichotillomania: results of a double-blind, placebo-controlled study. *J Clin Psychopharmacol.* 2014;34(1):134–138.

199. Grant JE, Odlaug BL, Kim SW. N-acetylcysteine, a glutamate modulator, in the treatment of trichotillomania: a double-blind, placebo-controlled study. *Arch Gen Psychiatry.* 2009;66(7):756–763.

200. Bloch MH, Panza KE, Grant JE, Pittenger C, Leckman JF. N-acetylcysteine in the treatment of pediatric trichotillomania: a randomized, double-blind, placebo-controlled add-on trial. *J Am Acad Child Adolesc Psychiatry.* 2013;52(3):231–240.

201. Panza KE, Pittenger C, Bloch MH. Age and gender correlates of pulling in pediatric trichotillomania. *J Am Acad Child Adolesc Psychiatry.* 2013;52(3):241–249.

202. Simeon D, Stein DJ, Gross S, Islam N, Schmeidler J, Hollander E. A double-blind trial of fluoxetine in pathologic skin picking. *J Clin Psychiatry.* 1997;58(8):341–347.

203. Bloch MR, Elliott M, Thompson H, Koran LM. Fluoxetine in pathologic skin-picking: open-label and double-blind results. *Psychosomatics.* 2001;42(4):314–319.

204. Arnold LM, Mutasim DF, Dwight MM, Lamerson CL, Morris EM, McElroy SL. An open clinical trial of fluvoxamine treatment of psychogenic excoriation. *J Clin Psychopharmacol.* 1999;19(1):15–18.

205. Keuthen NJ, Jameson M, Loh R, Deckersbach T, Wilhelm S, Dougherty DD. Open-label escitalopram treatment for pathological skin picking. *Int Clin Psychopharmacol.* 2007;22(5):268–274.

206. Arbabi M, Farnia V, Balighi K, et al. Efficacy of citalopram in treatment of pathological skin picking: a randomized double blind placebo controlled trial. *Acta Medica Iranica.* 2008;46(5):367–372.

207. Grant JE, Chamberlain SR, Redden SA, Leppink EW, Odlaug BL, Kim SW. N-acetylcysteine in the treatment of excoriation disorder: a randomized clinical trial. *JAMA Psychiatry.* 2016;73(5):490–496.

208. Morgan JR, Storch EA, Woods DW, Bodzin D, Lewin AB, Murphy TK. A preliminary analysis of the phenomenology of skin-picking in Prader-Willi syndrome. *Child Psychiatry Hum Dev.* 2010;41(4):448–463.

209. Grant JE, Odlaug BL, Kim SW. Lamotrigine treatment of pathologic skin picking: an open-label study. *J Clin Psychiatry.* 2007;68(9):1384–1391.

210. Grant JE, Odlaug BL, Chamberlain SR, Kim SW. A double-blind, placebo-controlled trial of lamotrigine for pathological skin picking: treatment efficacy and neurocognitive predictors of response. *J Clin Psychopharmacol.* 2010;30(4):396–403.

211. Benjamin E, Buot-Smith T. Naltrexone and fluoxetine in Prader-Willi syndrome. *J Am Acad Child Adolesc Psychiatry.* 1993;32(4):870–873.

212. Brakoulias V. The future of pharmacotherapy for obsessive-compulsive disorder may lie in a better understanding of its heterogeneity. *Expert Opin Pharmacother.* 2014;15(10):1321–1323.

213. Phillips KA, Hollander E, Rasmussen SA, Aronowitz BR, Decaria C, Goodman WK. A severity rating scale for body dysmorphic disorder: development, reliability, and validity of a modified version of the Yale-Brown Obsessive Compulsive Scale. *Psychopharmacol Bull.* 1997;33(1):17–22.

214. Abramowitz JS, Deacon BJ, Olatunji BO, et al. Assessment of obsessive-compulsive symptom dimensions: development and evaluation of the Dimensional Obsessive-Compulsive Scale. *Psychol Assess.* 2010;22(1):180–198.

215. Keuthen NJ, O'Sullivan RL, Ricciardi JN, et al. The Massachusetts General Hospital (MGH) Hairpulling Scale: 1. development and factor analyses. *Psychother Psychosom.* 1995;64(3–4):141–145.

216. Tolin DF, Frost RO, Steketee G. A brief interview for assessing compulsive hoarding: the Hoarding Rating Scale-Interview. *Psychiatry Res.* 2010;178(1):147–152.

217. Foa EB, Huppert JD, Leiberg S, et al. The Obsessive-Compulsive Inventory: development and validation of a short version. *Psychol Assess.* 2002;14(4):485–496.

218. Winchel RM, Jones JS, Molcho A, Parsons B, Stanley B, Stanley M. The Psychiatric Institute Trichotillomania Scale (PITS). *Psychopharmacol Bull.* 1992;28(4):463–476.

219. Frost RO, Steketee G, Grisham J. Measurement of compulsive hoarding: saving inventory-revised. *Behav Res Ther.* 2004;42(10):1163–1182.

220. Keuthen NJ, Wilhelm S, Deckersbach T, et al. The Skin Picking Scale: scale construction and psychometric analyses. *J Psychosom Res.* 2001;50(6):337–341.

221. Stanley MA, Breckenridge JK, Snyder AG, Novy DM. Clinician-rated measures of hair pulling: a preliminary psychometric evaluation. *J Psychopathol Behav Assess.* 1999;21(2):157–170.

222. Stanley MA, Prather RC, Wagner AL, Davis ML, Swann AC. Can the Yale-Brown Obsessive Compulsive Scale be used to assess trichotillomania? A preliminary report. *Behav Res Ther.* 1993;31(2):171–177.

223. Rosario-Campos MC, Miguel EC, Quatrano S, et al. The Dimensional Yale-Brown Obsessive-Compulsive Scale (DY-BOCS): an instrument for assessing obsessive-compulsive symptom dimensions. *Mol Psychiatry.* 2006;11(5):495–504.

224. LeBeau RT, Mischel ER, Simpson HB, et al. Preliminary assessment of obsessive–compulsive spectrum disorder scales for DSM-5. *J Obsessive-Compuls Relat Disord.* 2013;2(2):114–118.

Chapter 16

Psychological Treatment of Obsessive-Compulsive Disorder: Efficacy, Mechanisms and Transdiagnostic Implications

Jennifer L. Buchholz, Lillian Reuman, Shannon M. Blakey and Jonathan S. Abramowitz

Introduction

With the publication of the fifth edition of the *Diagnostic and Statistical Manual of Mental Disorders* (DSM-5) [1], obsessive-compulsive disorder (OCD) was moved from the anxiety disorders category (where it had been since DSM-III [2]) to a newly created diagnostic category, the obsessive-compulsive and related disorders (OCRDs). The OCRDs include body dysmorphic disorder (BDD), hoarding disorder, hair-pulling disorder (also known as trichotillomania) and skin-picking disorder (also known as excoriation disorder). Although this reclassification is based on putative overlaps in presenting symptoms (i.e., all OCRDs involve repetitive thinking and behavior), etiologically relevant factors (e.g., brain circuitry, neurotransmitter abnormalities) and treatment response [3], the empirical basis for such "overlaps" (and indeed for the DSM-5's reclassification) is not without criticism [4].

With regard to treatment, proponents of the OCRD approach argue that the new category is justified given that the OCRDs all share similar response profiles to "anti-obsessional behavioral therapies" [5]. In the present chapter, we challenge this claim and discuss the application and efficacy of exposure-based therapy in the treatment of OCD, the mechanisms of action of this intervention and its applicability to other OCRDs. We then turn to the implications of treatment response for understanding and classifying OCD and the other OCRDs.

Background and Recent Research Findings

Cognitive behavior therapy (CBT), a collection of experimentally established procedures based on the principles of thinking and learning, is the first-line psychological treatment for OCD. Cognitive models of OCD hold that obsessional fear arises from overestimates of the probability and costs of negative outcomes associated with certain external or internal stimuli (e.g., "I will likely become deathly ill if I use a public toilet" [6]). Behavioral models rely on operant and classical conditioning to understand the persistence of ritualistic behaviors that reduce or neutralize obsessional fear (e.g., washing and checking) [7]. CBT is used to weaken (or eliminate) inappropriate or maladaptive thinking and behavior patterns. Thus, planning an effective trial of CBT for an individual with OCD relies on precise information about the antecedents and consequences of the responses to be eliminated, as well as the cognitive basis for the emotion (e.g., what is the person fearful of and why?). Collecting this information is critical to the success of CBT, because it helps therapists to tailor treatment appropriately to the patient's specific fears.

Research shows that in OCD, obsessional stimuli (e.g., "contaminated" toilets) are associated with *increases* in anxiety, whereas compulsive rituals (e.g., hand washing) are associated with *reductions* in anxiety. In other words, as compulsive rituals provide an escape from anxiety they are negatively reinforced, leading to their repetitive use in similar situations (e.g., using any bathroom). Moreover, this immediate reduction in anxiety (as a result of ritualistic behavior) prevents the natural extinction of the anxiety response and urge to perform rituals. Thus, rituals maintain obsessional fear. Effective CBT for reducing OCD symptoms must therefore extinguish the associations between (a) obsessional stimuli and excessive anxiety and (b) compulsive rituals and the accompanying relief from anxiety. The most effective CBT techniques for accomplishing these goals are *exposure* and *response prevention* (ERP). We next turn to a discussion of the efficacy mechanisms by which these techniques operate before considering implications for transdiagnostic treatment.

What Are the Techniques of Exposure and Response Prevention?

Before the 1960s, OCD was considered to be a treatment-resistant condition. The most widely used intervention was psychodynamic psychotherapy, in which the therapist attempted to determine the cause of the patient's obsessions and compulsions by uncovering unconscious conflicts. Although the other OCRDs did not exist as official diagnoses until more recent publications of the DSM, unrealistic concerns about appearance (which we now refer to as BDD) and urges to engage in impulsive behaviors (such as hair pulling and skin picking) were addressed in a similar fashion. Unfortunately, there is little systematic research on the efficacy of psychodynamic treatment approaches for OCRDs. However, the fact that OCD (and what we now call the OCRDs) was considered treatment refractory suggests that psychodynamic therapy was generally ineffective in producing long-term treatment gains.

Disappointed by the poor results of psychodynamic treatments, behaviorally oriented researchers in the 1960s and 1970s began to apply learning and conditioning models to the treatment of fear-based problems such as OCD. Victor Meyer [8] first reported on the effects of an early (yet highly recognizable) form of ERP for OCD that included deliberately confronting (for two hours each day) fear-provoking situations and stimuli (e.g., floors, door knobs) to induce urges to ritualize. Patients were instructed to refrain from performing rituals such as washing or cleaning. Ten of Meyer's 15 patients responded extremely well to this therapy, and the remainder showed partial improvement. Follow-up studies found that most patients maintained their gains over several years [9].

Contemporary ERP entails therapist-guided systematic, repeated and prolonged exposure to the fear triggers. Abstinence from compulsive and ritualistic behaviors (i.e., response prevention) is also required. This might occur in the form of repeated (a) actual confrontation with feared but objectively low-risk situations (i.e., in vivo exposure), or (b) imaginal confrontation with anxiety-provoking intrusive thoughts and images (i.e., imaginal exposure). In the case of an individual who has obsessions about harm triggered by driving on crowded city streets, they would practice driving in places where pedestrians were walking nearby and frequently crossing the street. Response prevention is vital because rituals to reduce fear would prematurely discontinue exposure and consequently prevent the patient from learning that (a) the fear trigger is not realistically dangerous; (b) anxiety subsides on its own even if the ritual is not performed and (c) the temporary feelings of fear and anxiety are manageable. Thus, successful exposure requires that the patient remain in the feared situation despite experiencing anxiety or distress and without using rituals to artificially reduce the distress via avoidance or escape. Continuing on with the earlier example, the person with OCD would refrain from checking the roadside for accidents she might have caused. Although ERP can be considered as a behavioral technique, it is also thought to produce cognitive change (i.e., modifications of mistaken beliefs) via learning about the threat posed by feared situations.

How Does Exposure and Response Prevention Work?

From a learning (conditioning) perspective, ERP provides an opportunity for the extinction of conditioned fear responses. Extinction occurs when the once-feared obsessional stimulus is repeatedly paired with the nonoccurrence of feared consequences and eventual anxiety reduction. Research suggests that fear associations are not removed during extinction, but rather the associations remain intact as new learning about the feared stimulus occurs [10]. That is, following successful exposure, the feared stimulus is thought to possess two meanings: the original excitatory (i.e., fear-based) meaning as well as an inhibitory ("safety-based") meaning. Thus, even if fear subsides following successful exposure, the original excitatory meaning is retained and may be recovered under certain circumstances such as a change in context, the passage of time and reacquisition of the original association [11]. Accordingly, the extinction that occurs during exposure is the result of *inhibitory learning* – patients learn new, nonthreat associations and ways of enhancing the accessibility of these new associations (relative to the older threat associations) in different contexts and over time.

Another way to understand the way that exposure works is by considering its effects on beliefs that underlie fear and anxiety. Exposure presents the patient with disconfirmatory evidence, leading to modifications in overestimates of threat. Specifically, when patients confront feared situations and refrain from rituals, they find out that fear/anxiety is manageable (and often declines naturally) and that the anticipated negative consequences of confrontation with the feared stimulus are unlikely. This evidence is processed and incorporated into the patient's belief system. Thus, rituals to reduce anxiety and prevent feared disasters become unnecessary. Although level of fear throughout exposure trials is often construed as an index of corrective learning, evidence indicates that neither the degree of fear reduction, nor the ending fear level predict therapeutic outcome [10]. Developments in the theory and science of fear learning, fear extinction and memory indicate that "performance during training" is not commensurate with learning at the process level.

How Effective is Exposure and Response Prevention?

Studies evaluating the effectiveness of ERP for OCD consistently show that patients who complete this treatment achieve clinically significant and durable improvement. Average improvement rates typically range from 50% to 70% in these studies [12]. A review of 16 trials (involving 756 patients) indicated that ERP was substantially more efficacious than comparison treatments (e.g., relaxation, anxiety management training, waiting list, medication) immediately following therapy (effect size 1.39), and moderately more effective at long-term follow-up (effect size 0.43) [12]. Moreover, these trials indicate that the effects are due to the specific techniques of ERP over and above the factors common to all interventions, such as the therapeutic relationship, passage of time, expectations of improvement and spontaneous remission. Importantly, the effects of ERP are not limited to highly selected research samples or to treatment as delivered in specialty clinics. Effectiveness studies conducted with non-research patients [13] show that over 80% of patients who complete ERP achieve clinically significant improvement. Although ERP is effective in both the short and long terms for most people with OCD, about 20% do not respond, and about 25–30% drop out of therapy. A recent meta-analysis of 13 randomized controlled trials directly comparing ERP to serotonergic medications, which are considered the first-line pharmacological treatment of OCD, revealed that ERP is at least as effective (if not more so) than these medications [14]. Indeed, it is widely acknowledged that CBT is the first-line treatment for OCD (before SSRIs in most cases [15,16]).

Applying Exposure and Response Prevention to Other Obsessive-Compulsive and Related Disorders

As we have discussed, the use of ERP for OCD is derived from the unique relationship between obsessional fear and compulsive behavior. Specifically, obsessional fear is triggered by thoughts and feared situations that are not objectively dangerous. Performed deliberately with the intent of reducing obsessional anxiety, compulsive rituals and other neutralizing behaviors reduce anxiety in the moment, yet serve to maintain the anxiety in the long term. Despite the fact that anxiety and fear would decrease naturally even if no ritual was performed, individuals with OCD perform such behaviors compulsively as a way of ensuring anxiety reduction. The purpose of ERP is to teach the patient that obsessive fears are excessive, compulsive behaviors are unnecessary to maintain safety, and that anxiety and obsessional thoughts are safe and tolerable. Importantly, the use of these particular interventions is tied to cognitive and behavioral theories of OCD. Thus, when considering the transdiagnostic applicability of ERP, it is necessary to examine the relationship between cognitive factors and behavioral factors in the other OCRDs.

Body Dysmorphic Disorder

Prior to the publication of DSM-5, BDD was classified as a somatoform disorder. As an OCRD, BDD is characterized by preoccupation with one or more perceived defects or flaws in physical appearance (e.g., my ears are too large for my face), excessive behaviors in response to appearance concerns (e.g., repetitive mirror checking, concealment, plastic surgery), significant distress and impaired functioning. Research and clinical observations show that, as in OCD, appearance-related cognitions in BDD are experienced as intrusive, unwanted and distressing, and the repetitive behaviors function to reduce appearance-related anxiety [17]. Indeed, these behaviors are negatively reinforced. This process parallels the function of compulsive rituals in OCD [17,18,19].

Neziroglu, Roberts and Yaryura-Tobias [20] offer a cognitive-behavioral model of BDD, derived from Mowrer's two-factor theory [21], which provides a basis for the use of ERP. According to this conceptualization, classical conditioning occurs when negative emotions (e.g., shame, disgust) become associated with social trauma (e.g., teasing) related to one's body parts [22]. Veale [23] offered an alternative explanation for how BDD is maintained from a cognitive perspective, proposing that the chain of events begins with an "external representation" of the individual's appearance, such as seeing one's reflection, which triggers a defective mental image. Through selective attention, the individual experiences heightened awareness of specific characteristics within the image. Next, the individual negatively appraises their appearance, turning toward their existing values and assumptions about the importance of physical appearance (e.g., "If I am unattractive, then life is not worth living"). The person then engages in various "safety behaviors," such as avoidance or compulsive-like rituals (e.g., mirror checking, grooming) with the aim of preventing feared outcomes (e.g., social rejection) and reducing distress. Although these safety behaviors might temporarily alleviate distress (and are thereby negatively reinforced), they ultimately increase self-consciousness, preoccupation with the imagined defect and negative appraisals of oneself. Moreover, they prevent the unlearning of the initial emotional reaction, thereby strengthening the avoidance and compulsive behavior. This model has clear implications for treatment and generally leads to the use of exposure-based interventions.

ERP is implemented for BDD in much the same way that it is used in OCD [24]. In BDD, exposure helps the patient to learn that (a) the fear that others will notice and respond negatively to the imagined physical defect is excessive and unrealistic and (b) that anxiety and feelings of embarrassment are temporary and tolerable. The following behavioral experiments might be incorporated into exposure for BDD: going out in public without makeup, enhancing rather than concealing an imagined defect using makeup and wearing pants that reveal or accentuate certain parts of the body. Response prevention incorporates abstinence from behaviors such as prolonged mirror-gazing and self-inspection, wearing clothing (e.g., hats) to conceal the hair or face and seeking assurances from others.

Only a handful of studies have examined the effects of ERP for BDD, yet the literature indicates that this approach produces large effects from pre to post treatment that are comparable to its effects for OCD [25,26,27]. Exposure-based CBT for BDD generally performs better than wait-list control treatment and is associated with not only BDD symptom reduction, but also improvement in related symptoms of functioning, depression, anxiety and delusional beliefs.

Hair Pulling and Skin Picking

Formerly identified as an impulse control disorder, hair-pulling disorder (i.e., trichotillomania) is characterized in DSM-5 by recurrent hair pulling resulting in hair loss, repeated attempts to stop hair pulling and associated distress or impairment. Although hair pulling resembles OCD-related compulsions in that it is often repetitive, it is not generally preceded by the types of obsessional thoughts that occur in OCD. Research indicates that instead, hair pulling is triggered by feelings of general tension, depression, anger, boredom, frustration, indecision or fatigue [28]. Hair pulling is also maintained in part by positive reinforcement: the person often experiences a sense of pleasure from pulling the hair [29]. Negative reinforcement also plays a role, as hair pulling may elicit a sense of escape from general distress or from boredom. This pattern of reinforcement, however, is notably distinct from OCD-related compulsions, which are maintained by negative reinforcement (i.e., the rituals functions to reduce the distress associated with an obsessional thought, and this distress reduction is rewarding). Research also supports a distinction between "focused" and "automatic" pulling styles in hair-pulling disorder [30]. Focused pulling has a compulsive quality, whereas automatic pulling is conducted outside of an individual's awareness and often in concert with a mindless task (e.g., reading, watching television). The lack of awareness of automatic pulling represents another functional difference between hair-pulling disorder and OCD-related compulsions. That is, in OCD, rituals are usually performed deliberately and according to self-prescribed rules [1].

Skin-picking disorder (i.e., excoriation disorder) is a new diagnosis in DSM-5, and criteria are identical to those for hair-pulling disorder, substituting "skin picking" for "hair pulling." As with hair-pulling disorder, skin-picking disorder does not involve obsessional thoughts, and the picking behavior serves a different function than do compulsive rituals in OCD. Skin picking can be precipitated by an array of antecedents, including general stress, apprehension, boredom, fatigue and anger [31,32]. Furthermore, unlike in OCD, emotion regulation difficulties and emotional reactivity have been shown to predict excoriation behavior even after controlling for depression, anxiety and worry [33]. As with hair pulling, skin picking can be either automatic or focused, and often begins without the individual's awareness but becomes more conscious after a period of time [34,35]. This differs from deliberate anxiety-reducing compulsive behavior characteristic of OCD.

Although the presence or absence of obsessions and differences in how negative and positive reinforcement, respectively, maintain compulsions in OCD and hair-pulling and skin-picking disorders might seem technical, they have important implications for the use of ERP. As we have discussed, this is because exposure is a procedure for helping patients with excessive fears (e.g., obsessions) to repeatedly confront anxiety-provoking stimuli in order to promote changes (i.e., corrections) in expectations of feared consequences (e.g., "If I were to touch the toilet, I would get sick;" "If I go to school without wearing a hat, people will laugh at my hair."). Accordingly, this approach does not apply to hair-pulling and skin-picking behaviors that do not involve obsession-like fears of disastrous consequences.

We have observed the occasional clinician attempting to engineer (or recommend) ERP for hair pulling and skin picking. For example, they might instruct patients to expose themselves to situations in which hair pulling occurs, such as standing with tweezers by a mirror, and resisting the urge to pull. This, however, represents a misunderstanding of the principles of exposure therapy. ERP is a treatment designed to ameliorate fear-based avoidance and prevent compulsive behaviors, but is not appropriate for all forms of repetitive behavior. As discussed above, urges to pull hair and pick skin can be maintained by positive reinforcement when there is a pleasurable element to performing these behaviors (even if they result in long-term guilt and shame). This is in contrast to compulsive rituals in OCD, which are largely maintained by *negative* reinforcement. That is, on a functional level, OCD rituals are escape (safety) behaviors. Hair pulling and skin picking are not fear based, and therefore will not respond to exposure-based techniques. That is, the urge to pull or pick is not expected to decline as a result of the type of exposure exercise described above.

Instead, research suggests that individuals with hair pulling and skin picking are best served by implementing techniques that alter the antecedents (i.e., cues) of the target behaviors and that teach alternative response strategies [36]. For example, avoiding high-risk situations (the very *opposite* of what would be prescribed in exposure therapy) and using stimulus control techniques (e.g., removal of any implements used to pull or pick, such as tweezers). To reduce urges to pull, individuals with hair pulling or skin picking behaviors need to learn not to pursue positive reinforcement from pulling or picking. Habit reversal training, which principally involves learning to engage in an alternative action that is not compatible with pulling, is derived from this conceptualization. This approach is described in manual format by Grant, Donahue and Odlaug, and is one of the most effective and commonly used interventions [37].

Hoarding Disorder

After being considered a subtype of OCD for several decades [38], hoarding symptoms now comprise a unique disorder in DSM-5. This condition includes (a) persistent difficulty parting with possessions as a result of distress associated with discarding them and (b) a perceived need to save the items, regardless of the value of the possessions. Clinical hoarding behavior results in the accumulation of items that clutter living spaces and compromise the use of such areas, and can lead to emotional, social, financial and legal ramifications for both the individual and their family members. Research indicates important differences between hoarding and OCD symptoms [39]. More than 80% of individuals who demonstrate hoarding behaviors do not meet diagnostic criteria for OCD [40], and hoarding is more strongly related to other conditions (e.g., personality disorders) than to OCD [41].

Although some of the symptoms of hoarding disorder include recurring thoughts of acquiring and saving possessions, these thoughts are not generally experienced as intrusive or unwanted in the same way that obsessions are experienced in people with OCD [39,42]. Individuals with hoarding problems assign greater instrumental, sentimental and intrinsic value to possessions, feel greater responsibility and need to control possessions, and have deficits in information processing and memory that are not present in people with OCD [43]. Despite the inclusion of hoarding in the OCRDs category in DSM-5, hoarding behavior is present across a wide range of psychological conditions such as obsessive-compulsive personality disorder, schizophrenia and dementia [44]. Researchers have also proposed similarities between hoarding and impulse control disorders [45]. Saving or collecting behaviors in hoarding also do not belong to the same class of behavior as compulsive rituals in

OCD on a conceptual level, as hoarding behavior is not a response to obsessional fear in the same way that ritualized washing, checking or mental neutralizing serve to control anxiety about feared disastrous consequences.

Because there is no specific obsessional fear that serves as a trigger for hoarding behaviors in the way that obsessions provoke compulsive rituals in OCD (although patients with hoarding might report subjective anxiety in general), exposure-based therapy that facilitates the extinction of a conditioned fear response is not applicable to the treatment of hoarding. Indeed, research with OCD patients shows that when hoarding symptoms dominate the clinical picture, ERP outcomes are attenuated [39,46,47,48]. This provides further evidence that OCD and hoarding involve separate psychological mechanisms and demand distinct cognitive-behavioral treatments.

People with hoarding most likely respond poorly to ERP for several reasons. First, as mentioned above, there is no specific target for exposure – that is, there is no pathological fear or fear-induced ritualistic behavior. Second, individuals with hoarding often do not subjectively resist their urges to collect objects (i.e., these urges are ego-syntonic [45]). Instead, patients may consider their possessions to be an extension of themselves, to have human-like qualities and to provide comfort and security [43]. This is in stark contrast with obsessional thoughts and rituals, which are typically resisted in OCD and considered to be inconsistent with one's identity or true desires (i.e., ego-dystonic). Third, individuals with hoarding demonstrate excessive emotional attachment to possessions, and these distorted ideas about discarding similarly interfere with the success of exposure treatments [49]. Fourth, the associated information processing deficits that maintain hoarding behavior (e.g., poor categorization/organizational skills, deficits in decision making, difficulties with memory) are not addressed with ERP and instead require other types of interventions. Finally, relative to patients with OCD, those with primary hoarding symptoms tend to have higher rates of dependent and schizotypal personality disorder traits, which are likely to interfere with treatment [50].

Instead of using exposure, current cognitive behavioral treatment programs for hoarding [51] emphasize principles of motivational interviewing given that patients with this problem often have strong ambivalence about treatment and change. Treatment for hoarding also involves the development of attention, organization, decision making and problem solving skills. The process of helping the patient to organize and discard acquired materials is also conducted in a manner that is quite distinct from exposure. The sorting of possessions involves developing an understanding of *why* the patient saves possessions and is considered to be a process of discovery, in contrast to the emphasis on fear extinction in ERP. Behavioral experiments are sometimes used in the treatment for compulsive hoarding, which are perhaps similar to response prevention techniques in ERP. For example, patients are asked to visit locations in which acquisition is a particular problem to increase tolerance of urges to acquire possessions without giving into them. These exercises are more focused on learning to tolerate strong emotions (including, but not limited to anxiety) as opposed to modifying exaggerated estimates of threat.

Implications for Classification and Diagnosis

Parallels among the OCRDs can be observed at two levels. On one level, phenomena such as appearance concerns, hair pulling, skin picking and collecting can all be considered repetitive behaviors, not unlike obsessions and compulsive rituals in OCD. Yet, similarities at this *descriptive* level are not helpful in delineating OCRDs because many normal and pathological behaviors can be repetitive. Consider binging and purging, excessive smoking behavior, or even the repetitive casts of an avid fisherman. At a level of the *function* of these behaviors, however, we gain a more nuanced understanding of the purpose of these repetitive actions and can observe key differences among them. Indeed, understanding the function of repetitive behavior also reveals similarities and differences among the OCRDs. Whereas the repetitive behavior present in OCD and BDD is provoked by the perception of threat and is reinforced by a temporary reduction in fear, this mechanism is not present in hair pulling, skin picking and hoarding.

An important aspect of CBT is that it is derived from functional models of psychopathology (rather than etiological models) that have a sound empirical basis, as described above. The use of ERP for OCD and BDD, for example, is guided by a literature of experimental research demonstrating that these conditions are characterized by irrational (obsessional) fears that are maintained by avoidance, compulsive rituals and other neutralizing responses that temporarily reduce fear but impede long-term fear extinction [18,52]. ERP is therefore implemented as a fear extinction procedure intended to reduce maladaptive rituals that interfere with the extinction process.

There is a conceptually relevant (and thought-provoking) contrast to be made between the development of ERP for OCD and the development of medications – most notably, the serotonin reuptake inhibitors (SRIs) – in the treatment of OCRDs. Whereas ERP procedures were derived from empirically established psychological (cognitive and behavioral) models of obsessional fear and compulsive behavior, the SRIs were discovered serendipitously and only subsequently gave rise to (*post hoc ergo propter hoc*) etiological theories about the role of serotonin in OCD (and the OCRDs), which have turned out to lack empirical support [53]. Accordingly, whereas response to pharmacotherapy does not meaningfully inform the classification of OCRDs, ERP response has a better chance of identifying useful (i.e., treatment relevant) classes of psychological problems because it targets empirically established processes of psychopathology.

Whereas OCD and BDD respond preferentially to ERP [14,27], ERP is not appropriate for the treatment of other OCRDs such as hair pulling and skin picking that do not involve obsessional fears and are not maintained by avoidance and rituals. In other words, they are a conceptual mismatch with ERP. Instead, these problems are addressed using habit reversal, awareness training (identifying "high-risk" situations), developing a competing response until the urge to pull or pick passes (e.g., wearing gloves, holding an object), and stimulus control [54,55]. CBT for hoarding involves a mix of some strategies similar to habit reversal, and some cognitive therapy strategies to help patients modify exaggerated beliefs about their own possessions [41]. Again, exposure therapy is conceptually incongruent with the psychopathology of hoarding. Thus, we assert that OCD and BDD are phenomenologically similar – or to use the DSM-5 terminology, they are "related". On the other hand, hoarding, hair pulling and skin picking appear to be phenomenologically distinct from OCD and BDD.

Importantly, ERP is also a key component of CBT for a number of syndromes not included among the OCRDs. Individuals with social anxiety and specific phobias, for example, are instructed to systematically confront their feared stimuli (e.g., conversing with strangers and needles, respectively) while giving up safety behaviors such as avoidance, distraction, alcohol use [56]. Patients with panic disorder and agoraphobia are helped to confront feared internal states that cue panic attacks (e.g., dizziness, racing heart) via interoceptive exposure and feared situations (e.g., shopping malls) via in vivo exposure while simultaneously eliminating safety behaviors such as using benzodiazepine medication or resting to reduce a rapid heart rate [57]. Individuals with post-traumatic stress disorder are helped to confront unwanted intrusive memories of their traumatic experiences using imaginal exposure (reliving) while ceasing avoidance of situational reminders of the trauma [58].

As has been described elsewhere [4,59], OCD, BDD and anxiety disorders share fundamental psychological processes such as overestimation of threat, avoidance and safety behaviors. Functionally, these conditions are maintained by the same cognitive and behavioral processes that serve to maintain OCD. These conditions only appear to differ from each other at a descriptive level and in terms of the *content* or *focus* of the fear and the *form* of the safety behavior used to deal with the perceived threat. Accordingly, the CBT procedures described above for OCD, BDD and the anxiety disorders target this common essential underlying maintenance process: a self-perpetuating mechanism of dysfunctional catastrophic beliefs that produce anxiety and responses to anxiety that reinforce the erroneous beliefs. This fundamental maintenance process is no different in OCD and BDD than in the anxiety disorders. Accordingly, we suggest that OCD and BDD are best considered as members of the anxiety disorders diagnostic class.

Clinical Implications of Cross-Diagnostic Approaches for Treatment

A primary criticism of the current DSM diagnostic system is the artificial delineation of boundaries between "disorders" that do not actually exist in nature [60]. This limitation is exemplified by the OCRD classification in that (a) the boundary between OCD and BDD is irrelevant when it comes to choosing an effective treatment approach; (b) OCD and BDD overlap with the anxiety disorders in several key ways and (c) hair-pulling disorder, skin-picking disorder and hoarding are not mechanistically similar to OCD, BDD, or the anxiety disorders. Pity the poor practitioner who uses the DSM to guide decisions about treatment! Indeed, in our OCD clinic we receive numerous referrals for the treatment of "OCD" involving hoarding, skin picking and hair pulling rituals that are "resistant" to ERP. It appears that lumping these putative OCRDs in the same category as OCD has led to the erroneous assumption that all can be treated the same way.

Accordingly, we believe that optimal clinical management of OCRDs depends much more on an accurate understanding of the psychological (i.e., cognitive and behavioral) processes and mechanisms involved in the problem than it does on accurate diagnosis or classification. As we have discussed, DSM diagnosis and classification is largely descriptive and atheoretical, as well as based primarily on criteria involving lists of signs and symptoms. Yet ERP (for example) is not a treatment for OCD itself; rather, it includes a set of procedures to extinguish fear. Habit reversal training is not a treatment for hair-pulling or skin-picking disorders, but rather a set of techniques for helping individuals change their behavior in response to antecedents of such habits. Knowledge of psychological processes provides a guide for assessment that is necessary for effective treatment. A list of the situations and stimuli that trigger undesirable behaviors and emotions must be obtained, along with information about the function and consequences of repetitive behavior. In other words, it is necessary to understand *why* patients perform repetitive behaviors – not simply *that* they do.

Future Directions

The process described above of using what we know about experimentally established cognitive and behavioral principles to identify the antecedents and maintenance factors of undesirable emotions and behaviors is called *functional analysis* [61]. Functional analysis is a tool that conceptually transcends DSM because it provides a patient specific roadmap of the problem that leads to the choice of procedures for implementing a solution. Thus, as we look to the future, the difficulties with the OCRD classification suggest that it would be useful to move away from the idea of *treatments* or *therapies* for DSM *disorders*, and instead conceptualize psychological interventions as empirically supported *procedures* that are effective for reducing particular (functionally defined) sorts of psychological signs and symptoms (e.g., irrational fear, positively reinforced behavior, negatively reinforced behavior, etc.). Although the DSM might provide some initial guidance for how to classify and choose a treatment for individuals with mental and behavioral health problems, no diagnostic manual can sufficiently address the innumerable complexities with which patients present. Training for mental health professionals should therefore emphasize the use of functional assessment rather than rely on DSM classifications to guide diagnostic decisions and treatment planning.

References

1. American Psychiatric Association. *Diagnostic and Statistical Manual of Mental Disorders,* 5th ed. Washington, DC: APA; 2013.
2. American Psychiatric Association. *Diagnostic and Statistical Manual of Mental Disorders,* 3rd ed. Washington, DC: APA; 1980.
3. Fineberg NA, Saxena S, Zohar J, Craig KJ. Obsessive-compulsive disorder: boundary issues. In: Hollander E, Zohar J, Sirovatka PJ, Regier DA, eds. *Obsessive-Compulsive Spectrum Disorders: Refining the Research Agenda for DSM-V* . Washington, DC: American Psychiatric Association; 2011:1–32.
4. Abramowitz JS, Jacoby RJ. Obsessive-compulsive and related disorders: a critical review of the new diagnostic class. *Annu Rev Clin Psychol.* 2015;11:165–186.
5. Hollander E, Friedberg JP, Wasserman S, Yeh C-C, Iyengar R. The case for the OCD spectrum. In: Abramowitz JS, Houts AC, eds. *Concepts and Controversies in Obsessive-Compulsive Disorder.* New York, NY: Springer; 2005:95–118.
6. Salkovskis PM. Understanding and treating obsessive–compulsive disorder. *Behav Res Ther.* 1999;37(Suppl 1):S29–S52.
7. Rachman SJ. A cognitive theory of compulsive checking. *Behav Res Ther.* 2002;40:624–639.
8. Meyer V. Modification of expectations in cases with obsessional rituals. *Behav Res Ther.* 1966;4:273–280.
9. Meyer V, Levy R, Schnurer A. The behavioral treatment of obsessive-compulsive disorders. In: Beech HR, ed. *Obsessional States.* London: Methuen; 1974:233–258.
10. Craske MG, Kircanski K, Zelikowsky M, Mystkowski J, Chowdhury N, Baker A. Optimizing inhibitory learning during exposure therapy. *Behav Res Ther.* 2008;46:5–27.
11. Bouton ME. Context, ambiguity, and unlearning: sources of relapse after behavioral extinction. *Biol Psychiatry.* 2002;52:976–986.

12. Olatunji BO, Davis ML, Powers MB, Smits JAJ. Cognitive-behavioral therapy for obsessive-compulsive disorder: a meta-analysis of treatment outcome and moderators. *J Psychiatr Res.* 2013;47:33–41.
13. Franklin ME, Abramowitz JS, Kozak MJ, Levitt JT, Foa EB. Effectiveness of exposure and ritual prevention for obsessive-compulsive disorder: randomized compared with nonrandomized samples. *J Consult Clin Psychol.* 2000;68:594–602.
14. Romanelli RJ, Wu FM, Gamba R, Mojtabai R, Segal JB. Behavioral therapy and serotonin reuptake inhibitor pharmacotherapy in the treatment of obsessive–compulsive disorder: a systematic review and meta-analysis of head-to-head randomized controlled trials. *Depress Anxiety.* 2014; 31(8):641–52.
15. Koran LM, Hanna GL, Hollander E, Nestadt G, Simpson HB, American Psychiatric Association. Practice guideline for the treatment of patients with obsessive-compulsive disorder. *Am J Psychiatry.* 2007;164(7 Suppl):5–53.
16. National Institute for Health and Care Excellence. *Obsessive-Compulsive Disorder: Core Interventions in the Treatment of Obsessive-Compulsive Disorder and Body Dysmorphic Disorder.* Clinical Guideline CG31. London: NICE; 2005.
17. Phillips KA, Wilhelm S, Koran LM, et al. Body dysmorphic disorder: some key issues for DSM-V. *Depress Anxiety.* 2010;27:573–591.
18. Veale D, Riley S. Mirror, mirror on the wall, who is the ugliest of them all? The psychopathology of mirror gazing in body dysmorphic disorder. *Behav Res Ther.* 2001;39:1381–1393.
19. Windheim K, Veale D, Anson M. Mirror gazing in body dysmorphic disorder and healthy controls: effects of duration of gazing. *Behav Res Ther.* 2011;49:555–564.
20. Neziroglu F, Roberts M, Yaryura-Tobias JA. A behavioral model for body dysmorphic disorder. *Psychiatr Ann.* 2004;34:915–920.
21. Mowrer OH. On the dual nature of learning – a re-interpretation of "conditioning" and "problem-solving." *Harv Educ Rev.* 1947;17:102–148.
22. Neziroglu F, Khemlani-Patel S, Jacofsky M. Body dysmorphic disorder: symptoms, models and treatment interventions. In: Simos G, ed. *Cognitive Behaviour Therapy: A Guide for the Practising Clinician.* New York: Routledge; 2009:243–260.
23. Veale D. Advances in a cognitive behavioural model of body dysmorphic disorder. *Body Image.* 2004;1:113–125.
24. Neziroglu F, Khemlani-Patel S. Therapeutic approaches to body dysmorphic disorder. *Brief Treat Crisis Interv.* 2003 1;3:307.
25. Cororve MB, Gleaves DH. Body dysmorphic disorder: a review of conceptualizations, assessment, and treatment strategies. *Clin Psychol Rev.* 2001;21:949–970.
26. Wilhelm S, Phillips KA, Didie E, et al. Modular cognitive-behavioral therapy for body dysmorphic disorder: a randomized controlled trial. *Behav Ther.* 2014;45:314–327.
27. Williams J, Hadjistavropoulos T, Sharpe D. A meta-analysis of psychological and pharmacological treatments for body dysmorphic disorder. *Behav Res Ther.* 2006;44:99–111.
28. Christenson GA, Ristvedt SL, Mackenzie TB. Identification of trichotillomania cue profiles. *Behav Res Ther.* 1993;31:315–320.
29. Stanley MA, Swann AC, Bowers TC, Davis ML, Taylor DJ. A comparison of clinical features in trichotillomania and obsessive-compulsive disorder. *Behav Res Ther.* 1992;30:39–44.
30. Flessner CA, Conelea CA, Woods DW, Franklin ME, Keuthen NJ, Cashin SE. Styles of pulling in trichotillomania: exploring differences in symptom severity, phenomenology, and functional impact. *Behav Res Ther.* 2008;46:345–357.
31. Arnold LM, Auchenbach MB, McElroy SL. Psychogenic excoriation: clinical features, proposed diagnostic criteria, epidemiology and approaches to treatment. *CNS Drugs.* 2001;15:351–359.
32. Neziroglu F, Rabinowitz D, Breytman A, Jacofsky M. Skin picking phenomenology and severity comparison. *Prim Care Companion J Clin Psychiatry.* 2008;10:306–312.
33. Snorrason I, Smári J, Olafsson RP. Emotion regulation in pathological skin picking: findings from a non-treatment seeking sample. *J Behav Ther Exp Psychiatry.* 2010;41:238–245.
34. Keuthen NJ, Deckersbach T, Wilhelm S, et al. Repetitive skin-picking in a student population and comparison with a sample of self-injurious skin-pickers. *Psychosomatics.* 2000;41:210–215.
35. Lochner C, Simeon D, Niehaus DJH, Stein DJ. Trichotillomania and skin-picking: a phenomenological comparison. *Depress Anxiety.* 2002;15:83–86.
36. Elliott AJ, Fuqua RW. Trichotillomania: conceptualization, measurement, and treatment. *Behav Ther.* 2000;31:529–545.
37. Flessner CA, Penzel F, Trichotillomania Learning Center–Scientific Advisory Board; Keuthen NJ. Current treatment practices for children and adults with trichotillomania: consensus among experts. *Cogn Behav Pr.* 2010;17:290–300.

38. Coles ME, Frost RO, Heimberg RG, Steketee GS. Hoarding behaviors in a large college sample. *Behav Res Ther*. 2003;41:179–194.
39. Wheaton MG, Abramowitz JS, Fabricant LE, Berman NC, Franklin JC. Is hoarding a symptom of obsessive-compulsive disorder? *Int J Cogn Ther*. 2011;4:225–238.
40. Mataix-Cols D, Frost RO, Pertusa A, et al. Hoarding disorder: a new diagnosis for DSM-V? *Depress Anxiety*. 2010;27:556–572.
41. Frost RO, Tolin DF. Compulsive hoarding. In: Abramowitz JS, McKay D, Taylor S, eds. *Clinical Handbook of Obsessive-Compulsive Disorder and Related Problems*. Baltimore, MD: Johns Hopkins University Press; 2008:76–94.
42. Rachman SJ, Elliott CM, Shafran R, Radomsky AS. Separating hoarding from OCD. *Behav Res Ther*. 2009;47:520–522.
43. Frost RO, Hartl TL. A cognitive-behavioral model of compulsive hoarding. *Behav Res Ther*. 1996;34:341–350.
44. Fontenelle LF, Mendlowicz MV, Soares ID, Versiani M. Patients with obsessive-compulsive disorder and hoarding symptoms: a distinctive clinical subtype? *Compr Psychiatry*. 2004;45:375–383.
45. Steketee G, Frost R. Compulsive hoarding: current status of the research. *Clin Psychol Rev*. 2003;23:905–927.
46. Abramowitz JS, Franklin ME, Schwartz SA, Furr JM. Symptom presentation and outcome of cognitive-behavioral therapy for obsessive-compulsive disorder. *J Consult Clin Psychol*. 2003;71:1049–1057.
47. Abramowitz JS, Wheaton MG, Storch EA. The status of hoarding as a symptom of obsessive-compulsive disorder. *Behav Res Ther*. 2008;46:1026–1033.
48. McKay D, Abramowitz JS, Calamari JE, et al. A critical evaluation of obsessive-compulsive disorder subtypes: symptoms versus mechanisms. *Clin Psychol Rev*. 2004;24:283–313.
49. Kozak MJ, Foa EB. *Mastery of Obsessive-Compulsive Disorder: A Cognitive-Behavioral Approach Therapist Guide*. New York, NY: Oxford University Press; 1997.
50. Frost RO, Steketee G, Williams LF, Warren R. Mood, personality disorder symptoms and disability in obsessive compulsive hoarders: a comparison with clinical and nonclinical controls. *Behav Res Ther*. 2000 1;38:1071–1081.
51. Steketee G, Frost RO. *Compulsive Hoarding and Acquiring*. Oxford University Press; 2006.
52. Rachman SJ, Hodgson RJ. *Obsessions and Compulsions*. Englewood Cliffs, NJ: Prentice-Hall; 1980.
53. Whitaker R. *Anatomy of an Epidemic: Magic Bullets, Psychiatric Drugs, and the Astonishing Rise of Mental Illness in America*. New York, NY: Broadway Books; 2011.
54. Azrin NH, Nunn RG. Habit-reversal: a method of eliminating nervous habits and tics. *Behav Res Ther*. 1973;11:619–628.
55. Odlaug BL, Grant JE. Pathological skin picking. In: Grant JE, Stein DJ, Woods DW, Keuthen NJ, eds. *Trichotillomania, Skin Picking, and Other Body-Focused Repetitive Behaviors*. Washington, DC: APA; 2012:21–41.
56. Barlow DH. *Clinical Handbook of Psychological Disorders: A Step-by-Step Treatment Manual*, 5th ed. New York, NY: Guilford Press; 2007.
57. Otto MW, Jones JC, Barlow DH, Craske MG. *Stopping Anxiety Medication: Panic Control Therapy for Benzodiazepine Discontinuation, Therapist Guide*. Oxford University Press; 2004.
58. Foa EB, Rothbaum BO. *Treating the Trauma of Rape: Cognitive-Behavioral Therapy for PTSD*. New York, NY: Guilford Press; 2001.
59. Abramowitz JS, Deacon BJ. Reply to Hollander et al. the OC spectrum: a closer look at the arguments and the data. In: Abramowitz JS, Houts AC, eds. *Concepts and Controversies in Obsessive-Compulsive Disorder*. New York, NY: Springer; 2005:141–149.
60. Deacon BJ. The biomedical model of mental disorder: a critical analysis of its validity, utility, and effects on psychotherapy research. *Clin Psychol Rev*. 2013;33:846–861.
61. Wolpe J. *The Practice of Behavior Therapy*, 2nd ed. Oxford: Pergamon; 1973.

Chapter 17

Innovative Cognitive Behavioral Treatments for Obsessive-Compulsive Disorder

Kieron P. O'Connor, Catherine Ouellet-Courtois and Frederick Aardema

Introduction

There is a consensus that current cognitive models of obsessive-compulsive disorder (OCD) do not contribute substantially to the debate on improving treatment methods, particularly for those who do not respond to exposure and response prevention (ERP) [1]. Although there is evidence for the clinical effectiveness of cognitive behavioral interventions [2], there is a sizable percentage of patients (40%) who do not improve significantly [3,4]. Furthermore, ERP is associated with high levels of treatment refusal and dropout rates of 25% because people are unwilling or unable to undergo exposure [5]. Clearly, there is a strong need to improve therapy options.

Apart from current cognitive models not contributing substantially to outcome, cognitive therapy for OCD alone is not widely used in the context of clinical practice [1]. The main treatment component of choice in cognitive behavioral therapy (CBT) remains ERP. Cognitive restructuring has been added over the years, which tends to focus on the pre-existing beliefs a person may hold which sensitize them to react adversely to intrusive thoughts [6]. However, there is speculation that cognitive therapy may be counterproductive as it encourages rationalization or intellectualization of obsessions, thereby producing a reduction in anxiety, and allegedly interfering with effective exposure [7].

Cognitive aspects are increasingly viewed as second-order factors and reframed in behavioral terms (e.g., expectancy violation as part of inhibition learning) [8], integrated into neurogenetic explanations [9], or returned to Skinnerian notions of cognitions as epiphenomena of compulsions. For example, Anholt [10] suggests reframing OCD as a compulsive-obsessional disorder to better reflect the primary causal chain. Considering that there is a core thinking component in OCD, the minimization of the role of cognitive factors in OCD is unwarranted, and calls for the need of a complete reconceptualization of cognitive processes contributing to OCD.

Recent Research Findings

The Inference-Based Approach

The inference-based approach (IBA) offers an alternative cognitive account of obsessions and focuses on the reasoning that produces the initial obsessional doubt (e.g., maybe I am contaminated). In this IBA model, obsessions begin at the point where the person crosses over from reality into the initial obsessional doubt (Figure 17.1). The IBA model is different from the cognitive appraisal model [11], which proposes that unwanted intrusive thoughts are an unproblematic universal experience, but that if they are appraised negatively with undue importance (e.g. "Having this thought means I'm a bad person"), the person will become preoccupied and will try to suppress the thought, thereby maintaining the preoccupation about the thought and creating obsessions. Rather, IBA considers the initial intrusion as an inference that is an intrinsic part of the obsession. Rather than viewing the content of all intrusions as unproblematic, IBA conceptualizes "intrusions" as inferences or propositions that are formed and reinforced through faulty inductive reasoning processes [12]. Although IBA was originally formulated in the context of OCD, it offers a transdiagnostic conceptualization of the obsessional doubt, thus extending its applicability to a range of obsessional disorders such as body dysmorphic, eating and hoarding disorders. Moreover, in light of the credence given to imaginary processes in IBA, the model also well applies to delusional disorders.

Obsessive-Compulsive Disorder as a Phobic Disorder

Both current cognitive and behavioral models adopt a phobic model of OCD and provide experimental

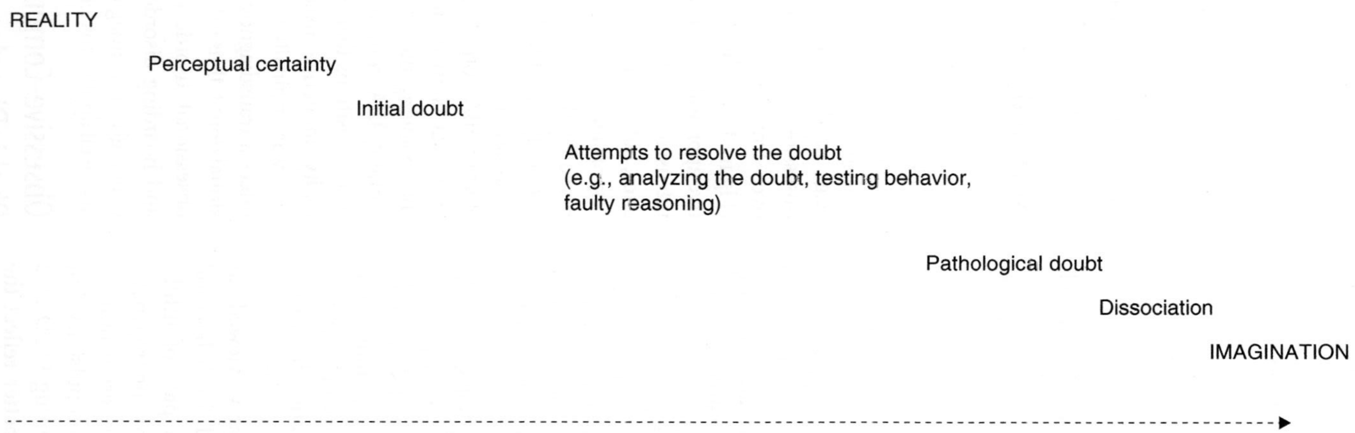

Figure 17.1 Doubting sequence.

support for behavioral techniques that are largely drawn from the experimental literature of phobia. The link made between phobias and OCD is sensible, given that the phobic model inspired Vic Meyer's first application of exposure to OCD [13]. However, a careful rereading of Meyer's seminal work reveals him to be critical of a simple application of a phobic model [13]. As his title and conclusions suggest, Meyer considered his approach rather centered on cognitive processes of expectancy and reality testing that are essential to fear reduction.

Phobias of spiders, open or closed spaces, insects, or blood are very efficiently treated by behavior therapy through exposing and reframing perceptual avoidance of the feared object. However, in these phobias, the person fears the attributes of the feared object. For instance, in the absence of a spider, there is no fear. The person may of course exaggerate the threat or may become anxious anticipating a spider and avoid places associated with spiders, and may even fear places where the object could be in the future (looming vulnerability) [14]. However, the fear is tied directly to the physical presence of the feared object and graded exposure exercises lead up to the handling of actual, real spiders.

On the other hand, in OCD, this fear sequence is reversed: obsessions only seem to occur when the feared object is not there. In other words, it is the possibility of an event or a state of affairs which elicits the fear, whereas the event or state of affairs as it occurs is frequently less anxiogenic. A woman cannot touch a red poster or a vampire Halloween mask because it could involve the presence of infected blood. However, when her son hurts his knee or has a nosebleed, she copes normally with actual blood: she is not blood phobic.

Another related fact is that, in OCD, the object of fear is selective. For example, a person who is afraid of the possibility of being exposed to one type of disease may not be afraid of another equally contagious disease. Similarly, a person unable to touch door handles for fear of contamination by germs will breathe in germs in the air without precaution. For whatever the object or event the person with OCD claims to fear, there will be a context where they will not fear this category of object. For example, some dirt (e.g., bus pole) may be feared, but other dirt of a slightly different nature or origin (e.g., dust) will not be feared. This selectivity is not the product of mere ignorance, as a client can be fully aware of other forms of toxicity or contamination in the environment, and yet remain indifferent (although aware of the contradiction). In a phobic model, the unlikely equivalent would be a person reporting a phobia of tarantulas, but not of black widow spiders. Furthermore, we can point to the existence of mental or symbolic contamination in OCD where the person fears ideas as well as magical and moral influences [15]. Accordingly, the feared object in OCD is not often prone to the behavioral exercises used in the context of phobias. In fact, most of the obsessional content in OCD is impossible to tackle and reproduce for the purpose of exposure. For instance, think of a man with homosexuality obsessions, who doubts about his own sexuality and fears the possibility of being attracted to men, although not being homophobic.[1] Exposing the man to homosexual pornography or to the actual presence of other men would not actually tackle the obsession, as the possibility would remain that he might not truly be heterosexual.

The experimental support for exposure is drawn largely from conditioning theory. Conditioning is one type of learning where pairing transforms an innately emotion-laden value to a neutral one. Recent developments in fear extinction theory emphasize the role of inhibitory learning [8]. ERP works in OCD by addressing the feared consequences of the obsession, which is purported to encourage individuals to rethink their obsessions. ERP does not usually eliminate the obsession but aims rather to make it more tolerable and to replace the anxiety response by new learning. However, redundant responses and irrelevant associations do play a part in OCD, and such associations do not need to be traced to classical conditioning, or to a change from a neutral signal to a feared one.

Some cases of OCD can be acquired through incidental learning. A person may hear on the radio that the number 5 is unlucky and thereafter avoidance of 5 becomes enshrined as a compulsive rule. Take the case of a patient who dislikes people or situations because symbolically she associates them with the number 5. Thereafter anything containing a number 5 is avoided for fear of remembering the event and contaminating the current activity. This may appear as a clear case of conditioned association; yet the

[1] In our experience, the vast majority of individuals with homosexual obsessions are not homophobic.

question remains as to why she associates people with numbers and not with some other neutral aspect of these situations. We could invoke second-order conditioning and say she has learned earlier to associate certain numbers with security and insecurity, but each number is fine tuned to a particular experience, and sometimes simply rethinking her belief and redefining her experience may change the number. This change can be affected casually without the need for elaborate exposure. In fact, she acquired the association with numbers through a chance conversation with a friend about numerology.

The emphasis on exposure as a core technique in CBT, as well as the deemed importance of elevated anxiety at the start of exposure to ensure a satisfactory reduction after exposure, assume that anxiety or fear activation is the principal mechanism at the origin of the obsession, rather than anxiety being a result of the individual's obsessional belief.

To use an analog example, if I mistakenly believe a relative is on board an aircraft that crashed, being informed that my belief is incorrect would justifiably alleviate my anxiety, and would do so more efficiently than repeated exposure to news of a plane crash. Few people would argue that correcting the belief is detrimental to subsequent anxiety reduction through exposure. If anxiety is a consequence of a belief, it is sensible to directly restructure the belief to alleviate the anxiety. This is distinct from the case where I become anxious simply at the thought of flying, where exposure may be warranted.

Current cognitive models also assume that OCD is essentially an anxiety disorder. The current cognitive model [16] is derived from Beck's two-stage model initially applied to depression [17] and later panic disorder [18], where cognitive factors are purported to influence the interpretation of thoughts or sensations. The model claims that intrusions are normal universal experiences, and that it is appraisals operationalized as a number of belief domains that convert normal intrusions into anxiogenic obsessions. This appraisal-based model of OCD led to the development of the Obsessive Compulsive Cognitions Working Group [11,19], which identified six OCD-relevant beliefs involved in the appraisal of intrusive cognitions, including inflated responsibility, the overestimation of threat, the over-importance given to thoughts, the importance of controlling one's thoughts, perfectionism, and intolerance of uncertainty.

The appraisal model includes many astute clinical observations, in particular the undue importance given to thoughts in increasing distress, which can certainly explain the vicious cycle that reinforces maintenance of thoughts, not just in OCD, but also in anxious and normal controls. However, a large proportion of individuals with OCD do not score high on obsessive beliefs as identified by the Obsessive Compulsive Cognitions Working Group [20,21,22]. Findings are also very mixed in terms of the role of obsessive beliefs in OCD in comparison with other clinical groups. Some studies have found significant differences in some belief domains, while others have not [23,24,25]. How can one explain these mixed findings?

The appraisal model claims that all obsessions pass through a kind of caterpillar phase where they are normal intrusions, universally experienced, before blooming into full-blown obsessions. However, although the content of intrusions may be sometimes universal, other parameters sustain emotional investment, and the vividness, context, and imaging of obsessions are distinct from normal obsessions. The two-stage appraisal model can be readily applied to depression where depressive beliefs clearly form an observable part of the problem. Indeed, depressive self-reports, such as "everything is hopeless"; "I see it all black"; "I always see the negative side", are typical narratives in depression [26]. However, it would be extremely atypical for a patient with OCD to spontaneously report: "I'm over responsible"; "I treat my thoughts too seriously"; "I'm intolerant of uncertainty", at least prior to cognitive therapy. More typically, the spontaneous self-reports concern wanting to get rid of the obsessions and of the fears that it will get worse. People with OCD may complain about being too perfectionist or not being able to control their thoughts, as a way of explaining their symptoms ("I check because I'm a perfectionist"; "my problem is not being able to control my thoughts"). While negative judgment and hopelessness are characteristic of depression; perfectionism, lack of controllability, and intolerance of uncertainty are found in many disorders (even to some extent in healthy individuals), and not specifically in OCD. Although it could be argued that these are transdiagnostic thinking styles, they fail to properly capture the phenomenology of OCD. As noted, metacognitions can be relevant to maintaining a disorder without explaining its etiology, and without being representative of its core phenomenology.

Reasoning in Obsessive-Compulsive Disorder

Looking more closely at the phenomenology of OCD, Bucarelli and Purdon [27,28] conducted a series of informative studies in an attempt to relate experimental findings to everyday experiences of distress and related cognitive events, such as sensory and cognitive doubt, and compulsion termination criteria. Patients with OCD kept a repeated actions diary for three consecutive days. The results indicated that repetitions of action and uncertainty were related to higher sensory and cognitive doubt. The authors suggested that once a compulsion is initiated, contextual factors may be more important in its persistence than triggering factors, and that the compulsion is not a series of repetitive actions, but rather a sequence that builds up over time. Notably, the authors also noted that participants with OCD were certain that the stove was off before they left, but that doubt struck once they left the kitchen. The authors suggested that it would be interesting to examine the reasoning processes leading to the doubt. If obsessions do not stem from normal intrusions, and people with OCD can have both normal intrusions and obsessions, where do obsessions come from?

One possibility is that obsessions are the product of faulty thinking and biases. There is certainly some evidence of information processing deficits or biases in OCD, but the evidence is inconsistent and it is not clear how such biases would account for the heterogeneity found in OCD [29]. An alternative hypothesis is that intrusions are a product of reasoning processes. Reasoning is a transparent process involving a sequence of steps resulting in an inference about a state of affairs. One arrives at a conclusion through a coherent chaining of ideas that both makes sense to the person and justifies their conclusion. The reasoning may appear logical or experiential, as reasoning is a real-time process, with a progression of arguments toward conclusions that are context dependent. One can reason differently in different situations because the reasoning steps rely on context in the here and now, and depend on the available sources of reasoning heuristics. Notably, the selective contextual aspect in reasoning fits well with OCD reasoning. Reasoning may offer an alternative, more readily observable device for studying cognitive processes than other information processing models. It is contextual, idiosyncratic, and transparent in revealing all stages in its evolution; allowing any stage to be targeted later in therapy. So can reasoning processes account for obsessions?

Reasoning Confusion

One consistent finding in the literature is a degree of reasoning confusion in OCD. This confusion manifests itself principally in confusion between a subjective, imagined possibility, and real probability. This reasoning principally involves inductive errors, but has several components. First, there are straightforward errors of reasoning. These are simply devices that misguide the person to conclusions. Keen, Brown and Wheatley [30], based on the work of Kahneman and Tversky [31], have identified a propensity to simulation heuristics, such that the individual is more likely to simulate and imagine negative possibilities, thereby influencing one's estimation of probability. Second, there is now considerable evidence that people with OCD, when presented with various options, invest in alternative possibilities at the expense of grounding themselves in an initial sensible conclusion. Particular sources of possibilities seem more influential, for example, when given externally or when contradicting initial conclusions. This could indicate suggestibility, but interestingly people with OCD are not so influenced by supporting alternatives [32].

Secondly, the investment could be due to an extensive imagination, and there is some evidence that individuals with OCD have greater imagery and immersion ability. In fact, many studies indicate that individuals with OCD show a reasoning style known as *inferential confusion*, whereby they confuse an imagined possibility (e.g., maybe the door is unlocked) with an actual, reality-based probability (e.g., I checked the door several times, therefore it should be locked). A key result of the research on inferential confusion is its association with dissociative absorption, which manifests itself mostly as derealization in a bubble [33], or, when more severe, as immersion in an alternative world, including confabulation and hallucinations [34]. This is one parameter that, as noted earlier, distinguishes obsessions from normal intrusions. In the case of normal intrusions, the individual remains grounded in reality and is fully aware of the absurdity of the intrusion, whereas in obsessional intrusions, the individual has crossed the bridge from reality to the imagination, and therefore buys into the obsession as if it was revealing a true state of affairs. Third, investment in alternative imaginary possibilities could be due to a distrust of the senses (e.g., I don't trust what I see and hear as I lock the door), or a general lack of confidence in both faculties and senses. Lack of *cognitive confidence* is a term that has been repeatedly employed in the research literature and that is closely intertwined with distrust of the senses, as it reflects a lack of confidence in one's attention, perception and memory.

Cognitive Confidence and Distrust of the Senses

The lack of strong empirical support for impaired memory processes in OCD [35], yet with the presence of repetitive checking or ritualistic behaviors that remained unexplained, led to the postulation that individuals with OCD may not have poor memory per se, but may have poor *confidence* in their memory. In support of this postulation, one study demonstrated that although individuals with OCD performed as well as non-anxious controls in a task that entailed recalling performed actions, they were more likely to report less confidence in their memory for these events, a phenomenon that was referred to as poor cognitive confidence [36]. The data from this study suggested that individuals with OCD's lower cognitive confidence extended beyond the realm of memory and was present on three specific levels, as these individuals displayed less confidence in: (i) their memory for actions; (ii) their ability to differentiate between actions and their imagination; and (iii) their attentional abilities. Later work from this research group has suggested that OCD may in fact entail lower confidence in attention and perception, in addition to lower confidence in memory [37]. As a result, the construct of cognitive confidence is now considered to be more comprehensive as it not only relates to confidence in memory, but also to confidence in other cognitive domains, such as attention and perception.

Research on cognitive confidence has employed different measures to assess the construct. Questionnaire-based studies on cognitive confidence have employed cross-sectional designs, comparing individuals with OCD with clinical and non-clinical control groups. This line of research demonstrates that, compared with non-clinical healthy controls, OCD individuals show lower cognitive confidence. On the other hand, when compared with individuals with other mental health disorders, such as schizophrenia [38,39], generalized anxiety disorder [40,41], or depression [40], the scores of individuals with OCD do not significantly differ, suggesting that low cognitive confidence is not specific to OCD. However, it is important to consider that these self-report questionnaires usually measure cognitive confidence as a trait that spreads across life events (e.g., confidence in one's general memory), rather than specific situations (e.g., memory for having locked the door).

Experimental studies have attempted to measure low cognitive confidence in a way that is more ecologically-valid and that taps into OCD-specific situations. For instance, van den Hout and colleagues [42] have employed a task with a virtual gas stove. After performing virtual checks, participants had to rate their memory regarding the task, as well as their confidence in their performance. It was found that the more participants checked, the less vivid and detailed were their recollections, and the more their memory confidence decreased. The same pattern of results was replicated by Radomsky, Gilchrist and Dussault [43], using a task involving a real stove in a laboratory kitchen. However, research has also demonstrated that repeated checking increases doubt (i.e., lowers cognitive confidence) in both individuals with OCD and non-clinical healthy controls [44], as well as in both high and low checkers [45,46]. Therefore, the finding that repeated checking lowers cognitive confidence seems to point to a normal process that is not OCD specific. The remaining question is thus what makes individuals with OCD doubt and check in the first place.

Findings from both questionnaire-based and experimental studies, taken together, suggest that individuals with OCD demonstrate low cognitive confidence, and that this distrust in their cognitive abilities seems to be OCD themed (e.g. I don't trust my memory for locking the door). These findings underline, as touched upon earlier, that OCD is selective and that dysfunctional cognitive processes only reveal themselves under specific circumstances that tap into the individual's obsession. It is therefore possible that much of the literature on cognitive confidence may rather be measuring the construct of distrust of the senses, as postulated in the IBA model. This concept seems more relevant to OCD as people do not initially lack confidence in their senses but only later doubt or distrust them. So how can reasoning lead to distrust of the senses?

Inductive reasoning can lead the person astray on the basis of experience and personal stories and heuristics rather than logic. Inductive reasoning involves past experience and drawing beyond the information that is out there to arrive at a reasoned conclusion. There are a number of ways one can be led astray. First, the information may be irrelevant or redundant, which can occur through mis-associations, heuristics, and faulty arguments. If one looks at how people with OCD justify their obsessions, generally they produce reasons that reflect all of the above. Furthermore, OCD thinking is chained thinking, such that it is generally dynamic and evolves exactly by chaining one perseverative thought to another [47].

The IBA model posits that the inductive reasoning in OCD includes various reasoning devices, such as inverse inference and attributing a real probability to subjective or hypothetical possibilities. Heuristic devices include misplaced representativeness, miss-associations, drawing on out-of-context facts, rhetorical devices, mislabeling experiences and immersion in a spiraling story. Clearly, a simple reality check would expose this inductive narrative as flawed and inaccurate. However, the power of the narrative lies in its ability to always question reality and perception, thus reinforcing the obsessional doubt. We noted earlier Bucarelli and Purdon's [28] observation that during the checking ritual, individuals with OCD are certain of what they are doing, but only once in a different context do they doubt their action. Distrust of the senses and investment in imaginary possibilities work in tandem to convince the individual to doubt reality and to rather give credence to the obsessional belief.

In light of the thought chaining or perseverative thinking [47] in OCD, we can consider the OCD reasoning chain as a narrative. The concept of the narrative is very helpful clinically, because it taps into several aspects relevant to OCD, namely immersion, absorption, and dissociation. Sarbin [48] noted that our beliefs are just stories we tell ourselves. A story has a power that simple, discrete words do not have – a story can capture a lived quality of the obsessional experience, making it more convincing and absorbing [49].

Inferential Confusion

Many of the aforementioned concepts come together in inferential confusion, which posits that its two components (i) distrust of the senses, combined with (ii) an overinvestment in imaginary possibilities, lead to obsessional doubt in OCD. These two processes operate in tandem and both seem necessary to induce doubt. It is still unclear whether one has priority, as both are closely intertwined. Distrust of the senses in OCD has been researched and empirically validated, although different terms have been employed to refer to the construct in the research literature. As noted earlier, poor cognitive confidence is a construct highly similar to distrust of the senses in inferential confusion, as the individual has difficulties trusting their memory for their actions – such as compulsions – and doubts whether they perceived or attended to a real action (and if they did, did they *correctly* perceive what there was to see?) or whether they only imagined it. However, it is important to note that the two constructs differ conceptually. While distrust of the senses pertains more to a state construct (e.g., "I don't trust what I see as I turn off the stove"), low cognitive confidence refers more to trait construct (e.g., "I am usually distracted, so I am not confident in my ability to pay attention when I turn off the stove"). Moreover, although distrust of the senses also involves suspicions toward oneself ("I don't trust my cognitive capacities"), it is more directed toward the outside world ("I don't trust the information my senses are telling me"; "I don't trust what is there before my eyes"). Individuals with OCD who distrust their senses believe that they cannot rely on their perception to judge whether their hands are covered with germs or not ("my hands look clean but there might be germs I can't see"), and invest into imaginary possibilities ("my hands may be covered with germs and I will contaminate myself and others") at the expense of trusting the information that is there before their eyes.

However, this fairly straightforward process of inferential confusion contains several components and can account for the phenomenology of OCD. Distrust of the senses and of cognitive faculties may involve overall a lack of confidence in the ability to detect memory or events, as noted earlier. Further, inferential confusion may be motivated by a desire to go beyond the senses to a deeper level of meaning and reality, as if one's senses was not providing enough information about the true state of affairs. There may

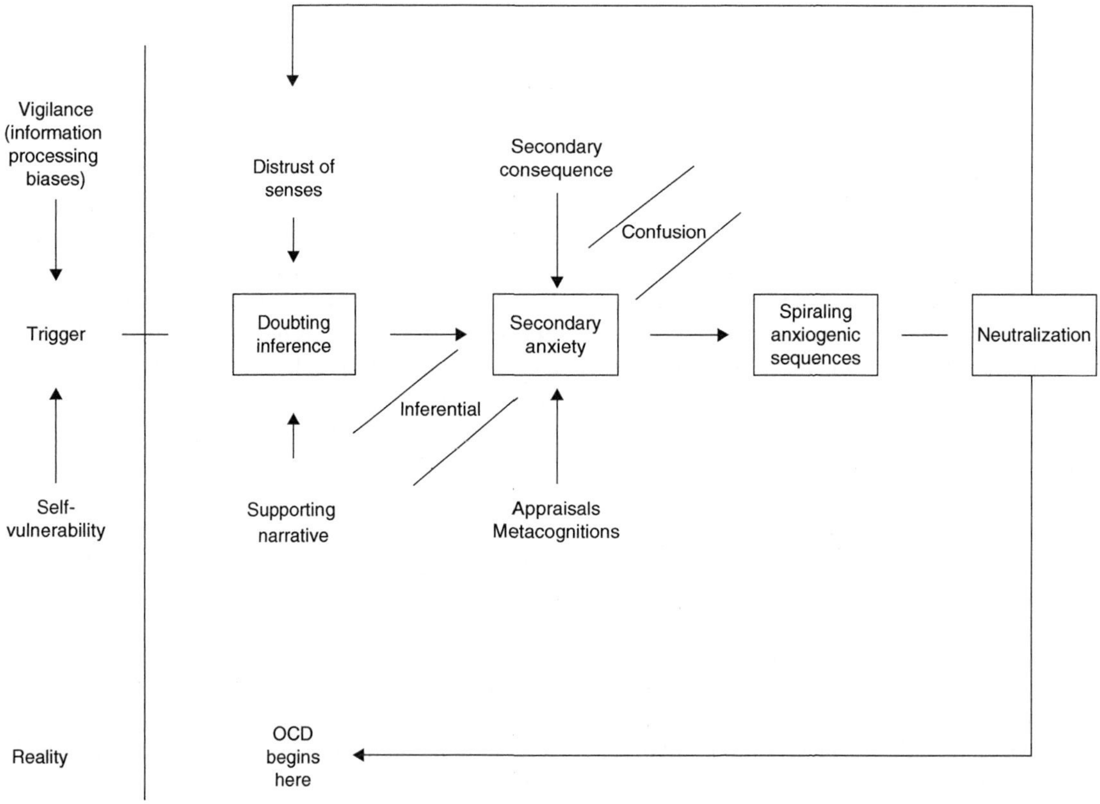

Figure 17.2 The inference-based approach sequence of obsessional thinking.

even be an element of paranoia in inferential confusion thinking (i.e., believing that things are not as they appear to be).

Clinical Validity of the Inference-Based Approach Model

Treatment outcome studies where inferential confusion is explicitly targeted have shown significant improvement in OCD symptoms, including an increased ability of treatment responders to resolve obsessional doubt [50,51,52]. Moreover, there is emerging evidence that treatment following the principles of IBA is able to overcome the treatment resistance of those with overvalued ideation, which refers to a greater investment and certainty in the obsession. Confirming earlier findings, a 2015 independent, multicenter, randomized controlled trial indicated significantly greater improvement in individuals with high levels of overvalued ideation who undertook IBA, with an effect size of 2.24 [53]. In contrast, patients with high levels of overvalued ideation showed a more attenuated response to CBT-as-usual, with most patients remaining symptomatic following treatment. More recently, an open trial has shown IBA to be equally effective for those with and without overvalued ideation [54].

Does the Inference-Based Approach Model Overlap With Other Treatment Approaches?

IBA can in practice be combined with ERP [55], but disagrees theoretically with current CBT, although supporting its clinical observations on the role of metacognitions (Figure 17.2). However, doubt is conceptually distinct from uncertainty since, as we noted earlier, people with OCD are often certain before they doubt. The other conceptual overlap appears with mindfulness techniques and its variants (e.g., acceptance and commitment therapy), where the IBA technique of making the bridge to reality appears to overlap with being in the here and now and connecting with the five senses.

However, when we steer the client toward reality in inference-based therapy via a grounded story, we appeal to consensual understanding of reality and not simply to a reliance on external cues. Therefore, the person is asked to rely on what appears before them as reality, using their senses, but also to rely on their common sense (an "internal" sense), which can be more persuasive than relying on appearance. In any case, as Michael Mahoney [56] once famously noted, there is no "immaculate perception", and there is always some imagination in perception, as both past and future horizons of an object need to come into view to contextualize the object and make it into a solid and continuous object in the present [57].

Therefore, IBA does not encourage people to get out of their minds, nor does it require any special skills or devices such as the matrix (as employed in acceptance and commitment therapy), or meditation, no matter how useful these techniques might be for other problems. Rather, clients are asked to accept reality without any effort because reality hits the person between the eyes, as in other non-OCD walks of life. For the same reason, reality sensing in IBA is distinct from reality testing and exposure, as IBA is not interested in testing reality or reconceptualizing experience. Rather, in IBA the client is simply asked to accept reality as it is without the additions of effort or new arguments. Yet, the client is invited to apply the insight gained in therapy about their reasoning and about their misleading stories telling them that there is more to do (i.e., compulsions and lengthy rituals).

Pathological Doubt as a Transdiagnostic Factor: the Relevance of the Inference-Based Approach Across Obsessional Disorders

Apart from successfully adapting IBA to other populations such as children and adolescents, we have explored pathological doubt in other disorders. It seems that obsessional doubt reveals itself across several distinct OCD spectrum disorders in different ways, namely: body dysmorphic disorder [58], eating disorders [59], delusional disorder [60,61], and hoarding disorder [62]. All of these groups score higher than controls on measures of inferential confusion and all benefit from IBA therapy. What they all have in common is a distrust of the senses, a reliance and investment on subjective possibilities at the expense of the senses, and a construction of incoherent justifying narratives.

Although the concept of inferential confusion and the IBA model were originally formulated in the context of OCD, research has demonstrated that they also apply to other psychopathologies with an obsessional nature. For example, an individual with an eating disorder who looks at herself in the mirror will not rely on her senses (e.g., "I don't see any fat on my body") in judging her body shape or weight, but will rely on possibility-based information from her imagination (e.g., "if I don't get to exercise enough today I will get fat"). Body image disturbance is considered to be a core feature of eating disorders [63], and entails an obsessional doubt about one's body shape or weight. In line with the IBA model that states that the obsessional doubt generates OCD symptoms and behaviors, body image disturbance has been found to be a predictor of eating disorder symptoms and disorder severity, and to impede recovery [64]. It is possible that body image disturbance is a consequence of inferential confusion, as it involves a distrust of the senses (e.g., "I doubt what I see in the mirror"; "I doubt what I feel when I touch my hips"), together with an overinvestment in the imagination and possibility-based information (for example, "What if I am fatter than what I may see, what if there is more fat on my hips than what I may feel?"). It thus appears that one important cognitive feature shared by individuals with OCD and eating disorders is the credibility given to imaginary processes, and the lack thereof, to reality-based information. Notably, there has been recent empirical attention devoted to the examination of cognitive confidence (i.e., doubting one's senses) in eating disorders. Some findings suggest that individuals with eating disorders, just like those with OCD, may also be prone to display poor cognitive confidence [65], suggesting that individuals with eating disorders also doubt their senses, namely their attention, perception and memory.

Although research examining inferential confusion in eating disorders is scarce to this day, the available evidence highlights that inferential confusion is a concept relevant to eating psychopathology. Notably, in one recent clinical trial, IBA was adapted for eating disorders, and it was demonstrated that the treatment produced significant reductions in body image disturbance and symptoms [59]. Once again, such findings support the idea that inferential confusion might be an important factor in the etiology and maintenance of eating disorders, thus highlighting the transdiagnostic nature of the construct.

Similarly, IBA is also relevant to other disorders where obsessional beliefs are strongly held contrary to evidence. In the case of BDD, the individual again distrusts their senses and common sense (e.g., "I doubt what people say when they say that my nose looks normal"), together with an overinvestment in the imagination (e.g., "What if my nose is deformed and ugly?"). In one study [58], ten patients with BDD completed IBA therapy and showed significant improvements, with large diminutions in symptoms. Pathological doubt is also prominent in hoarding disorder (e.g., "Maybe one day I will need this object"), and an open trial has shown that IBA therapy was effective in the treatment of compulsive hoarding [62].

Conclusion and Future Directions

The efficacy of IBA therapy in obsessional belief populations has been demonstrated. Nonetheless, further clinical trials are needed to compare the effectiveness of IBA therapy with other commonly administered therapies, such as CBT, in order to fully test the transdiagnostic value of IBA. Considering that IBA is relevant to all psychopathologies where imaginary and faulty reasoning processes are at play, IBA is a good fit for all disorders with obsessive profiles, where the individual is invested in the obsessional narrative at the expense of reality-based evidence.

References

1. Emmelkamp PMG. Commentary on treatment. In: RO Frost, G Steketee, eds. *Cognitive Approaches to Obsessions and Compulsions: Theory, Assessment, and Treatment*. Oxford: Elsevier Science; 2002;461–463.
2. Abramowitz JS. Does cognitive-behavioral therapy cure obsessive-compulsive disorder? A meta-analytic evaluation of clinical significance. *Behav Ther*. 1998;29:339–355.
3. Stanley MA, Turner SM. Current status of pharmacological and behavioural treatment of obsessive-compulsive symptoms. *Behav Ther*. 1995;26:163–186.
4. Whittal ML, Thordarson DS, McLean PD. Treatment of obsessive-compulsive disorder: cognitive behavior therapy vs. exposure and response prevention. *Behav Res Ther*. 2005;43:1559–1576.
5. Franklin ME, Abramowitz JS, Kozak MJ, Levitt JT, Foa EB. Effectiveness of exposure and ritual prevention for obsessive-compulsive disorder: randomized compared with nonrandomized samples. *J Consult Clin Psychol*. 2000;68:594–602.
6. Frost R, Steketee G. *Cognitive Approaches to Obsessions and Compulsions: Theory, Assessment, and Treatment*. Oxford: Elsevier Science; 2002.
7. Jacoby RJ, Abramowitz JS. Inhibitory learning approaches to exposure therapy: a critical review and translation to obsessive-compulsive disorder. *Clin Psychol Rev*. 2016;49:28–40.
8. Craske MG, Treanor M, Conway CC, Zbozinek T, Vervliet B. Maximizing exposure therapy: an inhibitory learning approach. *Behav Res Ther*. 2014;58:10–23.
9. Taylor S. Disorder-specific genetic factors in obsessive-compulsive disorder: a comprehensive meta-analysis. *Am J Med Genet B Neuropsychiatr Genet*. 2016;3:325–332.
10. Anholt G, Kalanthroff E. Do we need a cognitive theory for obsessive-compulsive disorder? *Clin Neuropsychiatry J Treat Eval*. 2014;11:194–196.
11. Obsessive Compulsive Cognitions Working Group. Cognitive assessment of obsessive-compulsive disorder. *Behav Res Ther*. 1997;35:667–681.
12. O'Connor K. Intrusions and inferences in obsessive compulsive disorder. *Clin Psychol Psychother*. 2002;9(1):38–46.
13. Meyer V. Modification of expectations in cases with obsessional rituals. *Behav Res Ther*. 1966;4:273–280.
14. Riskind JH. Looming vulnerability to threat: a cognitive paradigm for anxiety. *Behav Res Ther*. 1997;35(8):685–702.
15. Rachman S, Radomsky AS, Elliott CM, Zysk E. Mental contamination: the perpetrator effect. *J Behav Ther Exp Psychiatry*. 2012;43(1):587–593.
16. Salkovskis PM. Obsessional-compulsive problems: a cognitive-behavioural analysis. *Behav Res Ther*. 1985;23(5):571–583.
17. Clark DA, Beck AT, Brown G. Cognitive mediation in general psychiatric outpatients: a test of the content-specificity hypothesis. *J Pers Soc Psychol*. 1989;56:958–964.
18. Clark DM. Cognitive mediation of panic attacks induced by biological challenge tests. *Adv Behav Res Ther*. 1993;15(1):75–84.
19. Obsessive Compulsive Cognitions Working Group. Psychometric validation of the Obsessive Belief Questionnaire and Interpretation of Intrusions Inventory – Part 2: factor analyses and testing of a brief version. *Behav Res Ther*. 2005;43:1527–1542.
20. Calamari JE, Cohen RJ, Rector NA, Szacun-Shimizu K, Reimann BC, Norberg MM. Dysfunctional

belief-based obsessive-compulsive disorder subgroups. *Behav Res Ther*. 2006;44:1347–1360.

21. Polman A, O'Connor K, Huisman M. Dysfunctional belief-based subgroups and inferential confusion in obsessive–compulsive disorder. *Pers Individ Diff*. 2011;50:153–158.
22. Taylor S, Abramovitch JS, Makay D. Do dysfunctional beliefs play a role in all type of obsessive compulsive disorder? *J Anxiety Disord*. 2006;20:216–228.
23. Sica C, Cosadeschi D, Sanavio E. A study of the psychometric properties of the obsessive beliefs inventory and interpretations of intrusions inventory on clinical Italian individuals. *J Anxiety Disord*. 2004;188:291–307.
24. Tolin DF, Woods CM, Abramowitz JS. Relationship between obsessive beliefs and obsessive-compulsive symptoms. *Cognit Ther Res*. 2003;27:657–669.
25. Shams G, Milosevic I. A comparative study of obsessive beliefs in obsessive-compulsive disorder, anxiety disorder patients and a normal group. *Acta Med Iran*. 2015;53:301–310.
26. Ratcliffe M. *Experiences of Depression: A Study in Phenomenology*. Oxford University Press; 2015:318.
27. Bucarelli B, Purdon C. A diary study of the phenomenology and persistence of compulsions. *J Behav Ther Exp Psychiatry*. 2015; 49(Pt B):209–215.
28. Bucarelli B, Purdon C. Stovechecking behaviour in people with OCD vs anxious controls. *J Behav Ther Exp Psychiatry*. 2016;53:17–24.
29. Dèttore D, O'Connor K. OCD and cognitive illusions. *Cognit Ther Res*. 2012;37(1):109–121.
30. Keen N, Brown GP, Wheatley J. Obsessive compulsive symptoms and the simulation of future negative events. *Br J Clin Psychol*. 2008;47:265–279.
31. Kahneman D, Tversky K. The simulation heuristic. In: Kahnman D, Tversky K, eds. *Judgement Under Uncertainty: Heuristics and Biases*. New York, NY: Cambridge University Press; 1982:201–208.
32. Keen N, Brown G, Wheatley J. Obsessive compulsive symptoms and the simulation of future negative events. *Br J Clin Psychol*. 2008;47:265–279.
33. O'Connor K, Aardema F. Living in a bubble: dissociation, relational consciousness, and obsessive compulsive disorder. *J Consciousness Stud*. 2012;19(7–8):216–246.
34. Aardema F, Johansson P, Hall L, Paradisis S, Zidana M, Roberts S. Choice blindness, confabulatory introspection and obsessive compulsive symptoms: a new area of investigation. *Int J Cognit Ther*. 2014;7:88–102.
35. Abramovitch A, Abramowitz JS, Mittelman A. The neuropsychology of adult obsessive–compulsive disorder: a meta-analysis. *Clin Psychol Rev*. 2013;33:1163–1171.
36. Hermans D, Martens K, De Cort K, Pieters G, Eelen P. Reality monitoring and metacognitive beliefs related to cognitive confidence in obsessive–compulsive disorder. *Behav Res Ther*. 2003;41:383–401.
37. Hermans D, Engelen U, Grouwels L, Joos E, Lemmens J, Pieters G. Cognitive confidence in obsessive-compulsive disorder: distrusting perception, attention and memory. *Behav Res Ther*. 2008;46:98–113.
38. García-Montes JM, Pérez-Álvarez M, Balbuena CS, Garcelán SP, Cangas AJ. Metacognitions in patients with hallucinations and obsessive-compulsive disorder: the superstition factor. *Behav Res Ther*. 2006;44(8):1091–1104.
39. Moritz S, Peters MJ, Larøi F, Lincoln TM. Metacognitive beliefs in obsessive-compulsive patients: a comparison with healthy and schizophrenia participants. *Cogn Neuropsychiatry*. 2010;15:531–548.
40. Barahmand U. Meta-cognitive profiles in anxiety disorders. *Psychiatry Res*. 2009;169:240–243.
41. Cartwright-Hatton S, Wells A. Beliefs about worry and intrusions: the Meta-Cognitions Questionnaire and its correlates. *J Anxiety Disord*. 1997;11:279–296.
42. van den Hout M, Kindt M. Repeated checking causes memory distrust. *Behav Res Ther*. 2003;41:301–316.
43. Radomsky AS, Gilchrist PT, Dussault D. Repeated checking really does cause memory distrust. *Behav Res Ther*. 2006;44:305–316.
44. Dek EC, van den Hout MA, Engelhard IM, Giele CL, Cath DC. Perseveration causes automatization of checking behavior in obsessive-compulsive disorder. *Behav Res Ther*. 2015;71:1–9.
45. Ashbaugh AR, Radomsky AS. Attentional focus during repeated checking influences memory but not metamemory. *Cognit Ther Res*. 2007;31:291–306.
46. Harkin B, Kessler K. How checking breeds doubt: reduced performance in a simple working memory task. *Behav Res Ther*. 2009;47:504–512.
47. Giele C, Van Den Hout, Engelhard I, Elaine C., Dek C, Hopfmeier F. Obsessive compulsive like reasoning makes an unlikely catastrophe. *J Behav Ther Exp Psychiatry*. 2011;42:293–297.
48. Sarbin TR. Believed in imaginings: a narrative approach. In: J de Rivera, TR Sarbin, eds. *Believed In Imaginings: The Narrative Construction of Reality*. Washington, DC: American Psychiatric Association; 1998.
49. White M, Epston D. *Narrative Means to Therapeutic Ends*. New York, NY: Norton; 1990.

50. O'Connor K, Aardema F, Bouthillier D, et al. Evaluation of an inference-based approach to treating obsessive-compulsive disorder. *Cognit Behav Ther.* 2005;34:148–163.

51. Aardema F, O'Connor K. Dissolving the tenacity of obsessional doubt: implications for treatment outcome. *J Behav Ther Exp Psychiatry.* 2012;43:855–861.

52. Julien D, O'Connor KP, Aardema F. The inference-based approach to obsessive-compulsive disorder: a systematic review of its etiological model, treatment efficacy, and model of change. *J Affect Disord.* 2016;202:187–196.

53. Visser H, Van Megen H, Van Oppen P. The effectiveness of the inference based approach to treating obsessive-compulsive disorder with poor insight: results of a randomized multicentre trial. *Psychother Psychosom.* 2015;84:284–293.

54. Aardema F, O'Connor KP, Delorme ME, Audet JS. The inference-based approach (IBA) to the treatment of obsessive-compulsive disorder: an open trial across symptom subtypes and treatment-resistant cases. *Clin Psychol Psychother.* 2017;24(2):289–301.

55. van Niekerk J, Brown G, Aardema F, O'Connor K. Integration of inference-based therapy and cognitive-behavioral therapy for obsessive-compulsive disorder – a case series. *Int J Cognit Ther.* 2014;7(1):67–82.

56. Mahoney MJ. *Constructive Psychotherapy: Theory and Practice.* New York, NY: Guilford Press; 2006.

57. O'Connor K. *A Constructionist Clinical Psychology for Cognitive Behaviour Therapy.* Abingdon: Routledge; 2015.

58. Taillon A, O'Connor K, Dupuis G, Lavoie M. Inference-based therapy for body dysmorphic disorder. *Clin Psychol Psychother.* 2013;20:67–76.

59. Purcell-Lalonde M, O'Connor K, Aardema F, Coelho JS. Food for thought: ego-dystonicity and fear of self in eating disorders. *Eur Eat Disord Rev.* 2015;23:179–184.

60. Aardema F, O'Connor K, Emmelkamp P, Marchand A, Todorov C. Inferential confusion in obsessive-compulsive disorder: Inferential Confusion Questionnaire. *Behav Res Ther.* 2005;43:293–308.

61. O'Connor KP: Cognitive and meta-cognitive dimensions of psychoses. *Can J Psychiatry.* 54(3): 152–159, 2009.

62. Blais M, Bodryzlova Y, Aardema F, O'Connor K. Open trial of inference-based therapy in the treatment of compulsive hoarding. *J Psychol Clin Psychiatry.* 2016;6:403.

63. Farrell C, Shafran R, Fairburn CG. Body size estimation: testing a new mirror-based assessment method. *Int J Eat Disord.* 2003;34:162–171.

64. Cash TF, Deagle EA. The nature and extent of body-image disturbances in anorexia nervosa and bulimia nervosa: a meta-analysis. *Int J Eat Disord.* 1997;22:107–126.

65. Davenport E, Rushford N, Soon S, McDermott C. Dysfunctional metacognition and drive for thinness in typical and atypical anorexia nervosa. *J Eat Disord.* 2015;3:1.

Chapter 18

Drug Augmentation Strategies for Treatment-Resistant Obsessive-Compulsive and Related Disorders

Roseli Gedanke Shavitt and Juliana Belo Diniz

Introduction

First-line pharmacological treatment for obsessive-compulsive disorder (OCD) encompasses all selective serotonin reuptake inhibitors (SSRIs), at the maximum tolerated or recommended dosage, for at least 12 weeks (at least 8 weeks at maximum dosage) [1]. For the OCD-related disorders, a few clinical trials have associated the use of SSRIs with symptomatic improvement, like in body dysmorphic disorder (BDD) [2], trichotillomania (TTM) [3], skin-picking disorder and hoarding disorder [4]. The reported effect sizes are smaller than those observed in OCD, and there is no Food and Drug Administration approved pharmacological treatment for the OCRDs. Reviews and meta-analyses with patients suffering from OCRDs point to conflicting results for treatment with SSRIs, mood stabilizers/anticonvulsants, naltrexone and N-acetyl-cysteine (NAC), reaching the conclusion that more controlled trials are needed to establish the efficacy of these pharmacological agents in this context. For example, a meta-analysis that included seven studies, with a total of 92 participants that received pharmacological treatment for pathological hoarding, assessed the response not only to serotonin reuptake inhibitors (SRIs) but also to venlafaxine, methylphenidate, and augmentation of SRIs with quetiapine, minocycline and naltrexone [4]. The majority of participants met diagnostic criteria for OCD, and more than half of the participants responded. The authors concluded that new trials of pharmacotherapy for pathological hoarding are needed, in particular testing novel agents that target the unique neurobiological correlates of this disorder.

Results from a global, expert consensus regarding the conceptual and operational definitions of treatment response, remission, recovery and relapse for use in clinical trials of OCD [5], consider the conceptual definition of treatment response as a clinically meaningful reduction in symptoms (time, distress and interference associated with obsessions, compulsions and avoidance) relative to baseline severity in an individual who meets diagnostic criteria for OCD. The operational definition of treatment response would be a 35% reduction in Yale-Brown Obsessive-Compulsive Scale (Y-BOCS) scores plus clinical global impression – improvement rating of 1 (very much improved) or 2 (much improved), lasting for at least one week. Following the same criteria, a partial response would be considered for a reduction in Y-BOCS scores between 25% and 35%. These standardized criteria are relevant, among other aspects, for the improvement of the guidelines for evaluation of clinical efficacy of various treatments by regulatory agencies and the development of improved treatment guidelines for clinical practice. For the purposes of this chapter, we consider as resistance to pharmacological treatment in OCD the absence of a partial or full response to one or more first-line treatments for OCD. We do not refer to the term "treatment refractory OCD", leaving that to a condition where the patient remains symptomatic despite having received every treatment available, including cognitive behavioral therapy (CBT), pharmacological combination and augmentation strategies and the combination of CBT and pharmacological treatments.

Considering a main diagnosis of OCD, in a pragmatic clinical setting, only 30% of patients are expected to reach a satisfactory response in the first 12-week timeframe with pharmacological treatment [6]. However, the expected initial response to treatment is indeed a partial response. We only rarely observe the full remission of OCD symptoms in such a short period of time. In addition, the maintenance of SSRIs at the maximum tolerated dosage beyond 12 weeks has been associated with progressive improvement, even when no other active interventions are added [7,8]. Such progressive improvement of OCD with sustained SSRI treatment has not been reported for the OCRDs, which have been associated with loss of response after initial improvement [9].

In OCD, the absence of improvement or insufficient response with a first-line treatment may be overcome by the combination with CBT [10]. The effect sizes associated with the combination of SSRI and CBT are indeed larger than those reported for the augmentation of SSRIs with different classes of psychiatric drugs [11]. The combination with CBT has also been considered the main alternative for the pharmacological treatment resistance observed in the OCRDs [12,13]. In contrast, the lack of availability of CBT for OCD and OCRDs, or the non-acceptance or failure of CBT lead the clinician to consider other pharmacological alternatives, such as switching to another SSRI or to clomipramine (a non-selective SRI) [1], or even to use an SSRI in dosages above the usual limits [14]. The presence of a contraindication or intolerance to clomipramine or to higher SSRI dosages may prevent the adoption of such measures. As well, the failure of these alternatives may lead to the use of drug combination (within the same class of drugs, such as the combination of an SSRI with clomipramine) or augmentation (with different classes, such as adding an antipsychotic to clomipramine or an SSRI) [1]. This sequence of strategies is based on the treatment guidelines for obsessive and compulsive symptoms. The presence of other comorbid psychiatric disorders may indicate other lines of intervention, with earlier implementation of drugs combination or augmentation. Consequently, in the case of short-term SSRI failure, strategies like a pharmacological switch, combination or augmentation have to be considered on an individual basis, taking potential risks and benefits into account.

Before considering drug combination or augmentation, or the use of clomipramine, or prescribing unusually high dosages of SSRIs, treatment guidelines recommend switching to another SSRI [1]. However, there are no clinical trials that evaluated the efficacy of such strategy. The rationale for presenting this approach in the guidelines in the absence of sufficient evidence seems to be that drug combination or augmentation, the switch to clomipramine or to higher than usual SSRI dosages are all associated with a higher risk of severe adverse events. The switch to another SSRI seems an alternative to avoid such complications. In the case that the first SSRI has not been well tolerated, switching to a second SSRI has a higher chance to promote benefits if it is associated with fewer adverse effects, allowing for higher dosages to be reached.

Recent Research Findings

Given that the combination of an SSRI with CBT is not always feasible, the pharmacological combination or augmentation of SSRIs may be necessary for some OCD patients [15]. Notwithstanding, it is important to have in mind that while the effect size of SSRIs is only moderate as compared to placebo, for the combination or augmentation of an SSRI with other drugs this effect size is even smaller. Therefore, it is necessary to evaluate if the potential benefits with such measures overcome the risks that they represent. Pharmacological combination or augmentation are not routinely prescribed for patients with residual symptoms with none or only mild functional impairment [47]. These measures seem more adequate for patients whose symptoms are maintained at moderate and severe levels despite a good adherence to SSRI treatment.

Combining a Selective Serotonin Reuptake Inhibitors With Low-Dose Clomipramine

The combination of an SSRI with clomipramine up to 150 mg/day has been tested in case series (evidence level 3), open-label trials (evidence level 2) and in one double-blind randomized controlled trial (RCT; evidence level 1). Additional double-blind RCTs have not been published yet, precluding a meta-analysis on the subject. The following SSRIs have been tested in the combination with clomipramine: fluoxetine [7,16,17,18], sertraline [19] and citalopram [20,21]. The open-label trials have shown that clomipramine could be better tolerated if used in low dosages (up to 150 mg/day) combined with an SSRI than if used in the high dosages (150–300 mg/day) required to produce a significant effect in monotherapy. In the only double-blind RCT that compared the clomipramine–fluoxetine combination to the placebo–fluoxetine combination, there was a significant improvement after the addition of clomipramine, but this improvement was not significantly superior to that produced by placebo [7].

The greatest concern associated with the combination of clomipramine and an SSRI is that the increment in the blood levels of both drugs consequent to drug interaction may increase the risk of severe and potentially life-threatening adverse effects, such as seizures, heart arrhythmia and serotonergic overstimulation. In addition, pharmacodynamic interactions may increase the risk of cardiac arrhythmias when both drugs are independently associated with such events, which is the case for clomipramine and high-dose citalopram [22]. Close monitoring is advised when using any clomipramine–SRRI combination. Vital signs such as heart rate and arterial blood pressure may indicate the potential risk of arrhythmia and postural hypotension. Electrocardiograms should be performed at every dosage increase and the QTc interval should be calculated. QTc intervals equal to or superior to 440 ms are not safe and indicate drug discontinuation. Regarding the dosage of drug and metabolites blood levels, clomipramine and desmethylclomipramine combined blood levels should not exceed 450 ng/ml [22].

So far, the SSRI–clomipramine combination has been investigated in placebo-controlled RCTs exclusively in OCD. In a sequential trial that compared the effects of combining fluoxetine with clomipramine, fluoxetine with quetiapine and fluoxetine with placebo as a second step in patients with OCD who did not respond to initial treatment with fluoxetine, the presence of comorbid BDD predicted a worse response to the combination fluoxetine–clomipramine [23]. Of note, in major depressive disorder, the combination of antidepressants of different pharmacological classes has also been investigated for the treatment of resistant and refractory cases. However, for major depressive disorder, the specific combination of SSRI and clomipramine has been avoided, owing to the potential risks compared with other possible drug combinations [24].

Augmentation of Selective Serotonin Reuptake Inhibitors or Clomipramine With First- and Second-Generation Antipsychotics

Although monotherapy with antipsychotics has been associated with the appearance of new OCD symptoms [25,26], preliminary evidence suggests that specific antipsychotics may be effective in OCD treatment [27]. In addition, the augmentation of SSRIs with antipsychotics is one of the most commonly used pharmacological strategies for patients with OCD who are resistant to SSRIs [28,29]. The neurophysiologic bases of this apparent paradox are not completely understood. The dopaminergic and serotonergic systems are highly interconnected and participate in the prefrontal cortex control of basal ganglia activity.

Studies using single photon emission computed tomography have found that, when compared with healthy people, patients with OCD present an increased ratio of specific to non-specific binding to the dopamine transporter in the basal ganglia [30,31]. The same finding has been reported for drug-naïve children with Tourette's disorder [32]. In degenerative disorders such as Parkinson's disease, this ratio is found to be decreased [33]. Therefore, the increased ratio of specific to non-specific binding to the dopamine transporters might indicate that, as compared with healthy people, those with OCD have an upregulated expression of dopamine transporters. Dopamine neurotransmission plays a major role in the pathophysiology of Tourette's disorder and probably also participate in the mechanisms that lead to TTM, skin-picking disorder and behavioral addictions [34].

In a preclinical trial that evaluated the association of quetiapine with fluvoxamine, the antipsychotic augmentation of fluvoxamine led to a synergic effect with significant increase of dopamine availability in the prefrontal and thalamic brain regions in mice [35]. The same effect has been described with the augmentation of fluoxetine with olanzapine [36]. These findings can help to explain the paradoxical effects of atypical antipsychotics in obsessive-compulsive symptoms: when used in monotherapy, atypical antipsychotics act on the $5HT_{2A}$ receptors and lead to increased dopaminergic neurotransmission in the basal ganglia; when atypical antipsychotics are combined to SSRIs, there is an additional increase of dopaminergic neurotransmission in the prefrontal cortex, and this later effect may counterbalance the hyperactivation of the basal ganglia.

The first reports of the potential benefit of the augmentation of SSRIs with antipsychotics came from studies that evaluated typical (first-generation) antipsychotics, which are drugs that carry as their main effect the blockade of dopaminergic activity through the antagonism of D_2 dopamine receptors. Haloperidol and pimozide were tested in patients with OCD and comorbid tic disorders in two randomized controlled trials [37,38]. Both haloperidol and pimozide were more effective than placebo in the augmentation of fluvoxamine treatment for OCD. However, the benefit of the augmentation was smaller than that reported for SSRI monotherapy.

Monotherapy with haloperidol and pimozide has been shown to be effective for the treatment of tic disorders regardless of their comorbidity with OCD [39]. However, such treatments rarely result in the remission of tics and, given their adverse-effect profile, they are reserved to more severe cases. Haloperidol has also been considered for the treatment of TTM. However, preliminary results still warrant confirmation [40].

The pharmacological profile of the atypical antipsychotics varies widely. However, it is a shared characteristic of these drugs that they induce less extrapyramidal symptoms than their typical counterparts. One of the characteristics of some atypical antipsychotics that may be related to this protective effect is the counterbalance of dopamine antagonism in the basal ganglia by the dopaminergic effect of blocking 5-HT_{2A} and 5-HT_{2C} receptors. The efficacy of add-on of atypical antipsychotics to SSRI pharmacotherapy has been evaluated in patients with OCD with or without comorbid tic disorders in several double-blind placebo-controlled trials.

In a 2015 meta-analysis on the subject [41], 14 placebo-controlled RCTs were included. The authors of this meta-analysis concluded that there was sufficient evidence of the efficacy of adding risperidone (0.5–6 mg/day, 4 studies, 132 patients) and aripiprazole (10–15 mg/day, 2 studies, 79 patients) to an SSRI. However, the atypical antipsychotic most frequently used in the studies included in this meta-analysis was quetiapine (4 studies, 142 patients), for which there was no evidence of efficacy when compared with placebo. For the remaining atypical antipsychotics, additional studies are needed [41].

In a previous meta-analysis in 2006, Bloch et al. [28] had reported that patients with OCD and comorbid tic disorders achieved a better outcome after treatment with the augmentation of SSRI with risperidone than those without tics. Notwithstanding, in the more recent 2015 meta-analysis conducted by Dold et al. [41], the exclusion of studies that recruited patients with OCD with comorbid tic disorders did not alter the effect size of augmentation of SSRIs with antipsychotics.

Monotherapy with atypical antipsychotics has been employed in the treatment of tic disorders and TTM. As in the case of typical antipsychotics and tic disorders, atypical antipsychotics are associated with partial improvement and severe adverse effects, being reserved for the most severe cases of Tourette's disorder and chronic motor tic disorders [39]. The atypical antipsychotic olanzapine has been tested in monotherapy for the treatment of TTM in one placebo-controlled RCT, with positive results [42]. Several open-label trials and case reports have described that the augmentation of SSRI with olanzapine may be effective for reducing TTM symptoms [43]. These later results still warrant replication in longer-term RCTs.

With regard to pathological skin picking, one case report describes the successful use of venlafaxine augmentation of aripiprazole in a 21-year-old woman [44], whereas another case report describes the successful haloperidol augmentation of fluvoxamine after partial response to fluvoxamine plus oxcarbazepine in a 59-year-old woman [45]. As for BDD, a controlled trial of pimozide augmentation of fluoxetine revealed that pimozide was not more effective than placebo, with no significant effect of baseline delusionality on endpoint severity of BDD [46]. Similar results were reported for a case series where six patients received augmentation of fluoxetine with olanzapine [47]. Only one case report described a successful augmentation of paroxetine with olanzapine in a 26-year-old woman with a 10-year history of BDD [48]. Finally, there is some evidence of successful augmentation of SSRIs with quetiapine for hoarding disorder [4].

The potential for antipsychotics to induce a metabolic syndrome, to induce severe motor symptoms such as tardive dyskinesia, and to accelerate cortical atrophy has raised the concern among some authors regarding the long-term use of antipsychotics as augmenters of SSRIs in non-psychotic disorders. Although SSRIs are associated with sedation and weight gain, these effects are usually more pronounced with the augmentation with antipsychotics [49]. In addition, as mentioned earlier, the combination of SSRIs with psychotherapy has been associated with higher effect sizes than the augmentation with antipsychotics [11]. Therefore, for OCD and other OCRDs, augmentation with antipsychotics is only indicated for those patients that do not accept or that have not benefited from combining CBT with SSRI treatment.

Augmentation of Selective Serotonin Reuptake Inhibitors with Glutamatergic Agents

Glutamate is the main excitatory neurotransmitter of the central nervous system. It is, at least to some extent, involved with all brain circuits that have been described so far, including the corticostriatothalamocortical circuit [50]. Hyperactivation of the latter has been consistently associated with OCD, according to previous studies comparing OCD patients and healthy controls [51]. In addition, specific genetic polymorphisms related to the glutamatergic system, such as those found in the gene that encodes the glutamate transporter known as *Slc1A1* [52] and in the gene that encodes the N-methyl-D-aspartate (NMDA) receptor subunits known as *Grin2B* [53], have been consistently found to be overrepresented in patients with OCD when compared with healthy controls. These findings have helped to build the grounds for the hypothesis that modulation of glutamatergic activity could result in obsessive-compulsive symptomatic improvement [51].

The following glutamatergic agents have been tested in a placebo-controlled RCT as augmenters of SSRIs: NAC, topiramate, riluzole, lamotrigine, memantine and ketamine [54]. Other glutamatergic agents that have been evaluated only in case series and open-label trials are not covered in this chapter, as there is not sufficient evidence of likelihood that they are indicated for OCD treatment. The glutamatergic agents studied so far, are, as a class, associated with weaker evidence of efficacy as augmenters of SSRIs in OCD than antipsychotics such as risperidone and aripiprazole [54]. In the following paragraphs we describe the glutamatergic agents that have been associated with promising initial findings but still need to be tested in additional trials to confirm their efficacy in OCD treatment.

N-Acetyl Cysteine

NAC is the N-acetyl derivative of the amino acid L-cysteine, which is a precursor of the antioxidant glutathione in the brain. NAC is best known for its mucolytic effects and for its use as a treatment for acetaminophen intoxication. The ingestion of high doses (up to 3 g/day) of NAC increases the availability of cysteine in the brain. Cysteine acts as the substrate of the cysteine–glutamate antiporter. The increase in cysteine availability thus results in increased extra-synaptic concentration of glutamate. The excess of extra-synaptic glutamate then activates metabotropic receptors that diminish the release of glutamate at the nucleus accumbens. Hypothetically, this latter effect could compensate for the baseline hyperactivation of the corticostriatothalamocortical circuit in OCD [54].

NAC up to 3 g/day has been tested as an augmenter of SSRIs for OCD treatment in four placebo-controlled RCTs [9,55,56,57]. In two of these four RCTs, NAC augmentation was not superior to placebo augmentation of SSRI, while in the remaining two studies, NAC augmentation showed some evidence of superior efficacy to placebo. NAC is sold over the counter, because of its benign adverse-effect profile and high safety profile. Such a benign profile indicates that NAC may play a role in OCD treatment even if it is associated with a small effect size. For some OCRDs such as TTM and skin picking, NAC has been shown to be effective when used as monotherapy [58,59]. The lack of a strong support for NAC efficacy in OCD has led some researchers to raise questions about how OCD and OCRDs may behave as a group in response to treatment characteristics [9].

Topiramate

Topiramate is an inhibitor of glutamatergic activity with anti-epileptic properties that has also been shown to prevent migraine, stabilize mood and reduce impulsivity [60]. It interferes with glutamatergic activity through several mechanisms of action, including the inhibition of voltage-dependent sodium channels, negative modulation of α-amino-3-hydroxy-5-methyl-4-isoxazolepropionic acid glutamate receptors, inhibition of L-type calcium channels and limitation of calcium-dependent second messenger systems [61]. Topiramate is also a weak inhibitor of carbonic anhydrase isoenzymes. This latter effect is responsible for some of topiramate's well-known adverse effects, which increase the likelihood of acidosis and the formation of renal stones [61].

In one placebo-controlled RCT, SSRI augmentation with topiramate up to 400 mg/day was shown to be more effective than placebo augmentation to reduce compulsive rituals in patients with OCD, although no difference was found regarding total Y-BOCS scores [62]. In addition, 5 of the 18 patients with OCD included in the topiramate group interrupted treatment because of adverse effects, and 7 of the remaining 12 patients could not reach the maximum dosage of 400 mg/day, also as a consequence of intolerable adverse effects. Thus, even if shown to be effective in larger samples, topiramate may have a restricted role in the treatment of OCD because of its safety and tolerance profile [62].

Topiramate in monotherapy or in combination with other agents is regarded as a second-line treatment for chronic tic disorders. This indication is based on the results of one placebo-controlled RCT that evaluated 29 patients with Tourette's disorder [63]. Topiramate in monotherapy has been tested for TTM treatment in one open-label trial [64]. As was the case for OCD treatment, one-third of patients with TTM did not tolerate topiramate. However, most of the patients that continued with treatment have reported some symptomatic improvement [64]. There are also case reports and case series that have described benefits from topiramate monotherapy for treating skin-picking disorder alone [65] or associated with pervasive developmental disorders [66].

Riluzole

Riluzole is a modulator of glutamatergic activity that inhibits the progression of amyotrophic lateral sclerosis. It modulates glutamatergic activity through two main mechanisms: inhibition of voltage-dependent sodium channels and potentiation of glutamate reuptake by glial cells, reducing glutamatergic toxicity and neuronal loss [67].

After promising results had been reported in a few case series, open-label trials and a pilot study [68], riluzole augmentation of SSRIs was tested in two placebo-controlled RCTs including patients with OCD [69,70]. In children with early-onset OCD, riluzole augmentation was not more effective than placebo [70]. In adults with OCD, in an eight-week trial in which the SSRI fluvoxamine plus riluzole or placebo were initiated concomitantly (with no prior SSRI monotherapy stabilization), the group under riluzole augmentation achieved higher symptomatic improvement than the group under placebo augmentation [69].

Riluzole monotherapy was also tested in children with Tourette's disorder in a small placebo-controlled RCT with negative results [71]. For OCRDs, there are only single-case reports of beneficial treatment of TTM and skin-picking disorder with riluzole [72,73]. Given its high cost and adverse-effect profile, it is unlikely that riluzole will play an important role in OCRDs treatment used as monotherapy or before SSRI non-response is established [54].

Lamotrigine

Lamotrigine is an inhibitor of glutamatergic activity best known for its anti-epileptic properties. It is also a Food and Drug Administration-approved drug for the treatment of bipolar disorder. In addition, lamotrigine may be recommended for the treatment of refractory major depression and as an augmenter of antipsychotics in refractory schizophrenia. Its effects on glutamatergic activity are probably related to the inhibition of voltage-dependent sodium channels [74].

In one placebo-controlled RCT, the augmentation of SSRIs with lamotrigine (up to 100 mg/day) was superior to placebo augmentation regarding improvement of both OCD and depressive symptoms [75]. Further replication of these findings is still warranted. Lamotrigine is promising as an augmentation agent given its moderate costs, tolerability and availability. The most concerning of lamotrigine's adverse effects, which is Steven–Johnsons syndrome, may have its risks dramatically reduced by slow titration of initial dosages [76].

Memantine

Memantine is a NMDA receptor antagonist used to slow the progression of Alzheimer's disease. Memantine reduces glutamate toxicity by interfering with calcium influx mediated by NMDA extrasynaptic receptors [77]. In a placebo-controlled RCT in patients with OCD who had moderate and severe symptoms, SSRI augmentation with memantine (up to 20 mg/day) was more effective than placebo augmentation [78]. These results still warrant replication. Given memantine's benign adverse-effect profile and moderate costs, it seems a promising agent for OCD treatment as an augmenter of SSRIs.

Ketamine

Ketamine is a non-competitive and non-selective NMDA receptor antagonist with anesthetic and psychotomimetic properties that has been recently included among potential agents for the treatment of refractory depression and suicidal ideation. Differently from the glutamatergic agents previously described in this chapter, ketamine has been associated with acute and transient effects after intravenous or intranasal administration of single dosages [79].

In a small placebo-controlled RCT, a single ketamine injection was superior to a single placebo injection in reducing OCD symptoms in the very short term, but sustainable improvement was not observed [80]. The same authors of this initial study suggested that adding CBT after ketamine injection could extend the symptomatic improvement. However, the first study that investigated this possibility was inconclusive about this possible effect [81]. Ketamine has not yet been tested for the treatment of any other OCDRD.

Augmentation of Selective Serotonin Reuptake Inhibitors With Other Pharmacological Agents

Some other agents that are unrelated to antipsychotic effects or glutamatergic activity have been reported to benefit patients with OCD when combined with SSRIs, according to placebo-controlled RCTs. Two inhibitors of type 3 serotonin receptors (5-HT_3) – ondansetron and granisetron – have been tested in one trial each [82,83]. In addition, there was one trial in which the non-steroid anti-inflammatory celecoxib [84] was tested, and another in which a weekly dose of morphine was tested [85]. The positive results from those trials still warrant replication. At this moment, the small amount of information on these agents precludes further conclusions about how promising they might be as SSRI augmenters for the treatment of OCD.

Cross-Diagnostic Approaches and Their Implications for Classification and Diagnosis

Why do Obsessive-Compulsive Disorder and Related Disorders Seem so Different in their Responses to Pharmacological Treatment Despite Belonging to the Same Diagnostic Category?

First, we need to consider that most of the available pharmacological treatments were not developed to target known etiological mechanisms of specific psychiatric disorders [86]. It seems that the serotonin transporter became the main target of pharmacological interventions for depression and anxiety, mostly because serotonin is a broad-range regulatory neurotransmitter, rather than a specific excitatory or inhibitory neurotransmitter. Hence, when acting on serotonin availability on the synaptic cleft, SRIs interfere with several other neurotransmitter systems, without being disruptive or completely shutting down the system [87].

Indeed, the exact pathway through which SRIs or their combination with different pharmacological agents result in measurable symptomatic improvement is mostly unknown for OCD [88]. In addition, SRIs are helpful to some but not all patients with either OCD or OCRDs. Heterogeneity of the pharmacological response may be the reflex of complex interactions between neurotransmitters and also the result of psychological heterogeneity between patients placed under the same psychiatric diagnosis [9]. Therefore, the lack of similarity between OCD and OCRDs regarding treatment response to pharmacological interventions does not necessarily indicate that these disorders do not share any common psychopathology.

Second, differently from pharmacological interventions, CBT protocols have been shown effective not only for OCD but also for OCRDs, encompassing similar techniques, known as exposure and response prevention. The main objective of such interventions is to obtain a continuous effect of habituation. The reason for using common techniques across disorders is that those techniques can be applied for any behavior that is maintained by negative reinforcement [89].

Resistance to negatively reinforced behaviors leads to increased discomfort, which is commonly manifested as anxiety. To prevent discomfort, patients can avoid situations that might trigger fear, can anticipate rituals before the discomfort arises, or they may fail to resist repetitive behaviors known to alleviate discomfort once preemptive avoidance failed [90]. The tendency to avoid discomfort and the lack of resistance to responses that may immediately alleviate distress despite potential collateral damage represent a common ground for many psychiatric disorders, including anxiety related disorders, OCRDs and addictions. These phenomena are also known as low distress tolerance [91].

Pharmacological treatments might reduce distress and facilitate the resistance to ritualize. However, if preemptive avoidance is being effective, patients might not benefit from this effect, as they would not risk feeling any discomfort in the first place [91,92]. The lower the tolerance to distress, the harder patients will work to avoid uncomfortable feelings. Since the behavioral treatment usually triggers uncomfortable feelings, it is likely that a stronger avoidant behavior will reduce the chance of benefiting from treatment [91]. The lack of satisfactory treatment response in

OCRDs could be associated to higher levels of intolerance to distress and, consequently, greater avoidance. BDD, for example, is more frequently associated with social phobia and avoidant personality than OCD [93,94], which could contribute to a different pattern of response to treatment when compared with that of OCD.

Importantly, increasing distress tolerance seems insufficient to reduce the frequency of behaviors that are maintained through negative reinforcement. The management of the response control is also necessary. To be able to control behavior, patients need to discriminate the triggers of the behavioral response. In other words, to prevent the response from being performed, patients need to know when it is going to happen [89]. Patients with behavioral addictions often describe that they are "caught" while performing the addictive behavior. They frequently cannot tell how and when exactly it started. This sensation of lack of control, also known as lack of inhibitory control, is characteristic of the impulse control disorders. Interestingly, TTM had been placed under the umbrella of impulse control disorders before being diverted to the group of OCRDs in the *Diagnostic and Statistical Manual of Mental Disorders*, 5th edition [95], together with skin-picking disorder [96,97].

TTM may have a different pattern of treatment response in relation to OCD because hair pulling might impose a greater difficulty for patients to gain control of their compulsive behavior [98]. These patients may also exhibit a greater difficulty in discriminating the triggers for their compulsive behavior, as may also happen with excoriations from skin-picking disorder [99]. Consequently, it is possible to place BDD in an extreme of avoidance in the obsessive-compulsive spectrum, while TTM and skin-picking disorder lie on the impulsive extreme of the same spectrum. Being more heterogeneous than BDD with regard to avoidance, and being more heterogeneous than TTM and skin-picking disorder with regard to inhibitory control, OCD may be associated with a broader range of effective pharmacological and behavioral targets. Still, this hypothesis needs to be taken with caution. There are far fewer pharmacological controlled trials for BDD, TTM and skin-picking disorder than for OCD. Hence, our understanding of the differences in response to treatment between OCD and OCDRDs is currently based on scarce evidence, suggesting a higher resistance to treatment for OCDRDs which may be later proved to be an artifact of trial selectivity. Notwithstanding, pharmacological treatment resistance in OCD and OCRDs reinforces the need of further investigation of more specific treatment targets.

Lastly, there has been great effort employed at improving CBT outcomes in OCD with the use of cognitive enhancers during exposure treatment [100]. Enhancers aim to improve extinction retention (habituation). Results have been inconsistent so far, but several new potential extinction enhancers (such as cannabidiol [101,102] and fatty acid amide hydrolase inhibitors [103]) are being considered to enter the pipeline for clinical use. We might have positive surprises from this line of research in the near future. Meanwhile, we are trying to better understand how distress tolerance and inhibitory control can be improved so that newer treatments can be developed to target specific aspects of OCD and OCRDs.

Conclusions and Future Directions

From the evidence compiled above, we can observe a difference between OCD and the OCRDs with regard to the degree of consensus about the treatment sequence in face of non-response to first-line treatments. In fact, at present, there is insufficient evidence to support the choice of a first-line pharmacological treatment for the OCRDs. In addition, the available evidence for the pharmacological treatment of the different OCRDs suggests different patterns of response to the SSRIs across diagnoses. Therefore, whereas for OCD it is well established that the lack of response to an SSRI can be successfully managed by switching to another SSRI, combining CBT or certain antipsychotics, for the OCRDs further studies are needed to guide our decisions in the face of non-response to initial treatment. For example, instead of adding an antipsychotic to an SSRI, we may find that a mood stabilizer or an opioid antagonist is more effective in these disorders. In this context, we could argue that the evidence to come regarding the augmentation strategies for OCD and the OCRDs could inform us about a new diagnostic organization. If future RCTs demonstrate a positive response to augmentation and combination strategies for the OCRDs that are different from those that work for OCD, a diagnostic organization more oriented toward the impulsivity–compulsivity spectrum may be needed.

References

1. Bandelow B, Zohar J, Hollander E, et al. World Federation of Societies of Biological Psychiatry (WFSBP) guidelines for the pharmacological treatment of anxiety, obsessive-compulsive and post-traumatic stress disorders – first revision. *World J Biol Psychiatry.* 2008;9(4):248–312.
2. Hollander E, Allen A, Kwon J, et al. Clomipramine vs desipramine crossover trial in body dysmorphic disorder: selective efficacy of a serotonin reuptake inhibitor in imagined ugliness. *Arch Gen Psychiatry.* 1999;56(11):1033–1039.
3. Johnson J, El-Alfy AT. Review of available studies of the neurobiology and pharmacotherapeutic management of trichotillomania. *J Adv Res.* 2016;7(2):169–184.
4. Brakoulias V, Eslick GD, Starcevic V. A meta-analysis of the response of pathological hoarding to pharmacotherapy. *Psychiatry Res.* 2015;229(1–2):272–276.
5. Mataix-Cols D, Fernández de la Cruz L, Nordsletten AE, Lenhard F, Isomura K, Simpson HB. Towards an international expert consensus for defining treatment response, remission, recovery and relapse in obsessive-compulsive disorder. *World Psychiatry.* 2016;15(1):80–81.
6. Belotto-Silva C, Diniz JB, Malavazzi DM, et al. Group cognitive-behavioral therapy versus selective serotonin reuptake inhibitors for obsessive-compulsive disorder: a practical clinical trial. *J Anxiety Disord.* 2012;26(1):25–31.
7. Diniz JB, Shavitt RG, Fossaluza V, Koran L, de Braganca Pereira CA, Miguel EC. A double-blind, randomized, controlled trial of fluoxetine plus quetiapine or clomipramine versus fluoxetine plus placebo for obsessive-compulsive disorder. *J Clin Psychopharmacol.* 2011;31(6):763–768.
8. Jakubovski E, Diniz JB, Valério C, et al. Clinical predictors of long-term outcome in obsessive-compulsive disorder. *Depress Anxiety.* 2013;30(8):763–772.
9. Costa DL, Diniz JB, Miguel EC. How similar are the disorders included under the umbrella of obsessive-compulsive disorder and related disorders? *JAMA Psychiatry.* 2016;73(8):877.
10. Foa EB, Simpson HB, Liebowitz MR, et al. Six-month follow-up of a randomized controlled trial augmenting serotonin reuptake inhibitor treatment with exposure and ritual prevention for obsessive-compulsive disorder. *J Clin Psychiatry.* 2013;74(5):464–469.
11. Simpson HB, Foa EB, Liebowitz MR, et al. Cognitive-behavioral therapy vs risperidone for augmenting serotonin reuptake inhibitors in obsessive-compulsive disorder: a randomized clinical trial. *JAMA Psychiatry.* 2013; 70(11):1190–1199.
12. Keuthen NJ, Tung ES, Reese HE, Raikes J, Lee L, Mansueto CS. Getting the word out: cognitive-behavioral therapy for trichotillomania (hair-pulling disorder) and excoriation (skin-picking) disorder. *Ann Clin Psychiatry.* 2015;27(1):10–15.
13. Williams M, Viscusi JA. Hoarding disorder and a systematic review of treatment with cognitive behavioral therapy. *Cogn Behav Ther.* 2016;45(2):93–110.
14. Pampaloni I, Sivakumaran T, Hawley C, et al. High-dose selective serotonin reuptake inhibitors in OCD: a systematic retrospective case notes survey. *J Psychopharmacol.* 2010; 24(10):1439–1445.
15. Math S, Janardhan Reddy Y. Issues in the pharmacological treatment of obsessive-compulsive disorder. *Int J Clin Pract.* 2007;61(7):1188–1197.
16. Simeon J, Thatte S, Wiggins D. Treatment of adolescent obsessive-compulsive disorder with a clomipramine-fluoxetine combination. *Psychopharmacol Bull.* 1990;26(3):285–290.
17. Browne M, Horn E, Jones T. The benefits of clomipramine-fluoxetine combination in obsessive compulsive disorder. *Can J Psychiatry.* 1993;38(4):242–243.
18. Diniz JB, Shavitt RG, Pereira CAB, et al. Quetiapine versus clomipramine in the augmentation of selective serotonin reuptake inhibitors for the treatment of obsessive-compulsive disorder: a randomized, open-label trial. *J Psychopharmacol.* 2010;24(3):297–307.
19. Ravizza L, Barzega G, Bellino S, Bogetto F, Maina G. Drug treatment of obsessive-compulsive disorder (OCD): long-term trial with clomipramine and selective serotonin reuptake inhibitors (SSRIs). *Psychopharmacol Bull.* 1996;32(1):167–173.
20. Pallanti S, Quercioli L, Paiva R, Koran L. Citalopram for treatment-resistant obsessive-compulsive disorder. *Eur Psychiatry.* 1999;14(2):101–106.
21. Marazziti D, Golia F, Consoli G, et al. Effectiveness of long-term augmentation with citalopram to clomipramine in treatment-resistant OCD patients. *CNS Spectr.* 2008;13(11):971–976.
22. Andrade C. Augmenting selective serotonin reuptake inhibitors with clomipramine in obsessive-compulsive disorder: benefits and risks. *J Clin Psychiatry.* 2013;74(12):e1128–e1133.
23. Diniz JB, Costa DL, Cassab RC, Pereira CA, Miguel EC, Shavitt RG. The impact of comorbid body dysmorphic disorder on the response to sequential pharmacological trials for obsessive-compulsive disorder. *J Psychopharmacol.* 2013;28(6):603–611.

24. Trivedi MH, Fava M, Wisniewski SR, et al. Medication augmentation after the failure of SSRIs for depression. *N Engl J Med*. 2006;354(12):1243–1252.
25. Alevizos B, Lykouras L, Zervas I, Christodoulou G. Risperidone-induced obsessive-compulsive symptoms: a series of six cases. *J Clin Psychopharmacol*. 2002;22(5):461–467.
26. Alevizos B, Papageorgiou C, Christodoulou G. Obsessive-compulsive symptoms with olanzapine. *Int J Neuropsychopharmacol*. 2004;7(3):375–377.
27. Ercan ES, Ardic UA, Ercan E, Yuce D, Durak S. A promising preliminary study of aripiprazole for treatment-resistant childhood obsessive-compulsive disorder. *J Child Adolesc Psychopharmacol*. 2015;25(7):580–584.
28. Bloch M, Landeros-Weisenberger A, Kelmendi B, Coric V, Bracken M, Leckman J. A systematic review: antipsychotic augmentation with treatment refractory obsessive-compulsive disorder. *Mol Psychiatry*. 2006;11(7):622–632.
29. Albert U, Carmassi C, Cosci F, et al. Role and clinical implications of atypical antipsychotics in anxiety disorders, obsessive-compulsive disorder, trauma-related, and somatic symptom disorders: a systematized review. *Int Clin Psychopharmacol*. 2016;31(5):249–258.
30. Kim C, Koo M, Cheon K, Ryu Y, Lee J, Lee H. Dopamine transporter density of basal ganglia assessed with [123I]IPT SPET in obsessive-compulsive disorder. *Eur J Nucl Med Mol Imaging*. 2003;30(12):1637–1643.
31. van der Wee N, Stevens H, Hardeman J, et al. Enhanced dopamine transporter density in psychotropic-naive patients with obsessive-compulsive disorder shown by [123I]{beta}-CIT SPECT. *Am J Psychiatry*. 2004;161(12):2201–2206.
32. Cheon KA, Ryu YH, Namkoong K, Kim CH, Kim JJ, Lee JD. Dopamine transporter density of the basal ganglia assessed with [123I]IPT SPECT in drug-naïve children with Tourette's disorder. *Psychiatry Res*. 2004;130(1):85–95.
33. Winogrodzka A, Bergmans P, Booij J, van Royen EA, Stoof JC, Wolters EC. [(123)I]beta-CIT SPECT is a useful method for monitoring dopaminergic degeneration in early stage Parkinson's disease. *J Neurol Neurosurg Psychiatry*. 2003;74(3):294–298.
34. Dell'Osso B, Altamura AC, Allen A, Marazziti D, Hollander E. Epidemiologic and clinical updates on impulse control disorders: a critical review. *Eur Arch Psychiatry Clin Neurosci*. 2006;256(8):464–475.
35. Denys D, Klompmakers A, Westenberg H. Synergistic dopamine increase in the rat prefrontal cortex with the combination of quetiapine and fluvoxamine. *Psychopharmacology (Berl)*. 2004;176(2):195–203.
36. Zhang W, Perry K, Wong D, et al. Synergistic effects of olanzapine and other antipsychotic agents in combination with fluoxetine on norepinephrine and dopamine release in rat prefrontal cortex. *Neuropsychopharmacology*. 2000;23(3):250–262.
37. McDougle C, Goodman W, Leckman J, Lee N, Heninger G, Price L. Haloperidol addition in fluvoxamine-refractory obsessive-compulsive disorder. A double-blind, placebo-controlled study in patients with and without tics. *Arch Gen Psychiatry*. 1994;51(4):302–308.
38. McDougle C, Goodman W, Price L, et al. Neuroleptic addition in fluvoxamine-refractory obsessive-compulsive disorder. *Am J Psychiatry*. 1990;147(5):652–654.
39. Srour M, Lespérance P, Richer F, Chouinard S. Psychopharmacology of tic disorders. *J Can Acad Child Adolesc Psychiatry*. 2008;17(3):150–159.
40. Van Ameringen M, Mancini C, Oakman JM, Farvolden P. The potential role of haloperidol in the treatment of trichotillomania. *J Affect Disord*. 1999;56(2–3):219–226.
41. Dold M, Aigner M, Lanzenberger R, Kasper S. Antipsychotic augmentation of serotonin reuptake inhibitors in treatment-resistant obsessive-compulsive disorder: an update meta-analysis of double-blind, randomized, placebo-controlled trials. *Int J Neuropsychopharmacol*. 2015;18(9) pii: pyv047.
42. Van Ameringen M, Mancini C, Patterson B, Bennett M, Oakman J. A randomized, double-blind, placebo-controlled trial of olanzapine in the treatment of trichotillomania. *J Clin Psychiatry*. 2010;71(10):1336–1343.
43. Rothbart R, Stein DJ. Pharmacotherapy of trichotillomania (hair pulling disorder): an updated systematic review. *Expert Opin Pharmacother*. 2014;15(18):2709–2719.
44. Turner GA, Sutton S, Sharma A. Augmentation of venlafaxine with aripiprazole in a case of treatment-resistant excoriation disorder. *Innov Clin Neurosci*. 2014;11(1–2):29–31.
45. Luca M, Vecchio C, Luca A, Calandra C. Haloperidol augmentation of fluvoxamine in skin picking disorder: a case report. *J Med Case Rep*. 2012;6:219.
46. Phillips KA. Placebo-controlled study of pimozide augmentation of fluoxetine in body dysmorphic disorder. *Am J Psychiatry*. 2005;162(2):377–379.
47. Phillips KA. Olanzapine augmentation of fluoxetine in body dysmorphic disorder. *Am J Psychiatry*. 2005;162(5):1022–1023.
48. Nakaaki S, Murata Y, Furukawa TA. Efficacy of olanzapine augmentation of paroxetine therapy in patients with severe body dysmorphic disorder. *Psychiatry Clin Neurosci*. 2008;62(3):370.

49. Matsunaga H, Nagata T, Hayashida K, Ohya K, Kiriike N, Stein D. A long-term trial of the effectiveness and safety of atypical antipsychotic agents in augmenting SSRI-refractory obsessive-compulsive disorder. *J Clin Psychiatry*. 2009;70(6):863–868.

50. Cortese B, Phan K. The role of glutamate in anxiety and related disorders. *CNS Spectr*. 2005;10(10):820–830.

51. Bhattacharyya S, Chakraborty K. Glutamatergic dysfunction: newer targets for anti-obsessional drugs. *Recent Pat CNS Drug Discov*. 2007;2(1):47–55.

52. Stewart S, Fagerness J, Platko J, et al. Association of the SLC1A1 glutamate transporter gene and obsessive-compulsive disorder. *Am J Med Genet B Neuropsychiatr Genet*. 2007;144B(8):1027–1033.

53. Qin H, Samuels JF, Wang Y, et al. Whole-genome association analysis of treatment response in obsessive-compulsive disorder. *Mol Psychiatry*. 2016;21(2):270–276.

54. Pittenger C. Glutamate modulators in the treatment of obsessive-compulsive disorder. *Psychiatr Ann*. 2015;45(6):308–315.

55. Afshar H, Roohafza H, Mohammad-Beigi H, et al. N-acetylcysteine add-on treatment in refractory obsessive-compulsive disorder: a randomized, double-blind, placebo-controlled trial. *J Clin Psychopharmacol*. 2012;32(6):797–803.

56. Paydary K, Akamaloo A, Ahmadipour A, Pishgar F, Emamzadehfard S, Akhondzadeh S. N-acetylcysteine augmentation therapy for moderate-to-severe obsessive-compulsive disorder: randomized, double-blind, placebo-controlled trial. *J Clin Pharm Ther*. 2016;41(2):214–219.

57. Sarris J, Oliver G, Camfield DA, et al. N-acetyl cysteine (NAC) in the treatment of obsessive-compulsive disorder: a 16-week, double-blind, randomised, placebo-controlled study. *CNS Drugs*. 2015;29(9):801–809.

58. Grant JE, Odlaug BL, Kim SW. N-acetylcysteine, a glutamate modulator, in the treatment of trichotillomania: a double-blind, placebo-controlled study. *Arch Gen Psychiatry*. 2009;66(7):756–763.

59. Grant JE, Chamberlain SR, Redden SA, Leppink EW, Odlaug BL, Kim SW. N-acetylcysteine in the treatment of excoriation disorder: a randomized clinical trial. *JAMA Psychiatry*. 2016;73(5):490–496.

60. Donegan S, Dixon P, Hemming K, Tudur-Smith C, Marson A. A systematic review of placebo-controlled trials of topiramate: how useful is a multiple-indications review for evaluating the adverse events of an antiepileptic drug? *Epilepsia*. 2015;56(12):1910–1920.

61. Shank RP, Gardocki JF, Streeter AJ, Maryanoff BE. An overview of the preclinical aspects of topiramate: pharmacology, pharmacokinetics, and mechanism of action. *Epilepsia*. 2000;41 Suppl 1:S3–S9.

62. Berlin H, Koran L, Jenike M, et al. Double-blind, placebo-controlled trial of topiramate augmentation in treatment-resistant obsessive-compulsive disorder. *J Clin Psychiatry*. 2011;72(5):716–721.

63. Jankovic J, Jimenez-Shahed J, Brown LW. A randomised, double-blind, placebo-controlled study of topiramate in the treatment of Tourette syndrome. *J Neurol Neurosurg Psychiatry*. 2010;81(1):70–73.

64. Lochner C, Seedat S, Niehaus DJ, Stein DJ. Topiramate in the treatment of trichotillomania: an open-label pilot study. *Int Clin Psychopharmacol*. 2006;21(5):255–259.

65. Jafferany M, Osuagwu FC. Use of topiramate in skin-picking disorder: a pilot study. *Prim Care Companion CNS Disord*. 2017;19(1): doi: 10.4088/PCC.16m01961.

66. Jafferany M, Shireen F, Ibrahim A. An open-label trial of topiramate in the treatment of skin picking in pervasive developmental disorder not otherwise specified. *Prim Care Companion J Clin Psychiatry*. 2010;12(2): pii: PCC.09l00829.

67. Katoh-Semba R, Asano T, Ueda H, et al. Riluzole enhances expression of brain-derived neurotrophic factor with consequent proliferation of granule precursor cells in the rat hippocampus. *FASEB J*. 2002;16(10):1328–1330.

68. Pittenger C, Bloch MH, Wasylink S, et al. Riluzole augmentation in treatment-refractory obsessive-compulsive disorder: a pilot randomized placebo-controlled trial. *J Clin Psychiatry*. 2015;76(8):1075–1084.

69. Emamzadehfard S, Kamaloo A, Paydary K, et al. Riluzole in augmentation of fluvoxamine for moderate to severe obsessive compulsive disorder: randomized, double-blind, placebo-controlled study. *Psychiatry Clin Neurosci*. 2016;70(8):332–341.

70. Grant PJ, Joseph LA, Farmer CA, et al. 12-week, placebo-controlled trial of add-on riluzole in the treatment of childhood-onset obsessive-compulsive disorder. *Neuropsychopharmacology*. 2014;39(6):1453–1459.

71. Lemmon ME, Grados M, Kline T, Thompson CB, Ali SF, Singer HS. Efficacy of glutamate modulators in tic suppression: a double-blind, randomized control trial of d-serine and riluzole in Tourette syndrome. *Pediatr Neurol*. 2015;52(6):629–634.

72. Coric V, Kelmendi B, Pittenger C, Wasylink S, Bloch MH, Green J. Beneficial effects of the antiglutamatergic agent riluzole in a patient diagnosed with trichotillomania. *J Clin Psychiatry*. 2007;68(1):170–171.

73. Sasso DA, Kalanithi PS, Trueblood KV, et al. Beneficial effects of the glutamate-modulating agent

riluzole on disordered eating and pathological skin-picking behaviors. *J Clin Psychopharmacol.* 2006;26(6):685–687.

74. Reid JG, Gitlin MJ, Altshuler LL. Lamotrigine in psychiatric disorders. *J Clin Psychiatry.* 2013;74(7):675–684.

75. Bruno A, Micò U, Pandolfo G, et al. Lamotrigine augmentation of serotonin reuptake inhibitors in treatment-resistant obsessive-compulsive disorder: a double-blind, placebo-controlled study. *J Psychopharmacol.* 2012;26(11):1456–1462.

76. Bloom R, Amber KT. Identifying the incidence of rash, Stevens–Johnson syndrome and toxic epidermal necrolysis in patients taking lamotrigine: a systematic review of 122 randomized controlled trials. *An Bras Dermatol.* 2017;92(1):139–141.

77. Plosker GL, Lyseng-Williamson KA. Memantine: a pharmacoeconomic review of its use in moderate-to-severe Alzheimer's disease. *Pharmacoeconomics.* 2005;23(2):193–206.

78. Ghaleiha A, Entezari N, Modabbernia A, et al. Memantine add-on in moderate to severe obsessive-compulsive disorder: randomized double-blind placebo-controlled study. *J Psychiatr Res.* 2013;47(2):175–180.

79. Bartoli F, Riboldi I, Crocamo C, Di Brita C, Clerici M, Carrà G. Ketamine as a rapid-acting agent for suicidal ideation: a meta-analysis. *Neurosci Biobehav Rev.* 2017;77:232–236.

80. Rodriguez CI, Kegeles LS, Levinson A, et al. Randomized controlled crossover trial of ketamine in obsessive-compulsive disorder: proof-of-concept. *Neuropsychopharmacology.* 2013;38(12):2475–2483.

81. Rodriguez CI, Wheaton M, Zwerling J, et al. Can exposure-based CBT extend the effects of intravenous ketamine in obsessive-compulsive disorder? an open-label trial. *J Clin Psychiatry.* 2016;77(3):408–409.

82. Andrade C. Ondansetron augmentation of serotonin reuptake inhibitors as a treatment strategy in obsessive-compulsive disorder. *J Clin Psychiatry.* 2015;76(1):e72–e75.

83. Askari N, Moin M, Sanati M, et al. Granisetron adjunct to fluvoxamine for moderate to severe obsessive-compulsive disorder: a randomized, double-blind, placebo-controlled trial. *CNS Drugs.* 2012;26(10):883–892.

84. Shalbafan M, Mohammadinejad P, Shariat SV, et al. Celecoxib as an adjuvant to fluvoxamine in moderate to severe obsessive-compulsive disorder: a double-blind, placebo-controlled, randomized trial. *Pharmacopsychiatry.* 2015;48(4–5):136–140.

85. Koran L, Aboujaoude E, Bullock K, Franz B, Gamel N, Elliott M. Double-blind treatment with oral morphine in treatment-resistant obsessive-compulsive disorder. *J Clin Psychiatry.* 2005;66(3):353–359.

86. Hamon M, Blier P. Monoamine neurocircuitry in depression and strategies for new treatments. *Prog Neuropsychopharmacol Biol Psychiatry.* 2013;45:54–63.

87. Kennedy SH, Rizvi SJ. Emerging drugs for major depressive disorder. *Expert Opin Emerg Drugs.* 2009;14(3):439–453.

88. Grados M, Prazak M, Saif A, Halls A. A review of animal models of obsessive-compulsive disorder: a focus on developmental, immune, endocrine and behavioral models. *Expert Opin Drug Discov.* 2016;11(1):27–43.

89. Cobb J. Behaviour therapy in phobic and obsessional disorders. *Psychiatr Dev.* 1983;1(4):351–365.

90. Manos RC, Cahill SP, Wetterneck CT, Conelea CA, Ross AR, Riemann BC. The impact of experiential avoidance and obsessive beliefs on obsessive-compulsive symptoms in a severe clinical sample. *J Anxiety Disord.* 2010;24(7):700–708.

91. Katz D, Rector NA, Laposa JM. The interaction of distress tolerance and intolerance of uncertainty in the prediction of symptom reduction across CBT for social anxiety disorder. *Cogn Behav Ther.* 2017:1–19.

92. Costa DLDC, Barbosa VS, Requena G, Shavitt RG, Pereira CAB, Diniz JB. Dissecting the Yale-Brown Obsessive-Compulsive Scale severity scale to understand the routes for symptomatic improvement in obsessive-compulsive disorder. *J Psychopharmacol.* 2017:31(10):1312–1322.

93. Conceição CDL, Chagas AM, Arzeno FY, et al. Body dysmorphic disorder in patients with obsessive-compulsive disorder: prevalence and clinical correlates. *Depress Anxiety.* 2012;29(11):966–975.

94. Kelly MM, Walters C, Phillips KA. Social anxiety and its relationship to functional impairment in body dysmorphic disorder. *Behav Ther.* 2010;41(2):143–153.

95. American Psychiatric Association. *Diagnostic and Statistical Manual of Mental Disorders.* 5th ed. Washington, DC: APA; 2013.

96. Bohne A, Savage CR, Deckersbach T, Keuthen NJ, Wilhelm S. Motor inhibition in trichotillomania and obsessive-compulsive disorder. *J Psychiatr Res.* 2008;42(2):141–150.

97. Chamberlain S, Odlaug B, Boulougouris V, Fineberg N, Grant J. Trichotillomania: neurobiology and treatment. *Neurosci Biobehav Rev.* 2009;33(6):831–842.

98. Christenson GA, Mackenzie TB. Trichotillomania, body dysmorphic disorder, and obsessive-compulsive disorder. *J Clin Psychiatry.* 1995;56(5):211–212.

99. Arnold L, Auchenbach M, McElroy S. Psychogenic excoriation. Clinical features, proposed diagnostic criteria, epidemiology and approaches to treatment. *CNS Drugs*. 2001;15(5):351–359.

100. McGuire JF, Wu MS, Piacentini J, McCracken JT, Storch EA. A meta-analysis of d-cycloserine in exposure-based treatment: moderators of treatment efficacy, response, and diagnostic remission. *J Clin Psychiatry*. 2017;78(2):196–206.

101. Song C, Stevenson CW, Guimarães FS, Lee JL. Bidirectional effects of cannabidiol on contextual fear memory extinction. *Front Pharmacol.* 2016;7:493.

102. Jurkus R, Day HL, Guimarães FS, Lee JL, Bertoglio LJ, Stevenson CW. Cannabidiol regulation of learned fear: implications for treating anxiety-related disorders. *Front Pharmacol.* 2016;7:454.

103. Wang Y, Zhang X. FAAH inhibition produces antidepressant-like efforts of mice to acute stress via synaptic long-term depression. *Behav Brain Res.* 2017;324:138–145.

Chapter 19

Integrating Cognitive Behavioral Therapy and Medications for the Treatment of Obsessive-Compulsive Disorder

Yael R. Stovezky, Marina Gershkovich, Reilly Kayser and H. Blair Simpson

Introduction

Obsessive-compulsive disorder (OCD) is a disabling condition with a lifetime prevalence of 2–3% (i.e., two to three times more common than schizophrenia) [1]. There are two first-line treatments for OCD: pharmacotherapy with serotonin reuptake inhibitors (SRIs) and cognitive behavioral therapy (CBT) consisting of exposure and response prevention (ERP; see Chapters 15 and 16). Either alone or in combination, SRIs and ERP can help up to half of patients to achieve minimal symptoms and improved quality of life [2,3,4]. Nonetheless, many patients continue to experience clinically significant symptoms that impair their functioning and compromise their overall wellbeing.

This chapter reviews empirical evidence for combining pharmacotherapy and ERP in the treatment of OCD. First, we summarize randomized controlled trials (RCTs) that combined SRIs and ERP in treatment and consider the clinical conditions under which combined treatments can be effective. Second, we present novel pharmacological strategies for enhancing fear extinction learning that may be used to augment ERP.

In recent years, psychiatry has deemphasized observable phenomenology in favor of underlying neurobiological processes as a framework for conceptualizing psychiatric disorders. This transdiagnostic approach, as epitomized by the Research Domain Criteria (RDoC) project, proposes that dysfunction in distinguishable neurobehavioral domains underlies various forms of psychopathology. Focusing on domains of dysfunction rather than the traditional categorical diagnostic system provides a new perspective with which to investigate disorders such as OCD with the goal of moving toward a future of tailored psychiatric interventions. Of note, the studies documented in the literature and reviewed here focus on the treatment of OCD as a single categorical disorder. However, where possible, we will also reflect on combination strategies in the context of transdiagnostic approaches and their implications for the treatment of OCD.

Recent Research Findings

Combining Serotonin Reuptake Inhibitors and Cognitive Behavioral Therapy (Exposure and Response Prevention Based)

Overview

Several RCTs have examined the efficacy of combining SRIs and ERP treatments in individuals with OCD. These studies address two important questions. First, whether the simultaneous combination of an SRI and ERP is more effective than either treatment alone. Second, whether the sequential addition of ERP to an SRI trial is superior to continued SRI monotherapy or other augmentation strategies. This section briefly reviews these trials and highlights the main findings, which are summarized in Tables 19.1 and 19.2.

Randomized Controlled Trials that Simultaneously Combined Serotonin Reuptake Inhibitors and Cognitive Behavioral Therapy (Exposure and Response Prevention Based)

Several RCTs have examined whether the simultaneous delivery of SRIs and ERP (i.e., concurrent instigation of both treatments) is superior to either treatment alone (Table 19.1). Marks et al. [5] compared the outcome of 55 adults assigned to one of four groups: 6 months of the SRI clomipramine with: (i) instructions to not engage in exposures for 23 weeks; (ii) self-guided ERP for 23 weeks; (iii) self-guided ERP for 8 weeks followed

Table 19.1 Randomized controlled trials that simultaneously combined serotonin reuptake inhibitors and cognitive behavioral therapy in obsessive-compulsive disorder.

Study	Patients		Treatment arms		Study Duration (weeks)	Y-BOCS total score			Main Findings
	Population	Entered Study (*n*)	Treatments	Entered Study (*n*)		Pre-treatment Mean (SD)	Post-treatment Mean (SD)	Type of Data Analysis	
Marks et al., 1988	Adults	55	CMI + ERP (s)	12[a]	23	–	–	n/a	At week 8: CMI+ ERP (s) > CMI+ AE CMI+ ERP (s) > PBO+ ERP (s) At week 23: CMI+ ERP (s & t) = PBO + ERP (s & t)
			CMI + AE	12[a]					
			CMI + ERP (s &t)	13[a]					
			PBO + ERP (s & t)	12[a]					
Cottraux et al., 1990	Adults	60	FLV + ERP	20	24	–	–	n/a	FLV + ERP = PBO + ERP= FLV + AE FLV + ERP > PBO + ERP on measures of depression
			PBO – ERP	20					
			FLV + AE	20					
Hohagen et al., 1998	Adults	60	FLV + BT (including ERP)	30	9	27.9 (2.9) CM	12.4 (6.8)	CM	At week 9: FLV + BT (including ERP) = PBO + BT (including ERP) (Total Y-BOCS score) FLV + BT (including ERP) > PBO + BT (including ERP) (Y-BOCS obsession subscale) Patients with comorbid depression fared better with FLV + BT (including ERP) than with PBO + BT (including ERP)
			PBO – BT (including ERP)	30		28.4 (3.8) CM	15.9 (7.9)		
Foa et al., 2005	Adults	122	CMI + ERP	31	12	25.4 (4.6)	10.5 (8.2)	OM	CMI + ERP = ERP > CMI
			CMI	36		26.3 (4.4)	18.2 (7.8)		
			ERP	29		24.6 (4.8)	11.0 (7.9)		
			PBO	26		25.0 (4.0)	22.2 (6.4)		
POTS, 2004	Children	112	CBT	28	12	26.0 (4.6)[b]	14.0 (9.5)[b]	EM(LOCF)	CBT + SER > CBT = SER
			SER	28		23.5 (4.7)[b]	16.5 (9.1)[b]		
			CBT + SER	28		23.8 (3.0)[b]	11.2 (8.6)[b]		
			Placebo	28		25.2 (3.3)[b]	21.5 (5.4)[b]		

[a] Numbers were provided only for patients who completed treatment.
[b] The Children's Yale-Brown Obsessive-Compulsive Scale (CY-BOCS) means (and standard deviations) are presented.
AE, anti-exposure instructions; BT, behavioral therapy; CM, completers means; CMI, clomipramine; CT, cognitive therapy; EM(LOCF), estimated means (last observation carried forward); ERP, exposure and response prevention; FLV, fluvoxamine; OM, observed means; PBO, pill placebo; R, relaxation therapy; s, self-controlled; SER, sertraline; t, therapist-aided; Y-BOCS, Yale-Brown Obsessive Compulsive Scale.

Table 19.2 Randomized controlled trials that sequentially combined serotonin reuptake inhibitors and cognitive behavioral therapy in obsessive-compulsive disorder.

Study	Patients		Treatment Arms		Duration (weeks)	Y-BOCS Total Score			Main Findings
	Population	Entered Study (*n*)	Treatment	Entered Study (*n*)		Pre-treatment mean (SD)	Post-treatment mean (SD/CI)	Type of Data Analysis	
Marks et al., 1980	Adults	50	CMI → + ERP	10[a]	10	–	–	n/a	At week 7 (improvement in rituals): CMI + ERP > PBO + ERP CMI + ERP > CMI + R
			CMI → + R → + ERP	10[a]					
			PBO → + ERP	10[a]					
			PBO → + R→ + ERP	10[a]					
Van Balkom et al., 1998	Adults	117	FLV → + CT	24	16	27.2 (5.7)	15.6 (5.4)	CM	FLV + CT = FLV + ERP =ERP=CT
			FLV → + ERP	28		24.7 (7.9)	12.6 (6.6)		
			CT	25		25.3 (6.6)	13.5 (9.7)		
			ERP	22		25.0 (7.9)	17.1 (8.4)		
			WT	18		26.8 (6.4)	n/a		
Tenneij et al., 2005	Adults	96	SRI → + ERP	47	24	14.47 (4.93)	10.56 (7.77)	CM	SRI + ERP > SRI SRI + ERP starting at 3 months > SRI + ERP starting at 9 months
			SRI → → → +ERP	49		14.5 (6.17)	18.36 (7.95)		
Simpson et al., 2008	Adults	108	SRI → + ERP	54	8	25.4 (4.7)	14.2 (6.6)	OM	SRI + ERP > SRI+ SMT
			SRI → + SMT	54		26.2 (4.4)	22.6 (6.3)		
Simpson et al., 2013	Adults	100	SRI → + ERP	40	8	27.2 (3.9)	13.0 (6.1)	OM	SRI + ERP > SRI+ RSP = SRI+ PBO
			SRI → + RSP	40		26.1 (4.3)	22.6 (8.8)		
			SRI → + PBO	20		25.9 (6.9)	23.1 (6.9)		
Franklin et al., 2011	Children	124	SRI → + CBT-I	40	12	27.4 (4.75)[b]	20.05 (95%CI:17.45, 22.65)[b]	EM(MEM)	SRI+ CBT > SRI SRI+ CBT > SRI + CBT-I
			SRI → + CBT	42		25.45 (5.18)[b]	14.23 (95%CI:11.85, 16.62)[b]		
			SRI	42		26.08 (5.12)[b]	21.35 (95%CI:18.89, 23.80)[b]		

[a] Numbers were provided only for patients who completed treatment.
[b] The Children's Yale-Brown Obsessive-Compulsive Scale (CY-BOCS) means (and standard deviations) are presented.
AE, anti-exposure instructions; BT, behavioral therapy; CBT-I, CBT instructions; CM, completers means; CMI, clomipramine; CT, cognitive therapy; EM(MEM), estimated means (mixed effects models); ERP, exposure and response prevention; FLV, fluvoxamine; OM, observed means; PBO, pill placebo; R, relaxation therapy; RSP, risperidone; SMT, stress management training; WL, wait list control; Y-BOCS, Yale-Brown Obsessive Compulsive Scale.

by therapist-guided exposure for 15 weeks or iv) 6 months of placebo and 8 weeks of self-guided ERP followed by therapist-guided exposure for 15 weeks. Self-guided ERP consisted of instructions to make contact with feared stimuli and to refrain from ritualizing for increasingly longer periods. Therapist-guided exposure consisted of two-hour weekly sessions, though the number of sessions varied from 5 to 15. Evaluators blind to treatment assignment assessed OCD symptom severity and mood throughout the study using measures of ritual severity (e.g., time) and depression (e.g., Hamilton Depression Rating Scale, HAM-D) [6]). At week 8, among the 49 patients who completed the study, clomipramine plus self-guided ERP produced significantly greater improvements in symptoms of OCD and depression than placebo plus self-guided ERP. However, at week 23, clomipramine plus ERP (self-guided and therapist-aided) showed no superiority over placebo plus ERP (self-guided and therapist-aided). The authors concluded that the combination of clomipramine and ERP had a small short-term additive effect compared with placebo plus ERP. However, given the complexity of the study design, lack of standardized OCD measures and suboptimal clomipramine doses (mean dose for clomipramine groups was 127–157 mg), further research was needed.

Cottraux et al. [7] compared the efficacy of fluvoxamine plus ERP, fluvoxamine plus anti-ERP (i.e., instructions not to engage in exposures) and placebo plus ERP for a period of 24 weeks in 60 adults with OCD, many with major depressive or dysthymic disorder at baseline (43% of study completers). ERP consisted of eight weekly sessions that included imaginal exposure with a therapist and self-controlled exposure between sessions followed by 16 weeks of therapist-guided exposure. Raters blind to treatment assignment evaluated severity of rituals (e.g., duration of rituals per day) and depression (HAM-D) at baseline and post-treatment. Among the 44 treatment completers, all groups improved on some measures of rituals and depression from week 0 to week 24, but only the fluvoxamine plus ERP group showed improvements in all symptom domains. This group had the largest percentage reduction in the duration of rituals per day (fluvoxamine plus ERP = 46%; fluvoxamine plus anti-ERP = 42%; placebo plus ERP = 25%; not significant). Despite methodological limitations (e.g., heterogeneity of sample with regard to comorbid depression, full data only presented for treatment completers), the findings suggest that combination treatment may be somewhat superior to monotherapy in adults with OCD and comorbid depression.

Hohagen and colleagues [8] compared the efficacy of behavioral therapy plus fluvoxamine or behavioral therapy plus placebo in 60 adults with OCD. Behavioral therapy consisted of ERP, cognitive restructuring and development of alternative behaviors, and was delivered weekly for nine weeks. Evaluators blind to treatment assignment conducted weekly assessments of OCD symptoms and mood using the Yale-Brown Obsessive Compulsive Scale (Y-BOCS) [9,10] and the HAM-D, respectively. After nine treatment weeks, the 49 patients who completed treatment and were included in the final analysis showed significant Y-BOCS reductions. However, there were significantly more responders (i.e., Y-BOCS reduction 35% or greater) in the behavioral therapy plus fluvoxamine group (87.5%) than in the behavioral therapy plus placebo group (60%). A secondary analysis revealed that the two groups produced comparable reductions in compulsions, but the behavioral therapy plus fluvoxamine group significantly reduced obsessions. Furthermore, patients with co-occurring depression at baseline who received behavioral therapy plus placebo experienced significantly worse treatment outcome than all other groups. One study limitation is that patients with a previous history of ERP non-response were included, but their distribution in the two treatment groups was not reported; moreover, the therapy was multimodal and therapist adherence to the treatment manual was not formally assessed. Nonetheless, the authors concluded that behavioral therapy combined with fluvoxamine could produce greater gains when obsessions are primary or when comorbid depression is present.

Foa, Liebowitz and colleagues [2] conducted a multisite RCT in 122 non-depressed adult outpatients with OCD, comparing ERP, clomipramine, their combination and pill placebo for 12 weeks. The ERP was a manual-based, empirically validated intervention consisting of 17 sessions delivered intensively over four weeks of therapist-guided and homework exposures followed by eight weekly maintenance sessions. Evaluators blind to treatment assignment assessed OCD severity using the Y-BOCS. An intent-to-treat analysis indicated that combined treatment (clomipramine plus ERP) was superior to clomipramine alone but not over ERP alone. One study limitation is that the simultaneous instigation of ERP and slow upward titration of clomipramine meant that the intensive phase of ERP (the first four weeks) was completed before the full impact of the drug could be realized, and significantly fewer patients in the combined group than the clomipramine only group achieved the maximum drug dose at week 12 (37.5% vs. 77% of treatment completers). Thus, the sensitivity of this design to the effects of combining clomipramine with ERP may have been compromised in favor of the effects of ERP. Second, data on patients who withdrew participation after randomization but before any treatment commenced was not collected. Despite these limitations, these data demonstrate that clomipramine, ERP and their combination are all efficacious treatments for OCD. The authors concluded that intensive ERP may be superior to clomipramine and, by implication, to monotherapy with the other SRIs, when delivered intensely to patients with OCD without comorbid depression by skilled therapists. This was the largest RCT to date to investigate the efficacy of a simultaneous delivery of SRIs and ERP in adults with OCD.

The comparative efficacy of CBT consisting of ERP, SRIs and their combination has also been studied in children and adolescents with OCD. Paralleling the study design of Foa et al. in adults [2], the Pediatric OCD Treatment Study [11] compared CBT alone, SRI alone (sertraline), their combinations and a pill placebo in 112 patients aged 7–17 years for 12 weeks. CBT treatment consisted of 14 visits of approximately one hour in length over 12 weeks, which involved ERP, psychoeducation and cognitive training. Raters blind to treatment assignment evaluated OCD severity using the Children's Yale-Brown Obsessive-Compulsive Scale (CY-BOCS) [12]. In an intention to treat analysis, all treatments were superior to placebo, and combination treatment was superior to CBT or SRI alone. Importantly, there was significant site × treatment interaction: the effects of CBT alone were greater at one of the sites, whereas no site effect was found for the combined treatment. One interpretation of this interaction is that the effects of ERP vary depending on who delivers it. The authors concluded that treatment of children and adolescents with OCD should begin with either the combination of SRIs and CBT (including ERP) or with CBT alone.

In summary, a few RCTs examined the effects of simultaneously combining SRIs with ERP compared with either treatment alone. The evidence suggests that simultaneous instigation of ERP and SRIs might be superior to monotherapy in some patients with OCD, but is not necessary for all. Specifically, the data indicate that combination therapy can be superior to: (i) ERP monotherapy in adult patients with OCD with comorbid depression [8]; (ii) SRI monotherapy in adult patients with OCD without comorbid depression [2]; and (iii) ERP and SRI monotherapies in children and adolescents without comorbid depression [11]. However, when compared to ERP alone when optimally delivered in adult patients with OCD without comorbid depression, combined treatment produced no additive gains [2].

Several factors complicate direct comparisons between these studies and highlight the need for nuanced conclusions. First, the studies differed in their specific designs as well as in patient selection criteria (OCD severity, comorbid disorders) and outcome measures. Second, while ERP was delivered in all studies, key features of the treatment such as frequency and length of sessions, therapist adherence to the treatment protocol, and patient compliance with homework assignments, either clearly varied among the studies or were not formally assessed. Yet, data show that for optimal effect, ERP requires delivery by a skilled therapist and a high level of patient engagement with treatment procedures both in and outside of therapy sessions [13,14]. Finally, there are limited data on long-term benefits after acute treatment and the data that do exist are often confounded by the lack of blind ratings and/or inconsistencies in whether additional treatment was received during follow-up [5,15]. Of all studies in the review above, only Foa and colleagues provide follow-up data after sustained treatment discontinuation using evaluators who were blind to treatment assignment [16]. Their findings show that, 12 weeks after treatment discontinuation, those who responded to ERP with or without concomitant clomipramine ($n = 33$) compared with those who responded to clomipramine only ($n = 11$) had a significantly lower relapse rate (12% vs. 45%) and a significantly longer time to relapse. More research is needed to further characterize the long-term benefits of combination treatments.

Globally, these data from RCTs demonstrate that SRIs, CBT and their combinations are all effective treatments for OCD. At the same time, the ideal treatment choice for any patient is the one that not only has empirical support, but is also safe and acceptable for that individual. Patients with OCD have strong treatment preferences [17,18], some refusing medication, and others having difficulty engaging in psychotherapy. These preferences, alongside safety and cost effectiveness, contribute to the patient's unique clinical profile and should guide the treatment plan most suitable for the individual. Recognizing this complexity, the American Psychiatric Association practice guidelines for the treatment of OCD [19,20] recommend SRIs, ERP or their combination as first-line interventions.

Randomized Controlled Trials that Sequentially Combined Serotonin Reuptake Inhibitors and Exposure and Response Prevention Based Cognitive Behavioral Therapy

An alternative approach to combining SRIs and CBT involves the addition of ERP after SRI treatment has already been initiated. Several RCTs have examined this strategy (Table 19.2). Marks et al. [21] compared the efficacy of a sequential combination of ERP and an SRI in 50 adults with OCD with varying degrees of depression. Patients were randomly assigned to clomipramine or placebo for eight months. During weeks 4–7, these two groups were each randomly assigned to ERP or relaxation training. Subsequently, through weeks 7–10, all patients received ERP, which consisted of daily 45-minute sessions of in-vivo ERP. Relaxation training consisted of daily 45-minute sessions of therapist instruction on how to tense and relax different parts of the body. Evaluators blind to treatment assignment assessed obsessive-compulsive symptom severity and mood throughout the study using measures of ritual severity (e.g., time) and depression (e.g., HAM-D). At week 7, among the 40 patients who completed treatment, clomipramine plus ERP was associated with greater reductions in rituals compared with clomipramine plus relaxation training or placebo plus ERP. In addition, patients receiving clomipramine demonstrated better compliance with exposure instructions both during and between sessions than patients receiving placebo plus ERP. Owing to the study's design, direct comparisons of the four treatments were not possible beyond week 7. Study limitations include the lack of standardized measures, small sample and complex study design. Nonetheless, the authors concluded that the sequential addition of ERP to clomipramine had a small additive effect at week 7 and that clomipramine enhanced compliance with ERP.

In another study, Van Balkom et al. [22] randomized 112 adult patients to one of five conditions: (i) cognitive therapy for weeks 1–16; (ii) ERP for weeks 1–16; (iii) fluvoxamine for weeks 1–16 plus cognitive therapy in weeks 9–16 (ten sessions); (iv) fluvoxamine for weeks 1–16 plus ERP in weeks 9–16 (ten sessions); or (v) waiting list control condition for 8 weeks. Cognitive therapy consisted of identifying anxiety evoking automatic thoughts and replacing them with alternative, non-distressing thoughts. ERP consisted of gradual self-controlled exposure in-vivo with gradual response prevention. All therapy sessions were 45 minutes long. Evaluators blind to treatment assignment assessed OCD severity with the Y-BOCS. Among treatment completers (n = 86), all active treatments led to a significant decrease in obsessive-compulsive symptoms with no significant differences between them. Study limitations include the fact that while patients in the psychotherapy only groups (cognitive therapy or ERP) received a total of 16 therapy sessions, the patients in the fluvoxamine groups received only 10 sessions. Additionally, the ERP protocol included self-controlled rather than therapist-guided exposures. Lastly, the fluvoxamine dosing was not optimized (mean dose at week 16 in both fluvoxamine conditions was 197.1 mg (standard deviation 82.0 mg)). Despite these limitations, the authors concluded that the sequential combination of fluvoxamine with cognitive therapy or ERP was not superior to either cognitive therapy or ERP alone.

Tenneij et al. [23] randomized 96 adult patients who had a partial response to 3 months of SRI treatment to receive either an addition of ERP or continue pharmacotherapy alone for 6 months. Those who continued pharmacotherapy ultimately received the addition of ERP at the end of the study for an additional period of 6 months. The ERP consisted of 18 45-minute sessions of self-controlled in-vivo exposure with response prevention. Raters blind to treatment assignment assessed OCD severity and mood using the Y-BOCS and the HAM-D, respectively. Intention to treat analyses found sequential treatment to be superior to pharmacotherapy alone in reducing OCD symptoms. Significantly more patients receiving ERP achieved remission (i.e., a Y-BOCS score ≤ 8) compared with patients on medication alone (40% versus 15%). However, the authors also found that adding ERP after nine months of medication led to a nonsignificant reduction in obsessive-compulsive symptoms. In addition, the dropout rate in the combined treatment group (30%) was substantially higher than in the medication alone condition

(6%). Despite several limitations (suboptimal ERP session time, low mean Y-BOCS score at baseline), the authors concluded that ERP can effectively improve treatment gains for patients who respond to an SRI when added immediately after attaining SRI response, but not necessarily if the patient has been on the SRI for nine months.

Following this study, Simpson et al. [24] conducted a two-site RCT in 108 adult patients taking SRIs for at least three months who remained at least moderately ill (Y-BOCS score ≥ 16). Patients were randomized to receive either the addition of ERP or stress management training while continuing their SRI pharmacotherapy for eight weeks. The format of both CBT treatments was identical: 17 twice-weekly sessions (each 90–120 minutes), daily homework assignments and between-session phone calls (twice per week, each less than 20 minutes). Stress management training included training in relaxation techniques, assertiveness training and problem solving. Raters blind to treatment assignment evaluated OCD symptom severity and mood using the Y-BOCS and HAM-D, respectively. After 17 sessions (week 8), ERP was superior to stress management training in reducing OCD symptoms. Moreover, significantly more patients receiving ERP than patients receiving stress management training had a decrease in symptom severity of at least 25% (74% vs. 22%) and achieved minimal symptoms (Y-BOCS score ≤ 12; 33% versus 4%). Limitations include the lack of objective measures of SRI response prior to study entry. These data suggest that the addition of ERP to continuing SRI pharmacotherapy is an effective strategy for reducing obsessive-compulsive symptoms.

Simpson et al. [25] conducted another two-site RCT investigating the efficacy of ERP compared with risperidone in augmenting SRI treatment for OCD in 100 adults with moderate to severe obsessive-compulsive symptoms despite an SRI trial of at least three months at a stable dose (Y-BOCS score ≥ 16). SRI augmentation with antipsychotics has been shown to be effective in some RCTs in adults with OCD [26,27,28,29]. While continuing their SRI at the same dose, patients were randomized to eight weeks of risperidone ($n = 40$), ERP (17 sessions delivered twice weekly; $n = 40$) or pill placebo (n = 20). Raters blind to treatment assignment assessed OCD severity using the Y-BOCS. At week 8, patients on SRIs receiving ERP had significantly greater Y-BOCS reductions than those receiving risperidone or placebo using mixed effects models. Patients taking SRIs and receiving risperidone did not significantly differ from those receiving placebo. Moreover, significantly more patients on SRIs receiving ERP achieved minimal symptoms (Y-BOCS score ≤ 12: 43% for ERP, 13% for risperidone and 5% for placebo). These effects were maintained at six-month follow-up [30]. Factors like differential expectancy (patients receiving ERP knew they were receiving therapy, whereas those taking a pill understood they had a one-third chance of receiving placebo), and clinician contact (the ERP group had substantially more hours of clinical contact than the other two groups) may have affected the outcome. However, these data indicate that adding ERP to SRIs can produce superior results to both risperidone and pill placebo. With this in mind, the authors concluded that patients with OCD receiving SRIs who continue to have clinically significant symptoms should be offered ERP before augmenting with an antipsychotic agent, particularly given their known medical risks.

The effects of augmenting SRIs with CBT have also been examined in pediatric patients. Franklin et al. [31] conducted a 12-week multisite RCT in 7–17-year-old patients with clinically significant obsessive-compulsive symptoms despite an adequate SRI trial (CY-BOCS ≥ 16). Patients were randomly assigned to three treatment groups: (i) medication management only ($n = 42$), (ii) medication management plus CBT ($n = 42$) or (iii) medication management plus instructions in CBT (CBT-Instruction) ($n = 40$). CBT treatment included 14 one-hour visits involving ERP, psychoeducation and cognitive training. CBT-Instruction consisted of similar CBT components without therapist-assisted exposure, delivered by the pharmacotherapist assigned to manage medication. Raters blind to treatment assignment assessed OCD severity using the CY-BOCS. At 12 weeks, an intention to treat analysis revealed that 68.6% in the CBT group responded to treatment (defined as a CY-BOCS reduction of 30%), compared with 34.0% in the CBT-Instruction group, and 30.0% in the medication management only group. Despite differences in clinical contact time and intensity of treatment, these data suggest that medication combined with CBT is superior to medication monotherapy and to augmentation with CBT-Instruction and provide support for the use of ERP as an augmentative treatment for pediatric patients with OCD.

In conclusion, adding CBT, specifically ERP, to continuing SRI treatment can be beneficial for patients who remain symptomatic despite an adequate SRI trial. Three large RCTs in adults found ERP to be superior to continued SRIs monotherapy [23], stress-management training [24] and antipsychotic augmentation [25]. In all three studies, significantly more patients receiving ERP achieved minimal symptoms. In children and adolescents with OCD, adding CBT that included ERP to SRI medication alone also led to significantly greater response rates than SRIs alone [31]. Taken together, these findings strongly support using ERP as an initial SRI augmentation strategy in patients of all ages with OCD. What remains unclear is whether patients with OCD on SRIs who attain minimal symptoms after ERP is added can then safely discontinue their SRI and still maintain their wellness. Indeed, for many individuals, the side effects of SRIs (e.g., decreased sexual desire, headaches, insomnia, weight gain) become difficult to endure over time and some may for this reason wish to discontinue the medication. The collection of empirical data related to this question is under way [32,33].

Future Directions

As psychiatry continues to examine domains and constructs of relevance to OCD across different units of analysis (i.e., genes, circuits, behavior and others), we hope that our understanding of the pathogenesis, classification and treatment of OCD will become more nuanced. Few transdiagnostic treatment studies have yet been done. Moreover, the mapping of obsessive-compulsive symptoms (compulsions, obsessions and anxiety) to neurobehavioral domains of dysfunction remains a work in progress (as reviewed in Kalanthroff et al. [34]). Success in this approach may not only reveal why particular individuals respond differently to SRIs, ERP or their combination, but also lead to more specific treatment targets and novel interventions, including new ways to combine cognitive behavioral therapy and medications. To date, an association between compulsive behaviors and deficits in cognitive control and in reward processing has been documented in the literature. In addition, studies have found an association between anxiety and abnormal fear processing. Obsessions have been more difficult to map to the existing transdiagnostic domains and constructs. Pharmacological agents and behavioral approaches that act on specific dysfunctional domains, alone or in combination, may provide a path toward developing more precise treatments, such as interventions to increase cognitive control or to enhance extinction learning. Nonetheless, it is important to keep in mind that the domains and constructs of the RDoC matrix are unlikely to be independent of one another [34]. Examining the role of individual domains may lead to a fragmented understanding of compulsions, obsessions and anxiety. Multidimensional models may allow for more effective investigations into the underlying mechanisms that give rise to OCD symptomatology and elucidate shared mechanisms across disorders. This approach may pave the way to transdiagnostic treatments that target neurobiological processes and that address pathophysiology directly.

A Transdiagnostic Approach to Cognitive Behavioral Therapy Augmentation: Pharmacological Enhancement of Learning and Related Approaches

Overview

The studies discussed in the previous section focus on combining SRIs with ERP. Recent insights into the neural mechanisms of learning, including extinction learning, suggest that it may also be possible to use other medications to augment ERP. This work is briefly reviewed below. Findings are considered from the perspective of a transdiagnostic approach.

D-Cycloserine

D-cycloserine (DCS) is a partial agonist that increases excitatory neurotransmission by binding at the glycine/D-serine site on the N-methyl-D-aspartate (NMDA) receptor. One of several glutamate receptor subtypes, NMDA is a major player in the glutamatergic neurotransmitter system and is important for memory, learning and synaptic plasticity. Evidence from the animal literature suggests that pharmacological modulation of the NMDA receptor by DCS may enhance associative learning processes involved in fear extinction [35,36]. As such, DCS is an attractive agent with a transdiagnostic potential to augment exposure-based treatments for multiple disorders.

DCS has been tested as a psychotherapy adjuvant in the treatment of anxiety disorders including specific phobias [37,38,39], panic disorder [40,41] and social anxiety [42,43,44,45], with mixed results. In OCD, DCS augmentation studies have produced inconsistent results. Four RCTs have compared ERP with exposure augmented by DCS in adults with OCD. In two of these studies, DCS reduced the time to response, but did not result in an increased response by the end of the trial [46,47]. The other two RCTs found no group differences in symptom improvements at any point during or after treatment [48,49]. Paralleling findings in adults, the use of DCS as a psychotherapy adjuvant produced mixed results in the treatment of pediatric OCD. Three RCTs compared the efficacy of ERP with that of DCS-augmented exposure [50,51,52]. Only one study [49] found an additional benefit to DCS augmentation relative to placebo augmentation, with significantly greater improvements in OCD severity from post-treatment to one-month follow-up. As in the other pediatric RCTs, no significant differences were found at any other point during or after treatment.

Owing to these mixed results in OCD, DCS is not typically used in clinical practice. A recent meta-analysis found D-cycloserine to be associated with a small augmentation effect on exposure-based therapy for anxiety, obsessive-compulsive and posttraumatic stress disorders [53]. Whether DCS can indeed accelerate the rate of treatment response or can be used effectively in later periods of treatment by manipulating the dosage regimen remains to be answered. It may also be the case that the effect of DCS varies as a function of within-session learning experiences. Investigations in patients who do not have OCD suggest that DCS can exert its desired effects when applied after a successful exposure session and less so when inadequate fear attenuation has been achieved [53]. More research may provide clearer insight into the therapy conditions under which DCS may be effective and the patient profile for whom this intervention may be best suited.

Ketamine

Convergent evidence from genetic studies, imaging studies and animal models suggests that glutamatergic dysfunction contributes to OCD pathophysiology [54,55,56,57,58,59]. Ketamine is a noncompetitive antagonist of the NMDA glutamate receptor with powerful and often immediate therapeutic effects in depression and other disorders [60,61]. In addition, findings from the animal literature suggest that ketamine's effects on NMDA receptor-mediated neurotransmission and subsequent intracellular signaling pathways can impact plasticity and extinction learning [62,63,64].

The possibility of using ketamine in the treatment of OCD arose from a proof-of-concept crossover study by Rodriguez et al. in 2013, in which a single dose of intravenous ketamine (0.5 mg/kg) led to the rapid resolution of obsessions in unmedicated patients with OCD [65]. Adults with near-constant obsessions received two intravenous infusions of saline and ketamine spaced at least one week apart. One week post-infusion, 50% of those receiving ketamine met criteria for treatment response (≥ 35% Y-BOCS reduction) compared with none of those receiving placebo. In another 2016 open-label trial [66], Rodriguez and colleagues examined the possibility of using ketamine to enhance the extinction learning that occurs in ERP treatment. This study involved a single 40-minute intravenous infusion of ketamine (dose 0.5 mg/kg), followed by ten one-hour exposure sessions delivered over two weeks. In this open trial, the authors found that 63% of patients demonstrated treatment response (≥ 35% Y-BOCS reduction) at two weeks post-injection. Future research is required to inform the current debate surrounding ketamine's mechanism of action and to better evaluate its ability to potentiate ERP in OCD.

Other Fear Extinction Modulators

Many other pharmacological agents have been proposed to facilitate extinction processes in animals and humans, including noradrenergic drugs (propranolol), neuropeptides, glucocorticoids, GABA receptor antagonists, dopaminergic agents, histone acetylation modulators, endocannabinoids and others [67]. Some of these agents are thought to promote fear reduction by enhancing the plastic properties of associative learning, while others are believed to interfere with the protein-synthesis dependent process of feared memory reconsolidation. Considerable evidence in the animal literature demonstrates that it may indeed be possible to pharmacologically modulate both extinction and memory reconsolidation to reduce fear [67,68,69,70,71]. Given that both these processes are foundational to exposure-based treatments that cut across disorder categories, fear extinction modulators can potentially be beneficial as a transdiagnostic augmentation strategy for individuals with different anxiety disorders. Several studies in humans in other anxiety disorders [72,73,74] suggest that some of these agents may indeed enhance exposure-based treatments. Further research in OCD is necessary.

Conclusions

CBT consisting of ERP and SRIs are the first line of interventions for OCD. Either alone or in combination, these treatments effectively promote reductions in symptoms, allowing some but not all patients to achieve wellness. The data suggest that simultaneous delivery of CBT and SRIs as initial treatment (i.e., concurrent instigation of both treatments) generally produces little to no additive gains compared with CBT alone, when CBT is optimally delivered. However, sequential addition of CBT to pharmacotherapy with an SRI produces substantial benefits in patients who remain symptomatic after an SRI trial. Nonetheless, clinical issues such as other comorbid disorders, safety, cost effectiveness and patient preferences warrant careful consideration when establishing a treatment plan.

A recent wave of pharmacological research aims to enhance and accelerate the fear extinction learning that occurs in exposure-based therapies. To date, several agents have been proposed including glutamate modulators (DCS, ketamine) but data are inconclusive and more studies are needed in OCD. In addition, a variety of novel non-pharmacological approaches to enhancing fear-extinction learning are actively being studied [75,76,77,78]. More research is needed to clarify the neurobiological and clinical plausibility of ERP augmentation strategies.

As psychiatry continues to conceptualize disorders through an RDoC lens, the neurobiological processes that lead to the characteristic symptoms of OCD and the interaction between them are likely to become more clear. To date, few transdiagnostic treatment studies of relevance to patients with OCD have been documented. Furthermore, the link between OCD symptoms and neurobehavioral domains of dysfunction remains to be established. As animal investigations and human clinical trials continue to advance, treatments for OCD may become more targeted toward underlying pathophysiology. Finally, advances in our understanding of transdiagnostic genetic vulnerability and underlying neural processes have the potential to pave the way toward a precision medicine approach to the treatment of OCD. This may enable us one day to predict with accuracy how best to integrate CBT and medications in individuals with OCD based on the neurobiological domains implicated in the disorder so that more can attain and maintain wellness.

References

1. Ruscio AM, Stein DJ, Chiu WT, Kessler RC. The epidemiology of obsessive-compulsive disorder in the National Comorbidity Survey Replication. *Mol Psychiatry*. 2010;15(1):53–63.
2. Foa EB, Liebowitz MR, Kozak MJ, et al. Randomized, placebo-controlled trial of exposure and ritual prevention, clomipramine, and their combination in the treatment of obsessive-compulsive disorder. *Am J Psychiatry*. 2005;162(1):151–161.
3. Simpson HB, Foa EB, Liebowitz MR, et al. Cognitive-behavioral therapy vs risperidone for augmenting serotonin reuptake inhibitors in obsessive-compulsive disorder: a randomized clinical trial. *JAMA Psychiatry*. 2013;70(11):1190–1199.
4. Simpson HB, Huppert JD, Petkova E, Foa EB, Liebowitz MR. Response versus remission in obsessive-compulsive disorder. *J Clin Psychiatry*. 2006;67(2):269–276.
5. Marks IM, Lelliott P, Basoglu M, et al. Clomipramine, self-exposure and therapist-aided exposure for obsessive-compulsive rituals. *Br J Psychiatry*. 1988;152(4):522–534.
6. Hamilton M. A rating scale for depression. *J Neurol Neurosurg Psychiatry*. 1960;23(1):56–62.
7. Cottraux J, Mollard E, Bouvard M, et al. A controlled study of fluvoxamine and exposure in obsessive-compulsive disorder. *Int Clin Psychopharmacol*. 1990;5(1):17–30.
8. Hohagen F, Winkelmann G, Rasche-Räuchle H, et al. Combination of behaviour therapy with fluvoxamine in comparison with behaviour therapy and placebo: results of a multicentre study. *Br J Psychiatry*. 1998;(35):71–78.
9. Goodman WK, Price LH, Rasmussen SA, et al. The Yale-Brown obsessive compulsive scale: I. Development, use, and reliability. *Arch Gen Psychiatry*. 1989;46(11):1006–1011.
10. Goodman WK, Price LH, Rasmussen SA, et al. The Yale-Brown obsessive compulsive scale: II. Validity. *Arch Gen Psychiatry*. 1989;46(11):1012–1016.
11. Pediatric OCD Treatment Study (POTS) Team. Cognitive-behavior therapy, sertraline, and their combination for children and adolescents with obsessive-compulsive disorder: the Pediatric OCD

Treatment Study (POTS) randomized controlled trial. *JAMA*. 2004;292(16):1969–1976.

12. Scahill L, Riddle MA, McSwiggin-Hardin M, et al. Children's Yale-Brown obsessive compulsive scale: reliability and validity. *J Am Acad Child Adolesc Psychiatry*. 1997;36(6):844–852.
13. Simpson HB, Maher MJ, Wang Y, Bao Y, Foa EB, Franklin M. Patient adherence predicts outcome from cognitive behavioral therapy in obsessive-compulsive disorder. *J Consult Clin Psychol*. 2011;79(2):247.
14. Wheaton MG, Galfalvy H, Steinman SA, Wall MM, Foa EB, Simpson HB. Patient adherence and treatment outcome with exposure and response prevention for OCD: which components of adherence matter and who becomes well? *Behav Res Ther*. 2016;85:6–12.
15. Cottraux J, Mollard E, Bouvard M, Marks I. Exposure therapy, fluvoxamine, or combination treatment in obsessive-compulsive disorder: one-year followup. *Psychiatry Res*. 1993;49(1):63–75.
16. Simpson HB, Liebowitz MR, Foa EB, et al. Post-treatment effects of exposure therapy and clomipramine in obsessive–compulsive disorder. *Depress Anxiety*. 2004;19(4):225–233.
17. Patel SR, Galfavy H, Kimeldorf MB, Dixon LB, Simpson HB. Patient preferences and acceptability of evidence-based and novel treatments for obsessive-compulsive disorder. *Psychiatric Serv*. 2017;68(3):250–257.
18. Patel SR, Simpson HB. Patient preferences for OCD treatment. *J Clin Psychiatry*. 2010;71(11):1434.
19. Koran LM, Hanna GL, Hollander E, Nestadt G, Simpson HB. Practice guideline for the treatment of patients with obsessive-compulsive disorder. *Am J Psychiatry*. 2007;164(7):1.
20. Koran LM, Simpson HB. *Guideline Watch (March 2013): Practice Guideline for the Treatment of Patients with Obsessive-Compulsive Disorder*. Washington, DC: American Psychiatric Association; 2013.
21. Marks IM, Stern RS, Mawson D, Cobb J, McDonald R. Clomipramine and exposure for obsessive-compulsive rituals: I. *Br J Psychiatry*. 1980;136(1):1–25.
22. Van Balkom AJ, De Haan E, Van Oppen P, Spinhoven P, Hoogduin KA, Van Dyck R. Cognitive and behavioral therapies alone versus in combination with fluvoxamine in the treatment of obsessive compulsive disorder. *J Nerv Ment Dis*. 1998;186(8):492–499.
23. Tenneij NH, Van Megen HJ, Denys DA, Westenberg HG. Behavior therapy augments response of patients with obsessive-compulsive disorder responding to drug treatment. *J Clin Psychiatry*. 2005;66(9):1169–1175.
24. Simpson HB, Foa EB, Liebowitz MR, et al. A randomized, controlled trial of cognitive-behavioral therapy for augmenting pharmacotherapy in obsessive-compulsive disorder. *Am J Psychiatry*. 2008;165(5):621–630.
25. Simpson HB, Foa EB, Liebowitz MR, et al. Cognitive-behavioral therapy vs risperidone for augmenting serotonin reuptake inhibitors in obsessive-compulsive disorder: a randomized clinical trial. *JAMA Psychiatry*. 2013;70(11):1190–1199.
26. Bloch M, Landeros-Weisenberger A, Kelmendi B, Coric V, Bracken MB, Leckman JF. A systematic review: antipsychotic augmentation with treatment refractory obsessive-compulsive disorder. *Mol Psychiatry*. 2006;11(7):622–632.
27. Komossa K, Depping AM, Meyer M, Kissling W, Leucht S. Second-generation antipsychotics for obsessive compulsive disorder. *Cochrane Database Syst Rev*. 2010;(12):CD008141.
28. Dold M, Aigner M, Lanzenberger R, Kasper S. Antipsychotic augmentation of serotonin reuptake inhibitors in treatment-resistant obsessive-compulsive disorder: a meta-analysis of double-blind, randomized, placebo-controlled trials. *Int J Neuropsychopharmacol*. 2013;16(3):557–574.
29. Veale D, Miles S, Smallcombe N, Ghezai H, Goldacre B, Hodsoll J. Atypical antipsychotic augmentation in SSRI treatment refractory obsessive-compulsive disorder: a systematic review and meta-analysis. *BMC Psychiatry*. 2014;14(1):317.
30. Foa EB, Simpson HB, Rosenfield D, et al. Six-month outcomes from a randomized trial augmenting serotonin reuptake inhibitors with exposure and ritual prevention or risperidone in adults with obsessive-compulsive disorder. *J Clin Psychiatry*. 2015;76(4):440.
31. Franklin ME, Sapyta J, Freeman JB, et al. Cognitive behavior therapy augmentation of pharmacotherapy in pediatric obsessive-compulsive disorder: the Pediatric OCD Treatment Study II (POTS II) randomized controlled trial. *JAMA*. 2011;306(11):1224–1232.
32. New York State Psychiatric Institute. Attaining and maintaining wellness in obsessive-compulsive disorder. ClinicalTrials.gov Identifier NCT01686087. Available from: https://clinicaltrials.gov/ct2/show/NCT01686087 (accessed July 26, 2018).
33. Fanale MA, Horwitz SM, Forero-Torres A, et al. Brentuximab vedotin in the front-line treatment of patients with CD30+ peripheral T-cell lymphomas: results of a phase I study. *J Clin Oncol*. 2014;32(28):3137–3143.
34. Kalanthroff E, Anholt GE, Simpson HB. Research domain criteria and obsessive-compulsive disorder: an oxymoron? In: Pittenger C, ed. *Obsessive-Compulsive*

Disorder: Phenomenology, Pathophysiology, and Treatment. New York, NY: Oxford University Press; 2017:609–702.

35. Ledgerwood L, Richardson R, Cranney J. Effects of D-cycloserine on extinction of conditioned freezing. *Behav Neurosci*. 2003;117(2):341.
36. Walker DL, Ressler KJ, Lu KT, Davis M. Facilitation of conditioned fear extinction by systemic administration or intra-amygdala infusions of D-cycloserine as assessed with fear-potentiated startle in rats. *J Neurosci*. 2002;22(6):2343–2351.
37. Ressler KJ, Rothbaum BO, Tannenbaum L, et al. Cognitive enhancers as adjuncts to psychotherapy: use of D-cycloserine in phobic individuals to facilitate extinction of fear. *Arch Gen Psychiatry*. 2004;61(11):1136–1144.
38. Tart CD, Handelsman PR, DeBoer LB, et al. Augmentation of exposure therapy with post-session administration of D-cycloserine. *J Psychiatr Res*. 2013;47(2):168–174.
39. Nave AM, Tolin DF, Stevens MC. Exposure therapy, D-cycloserine, and functional magnetic resonance imaging in patients with snake phobia: a randomized pilot study. *J Clin Psychiatry*. 2012;73(9):1179–1186.
40. Otto MW, Tolin DF, Simon NM, et al. Efficacy of d-cycloserine for enhancing response to cognitive-behavior therapy for panic disorder. *Biol Psychiatry*. 2010;67(4):365–370.
41. Siegmund A, Golfels F, Finck C, et al. D-cycloserine does not improve but might slightly speed up the outcome of in-vivo exposure therapy in patients with severe agoraphobia and panic disorder in a randomized double blind clinical trial. *J Psychiatr Res*. 2011;45(8):1042–1047.
42. Hofmann SG, Meuret AE, Smits JA, et al. Augmentation of exposure therapy with D-cycloserine for social anxiety disorder. *Arch Gen Psychiatry*. 2006;63(3):298–304.
43. Guastella AJ, Richardson R, Lovibond PF, et al. A randomized controlled trial of D-cycloserine enhancement of exposure therapy for social anxiety disorder. *Biol Psychiatry*. 2008;63(6):544–549.
44. Hofmann SG, Smits JA, Rosenfield D, et al. D-Cycloserine as an augmentation strategy with cognitive-behavioral therapy for social anxiety disorder. *Am J Psychiatry*. 2013;170(7):751–758.
45. Sheerin CM. *Slope of Change through D-cycloserine Facilitation of Exposure Therapy in a Social Anxiety Population*. Dissertation, Western Michigan University; 2013.
46. Kushner MG, Kim SW, Donahue C, et al. D-cycloserine augmented exposure therapy for obsessive-compulsive disorder. *Biol Psychiatry*. 2007;62(8):835–838.
47. Wilhelm S, Buhlmann U, Tolin DF, et al. Augmentation of behavior therapy with D-cycloserine for obsessive-compulsive disorder. *Am J Psychiatry*. 2008;165(3):335–341.
48. Storch EA, Merlo LJ, Bengtson M, et al. D-cycloserine does not enhance exposure–response prevention therapy in obsessive–compulsive disorder. *Int Clin Psychopharmacol*. 2007;22(4):230–237.
49. Andersson E, Hedman E, Enander J, et al. D-cycloserine vs placebo as adjunct to cognitive behavioral therapy for obsessive-compulsive disorder and interaction with antidepressants: a randomized clinical trial. *JAMA Psychiatry*. 2015;72(7):659–667.
50. Farrell LJ, Waters AM, Boschen MJ, et al. Difficult-to-treat pediatric obsessive-compulsive disorder: feasibility and preliminary results of a randomized pilot trial of D-cycloserine-augmented behavior therapy. *Depress Anxiety*. 2013;30(8):723–731.
51. Mataix-Cols D, Turner C, Monzani B, et al. Cognitive-behavioural therapy with post-session D-cycloserine augmentation for paediatric obsessive-compulsive disorder: pilot randomised controlled trial. *Br J Psychiatry*. 2014;204(1):77–78.
52. Storch EA, Wilhelm S, Sprich S, et al. Efficacy of augmentation of cognitive behavior therapy with weight-adjusted D-cycloserine vs placebo in pediatric obsessive-compulsive disorder: a randomized clinical trial. *JAMA Psychiatry*. 2016;73(8):779–788.
53. Mataix-Cols D, de la Cruz LF, Monzani B, et al. D-cycloserine augmentation of exposure-based cognitive behavior therapy for anxiety, obsessive-compulsive, and posttraumatic stress disorders: a systematic review and meta-analysis of individual participant data. *JAMA Psychiatry*. 2017;74(5):501–510.
54. Pittenger C, Krystal JH, Coric V. Glutamate-modulating drugs as novel pharmacotherapeutic agents in the treatment of obsessive-compulsive disorder. *NeuroRx*. 2006;3(1):69–81.
55. Carlsson ML. On the role of prefrontal cortex glutamate for the antithetical phenomenology of obsessive compulsive disorder and attention deficit hyperactivity disorder. *Prog Neuropsychopharmacol Biol Psychiatry*. 2001;25(1):5–26.
56. Chakrabarty K, Bhattacharyya S, Christopher R, Khanna S. Glutamatergic dysfunction in OCD. *Neuropsychopharmacology*. 2005;30(9):1735–1740.
57. Rosenberg DR, Hanna GL. Genetic and imaging strategies in obsessive–compulsive disorder: potential implications for treatment development. *Biol Psychiatry*. 2000;48(12):1210–1222.

58. Rosenberg DR, MacMaster FP, Keshavan MS, Fitzgerald KD, Stewart CM, Moore GJ. Decrease in caudate glutamatergic concentrations in pediatric obsessive-compulsive disorder patients taking paroxetine. *J Am Acad Child Adolesc Psychiatry.* 2000;39(9):1096–1103.
59. Ting JT, Feng G. Glutamatergic synaptic dysfunction and obsessive-compulsive disorder. *Curr Chem Genomics.* 2008;2:62–71.
60. Berman RM, Cappiello A, Anand A, et al. Antidepressant effects of ketamine in depressed patients. *Biol Psychiatry.* 2000;47(4):351–354.
61. Kishimoto T, Chawla JM, Hagi K, et al. Single-dose infusion ketamine and non-ketamine N-methyl-D-aspartate receptor antagonists for unipolar and bipolar depression: a meta-analysis of efficacy, safety and time trajectories. *Psychol Med.* 2016;46(07):1459–1472.
62. Gideons ES, Kavalali ET, Monteggia LM. Mechanisms underlying differential effectiveness of memantine and ketamine in rapid antidepressant responses. *Proc Natl Acad Sci USA.* 2014;111(23):8649–8654.
63. Liu RJ, Lee FS, Li XY, Bambico F, Duman RS, Aghajanian GK. Brain-derived neurotrophic factor Val66Met allele impairs basal and ketamine-stimulated synaptogenesis in prefrontal cortex. *Biol Psychiatry.* 2012 Jun 1;71(11):996–1005.
64. Craske MG, Treanor M, Conway CC, Zbozinek T, Vervliet B. Maximizing exposure therapy: an inhibitory learning approach. *Behav Res Ther.* 2014;58:10–23.
65. Rodriguez CI, Kegeles LS, Levinson A, et al. Randomized controlled crossover trial of ketamine in obsessive-compulsive disorder: proof-of-concept. *Neuropsychopharmacology.* 2013;38(12):2475–2483.
66. Rodriguez CI, Wheaton M, Zwerling J, et al. Can exposure-based CBT extend the effects of intravenous ketamine in obsessive-compulsive disorder? an open-label trial. *J Clin Psychiatry.* 2016;77(3):408.
67. Fitzgerald PJ, Seemann JR, Maren S. Can fear extinction be enhanced? A review of pharmacological and behavioral findings. *Brain Res Bull.* 2014;105:46–60.
68. Nader K, Hardt O. A single standard for memory: the case for reconsolidation. *Nat Rev Neurosci.* 2009;10(3):224–234.
69. Nader K, Schafe GE, Le Doux JE. Fear memories require protein synthesis in the amygdala for reconsolidation after retrieval. *Nature.* 2000;406(6797):722–726.
70. Tronson NC, Taylor JR. Molecular mechanisms of memory reconsolidation. *Nat Rev Neurosci.* 2007;8(4):262–275.
71. Soeter M, Kindt M. Disrupting reconsolidation: pharmacological and behavioral manipulations. *Learn Mem.* 2011;18(6):357–366.
72. Kindt M, Soeter M, Vervliet B. Beyond extinction: erasing human fear responses and preventing the return of fear. *Nat Neurosci.* 2009;12(3):256.
73. Soeter M, Kindt M. An abrupt transformation of phobic behavior after a post-retrieval amnesic agent. *Biol Psychiatry.* 2015;78(12):880–886.
74. Brunet A, Orr SP, Tremblay J, Robertson K, Nader K, Pitman RK. Effect of post-retrieval propranolol on psychophysiologic responding during subsequent script-driven traumatic imagery in post-traumatic stress disorder. *J Psychiatr Res.* 2008;42(6):503–506.
75. Shiban Y, Pauli P, Mühlberger A. Effect of multiple context exposure on renewal in spider phobia. *Behav Res Ther.* 2013;51(2):68–74.
76. Vansteenwegen D, Vervliet B, Iberico C, Baeyens F, Van den Bergh O, Hermans D. The repeated confrontation with videotapes of spiders in multiple contexts attenuates renewal of fear in spider-anxious students. *Behav Res Ther.* 2007;45(6):1169–1179.
77. Balooch SB, Neumann DL, Boschen MJ. Extinction treatment in multiple contexts attenuates ABC renewal in humans. *Behav Res Ther.* 2012;50(10):604–609.
78. Dunsmoor JE, Campese VD, Ceceli AO, LeDoux JE, Phelps EA. Novelty-facilitated extinction: providing a novel outcome in place of an expected threat diminishes recovery of defensive responses. *Biol Psychiatry.* 2015;78(3):203–209.

Chapter 20

Deep Brain Stimulation, Transcranial Magnetic Stimulation and Transcranial Direct Current Stimulation for Obsessive-Compulsive Disorder

Rebecca A. Segrave, Joshua J. Hendrikse and Linden Parkes

Introduction

Obsessive-compulsive disorder (OCD) is a debilitating mental illness with an estimated lifetime prevalence rate of 2–3% [1]. Despite being typically viewed as the archetypal compulsive disorder, it has a highly heterogeneous clinical presentation [2]. Primary treatment strategies for OCD consist of selective serotonin reuptake inhibitors (SSRIs) and/or cognitive behavioral therapies, and for many individuals these treatments are very effective. However, for approximately 10–15% of patients they bring no, or only partial, symptomatic relief [3,4]. Two rapidly growing and complementary areas of clinical research are contributing to a new therapeutic approach: (i) the increasingly sophisticated understanding of the neurocircuitry that underlies OCD and (ii) a growing number of therapeutic brain stimulation techniques for psychiatric illnesses, beyond electroconvulsive therapy. Below we briefly outline current knowledge of the neurocircuitry of OCD before discussing emerging invasive and non-invasive brain stimulation approaches to treatment.

The prevailing neurobiological model of OCD implicates abnormalities in corticostriatal circuits [5,6]. For a detailed account of the field, we direct the reader to several reviews and meta-analyses in the literature [7,8,9,10]. In brief, the functional neuroimaging of OCD literature has converged upon a network involving the ventromedial prefrontal cortex, orbitofrontal cortex, head of the caudate nucleus (i.e., dorsal striatum), nucleus accumbens (i.e., ventral striatum), anterior cingulate cortex (ACC), as well as the thalamus and dorsal frontal cortical regions.

Early research into the neurobiology of OCD was conducted primarily using single photon emission computed tomography (SPECT), positron emission tomography (PET), and functional magnetic resonance imaging (fMRI) – imaging modalities that index brain function via regional cerebral blood flow, glucose metabolism, and changes in oxygenated and deoxygenated blood flow throughout the brain, respectively – and commonly involved examining patients with OCD during resting-state conditions or symptom provocation. Regarding the cortex, patients with OCD show dysfunction in the orbitofrontal and anterior cingulate cortices, as well as the dorsolateral and superior frontal cortices, relative to healthy controls [11,12,13,14,15,16,17,18,19,20,21,22,23,24]. Regarding the subcortex, dysfunction has been observed in the thalamus, caudate nucleus and putamen [11,12,24]. We note that the direction of dysfunction in the above regions has not always been consistent. However, meta-analytic work has since clarified some of the discrepancies and implicated hyperactivity in the bilateral head of the caudate and the left orbitofrontal cortex [10]. Critically, dysfunction in the orbitofrontal cortex and caudate nucleus appears to normalize following treatment with SSRIs or behavioral therapy [25,26,27]. However, Brody et al. [26] found that higher pretreatment activity in the orbitofrontal cortex was associated with greater response to behavioral therapy, whereas lower pretreatment activity was associated with a greater response to treatment with an SSRI. This suggests that the particular profile of corticostriatal dysfunction may determine from which treatment regime a patient is more likely to benefit.

In the late 2000s, the field shifted focus away from examining dysfunctional activity at the level of single brain regions and towards examining how regions within the corticostriatal circuits communicate, and how this so-called functional connectivity might be aberrant in OCD. Seminal work by Harrison et al. [28] using resting-state fMRI found that patients with OCD had increased functional connectivity between the ventral striatum (nucleus accumbens) and the medial orbitofrontal cortex, and that the strength of this dysconnectivity correlated positively with obsessive-compulsive symptoms. This finding has since been replicated [29,30], and has been shown to be independent of obsessive-compulsive symptom dimensions [31]. Specifically, Harrison et al. [31] found that the correlation between functional dysconnectivity between the ventral striatum and orbitofrontal cortex and symptom severity was common across patients with contamination/cleaning, aggression, sexual/religious, symmetry/ordering and hoarding related obsessions and compulsions. Furthermore, alongside this common biomarker, Harrison et al. [31] showed evidence of unique corticostriatal biomarkers for the aggression, sexual/religious and hoarding dimensions.

Targeted brain stimulation techniques are well positioned to provide therapeutic benefits to individuals with OCD through the modification of corticostriatal circuit dysfunction (Figure 20.1). In addition, results from the nascent functional connectivity literature [31] demonstrating partially distinct corticostriatal biomarkers across different symptom dimensions suggest a potential to tailor stimulation targets to individual patients. In this chapter, we review evidence for the efficacy of deep brain stimulation (DBS), repetitive transcranial magnetic stimulation (rTMS) and transcranial direct current stimulation (tDCS) for OCD, discuss future directions for the development of each technique and integrate this with broader emerging trends surrounding the neurobiology and classification of OCD in psychiatry.

Deep Brain Stimulation

DBS involves the surgical implantation of stimulating electrodes into the brain. The surgery comprises two stages: stereotaxic implantation of electrodes into highly precise sub-cortical neuroanatomical targets, and subcutaneous connection of the electrode leads to a pulse generator implanted in the chest. Electrodes are typically implanted bilaterally and most DBS devices comprise four stimulating electrodes at the tip of each lead. The pulse generator supplies persistent stimulation and thus persistent functional modification of local and downstream brain activity. Once a patient recovers from surgery stimulation is initiated and the parameters (voltage, frequency, pulse-width, electrode and reference montage) can be interrogated in an attempt to achieve maximal therapeutic outcomes.

DBS is a complex treatment that necessitates multidisciplinary care, but when provided by experienced clinical teams it is most often safe and well tolerated [32]. Risks fall into three categories: surgically induced adverse events (e.g. death, intracerebral hemorrhage), and device malfunction (e.g. lead fracture, device failure) which are relatively rare, and stimulation-induced adverse effects (e.g. agitation, insomnia, somatic or affective modulation) which are common during the DBS programming phase but typically reversible upon modification of stimulation parameters [32].

Over the past 15 years there has been growing interest in the application of DBS to treat OCD. This has stemmed from three convergent lines of evidence: historical use of lesional psychosurgery techniques (i.e. anterior capsulotomy, subcaudate tractotomy, limbic leucotomy) to disconnect cortical and sub-cortical nodes of OCD neurocircuitry, observation of reduced compulsivity in patients with Parkinson's disease post-DBS, and, as outlined above, an increasingly sophisticated understanding of the corticostriatal neurocircuits underlying OCD. While research into its efficacy continues, in 2008 the US Food and Drug Administration granted a humanitarian device exemption for DBS for severe refractory OCD, the first clinical regulatory approval of DBS for a psychiatric indication. European Conformity approval followed in 2009 and OCD is now the most common psychiatric indication for DBS.

To date, over 25 published reports describe DBS outcomes for over 130 patients with OCD (Tables 20.1 and 20.2). Given the expensive, clinically time consuming, and psychologically and medically complex nature of DBS reports inevitably describe outcomes from small cohorts ($n = 1$ to $n = 26$) and the majority are open-label case studies and case series. Outcomes from six implantation targets have been described and are outlined below.

Anterior Limb of the Internal Capsule

Selection of the anterior limb of the internal capsule (ALIC) as a target for OCD DBS was based on positive outcomes from ablative anterior capsulotomy.

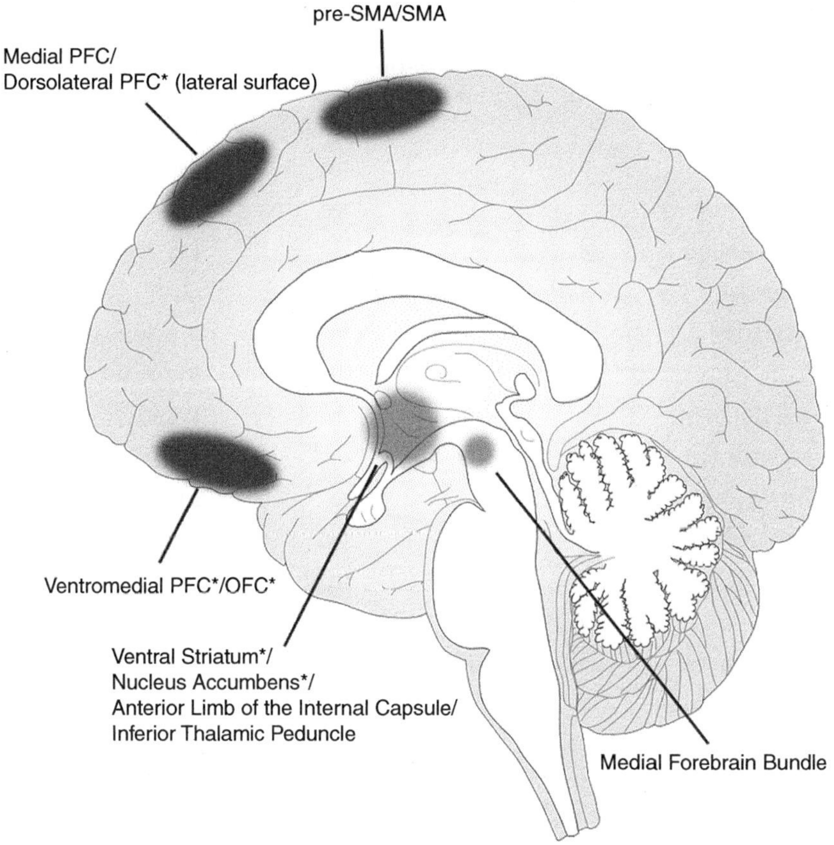

Figure 20.1 Corticostriatal regions to which deep brain stimulation, repetitive transcranial magnetic stimulation, and transcranial direct current stimulation have been trialed for obsessive-compulsive disorder.
Light gray circles indicate sub-cortical nodes and dark gray ovals represent cortical nodes. Targets marked with * are consistently implicated in neuroimaging literature as core nodes of OCD neurocircuitry. OFC, orbitofrontal cortex; PFC, prefrontal cortex; SMA, supplementary motor area.

The ALIC was the target of the first published report of DBS for OCD, with Nuttin et al. [33] describing unspecified "beneficial effects" for three of four patients with implants. Two subsequent open-label case reports also described substantial persistent reduction in symptom severity [34,35]. Two small investigations have included periods of blinded stimulation. While one observed reliable reduction in Yale-Brown Obsessive Compulsive Scale (Y-BOCS) scores during ON compared with OFF stimulation [36] the other did not [37]. Following longer-term open-label stimulation, however, both studies had a 50% response rate (i.e. patients who achieved ≥ 35% reduction in Y-BOCS).

Functional neuroimaging studies have documented normalization of neural activity in near and far nodes of OCD neurocircuitry following ALIC DBS. For example, a reduction in nucleus accumbens hyperactivity and normalization of this activity during reward processing has been documented post ALIC DBS [38], and therapeutic response has been associated with decreases in activity in the nucleus accumbens and orbitofrontal cortex [36,37,38].

Ventral Capsule/Ventral Striatum

Observations of positive outcome from Gamma Knife® capsulotomy of the ventral region of the ALIC impinging on the inferior ventral striatum contributed to subsequent targeting of the ventral capsule/ventral striatum (VC/VS) for OCD DBS [39]. Four open-label case series describing outcomes in a total of 19 patients have reported response rates between 40% and 100% [40,41,42,43]. One VC/VS investigation

Table 20.1 Open-label case reports and case series of deep brain stimulation for obsessive-compulsive disorder.

Target	Study (year)	Patients (*n*)	Follow-Up (months)	Responders (%)[a]	Follow-Up Y-BOCS Points Reduction (%)
Subthalamic nucleus	Mallet et al. (2002) [59][b]	2	6	100	↓ 20 (81.6)
	Fontaine et al. (2004) [60][b]	1	12	100	↓ 31 (96.9)
	Chabardes et al. (2013) [62][c]	4	6	75	↓ 18 (45.4)
Nucleus accumbens	Sturm et al. (2003) [48]	4	24–30	75	n/a
	Franzini et al. (2010) [49]	2	24–27	50	↓ 13 (38.2)
Anterior limb of internal capsule	Anderson and Ahmed (2003) [34]	1	10	100	↓ 27 (79.4)
	Choudhury et al. (2017) [35]	1	51	100	↓ 16 (43.2)
Ventral capsule/ventral striatum	Greenberg et al. (2006) [41]	10	36	40	↓ 12.3 (35.5)
	Tsai et al. (2014) [43]	4	15	50	↓ 12 (33.1)
	Roh et al. (2012) [42]	4	24	100	↓ 22 (59.5)
	Aouizerate et al. (2005) [40]	1	18	100	↓ 13 (52)
ALIC & VC/VS combined[d]	Nuttin et al. (1999) [33]	4	NA	NA	n/a
	Greenberg et al. (2010) [46][e]	26	3–36	62	↓ 13.1 (38.5)
Inferior thalamic peduncle	Jimenez-Ponce et al. (2009) [64]	5	12	100	↓ 17.2 (49.1)
Medial forebrain bundle	Coenen et al. (2017) [65]	2	12	100	↓ 9.5 (31.7)

n/a: not applicable or not reported; Y-BOCS, Yale-Brown Obsessive Compulsive Scale;
[a] Percentage of patients whose Y BOCS score was decreased by ≥ 35% from baseline at last follow-up.
[b] Patient/patients with Parkinson's disease and comorbid OCD.
[c] Includes two patients described in Mallet et al. (2002) [59].
[d] Combined outcomes from deep brain stimulation to anterior limb of the internal capsule and ventral capsule/ventral striatum.
[e] Includes five patients described in Greenberg et al. (2006) [41], five patients described in Goodman et al. (2010) [44], four patients described in Nuttin et al. (2003) [36].

included a sham component: Goodman et al. [44] employed a blinded staggering of stimulation onset contrasting initiation 30 days compared with 60 days post-surgery. No therapeutic benefit was observed prior to stimulation onset; four of the six patients met response criteria at 12-month post-surgery, and benefits were maintained at 6–9-year follow-up [45].

The largest case series of OCD DBS reported outcomes for 26 patients who underwent stimulation to the ALIC or VC/VS across four clinical research sites [46]. A cumulative response rate of 62% was reported, with only four patients obtaining no therapeutic benefit. For patients implanted at the VC/VS, acute stimulation was associated with increased regional cerebral blood flow to the orbitofrontal and anterior cingulate cortices, striatum, pallidum and thalamus [47]. An important outcome of this large series was the observation of greater therapeutic response following refinement of the implantation site more posteriorly than that used for lesional anterior capsulotomy; to the junction of the ALIC, anterior commissure and posterior ventral striatum.

Nucleus Accumbens

The nucleus accumbens, part of the ventral capsule located beneath the ventral ALIC, is a critical structure for reward and motivation processing that has been repeatedly implicated in OCD pathophysiology thus offering a promising target for OCD DBS. Unilateral stimulation of the right-hemisphere nucleus accumbens was initially trialed by Sturm et al. [48] with "nearly total recovery from both anxiety and OCD symptoms" described for three of four

Table 20.2 Deep brain stimulation for obsessive-compulsive disorder – studies with blinded component.

Target	Study (year)	Patients (*n*)	Follow-Up (months)	Responders (%)[a]	Follow-Up Y-BOCS Points Reduction (%)	Blinding ON/ OFF Protocol	Y-BOCS On vs. Off
Anterior limb of the internal capsule	Nuttin et al. (2003) [36]	6	3–31	n/a	n/a	3 months on, 5–10 weeks off (4 patients only)	19.8 vs. 32.3
	Abelson et al. (2005) [37]	4	4–24	50	↓ 9.8 (29.9)	4 blinded on/off periods (duration not reported)	26.5 vs. 29.3
Subthalamic nucleus	Mallet et al. (2008) [61]	16	3	n/a	↓ 8.9 (31)	3 months on, 3 months off	19.8 vs. 28.7
Ventral capsule/ ventral striatum	Goodman et al. (2010) [44]	6	12	67	↓ 15.7 (47.9)	Staggered stimulation onset: 30 or 60 days post-surgery	n/a
Nucleus accumbens	Huff et al. (2010) [50]	10	12	10	↓ 6.8 (21.1)	3 months on, 3 months off	27.9 vs. 31.1
	Denys et al. (2010) [51]	16	21	56	↓ 17.5 (51.9)	2 weeks on, 2 weeks off	8.3 pts difference

n/a, not applicable or not reported; Y-BOCS: Yale-Brown Obsessive-Compulsive Scale.
[a] Percentage of patients whose Y-BOCS score was decreased by ⩾ 35% from baseline at last follow-up.

implanted patients. Franzini et al. [49] tested bilateral DBS of the nucleus accumbens in two patients and described a slow progressive reduction in Y-BOCS scores, with one achieving and one approaching clinical response after two years.

Two studies have employed periods of blind stimulation. Minimal benefit was observed following right-hemisphere DBS of the nucleus accumbens, with no difference in response between periods of ON versus OFF stimulation and only one of ten patients achieving response following one year of open-label stimulation [50]. Greater benefit was described in 16 patients following bilateral DBS of the nucleus accumbens, with 9 patients responders eight-months post-DBS and ON stimulation associated with a 25% reduction in Y-BOCS scores compared with OFF [51].

DBS of the nucleus accumbens has been shown to modulate maladaptive activity and connectivity throughout compulsive neurocircuitry. Figee et al. [52] demonstrated that DBS of the nucleus accumbens normalizes nucleus accumbens activity, reduces excessive connectivity between the nucleus accumbens and the prefrontal cortex, and decreases frontal low-frequency neural oscillations during obsessive-compulsive symptom provocation. Incidental reduction in non-OCD compulsive behaviors have also been described following DBS of the nucleus accumbens, with patients with comorbid nicotine or alcohol addiction and OCD, Tourette's disorder or anxiety disorder experiencing a reduction in compulsive substance use [53,54]. This aligns with positive findings from a handful of case studies where patients received DBS of the nucleus accumbens specifically to treat other compulsive conditions (e.g., alcohol and heroin addiction or anorexia nervosa [55,56,57,58]).

Subthalamic Nucleus

The subthalamic nucleus is a key node in the corticostriatothalamocortical loop that governs motor inhibition. Targeting of the subthalamic nucleus to treat OCD arose from observation of reduced compulsivity and affective modulation in patients with comorbid OCD and Parkinson's disease who underwent DBS of the subthalamic nucleus to contain their motor symptoms. Mallett [59] and Fontaine [60] initially described remission from OCD following DBS of the subthalamic nucleus for three patients with comorbid Parkinson's disease.

A sham-controlled multi-site trial of DBS of the subthalamic nucleus has been conducted in 16 patients with OCD [61]. The trial employed a cross-over design to compare three-month periods of ON compared with OFF stimulation and found OCD severity significantly reduced and global functioning significantly increased following active stimulation. Outcomes from two further patients from the same protocol described persistent reduction in Y-BOCS following six months of stimulation, and electro-encephalogram source localization data indicated that therapeutic response was associated with downstream activation of the orbitobasal and prefrontal cortex [62]. This is consistent with prior observation that beneficial effects of DBS of the subthalamic nucleus for OCD are related to reduction in orbitofrontal hyperactivity [63].

Inferior Thalamic Peduncle

The inferior thalamic peduncle (ITP) connects the orbitofrontal cortex and the thalamus, two key nodes in OCD neurocircuitry. One research group has investigated DBS of the ITP for OCD; Jimenez-Ponce et al. [64] described open-label outcomes from six patients, three of whom had comorbid cocaine or alcohol addiction. While over a one- to three-year follow-up period, all six patients experienced marked reduction in OCD severity; compulsive substance use was unchanged for patients also experiencing addiction.

Medial Forebrain Bundle

The superolateral branch of the medial forebrain bundle (MFB) is the most recent anatomical target to be trialed for OCD. Its addition to the list of implantation sites followed reports of rapid onset of anti-depressant effects following DBS for refractory major depression. Coenen et al. [65] hypothesized that as the MFB has a regulating role effect within reward circuity, and is interconnected to other efficacious OCD DBS targets, it may also be an effective DBS target for OCD. They reported a 12-month open-label DBS outcome trajectory for two patients, with both responders at last follow-up.

Where Next With Deep Brain Stimulation?

Overall, the findings above suggest that approximately 50% of patients with severe refractory OCD who undergo DBS respond, irrespective of implantation target. This was borne out in a 2015 meta-analysis, which synthesized DBS outcomes from 116 patients across 31 studies, and found a 60% (95% confidence interval 49–69%) response rate and 45.1% estimated global Y-BOCS reduction [66]. While no difference in response was observed between stimulation targets, this may reflect the small numbers of patients in each study and substantial differences in cohort characteristics, stimulation parameters and electrode design.

Identifying the optimal target or targets for OCD is a critical next step for enhancing patient outcomes; there are a number of ways to approach this step. The most intuitive is via large prospective randomized controlled trials (RCTs) directly comparing therapeutic response with stimulation at different implantation sites. While there are numerous calls for such trials, given the expense and complexity of DBS and unique challenges of designing high-quality blinded RCTs (discussed below), it is unlikely that many such studies will be conducted.

An alternative approach is to refine electrode placement within a given target. DBS electrode placement is guided by neuroanatomical landmarks, coordinates derived from standard neuroimaging atlases and electrophysiological recordings. In patients undergoing DBS for major depression, differences in therapeutic outcome have not been associated with anatomical distribution of electrodes, but rather whether the active electrode rests within white-matter tracts that connect to key downstream nodes in depression neurocircuitry [67]. As our understanding of the functional connectivity within circuits that mediate compulsivity grows, individualized tractography guided implantation is another appealing proposition for OCD.

Given the clinical heterogeneity within OCD, the question is likely not "which is the most efficacious target for OCD DBS" but rather "which is the most efficacious target for this patient's OCD". Algorithms matching individual patients to specific stimulation targets are the holy grail of DBS research. While there are reports of differential response by symptom dimension [48,66] small patient numbers and lack of robust characterization measures render them inconclusive. Sub-typing and targeting by symptom dimension is appealing for its clinical ease, however evidence linking symptom clusters to specific corticostriatal neurocircuit profiles is preliminary [68,69], and the influence of symptom overlap and evolution over time unknown. Thus precision medicine approaches to DBS await identification of biologically valid phenotypes.

The need for large well-controlled RCTs of OCD DBS as a precursor to broad clinical uptake is often noted. However a number of features of DBS make it a poor fit with gold standard RCT design. A primary feature is how to administer periods of blinded stimulation. Inconsistent observation of response to ON/OFF stimulation at the same implantation site is an exemplar of this. For example, blinded studies of ALIC DBS for OCD have reported separable therapeutic effects for longer (i.e. months) periods of ON/OFF stimulation and no difference to shorter periods (i.e. weeks) [38,39]. How long is an adequate blinded phase for DBS? How much time "should" it take for clinical benefit to become apparent? It is clear from clinical observations that time to therapeutic response differs substantially between individuals, even those with comparable illness severity implanted at the same target. Similarly, effective stimulation parameters differ substantially between individuals and can take many months of trial and error to identify. This creates a choice between two unpalatable options: early evaluation of standardized (i.e. non-personalized) stimulation parameters, or later-stage evaluation of personalized settings. The first option produces poor quality evidence regarding efficacy, and the second requires withholding of effective treatment from severely unwell patients (indeed, many studies have reduced or abandoned blinded OFF phases due to acute clinical deterioration), and compromises the rigor of blinding, as prior experience of stimulation will enable many to differentiate between active and sham settings.

A related challenge is how best to program the DBS device post-surgery (i.e., what sequence of parameters to apply, how frequently to adjust them and how long to persist with the search for effective settings). It can take many months, even years, to determine whether efficacious parameters can be identified for a given patient, a highly impractical timeframe for clinical trials. For these reasons, the failure of large multicenter DBS studies for other psychiatric indications have been attributed by many to failed trials as opposed to a failed treatment [70,71], and there is a need to look to alternative research paradigms for high-quality clinical evidence [72].

The future of DBS for OCD will additionally be shaped by advances in device technology. In the last five years, implantable pulse generators have shifted to rechargeable models, extending their lifespan by a decade and reducing the need for frequent replacement surgeries. A host of further innovations are in development: novel electrode designs that allow precise control of the shape and size of tissue being stimulated and could target highly specific subregions of corticostriatal neurocircuits, integration of neuroimaging data and computational modeling of the DBS electric field to enable individual predictions of the neural response to DBS to different stimulation parameters, adaptive and closed-loop stimulation that could incorporate evidence of aberrant oscillatory activity in OCD [52] (for review see Kuhn and Volkmann [73]). Advances in device technology hold much promise, especially in developing efficient solutions for navigating the vast DBS parameter space.

Transcranial Magnetic Stimulation

Transcranial magnetic stimulation (TMS) is a non-invasive brain stimulation technique which uses time-varying magnetic fields to stimulate superficial areas of the cortex. It involves the use of a hand-held coil which is placed over a target region on the scalp and is capable of depolarizing underlying cortical neurons. TMS can be used to assess or modify the activity of brain networks depending on the parameters in which the stimulation is applied. Various coil types of different shape and size have been developed, which achieve different magnetic fields, with certain coil designs producing greater stimulation focality (i.e. figure-of-eight coil) or intracranial penetration (i.e. "deep TMS" H-coil and double cone coil). When multiple pulses are delivered in quick succession (i.e. at a frequency greater than 1 Hz, an approach known as repetitive TMS), TMS can induce changes to the excitability of cortical circuits that last beyond the period of stimulation. Through mechanisms akin to long-term potentiation and long-term depression, stimulation at or above 5 Hz (high-frequency rTMS) is applied to increase cortical excitability, while rTMS at or below a frequency of 1 Hz (low-frequency rTMS) is applied to reduce excitability. In this manner, rTMS can be used to selectively induce neural plasticity, and when the stimulation is applied across multiple sessions, long-lasting changes to the dynamics of brain networks can be achieved.

When delivered within established safety guidelines [74], rTMS is typically well tolerated and safe, and has Food and Drug Administration approval for the treatment of depression [75]. It is, however, associated with a number of potential risks. The rarest but most significant is inadvertent induction of a seizure [76]. Other adverse effects can include syncopal episodes (also uncommon) and transient headaches and/or stimulation site discomfort (more common) attributable to local scalp muscle contraction induced by TMS pulses [74].

Since 1997, 6 open-label and 15 randomized-controlled trials have been conducted to explore the efficacy of rTMS as a treatment for OCD (Table 20.3). Five rTMS stimulation targets have been investigated and outcomes are summarized below.

Dorsolateral Prefrontal Cortex

Initial investigation of the therapeutic potential of rTMS in OCD stimulated the dorsolateral prefrontal cortex (DLPFC). The selection of this target was derived from fMRI evidence associating OCD with prefrontal hyperactivity and rTMS treatment of depression, where stimulation of the DLPFC was known to elicit antidepressant effects. The first study conducted by Greenberg and colleagues [77] applied a single session of high-frequency rTMS to the left and right DLPFC, and an occipital control site over three separate days, in randomized order. rTMS applied to both hemispheres was accompanied by an immediate decrease in compulsive and depressive symptoms, but effects were largest and most durable following high-frequency rTMS to the right DLPFC.

Two open-label [77,78] and nine randomized-controlled trials [79,80,81,82,83,84,85,86,87] have been conducted to assess the efficacy of DLPFC rTMS for reduction of OCD symptoms. Overall, despite positive outcomes from initial open-label investigations, the results of subsequent RCTs have been equivocal. While some of the variability in RCT outcomes may be attributable to heterogeneity across protocols (Table 20.3), the largely negative findings suggest that the DLPFC is not an ideal therapeutic target for the treatment of OCD. This conclusion has been supported by a recent meta-analysis, which synthesized extant RCT data and reported no therapeutic benefit of DLPFC stimulation [88].

Aside from the DLPFC, other attempts to identify effective rTMS targets have focused on cortical regions directly implicated in corticostriatal models of OCD pathophysiology, including the orbitofrontal and medial prefrontal cortices, and pre-supplementary motor area (SMA).

Orbitofrontal Cortex

Functional neuroimaging studies have implicated hyperactivity of the orbitofrontal cortex in the pathophysiology of OCD [89]. Reducing orbitofrontal cortex metabolism through low-frequency rTMS may help to remediate dysfunction across functionally connected corticostriatal circuits, and alleviate associated OCD symptoms. To date, two trials of low-frequency rTMS in the orbitofrontal cortex have been conducted, one single-blind targeting the left orbitofrontal cortex [90] and one double-blind crossover trial targeting the right [91]. Both provided support for the efficacy of orbitofrontal cortex low-frequency rTMS, with significant reductions in Y-BOCS ratings following active, relative to sham, stimulation.

Medial Prefrontal Cortex

The medial prefrontal cortex (MPFC), situated slightly anterior of the pre-SMA, has also been implicated in the pathophysiology of OCD, with reduced gray matter volume [92] and altered resting-state functional connectivity [93] observed in OCD patients. Two studies have investigated the efficacy of MPFC stimulation [94,95]. Despite employing stimulation protocols of different frequency, coil type and treatment period, both open-label studies reported significant Y-BOCS reductions following active stimulation.

Pre-Supplementary Motor Area and Supplementary Motor Area

Neuroimaging evidence of hyperactivity across motor and pre-motor regions in OCD [96] has led to the investigation of the SMA as a therapeutic target. Normalizing hyperexcitability across motor and pre-motor networks may improve response inhibition and influence the ability for individuals with OCD to control urges, intrusive thoughts and repetitive motor actions [97]. To date, four RCTs have been conducted, applying low-frequency rTMS over the pre-SMA bilaterally. Three trials reported evidence of significant clinical benefit following low-frequency rTMS to the SMA [97,98,99], while the fourth did not find evidence of symptom reduction [100].

Where to Next for Repetitive Transcranial Magnetic Stimulation?

Determining rTMS targets on the basis of cortical-striatal models of OCD has significant therapeutic potential. However, while the majority of rTMS trials employing corticostriatal targets have reported group-level symptom reduction, there is substantial response variability at the individual level. Certain studies, such as that conducted by Dunlop et al. [94], report a clear bimodal response pattern, showing distinct sub-populations of individuals who either experienced a clinically meaningful reduction in obsessive-compulsive symptoms, or failed to respond to the treatment. This variability underscores a major challenge for the field of rTMS, with similar outcomes also noted in rTMS treatment of major depressive disorder, and also across experimental applications [103]. Hence, the next challenge for rTMS treatment of OCD will be to identify sources of, and methods to reduce, interindividual variability to maximize clinical benefit. While there are certain physiological traits known to influence the response to rTMS that are difficult to alter or control (e.g. genetics and age – see Ridding and Ziemann [104] for further discussion), the stimulation parameters in which rTMS is applied (i.e. method of target localization, stimulation frequency and intensity, total number of pulses and treatment duration), also influence the magnitude and durability of treatment outcomes and importantly, can be altered and optimized. While investigating and comparing the myriad of parameters presents a major challenge, it also affords a unique opportunity to develop methods of personalizing the application of rTMS, where parameters may, in future, be tailored to individual phenotypes.

Although experimental manipulation of rTMS parameters has led to the development of specific protocols thought to selectively increase (e.g., high-frequency rTMS) or decrease cortical excitability (e.g., low-frequency rTMS) [104], experimental evidence has shown that this assumption is commonly not met, with a large percentage of individuals demonstrating paradoxical outcomes with increased cortical excitability following protocols intending to reduce excitability, and vice versa [103,105]. Therapeutically, this presents a major issue, as treatment protocols routinely employ high-frequency rTMS to increase excitability within hypoactive brain networks, and low-frequency rTMS to reduce hyperactivity. Thus, there is a need to explore alternative rTMS parameters which may produce a more consistent physiological and behavioral response. Similarly, the stimulation intensity (i.e., percentage of resting motor threshold [106]), coil type [107], coil orientation [108] and interstimulus interval [109] also influence the plasticity response and should be considered in relation to the intended neurophysiological effects. The emergence of "burst" protocols, where one pattern of stimulation is superimposed on another (e.g., 50-Hz triplets delivered at a 5-Hz rhythm) [110] represents a step forward in the development of effective, novel rTMS parameters. Theta-burst TMS is delivered at lower stimulation intensities and enables a large number of pulses to be delivered over a short duration, increasing tolerability and clinical practicality. While these approaches are yet to be clinically trialed in OCD, a case study of theta-burst stimulation has reported clinically significant therapeutic benefit [111]. Electroencephalogram (EEG) linked approaches are another exciting method of optimizing treatment response, and have been employed in a 2014 double-blinded trial with positive results [84]. While computationally complex, this approach allows rTMS trains to be applied in synchrony with particular brain rhythms relevant to particular cognitive or affective states, which may in turn enhance therapeutic efficacy.

Clinical application of rTMS routinely involves multiple weeks of once-daily rTMS, with all sessions delivered on site at a treatment facility. The associated time and travel requirements limit access for many patients. In recent years, accelerated rTMS courses have been trialed where comparable total doses are consolidated into a much shorter period by delivering two or three treatment sessions per day. Preliminary results for patients with major depression have demonstrated comparable clinical efficacy and stimulation tolerability [112], indicating their potential to deliver rapid clinical response with similar risk profile and reduced logistical burden. Accelerated approaches have yet to be considered for OCD but may serve to expedite clinical response while reducing burden on patients and health care systems that may ultimately exert a positive influence on treatment adherence.

Ensuring accurate localization of the intended stimulation target is another important consideration

Table 20.3 Repetitive transcranial magnetic stimulation for obsessive-compulsive disorder.

Study (year)	Patients Total (n)	Female (%)	Target(s)/Coil Type	Frequency (Pattern of Stimulation)
		Open-label case series:		
		DLPFC		
Greenberg et al. (1997) [77]	12 OCD	50	R & L DLPFC, and mid-occipital control site. Figure eight-shaped coil	20 Hz (2s on, 58s off)
Sachdev et al. (2001) [78]	12 OCD	25	Randomized to either R or L DLPFC. Figure eight-shaped coil	10 Hz (5 s on, 25 s off)
		MPFC		
Dunlop et al. (2016) [94]	20 OCD + 40 healthy controls for fMRI comparison	80 + 57.5	L followed by R DMPFC, butterfly deep TMS coil	10 Hz (5 s on, 10 s off)
Modirrousta et al. (2015) [95]	10 OCD	n/a	MPFC, double-cone coil	1 Hz (2.5 min on, 2 min off with 10 min off between 4th and 5th train to prevent coil overheating)
		SMA		
Kumar et al. (2011) [101]	12 OCD	58.3	SMA, figure-eight coil	1 Hz (10 s on, 15 s off)
Mantovani et al. (2006) [102]	10 OCD and/or Tourette's disorder	20	Bilateral SMA, figure-eight coil	1 Hz (5 min on, 2 min off)
		Blinded trials		
		DLPFC		
Alonso et al. (2001) [79]	18 OCD (10 active rTMS, 10 sham)	67	R DLPFC, circular coil	1 Hz (on off NR, session time 20 mins)
Badawy et al. 2010 [80]	60 OCD (40 active: 20 monotherapy, 20 rTMS + SSRIs, 20 sham)	51.7	L DLPFC	20 Hz (NR)
Elbeh et al. (2016) [81]	45 OCD (30 active, 15 sham)	33	R DLPFC, figure-eight coil	1 Hz (8.3 min on, 40 s off; $n = 15$), 10 Hz (20 s on, 20 s off; $n = 15$)
Kang et al. (2009) [82]	20 OCD (10 active rTMS, 10 sham)	15	R DLPFC, followed by bilateral SMA, figure-eight coil	1 Hz (on/off NR, 10 min for each site)
Mansur et al. (2011) [83]	27 OCD (13 active, 14 sham)	51.9	R DLPFC, figure-eight coil	10 Hz (5 s on, 25 s off)
Ma et al. (2014) [84]	46 OCD (25 active, 21 sham)	34.7	Bilateral DLPFC, circular coil	Individual intrinsic αEEG-timed frequency (4 s on, 56 s off)

Total Pulses/ Session	RMT (%)[a]	Treatment Period	Responders (%)[b]	Results: Y-BOCS Change (%)
1600	80	1 session for each target, randomized order	NR	↓ following R DLPFC – effects persisted for 8 hours. No significant effects of L DLPFC, or mid-occipital TMS
1500	110	2 weeks (10 sessions)	33 overall (2 following R, 2 following L)	↓ across all subjects (–30.9 post treatment, –42 1-month follow-up). No difference between R and L DLPFC
3000/hemisphere, 6000 total	120	4 weeks (20 sessions); non-remitters offered additional 20 sessions	n/a[c]	↓ in OCD sample (–39.7)
1200	110	2 weeks (10 sessions)	NR	↓ post treatment (–39.4), and 1-month follow-up (NR)
1000	n/a[d]	3 weeks (15 sessions)	NR	↓ post treatment (–34.4)
1200	100	2 weeks (10 sessions)	n/a[e]	↓ post treatment (–28.6)
NR	110	6 weeks (3 sessions per week, 18 total)	20	No significant differences pre-/post-treatment, nor between active and sham stimulation conditions
n/a	n/a	3 weeks (15 sessions)	n/a[f]	No significant differences pre-/post-treatment for active stimulation as monotherapy (–8.2), or sham (–5.7) ↓ following active stimulation + SSRIs (–20.3)
2000	100	2 weeks (10 sessions)	NR	↓ following active (–35.3), but not sham stimulation (–5.6); larger reduction following 1 Hz (–44.9), relative to 10 Hz (-26.9) post-treatment; effects remained at 3-month follow-up
1200 each site, 2400 total	110	2 weeks (10 sessions)	n/a[g]	No significant differences pre- post treatment, nor between active and sham stimulation conditions
2000	110	6 weeks (30 sessions)	n/a[h]	↓ overall (–9.2), but no significant differences between active and sham stimulation conditions
Variable (648–872 per session)	80	2 weeks (10 sessions)	36 active 0 sham	↓ post-treatment; larger reduction following active (–34.4), compared with sham (–15.2) stimulation; effects of active stimulation present at 1-week follow-up (–32.2)

(*continued*)

Table 20.3 *(cont.)*

Study (year)	Patients Total (n)	Female (%)	Target(s)/Coil Type	Frequency (Pattern of Stimulation)
Prasko et al. (2006) [85]	33 OCD (18 active rTMS, 12 sham)	36	L DLPFC, figure-eight coil	1 Hz (on /off NR, session time 20 min)
Sachdev et al. (2007) [86]	18 OCD (10 active rTMS, 8 sham)	55.6	L DLPFC, figure-eight coil	10 Hz (5 s on, 25 s off)
Sarkhel et al. (2010) [87]	42 OCD (21 active rTMS, 21 sham)	45	R DLPFC, figure-eight coil	10 Hz (4 s on, off NR)
		OFC		
Ruffini et al. (2009) [90]	23 OCD (16 active rTMS, 7 sham)	NR	L OFC, figure-eight coil	1 Hz (on/off NR, session time 10 min)
Nauczyciel et al. (2014) [91]	15 OCD	79	R OFC, double-cone coil	1 Hz (NR)
		SMA		
Mantovani et al. (2010) [97]	21 OCD enrolled (18 completed trial: 9 active, 9 sham)	38	Pre-SMA, bilaterally, figure-eight coil	1 Hz (single 20 min train)
Gomes et al. (2012) [98]	22 OCD (12 active, 10 sham)	59	Pre-SMA, bilaterally, figure-eight coil	1 Hz (single 20-min train)
Hawken et al. (2016) [99]	22 OCD (10 active, 12 sham)	50	Pre-SMA, bilaterally, figure-eight coil	1 Hz (5 min on, 2 min off, 20 min total)
Pelissolo et al. (2016) [100]	40 OCD[l] (20 active, 19 sham)	57.5	Pre-SMA, bilaterally, figure-eight coil	1 Hz (4 min on, 2 min off, 26 min total)

DLPFC, dorsolateral prefrontal cortex; DMPFC, dorsomedial prefrontal cortex; EEG, electroencephalogram; fMRI, functional magnetic resonance imaging; L, left; min, minutes; MPFC, medial prefrontal cortex; n/a, not applicable; NR: not reported; OCD, obsessive-compulsive disorder; OFC, orbitofrontal cortex; R, right; rTMS, repetitive transcranial magnetic stimulation; s, seconds; SMA, supplementary motor area; SSRI, selective serotonin reuptake inhibitor; YBOCS, Yale-Brown Obsessive Compulsive Scale.

[a] Percentage resting motor threshold.

[b] Percentage of patients whose Y-BOCS score was decreased by ≥ 35% from baseline at last follow-up.

[c] 50% classified as responders by the authors, achieving a Y-BOCS reduction of ≥ 50% in score.

[d] rTMS delivered at 100% of patient's active motor threshold.

[e] 60% of "pure" OCD were classified as responders by the authors, achieving a Y-BOCS reduction of ≥ 40% in score.

[f] 55% rTMS + SSRI, 25% monotherapy and 5% sham were classified as responders by the authors, achieving a Y-BOCS reduction of ≥ 40% in score.

[g] 2 subjects from active and sham conditions were classified as responders by the authors, achieving a Y-BOCS reduction of ≥ 25% in score.

[h] 31% active, 14% sham were classified as responders by the authors, achieving a Y-BOCS reduction of ≥ 30% in score.

[i] Responder rates calculated for patients who completed trial only (3 non-completers).

[j] 41% active, 10% sham were classified as responders by the authors, achieving a Y-BOCS reduction of ≥ 25% in score.

[k] 80% active, 8% sham were classified as responders by the authors, achieving a Y-BOCS reduction of ≥ 25% in score.

[l] 40 patients were enrolled in the study, however one was excluded prior to randomization, and 36 were included in final analysis.

[m] 10.5% active, 20% sham were classified as responders by the authors, achieving a Y-BOCS reduction of ≥ 25% in score.

Total Pulses/ Session	RMT (%)[a]	Treatment Period	Responders (%)[b]	Results: Y-BOCS Change (%)
1800	110	2 weeks (10 sessions)	NR	↓ overall (−20.1%), but no significant differences between active and sham stimulation conditions
1500	110	2 weeks (10 sessions)	NR	↓ overall (non-significant when correcting for depression using MADRS scale scores); no significant differences between active and sham stimulation conditions
800	110	2 weeks (10 sessions)	NR	↓ overall (−8.5), but no significant differences between active and sham stimulation conditions
NR	80	3 weeks (15 sessions)	25 active 14 sham	↓ following active (−18.9), but not sham stimulation (−6.7); effects persisted for 10 weeks following treatment
1200	120	1 week (2 sessions per day, 10 total)	NR	↓ overall, non-significantly larger reduction for active compared with sham stimulation
1200	100	4 weeks double-blind treatment (20 sessions); non-responders to sham, or responders to active or sham stimulation offered additional 4 weeks open-label	67 active 22 sham[i]	↓ post-treatment; larger reduction following active (−25.4), compared with sham (−12) stimulation; responders to active stimulation showed −51 at 3-month follow-up, relative to baseline
1200	100	2 weeks (10 sessions)	n/a[j]	↓ post-treatment; larger reduction following active (−42), compared with sham (−16.7) stimulation; effects persisted for 14 weeks following treatment
NR	110	6 weeks (5 sessions/week for 4 weeks, 3 sessions in week 5, 2 sessions week 6;: 25 total)	n/a[k]	↓ post-treatment following active (−40) but not sham stimulation (NR); effects persisted for 6 weeks following treatment
1500	100	4 weeks (20 sessions)	NR[m]	No significant differences between active (−7.6) and sham (−3.5) stimulation conditions

for effective rTMS. Trials of different targeting methods have shown that greater precision equates to greater therapeutic efficacy [113]. However, precise targeting is challenging as, while the TMS coil is rested on the scalp, the intended stimulation site is cortical, and the relationship between scalp and cortical morphology is not consistent across individuals. There are a number of localization methods which have been developed including: the traditional "5-cm rule", where the TMS coil is simply placed 5 cm anterior of the M1 motor hotspot to localize the DLPFC – a method that cannot account for individual anatomical variability and has been shown to be therapeutically inferior in depression treatment trials; the 10–20 EEG system, where the coil is positioned in relation to standard EEG channel coordinates, allowing head shape and size to be incorporated; and image-guided stereotactic neuronavigation, which enables precise positioning in relation to individual brain anatomy. Neuronavigation systems use structural MRI scans and allow the TMS coil to be positioned and monitored in real-time in relation to individual sulcal and gyral configuration with millimeter accuracy. fMRI information may also be incorporated into these systems to further individualize treatment on the basis of brain function, as has been conducted for pre-SMA stimulation in past case studies, achieving significant symptom reduction (average 41% decrease in Y-BOCS, $n = 2$) [114]. While this technology circumvents the need for scalp-based positioning methods, the expense of these systems and requisite neuroimaging presents a major barrier for routine clinical use. Determining cortical targets in relation to the 10–20 EEG system (e.g. Fp1 to localize left orbitofrontal cortex) offers a low-cost alternative, balancing the trade-off between anatomical accuracy and clinical applicability, and is becoming standard clinical practice for treatment of depression [115].

Transcranial Direct Current Stimulation

tDCS is a non-invasive brain stimulation technique that involves application of a weak electrical current (generally 1–3 mA) via anodal and cathodal scalp electrodes. Unlike TMS, the strength of stimulation is not sufficient to directly induce neuronal firing. Rather, the weak surface stimulation produces a shift in the membrane potential of underlying cortical neurons. This results in partial depolarization (anode) or hyperpolarization (cathode) making the affected neurons more or less likely to fire when physiologically stimulated. Anodal stimulation can increase cortical excitability. Cathode stimulation tends to exert a more inhibitory effect, although its impact on cortical excitability is more variable.

tDCS is generally well tolerated and not associated with major adverse effects. Compared with rTMS and DBS research into its efficacy for OCD is in its infancy and the available data are exclusively from small open-label reports (Table 20.4). As with rTMS and DBS, tDCS has been applied to (i.e., scalp electrodes placed over) brain regions implicated in OCD neuropathology. However using the common two electrode montage tDCS is a far less focal method of stimulation and maximal effects can occur at cortical or subcortical sites remote from the electrodes. Nonetheless, we briefly describe therapeutic research outcome by the site of electrode placement and intended maximal neuromodulation.

Dorsolateral Prefrontal Cortex

A small pilot study and a single case report have described response to DLPFC stimulation. One applied anodal [116] and the other cathodal [117] stimulation and neither resulted in persistent change in OCD severity, though a prominent reduction in comorbid depression and anxiety was described in the case report. This is in keeping with predominantly poor efficacy of DLPFC rTMS for OCD but strong therapeutic response to DLPFC rTMS for major depression and highlights the need to target causal nodes within the neurocircuitry of the condition being treated.

Orbitofrontal Cortex

One small study and a case example have reported outcomes following tDCS of the orbitofrontal cortex. In eight patents with refractory OCD, cathodal stimulation of the left orbitofrontal cortex and anodal right cerebellar was associated with 28% reduction in Y-BOCS immediately following treatment, and three patients met response criteria at three-month follow-up [118]. A comparable reduction in symptom severity with delayed onset was reported in the case study [119].

Pre-Supplementary Motor Area

The largest study of tDCS for OCD conducted thus far used a partial crossover design to compare response to anodal versus cathodal midline pre-SMA tDCS

Table 20.4 Transcranial direct current stimulation for obsessive-compulsive disorder.

Study (year)	Patients (*n*)	Target	Electrode Montage	Current Density mA/cm^2	Sessions (*n*)	Final Assessment Timing post-tDCS	Symptom Change
Dinna et al. (2016) [116]	5	Anodal left DLPFC	Anode: F3 cathode: Fp2	0.057 anode and cathode	13–15	1 month	2% OCI ↑
Volpato et al. (2013) [117]	1	Cathodal left DLPFC[a]	Anode: neck Cathode: F3	0.057 anode and cathode	20	Immediate post-tDCS	Active tDCS[d]: no Y-BOCS change Sham tDCS[d]: no Y-BOCS change
Bation et al. (2016) [118]	8	Cathocal left OFC	Anode: right cerebellum Cathode: Fp1	0.057 anode and cathode	20	3 months	27% Y-BOCS ↓
Mondino et al. (2015) [119]	1	Cathodal left OFC	Anode: right occipital cortex Cathode: Fp1	0.02 anode 0.057 cathode	10	1 month	26% Y-BOCS ↓
D'Urso et al. (2016) [120]	11	Anodal versus cathodal bilateral pre-SMA	Anode/cathode: midline pre-SMA Anode/cathode: right deltoid	0.08 anode and cathode	10 anode pre-SMA[b] 10 cathode pre-SMA[b]	Immediate post-tDCS	Anode pre-SMA[d]: 3 Y-BOCS ↑ 1 Y-BOCS ↓ 1no Y-BOCS change Cathode pre-SMA[d]: 5 Y-BOCS ↓ 1 no Y-BOCS change
Narayanaswamy et al. (2015) [121]	2	Anodal left pre-SMA[c]	Anode: left pre-SMA Cathode: Fp2	0.057 anode and cathode	20	Immediate post-tDCS	43% Y-BOCS ↓
Silva et al. (2016) [122]	2	Cathodal bilateral pre-SMA	Anode: left deltoid Cathode: midline pre-SMA	0.08 anode and cathode	20	6 months	37% Y-BOCS ↓

DLPFC, dorsolateral prefrontal cortex; OCI, Obsessive Compulsive Inventory; OFC, orbitofrontal cortex; SMA, sensorimotor area; Y-BOCS, Yale-Brown Obsessive Compulsive Scale.
[a] Compared tDCS and rTMS in crossover design.
[b] Compared anode versus cathode over pre-SMA in crossover design, pre-crossover outcomes described.
[c] tDCS delivered with cognitive behavioral therapy.
[d] Y-BOCS scores not specified.

in 11 patients [120]. Anodal stimulation resulted in worsening of symptoms for three of five patients, which was reversed following subsequent anodal stimulation. The same dose of cathodal stimulation reduced symptom severity for five of six patients. This observation of clinical worsening following anodal pre-SMA stimulation is at odds with a description of therapeutic benefit for two patients who received anodal pre-SMA tDCS in conjunction with cognitive behavior therapy [121]. Pre- and post-tDCS fMRI data showed increased pre-SMA/SMA activity during a response inhibition task after tDCS.

Silva et al. [122] are conducting an RCT of cathodal pre-SMA tDCS in 44 patients with OCD and will investigate genetic markers of response and stimulation induced changes in cortical excitability and cognitive performance. Open-label piloting of the protocol for two patients resulted in a substantial but delayed reduction in OCD severity for one, and no response in the other.

Where Next With Transcranial Direct Current Stimulation for Obsessive-Compulsive Disorder?

Currently there are insufficient data to judge the therapeutic potential of tDCS for OCD. Across the range of psychiatric indications for which tDCS has been investigated, therapeutic outcomes are highly variable and frequently reflect statistically significant but clinically modest effects. This is likely due, in part, to the subtle non-depolarizing mechanisms of tDCS, complex often non-linear parameter space, and particular vulnerability to interindividual differences, all of which are only partially understood. As such, the next steps for tDCS for OCD are not specific to OCD, they are questions for the field.

A better understanding of the relationship between tDCS delivery protocols and neural and behavioral response is critical. The often cited model of anodal stimulation reliably exciting and cathodal stimulation reliably inhibiting underlying cortex has been disabused and numerous non-linear dose-response relationships, including reversal of the direction of excitatory/inhibitory tDCS after-effects following increases in stimulation intensity and duration identified [123–125]. In addition, electrode characteristics (i.e., size, proximity, number, montage) determine the strength and topography of neural response and their influence is only recently being systematically investigated [126]. High-definition tDCS arrays that increase focality and may induce stronger neuromodulation [127] are an intuitively promising next step for targeting cortical regions implicated in OCD psychopathology.

As with rTMS, application of identical tDCS protocols to different individuals can produce different responses [128,129]. For example, following motor cortex tDCS, there are individuals for whom cathodal stimulation has inhibitory after-effects and others for whom it produces an excitatory response, whereas anodal stimulation produces excitatory after-effects for some and has no neuromodulatory impact for others [128]. Sources of interindividual differences in response include baseline brain state, neurotransmitter balance, hormonal state, genotype, cognitive capacity and skull and cortical morphology [130]. The relative influence of and interplay between these variables is poorly understood and a topical area of investigation. In addition, most mechanistic studies (both into stimulation parameters and inter-individual differences) are based on motor cortex tDCS in healthy individuals where motor-evoked potentials provide a convenient and reliable outcome measure. An understanding of how these learnings translate to maladaptive brain states like OCD and the prefrontal regions most often targeted for therapeutic applications, which differ substantially in neuronal type, orientation and receptor availability, awaits dedicated investigations using non-motor outcomes, such as neuroimaging or TMS–EEG.

Finally, while available (albeit limited) evidence for the therapeutic impact of tDCS as a monotherapy is not compelling, there are a number of examples of concurrent tDCS augmenting therapeutic outcomes from pharmacological and cognitive therapies for other psychiatric indications [131,132]. Given its capacity to modulate neuroplasticity and enhance cognitive processing [127], combining tDCS with cognitive therapies for OCD is an appealing avenue that warrants investigation, and it may be that this technique is best suited to combined treatment approaches.

Transdiagnostic Future Directions for Brain Stimulation

The research discussed in this chapter has focused predominantly on the therapeutic benefits of stimulating corticostriatal circuits in patients with OCD.

However, corticostriatal dysfunction is not specific to OCD but rather is implicated in a broad range of both compulsive disorders, such as addictions [133], and non-compulsive conditions, such as Parkinson's disease [134], psychosis [135], bipolar [136] and major depression [137]. Furthermore, as previously mentioned, there is emerging evidence that corticostriatal dysfunction within OCD varies with the expression of primary OCD symptomatology [31]. Taken together with the still evolving understanding of brain stimulation mechanisms and methods, it is unsurprising that the therapeutic outcomes of intervention studies have thus far been heterogeneous. Thus, in addition to increasing our mechanistic understanding of the aforementioned brain stimulation techniques, clarifying the role of corticostriatal dysfunction within and between multiple disorders will likely yield insights into why stimulating certain targets is effective for some individuals and not others.

The Research Domain Criteria [138] serve as a promising framework for this endeavor because they recast the study of mental illness with a transdiagnostic focus, emphasizing the use of dimensional phenotypes and neurobiology to classify mental illness rather than traditional symptomatology. Within this framework, the therapeutic effects of brain stimulation may be examined according to certain corticostriatal biotypes and associated behavioral/cognitive phenotypes, rather than diagnostic labels [139]. In turn, differentiating individuals with OCD on such phenotypes (see below for examples) may help researchers to better understand the response rates for different brain stimulation techniques and targets in OCD and, by extension, help to tailor brain stimulation protocols to individuals.

Traditional views of OCD posited it as an anxiety disorder. However, the growing appreciation of the complexity of OCD led to it being separated into its own category in the current diagnostic systems. This change has given rise to many new ideas regarding the etiology of OCD. One perspective argues that OCD may be conceptualized as a behavioral addiction [140]. These arguments are born out of the observed clinical commonalities between the progression from hedonic pursuit to compulsive pursuit of a behavior in individuals who are both addicted and those who have OCD. Central to this transition are the phenotypes of impulsivity and compulsivity, which play a critical role in the clinical presentation of OCD and related disorders [140], and have been shown to be linked with poorer quality of life [141] and increased symptom severity [142]. Crucially, impulsivity and compulsivity are postulated to be governed by different subcomponents within the corticostriatal circuits. Fineberg et al. [143] suggest that the ventral striatum may drive impulsive behaviors and the anterior cingulate and ventromedial prefrontal cortices exert regulatory control, whereas the dorsal striatum drives compulsive behaviors, while the orbitofrontal cortex exerts regulatory control, although these ideas are yet to be confirmed in the human neuroimaging literature. Thus, the therapeutic benefits of stimulating nodes such as the ACC compared with the orbitofrontal cortex may depend upon an individual's profile of impulsivity and compulsivity.

A complementary account links OCD to deficits in goal directed behavioral control. Individuals with OCD have been shown to habitually avoid an electric shock (via lever press) even after the threat of shock has been explicitly removed (i.e., the source of the electric shock has been physically disconnected in full view of the patient) [144], which suggests that OCD is associated with excessive avoidance habits. Goal-directed and habitual behavior are associated with corticostriatal circuits that partially overlap with those implicated in this chapter. In particular, goal-directed behavior is thought to be subserved by a network involving the medial orbitofrontal cortex (i.e., ventromedial prefrontal cortex) and caudate nucleus while habitual behavior is controlled by a network involving the posterior putamen and pre-motor cortex [145,146]. Thus, dysfunction in the corticostriatal circuits that facilitate goal-directed behavior may cause an over-reliance on normally functioning habit circuits in OCD. As such, remediating activity in the orbitofrontal cortex, and connected regions, may be beneficial in patients showing dysfunctional goal-directed behavioral control.

In this section, we have not aimed to provide a comprehensive account or a prescriptive framework for the future direction of brain stimulation research. Rather, we highlight the potential for transdiagnostic approaches to improve therapeutic brain stimulation techniques by tailoring stimulation targets using phenotypes that cut across traditional diagnostic boundaries. As such, future work may benefit from the collection of rich phenotypic information alongside typically acquired clinical data to develop an evidence base for which phenotypes, and associated circuits, are most beneficial to OCD.

Conclusion

There is a pressing need for new effective treatments for OCD. Alongside pharmacotherapy and psychological interventions, brain stimulation is emerging as a third pillar of psychiatric treatment and holds huge promise for OCD. While development of therapeutic brain stimulation approaches for OCD are in early stages, growing evidence indicates that DBS and rTMS can be highly effective treatments. The therapeutic potency of tDCS is less clear, but will be informed by the rapidly increasing research into both its basic mechanisms and its application for OCD. For all three techniques, efforts to determine the most effective stimulation parameters and delivery methods and sources of interindividual variability in response to stimulation are intense areas of research focus. The future of brain stimulation for OCD will be guided by integration of insights from this work with the increasingly sophisticated nosology and neurocircuitry of OCD. And with the synthesis of these bodies of knowledge the future of brain stimulation for OCD looks bright.

References

1. Ruscio AM, Stein DJ, Chiu WT, Kessler RC. The epidemiology of obsessive-compulsive disorder in the National Comorbidity Survey Replication. *Mol Psychiatry*. 2010;15(1):53–63.
2. Mataix-Cols D, Rosario-Campos MC, Leckman JF. A multidimensional model of obsessive-compulsive disorder. *Am J Psychiatry*. 2005;162(2):228–238.
3. Denys D. Pharmacotherapy of obsessive-compulsive disorder and obsessive-compulsive spectrum disorders. *Psychiatr Clin North Am*. 2006;29(2):553–584, xi.
4. Skoog G, Skoog I. A 40-year follow-up of patients with obsessive-compulsive disorder [see commetns]. *Arch Gen Psychiatry*. 1999;56(2):121–127.
5. Saxena S, Bota RG, Brody AL. Brain-behavior relationships in obsessive-compulsive disorder. *Semin Clin Neuropsychiatry*. 2001;6(2):82–101.
6. Graybiel AM, Rauch SL. Toward a neurobiology of obsessive-compulsive disorder. *Neuron*. 2000;28(2):343–347.
7. Mataix-Cols D, van den Heuvel OA. Common and distinct neural correlates of obsessive-compulsive and related disorders. *Psychiatr Clin North Am*. 2006;29(2):391–410, viii.
8. Milad MR, Rauch SL. Obsessive-compulsive disorder: beyond segregated cortico-striatal pathways. *Trends Cogn Sci*. 2012;16(1):43–51.
9. Rotge JY, Guehl D, Dilharreguy B, et al. Provocation of obsessive-compulsive symptoms: a quantitative voxel-based meta-analysis of functional neuroimaging studies. *J Psychiatry Neurosci*. 2008;33(5):405–412.
10. Whiteside SP, Port JD, Abramowitz JS. A meta-analysis of functional neuroimaging in obsessive-compulsive disorder. *Psychiatry Res*. 2004;132(1):69–79.
11. Baxter LR, Jr, Phelps ME, Mazziotta JC, Guze BH, Schwartz JM, Selin CE. Local cerebral glucose metabolic rates in obsessive-compulsive disorder. A comparison with rates in unipolar depression and in normal controls. *Arch Gen Psychiatry*. 1987;44(3):211–218.
12. Baxter LR, Jr, Schwartz JM, Mazziotta JC, et al. Cerebral glucose metabolic rates in nondepressed patients with obsessive-compulsive disorder. *Am J Psychiatry*. 1988;145(12):1560–1563.
13. Breiter HC, Rauch SL, Kwong KK, et al. Functional magnetic resonance imaging of symptom provocation in obsessive-compulsive disorder. *Arch Gen Psychiatry*. 1996;53(7):595–606.
14. Lucey JV, Costa DC, Adshead G, et al. Brain blood flow in anxiety disorders. OCD, panic disorder with agoraphobia, and post-traumatic stress disorder on 99mTcHMPAO single photon emission tomography (SPET). *Br J Psychiatry*. 1997;171:346–350.
15. Lucey JV, Costa DC, Blanes T, et al. Regional cerebral blood flow in obsessive-compulsive disordered patients at rest. Differential correlates with obsessive-compulsive and anxious-avoidant dimensions. *Br J Psychiatry*. 1995;167(5):629–634.
16. Martinot JL, Allilaire JF, Mazoyer BM, et al. Obsessive-compulsive disorder: a clinical, neuropsychological and positron emission tomography study. *Acta Psychiatr Scand*. 1990;82(3):233–242.
17. Mataix-Cols D, Wooderson S, Lawrence N, Brammer MJ, Speckens A, Phillips ML. Distinct neural correlates of washing, checking, and hoarding symptom dimensions in obsessive-compulsive disorder. *Arch Gen Psychiatry*. 2004;61(6):564–576.
18. McGuire PK, Bench CJ, Frith CD, Marks IM, Frackowiak RS, Dolan RJ. Functional anatomy of obsessive-compulsive phenomena. *Br J Psychiatry*. 1994;164(4):459–468.
19. Nakao T, Nakagawa A, Yoshiura T, et al. Brain activation of patients with obsessive-compulsive disorder during neuropsychological and symptom provocation tasks before and after symptom improvement: a functional magnetic resonance imaging study. *Biol Psychiatry*. 2005;57(8):901–910.
20. Rauch SL, Jenike MA, Alpert NM, et al. Regional cerebral blood flow measured during symptom provocation in obsessive-compulsive disorder

using oxygen 15-labeled carbon dioxide and positron emission tomography. *Arch Gen Psychiatry.* 1994;51(1):62–70.

21. Rauch SL, Shin LM, Dougherty DD, Alpert NM, Fischman AJ, Jenike MA. Predictors of fluvoxamine response in contamination-related obsessive compulsive disorder: a PET symptom provocation study. *Neuropsychopharmacology.* 2002;27(5):782–791.
22. Schienle A, Schafer A, Stark R, Walter B, Vaitl D. Neural responses of OCD patients towards disorder-relevant, generally disgust-inducing and fear-inducing pictures. *Int J Psychophysiol.* 2005;57(1):69–77.
23. Shin YW, Kwon JS, Kim JJ, et al. Altered neural circuit for working memory before and after symptom provocation in patients with obsessive-compulsive disorder. *Acta Psychiatr Scand.* 2006;113(5):420–429.
24. Swedo SE, Schapiro MB, Grady CL, et al. Cerebral glucose metabolism in childhood-onset obsessive-compulsive disorder. *Arch Gen Psychiatry.* 1989;46(6):518–523.
25. Baxter LR, Jr, Schwartz JM, Bergman KS, et al. Caudate glucose metabolic rate changes with both drug and behavior therapy for obsessive-compulsive disorder. *Arch Gen Psychiatry.* 1992;49(9):681–689.
26. Brody AL, Saxena S, Schwartz JM, et al. FDG-PET predictors of response to behavioral therapy and pharmacotherapy in obsessive compulsive disorder. *Psychiatry Res.* 1998;84(1):1–6.
27. Saxena S, Brody AL, Maidment KM, et al. Localized orbitofrontal and subcortical metabolic changes and predictors of response to paroxetine treatment in obsessive-compulsive disorder. *Neuropsychopharmacology.* 1999;21(6):683–693.
28. Harrison BJ, Soriano-Mas C, Pujol J, et al. Altered corticostriatal functional connectivity in obsessive-compulsive disorder. *Arch Gen Psychiatry.* 2009;66(11):1189–1200.
29. Jung WH, Kang DH, Kim E, Shin KS, Jang JH, Kwon JS. Abnormal corticostriatal-limbic functional connectivity in obsessive-compulsive disorder during reward processing and resting-state. *Neuroimage Clin.* 2013;3:27–38.
30. Jung WH, Yucel M, Yun JY, et al. Altered functional network architecture in orbitofronto-striato-thalamic circuit of unmedicated patients with obsessive-compulsive disorder. *Hum Brain Mapp.* 2017;38(1):109–119.
31. Harrison BJ, Pujol J, Cardoner N, et al. Brain corticostriatal systems and the major clinical symptom dimensions of obsessive-compulsive disorder. *Biol Psychiatry.* 2013;73(4):321–328.
32. Appleby BS, Duggan PS, Regenberg A, Rabins PV. Psychiatric and neuropsychiatric adverse events associated with deep brain stimulation: a meta-analysis of ten years' experience. *Mov Disord.* 2007;22(12):1722–1728.
33. Nuttin B, Cosyns P, Demeulemeester H, Gybels J, Meyerson B. Electrical stimulation in anterior limbs of internal capsules in patients with obsessive-compulsive disorder. *Lancet.* 1999;354(9189):1526.
34. Anderson D, Ahmed A. Treatment of patients with intractable obsessive-compulsive disorder with anterior capsular stimulation. Case report. *J Neurosurg.* 2003;98(5):1104–1108.
35. Choudhury TK, Davidson JE, Viswanathan A, Strutt AM. Deep brain stimulation of the anterior limb of the internal capsule for treatment of therapy-refractory obsessive compulsive disorder (OCD): a case study highlighting neurocognitive and psychiatric changes. *Neurocase.* 2017;23(2):138–145.
36. Nuttin BJ, Gabriels LA, Cosyns PR, et al. Long-term electrical capsular stimulation in patients with obsessive-compulsive disorder. *Neurosurgery.* 2003;52(6):1263–1272; discussion 72–74.
37. Abelson JL, Curtis GC, Sagher O, et al. Deep brain stimulation for refractory obsessive-compulsive disorder. *Biol Psychiatry.* 2005;57(5):510–516.
38. Van Laere K, Nuttin B, Gabriels L, et al. Metabolic imaging of anterior capsular stimulation in refractory obsessive-compulsive disorder: a key role for the subgenual anterior cingulate and ventral striatum. *J Nucl Med.* 2006;47(5):740–747.
39. Greenberg BD, Rezai AR. Mechanisms and the current state of deep brain stimulation in neuropsychiatry. *CNS Spectr.* 2003;8(7):522–526.
40. Aouizerate B, Martin-Guehl C, Cuny E, et al. Deep brain stimulation for OCD and major depression. *Am J Psychiatry.* 2005;162(11):2192.
41. Greenberg BD, Malone DA, Friehs GM, et al. Three-year outcomes in deep brain stimulation for highly resistant obsessive-compulsive disorder. *Neuropsychopharmacology.* 2006;31(11):2384–2393.
42. Roh D, Chang WS, Chang JW, Kim CH. Long-term follow-up of deep brain stimulation for refractory obsessive-compulsive disorder. *Psychiatry Res.* 2012;200(2–3):1067–1070.
43. Tsai HC, Chang CH, Pan JI, et al. Acute stimulation effect of the ventral capsule/ventral striatum in patients with refractory obsessive-compulsive disorder – a double-blinded trial. *Neuropsychiatr Dis Treat.* 2014;10:63–69.
44. Goodman WK, Foote KD, Greenberg BD, et al. Deep brain stimulation for intractable obsessive compulsive disorder: pilot study using a blinded, staggered-onset design. *Biol Psychiatry.* 2010;67(6):535–542.

45. Fayad SM, Guzick AG, Reid AM, et al. Six–nine year follow-up of deep brain stimulation for obsessive-compulsive disorder. *PLoS One*. 2016;11(12):e0167875.
46. Greenberg BD, Gabriels LA, Malone DA, Jr, et al. Deep brain stimulation of the ventral internal capsule/ventral striatum for obsessive-compulsive disorder: worldwide experience. *Mol Psychiatry*. 2010;15(1):64–79.
47. Rauch SL, Dougherty DD, Malone D, et al. A functional neuroimaging investigation of deep brain stimulation in patients with obsessive-compulsive disorder. *J Neurosurg*. 2006;104(4):558–565.
48. Sturm V, Lenartz D, Koulousakis A, et al. The nucleus accumbens: a target for deep brain stimulation in obsessive-compulsive- and anxiety-disorders. *J Chem Neuroanat*. 2003;26(4):293–299.
49. Franzini A, Messina G, Gambini O, et al. Deep-brain stimulation of the nucleus accumbens in obsessive compulsive disorder: clinical, surgical and electrophysiological considerations in two consecutive patients. *Neurol Sci*. 2010;31:353–359.
50. Huff W, Lenartz D, Schormann M, et al. Unilateral deep brain stimulation of the nucleus accumbens in patients with treatment-resistant obsessive-compulsive disorder: outcomes after one year. *Clin Neurol Neurosurg*. 2010;112:137–143.
51. Denys D, Mantione M, Figee M, et al. Deep brain stimulation of the nucleus accumbens for treatment-refractory obsessive-compulsive disorder. *Arch Gen Psychiatry*. 2010;67(10):1061–1068.
52. Figee M, Luigjes J, Smolders R, et al. Deep brain stimulation restores frontostriatal network activity in obsessive-compulsive disorder. *Nat Neurosci*. 2013;16(4):386–387.
53. Kuhn J, Bauer R, Pohl S, et al. Observations on unaided smoking cessation after deep brain stimulation of the nucleus accumbens. *Eur Addict Res*. 2009;15(4):196–201.
54. Kuhn J, Lenartz D, Huff W, et al. Remission of alcohol dependency following deep brain stimulation of the nucleus accumbens: valuable therapeutic implications? *J Neurol Neurosurg Psychiatry*. 2007;78(10):1152–1153.
55. Lipsman N, Woodside DB, Giacobbe P, et al. Subcallosal cingulate deep brain stimulation for treatment-refractory anorexia nervosa: a phase 1 pilot trial. *Lancet*. 2013;381(9875):1361–1370.
56. Wu H, Van Dyck-Lippens PJ, Santegoeds R, et al. Deep-brain stimulation for anorexia nervosa. *World Neurosurg*. 2013;80(3–4):S29 e1–e10.
57. Muller UJ, Sturm V, Voges J, et al. Successful treatment of chronic resistant alcoholism by deep brain stimulation of nucleus accumbens: first experience with three cases. *Pharmacopsychiatry*. 2009;42(6):288–291.
58. Valencia-Alfonso CE, Luigjes J, Smolders R, et al. Effective deep brain stimulation in heroin addiction: a case report with complementary intracranial electroencephalogram. *Biol Psychiatry*. 2012;71(8):e35-7.
59. Mallet L, Mesnage V, Houeto JL, et al. Compulsions, Parkinson's disease, and stimulation. *Lancet*. 2002;360(9342):1302–1304.
60. Fontaine D, Mattei V, Borg M, et al. Effect of subthalamic nucleus stimulation on obsessive-compulsive disorder in a patient with Parkinson disease. Case report. *J Neurosurg*. 2004;100(6):1084–1086.
61. Mallet L, Polosan M, Nematollah Jaafari N, et al. Subthalamic nucleus stimulation in severe obsessive–compulsive disorder. *N Engl J Med*. 2008;359:2121–2134.
62. Chabardes S, Polosan M, Krack P, et al. Deep brain stimulation for obsessive-compulsive disorder: subthalamic nucleus target. *World Neurosurg*. 2013;80(3–4):S31 e1–e8.
63. Le Jeune F, Verin M, N'Diaye K, et al. Decrease of prefrontal metabolism after subthalamic stimulation in obsessive-compulsive disorder: a positron emission tomography study. *Biol Psychiatry*. 2010;68(11):1016–1022.
64. Jimenez-Ponce F, Velasco-Campos F, Castro-Farfan G, et al. Preliminary study in patients with obsessive-compulsive disorder treated with electrical stimulation in the inferior thalamic peduncle. *Neurosurgery*. 2009;65(6 Suppl):203–209.
65. Coenen VA, Schlaepfer TE, Goll P, et al. The medial forebrain bundle as a target for deep brain stimulation for obsessive-compulsive disorder. *CNS Spectr*. 2017;22(3):282–289.
66. Alonso P, Cuadras D, Gabriels L, et al. Deep brain stimulation for obsessive-compulsive disorder: a meta-analysis of treatment outcome and predictors of response. *PLoS One*. 2015;10(7):e0133591.
67. Riva-Posse P, Choi KS, Holtzheimer PE, et al. Defining critical white matter pathways mediating successful subcallosal cingulate deep brain stimulation for treatment-resistant depression. *Biol Psychiatry*. 2014;76(12):963–969.
68. van den Heuvel OA, Remijnse PL, Mataix-Cols D, et al. The major symptom dimensions of obsessive-compulsive disorder are mediated by partially distinct neural systems. *Brain*. 2009;132(Pt 4):853–868.
69. Koch K, Wagner G, Schachtzabel C, et al. White matter structure and symptom dimensions in obsessive-compulsive disorder. *J Psychiatr Res*. 2012;46(2):264–270.

70. Schlaepfer TE. Deep brain stimulation for major depression-steps on a long and winding road. *Biol Psychiatry*. 2015;78(4):218–219.

71. Fitzgerald PB. Deep brain stimulation in depression. *Aust N Z J Psychiatry*. 2016;50(1):94–95.

72. Frieden TR. Evidence for health decision making – beyond randomized, controlled trials. *N Engl J Med*. 2017;377(5):465–475.

73. Kuhn AA, Volkmann J. Innovations in deep brain stimulation methodology. *Mov Disord*. 2017;32(1):11–19.

74. Rossi S, Hallett M, Rossini PM, Pascual-Leone A. Safety, ethical considerations, and application guidelines for the use of transcranial magnetic stimulation in clinical practice and research. *Clin Neurophysiol*. 2009;120:2008–2039.

75. Gaynes BN, Lloyd SW, Lux L, et al. Repetitive transcranial magnetic stimulation for treatment-resistant depression: a systematic review and meta-analysis. *J Clin Psychiatry*. 2014;75:477–489.

76. Perera T, George MS, Grammer G, Janicak PG, Pascual-leone A, Wirecki TS. Brain stimulation the clinical TMS Society consensus review and treatment recommendations for TMS therapy for major depressive disorder. *Brain Stimul*. 2016;9:336–346.

77. Greenberg BD, George MS, Martin JD, et al. Effect of prefrontal repetitive transcranial magnetic stimulation in obsessive-compulsive disorder: a preliminary study. *Am J Psychiatry*. 1997;1546:867–869.

78. Sachdev PS, McBride R, Loo CK, Mitchell PB, Malhi GS, Croker VM. Right versus left prefrontal transcranial magnetic stimulation for obsessive-compulsive disorder: a preliminary investigation. *J Clin Psychiatry*. 2001;62:981–984.

79. Alonso P, Pujol J, Cardoner N, et al. Right prefrontal repetitive transcranial magnetic stimulation in obsessive-compulsive disorder: a double-blind, placebo-controlled study. *Am J Psychiatry*. 2001;158:1143–1145.

80. Badawy AA, Sawy HE, Abd M, Hay E. Efficacy of repetitive transcranial magnetic stimulation in the management of obsessive compulsive disorder. *Egypt J Neurol Pscyhiat Neurosurg*. 2010;47:393–398.

81. Elbeh KAM, Elserogy YMB, Khalifa HE, Ahmed MA, Hafez MH, Khedr EM. Repetitive transcranial magnetic stimulation in the treatment of obsessive-compulsive disorders: double blind randomized clinical trial. *Psychiatry Res*. 2016;238:264–269.

82. Kang JI, Kim C-H, Namkoong K, Lee C-i, Kim SJ. A randomized controlled study of sequentially applied repetitive transcranial magnetic stimulation in obsessive-compulsive disorder. *J Clin Psychiatry*. 2009;70:1645–1651.

83. Mansur CG, Myczkowki ML, de Barros Cabral S, et al. Placebo effect after prefrontal magnetic stimulation in the treatment of resistant obsessive-compulsive disorder: a randomized controlled trial. *Int J Neuropsychopharmacol*. 2011; 14:1389–1397.

84. Ma XY, Huang YQ, Liao LW, Jin Y. A randomized double-blinded sham-controlled trial of α electroencephalogram-guided transcranial magnetic stimulation for obsessive-compulsive disorder. *Chin Med J (Engl)*. 2014;127:601–606.

85. Prasko J, Pasková B, Záleský R, et al. The effect of repetitive transcranial magnetic stimulation (rTMS) on symptoms in obsessive compulsive disorder. A randomized, double blind, sham controlled study. *Neuro Endocrinol Lett*. 2006;27:327–332.

86. Sachdev PS, Loo CK, Mitchell PB, Mcfarquhar TF, Malhi GS. Repetitive transcranial magnetic stimulation for the treatment of obsessive compulsive disorder: a double blind controlled investigation. *Psychol Med*. 2007;37:1645–1649.

87. Sarkhel S, Sinha VK, Praharaj SK. Adjunctive high-frequency right prefrontal repetitive transcranial magnetic stimulation (rTMS) was not effective in obsessive-compulsive disorder but improved secondary depression. *J Anxiety Disord*. 2010;24:535–539.

88. Berlim MT, Neufeld NH, Van den Eynde F. Repetitive transcranial magnetic stimulation (rTMS) for obsessive-compulsive disorder (OCD): an exploratory meta-analysis of randomized and sham-controlled trials. *J Psychiatric Res*. 2013;47:999–1006.

89. Chamberlain SR, Menzies L, Hampshire A, et al. Orbitofrontal dysfunction in patients with obsessive-compulsive disorder and their unaffected relatives. *Science (NY)*. 2008;321:421–422.

90. Ruffini C, Locatelli M, Lucca A, Benedetti F, Insacco C, Smeraldi E. Augmentation effect of repetitive transcranial magnetic stimulation over the orbitofrontal cortex in drug-resistant obsessive-compulsive disorder patients. *Prim Care Companion J Clin Psychiatry*. 2009;11:226–230.

91. Nauczyciel C, Le Jeune F, Naudet F, et al. Repetitive transcranial magnetic stimulation over the orbitofrontal cortex for obsessive-compulsive disorder: a double-blind, crossover study. *Transl Psychiatry*. 2014;4:e436.

92. Radua J, van den Heuvel OA, Surguladze S, Mataix-Cols D. Meta-analytical comparison of voxel-based morphometry studies in obsessive-compulsive disorder vs other anxiety disorders. *Arch Gen Psychiatry*. 2010;67:701–711.

93. Stern ER, Fitzgerald KD, Welsh RC, Abelson JL, Taylor SF. Resting-state functional connectivity between fronto-parietal and default mode networks in obsessive-compulsive disorder. *PLoS ONE.* 2012;7:e36356.

94. Dunlop K, Woodside B, Olmsted M, Colton P, Giacobbe P, Downar J. Reductions in cortico-striatal hyperconnectivity accompany successful treatment of obsessive-compulsive disorder with dorsomedial prefrontal rTMS. *Neuropsychopharmacology.* 2016;41:1395–1403.

95. Modirrousta M, Shams E, Katz C, et al. The efficacy of deep repetitive transcranial magnetic stimulation over the medial prefrontal cortex in obsessive compulsive disorder: results from an open-label study. *Depress Anxiety.* 2015;32:445–450.

96. Yücel M, Harrison BJ, Wood SJ, et al. Functional and biochemical alterations of the medial frontal cortex in obsessive-compulsive disorder. *Arch Gen Psychiatry.* 2007;64:946–955.

97. Mantovani A, Simpson HB, Fallon BA, Rossi S, Lisanby SH. Randomized sham-controlled trial of repetitive transcranial magnetic stimulation in treatment-resistant obsessive–compulsive disorder. *Int J Neuropsychopharmacol.* 2010;13:217–227.

98. Gomes PVO, Brasil-Neto JP, Allam N, Rodrigues de Souza E. A randomized, double-blind trial of repetitive transcranial magnetic stimulation in obsessive-compulsive disorder with three-month follow-up. *J Neuropsychiatry Clin Neurosci* 2012;24:437–443.

99. Hawken ER, Dilkov D, Kaludiev E, Simek S, Zhang F, Milev R. Transcranial magnetic stimulation of the supplementary motor area in the treatment of obsessive-compulsive disorder: a multi-site study. *Int J Mol Sci.* 2016;17:420.

100. Pelissolo A, Harika-Germaneau G, Rachid F, et al. Repetitive transcranial magnetic stimulation to supplementary motor area in refractory obsessive-compulsive disorder treatment: a sham-controlled trial. *Int J Neuropsychopharmacol.* 2016;19:1–6.

101. Kumar, N, Chadda, RK. Augmentation effect of repetitive transcranial magnetic stimulation over the supplementary motor cortex in treatment refractory patients with obsessive compulsive disorder. *Indian J Psychiatry.* 2011;53(4):340–342.

102. Mantovani A, Lisanby SH, Pieraccini F, Ulivelli M, Castrogiovanni P, Rossi S. Repetitive transcranial magnetic stimulation (rTMS) in the treatment of obsessive–compulsive disorder (OCD) and Tourette's syndrome (TS). *Int J Neuropsychopharmacol.* 2006;9(1):95.

103. López-Alonso V, Cheeran B, Río-Rodríguez D, Fernández-Del-Olmo M. Inter-individual variability in response to non-invasive brain stimulation paradigms. *Brain Stimulation.* 2014;7:372–380.

104. Ridding MC, Ziemann U. Determinants of the induction of cortical plasticity by non-invasive brain stimulation in healthy subjects. *J Physiol.* 2010;588:2291–2304.

105. Houdayer E, Degardin A, Cassim F, Bocquillon P, Derambure P, Devanne H. The effects of low- and high-frequency repetitive TMS on the input/output properties of the human corticospinal pathway. *Exp Brain Res.* 2008;187(2):207–217.

106. Fitzgerald PB, Brown T, Daskalakis ZJ, Chen R, Kulkarni J. Intensity-dependent effects of 1 Hz rTMS on human corticospinal excitability. *Clin Neurophysiol.* 2002;113:1136–1141.

107. Lang N, Harms J, Weyh T, et al. Stimulus intensity and coil characteristics influence the efficacy of rTMS to suppress cortical excitability. *Clin Neurophysiol.* 2006;117:2292–2301.

108. Thomson RH, Cleve TJ, Bailey NW, et al. Blood oxygenation changes modulated by coil orientation during prefrontal transcranial magnetic stimulation. *Brain Stimul.* 2013;6:576–581.

109. Cash RFH, Dar A, Hui J, et al. Influence of inter-train interval on the plastic effects of rTMS. *Brain Stimul.* 2017;10:630–636.

110. Huang Y-Z, Edwards MJ, Rounis E, Bhatia KP, Rothwell JC. Theta burst stimulation of the human motor cortex. *Neuron.* 2005;45:201–206.

111. Wu C-C, Tsai C-H, Lu M-K, Chen C-M, Shen W-C, Su K-P. Theta-burst repetitive transcranial magnetic stimulation for treatment-resistant obsessive-compulsive disorder with concomitant depression. *J Clin Psychiatry.* 2010;71:504–506.

112. Holtzheimer PE, McDonald WM, Mufti M, et al. Accelerated repetitive transcranial magnetic stimulation for treatment-resistant depression. *Depress Anxiety.* 2010;27:960–963.

113. Fitzgerald PB, Hoy K, McQueen S, et al. A randomized trial of rTMS targeted with MRI based neuro-navigation in treatment-resistant depression. *Neuropsychopharmacology.* 2009;34:1255.

114. Mantovani A, Westin G, Hirsch J, Lisanby SH. Functional magnetic resonance imaging guided transcranial magnetic stimulation in obsessive-compulsive disorder. *Biol Psychiatry.* 2010;67:e39–e40.

115. McClintock S, Reti I, Carpenter L, et al. Consensus recommendations for the clinical application of repetitive transcranial magnetic stimulation (rTMS)

in the treatment of depression. *J Clin Psychiatry.* 2017; pii: 16cs10905.

116. Dinna WM, Aycicegi-Dinna A, Göralb F, et al. Treatment-resistant obsessive-compulsive disorder: insights from an open trial of transcranial direct current stimulation (tDCS) to design a RCT. *Neurol Psychiatry Brain Res.* 2016;22:124–154.

117. Volpato C, Piccione F, Cavinato M, et al. Modulation of affective symptoms and resting state activity by brain stimulation in a treatment-resistant case of obsessive-compulsive disorder. *Neurocase.* 2013;19(4):360–370.

118. Bation R, Poulet E, Haesebaert F, Saoud M, Brunelin J. Transcranial direct current stimulation in treatment-resistant obsessive-compulsive disorder: an open-label pilot study. *Prog Neuropsychopharmacol Biol Psychiatry.* 2016;65:153–157.

119. Mondino M, Haesebaert F, Poulet E, Saoud M, Brunelin J. Efficacy of cathodal transcranial direct current stimulation over the left orbitofrontal cortex in a patient with treatment-resistant obsessive-compulsive disorder. *J ECT.* 2015;31(4):271–272.

120. D'Urso G, Brunoni AR, Mazzaferro MP, Anastasia A, de Bartolomeis A, Mantovani A. Transcranial direct current stimulation for obsessive-compulsive disorder: a randomized, controlled, partial crossover trial. *Depress Anxiety.* 2016;33(12):1132–1140.

121. Narayanaswamy JC, Jose D, Chhabra H, et al. Successful application of add-on transcranial direct current stimulation (tDCS) for treatment of SSRI resistant OCD. *Brain Stimul.* 2015;8(3):655–657.

122. Silva RM, Brunoni AR, Miguel EC, Shavitt RG. Transcranial direct current stimulation for treatment-resistant obsessive-compulsive disorder: report on two cases and proposal for a randomized, sham-controlled trial. *Sao Paulo Med J.* 2016;134(5):446–450.

123. Jamil A, Batsikadze G, Kuo HI, et al. Systematic evaluation of the impact of stimulation intensity on neuroplastic after-effects induced by transcranial direct current stimulation. *J Physiol.* 2017;595(4):1273–1288.

124. Monte-Silva K, Kuo MF, Hessenthaler S, et al. Induction of late LTP-like plasticity in the human motor cortex by repeated non-invasive brain stimulation. *Brain Stimul.* 2013;6(3):424–432.

125. Batsikadze G, Moliadze V, Paulus W, Kuo MF, Nitsche MA. Partially non-linear stimulation intensity-dependent effects of direct current stimulation on motor cortex excitability in humans. *J Physiol.* 2013;591(7):1987–2000.

126. Shahid SS, Bikson M, Salman H, Wen P, Ahfock T. The value and cost of complexity in predictive modelling: role of tissue anisotropic conductivity and fibre tracts in neuromodulation. *J Neural Eng.* 2014;11(3):036002.

127. Hill AT, Rogasch NC, Fitzgerald PB, Hoy KE. Effects of prefrontal bipolar and high-definition transcranial direct current stimulation on cortical reactivity and working memory in healthy adults. *Neuroimage.* 2017;152:142–157.

128. Strube W, Bunse T, Nitsche MA, et al. Bidirectional variability in motor cortex excitability modulation following 1 mA transcranial direct current stimulation in healthy participants. *Physiol Rep.* 2016;4(15).

129. Krause B, Cohen Kadosh R. Not all brains are created equal: the relevance of individual differences in responsiveness to transcranial electrical stimulation. *Front Syst Neurosci.* 2014;8:25.

130. Li LM, Uehara K, Hanakawa T. The contribution of interindividual factors to variability of response in transcranial direct current stimulation studies. *Front Cell Neurosci.* 2015;9:181.

131. Segrave RA, Arnold S, Hoy K, Fitzgerald PB. Concurrent cognitive control training augments the antidepressant efficacy of tDCS: a pilot study. *Brain Stimul.* 2014;7(2):325–331.

132. Brunoni AR, Valiengo L, Baccaro A, et al. The sertraline vs. electrical current therapy for treating depression clinical study: results from a factorial, randomized, controlled trial. *JAMA Psychiatry.* 2013;70(4):383–391.

133. Everitt BJ, Robbins TW. From the ventral to the dorsal striatum: devolving views of their roles in drug addiction. *Neurosci Biobehav Rev.* 2013;37(9 Pt A):1946–1954.

134. DeLong MR, Wichmann T. Circuits and circuit disorders of the basal ganglia. *Arch Neurol.* 2007;64(1):20–24.

135. Fornito A, Harrison BJ, Goodby E, et al. Functional dysconnectivity of corticostriatal circuitry as a risk phenotype for psychosis. *JAMA Psychiatry.* 2013;70(11):1143–1151.

136. Liu J, Blond BN, van Dyck LI, Spencer L, Wang F, Blumberg HP. Trait and state corticostriatal dysfunction in bipolar disorder during emotional face processing. *Bipolar Disord.* 2012;14(4):432–441.

137. Price JL, Drevets WC. Neural circuits underlying the pathophysiology of mood disorders. *Trends Cogn Sci.* 2012;16(1):61–71.

138. Insel T, Cuthbert B, Garvey M, et al. Research domain criteria (RDoC): toward a new classification

framework for research on mental disorders. *Am J Psychiatry*. 2010;167(7):748–751.

139. American Psychiatric Association. *Diagnostic and Statistical Manual of Mental Disorders*, 5th ed. Washington, DC: APA; 2013.

140. Fontenelle LF, Oostermeijer S, Harrison BJ, Pantelis C, Yucel M. Obsessive-compulsive disorder, impulse control disorders and drug addiction: common features and potential treatments. *Drugs*. 2011;71(7):827–840.

141. Chamberlain SR, Stochl J, Redden SA, Grant JE. Latent traits of impulsivity and compulsivity: toward dimensional psychiatry. *Psychol Med*. 2017:1–12.

142. Prochazkova L, Parkes L, Dawson A, et al. Unpacking the role of self-reported compulsivity and impulsivity in obsessive-compulsive disorder. *CNS Spectr*. 2017:1–8.

143. Fineberg NA, Chamberlain SR, Goudriaan AE, et al. New developments in human neurocognition: clinical, genetic, and brain imaging correlates of impulsivity and compulsivity. *CNS Spectr*. 2014;19(1):69–89.

144. Gillan CM, Morein-Zamir S, Urcelay GP, et al. Enhanced avoidance habits in obsessive-compulsive disorder. *Biol Psychiatry*. 2014;75(8):631–638.

145. Balleine BW, O'Doherty JP. Human and rodent homologies in action control: corticostriatal determinants of goal-directed and habitual action. *Neuropsychopharmacology*. 2010;35(1):48–69.

146. de Wit S, Watson P, Harsay HA, Cohen MX, van de Vijver I, Ridderinkhof KR. Corticostriatal connectivity underlies individual differences in the balance between habitual and goal-directed action control. *J Neurosci*. 2012;32(35):12066–12075.

Chapter 21

Neurosurgery for Obsessive-Compulsive Disorder: Indications and Procedures

Antonio Carlos Lopes

Introduction

Obsessive-compulsive disorder (OCD) is usually characterized by a low rate of remission and a chronic course. Especially in its more severe and untreatable forms, the disabling symptoms may carry a high risk of suicide and severe psychosocial impairment [1,2]. The therapeutic options for OCD often include the use serotonin reuptake inhibitors (SRIs; selective, SSRIs or not, e.g., clomipramine), as well as exposure and response prevention (ERP) behavior therapy. In the majority of patients, conventional treatments are efficacious and safe. However, probably up to 20% of patients remain refractory to multiple treatment trials [3,4]. For this subgroup of individuals, neurosurgery is an option. Different neurosurgical techniques have been developed so far, including both ablative techniques (stereotactic neurosurgeries or radiosurgery) and deep brain stimulation. Modern surgical techniques now provide a relatively low incidence of severe adverse events or permanent complications. However, there are no risk-free neurosurgical interventions. Eligible patients for surgery must always be carefully selected beforehand.

Since the 1990s, most studies have set somewhat similar inclusion and exclusion criteria for OCD surgery. Briefly speaking, eligible patients should have a long history of OCD as the primary diagnosis, with marked psychosocial impairment, as well as a documented use of several SRIs, drug augmentation strategies and adequately conducted behavior therapy (Table 21.1). There is also some consensus regarding exclusion criteria (or contraindications) for surgery, and usually psychotic disorders, current or unstably

Table 21.1 Commonly used inclusion and exclusion criteria for surgical procedures in refractory obsessive-compulsive disorder.

Inclusion Criteria	Exclusion Criteria
Age between 18 and 65 years	Comorbid psychotic disorders
OCD as the primary diagnosis	Cognitive deficits
OCD duration of more than five years	Neurological disorder or medical illness (except tic disorder)
Marked functional impairment associated to the OCD severity	Pregnancy or lack of use of contraceptives
Minimum Yale-Brown Obsessive Compulsive Scale (Y-BOCS) scores of 25	Imminent risk of suicide
Adequate trials of SRIs (one of which should be clomipramine), for a minimum of three months, at the maximum recommended or tolerated doses)	Substance disorder
Augmentation drugs associated (e.g., a neuroleptic or benzodiazepine)	In some studies: comorbid recent manic episode, or severe personality disorder (especially DSM-IV clusters A or B)
A minimum of 20 sessions of behavior therapy (exposure and response prevention techniques)	
Null or minimum improvement after repetitive treatment trials	

DSM-IV, *Diagnostic and Statistical Manual of Mental Disorders*, 4th edition; OCD, obsessive-compulsive disorder; SRI, serotonin reuptake inhibitor; Y-BOCS, Yale-Brown Obsessive Compulsive Scale.

remitted substance disorder, neurological/general medical conditions or pregnancy have precluded the indications of surgery.

The Advent of Stereotactic Neurosurgeries for Mental Disorders and Ablative Neurosurgical Procedures for Obsessive-Compulsive Disorder

In 1936, Antonio Egas Moniz and Almeida Lima reported the employment of a neurosurgical intervention in the frontal lobes of 20 psychiatric patients with relatively good results for those times, in a technique called "frontal leucotomy" [5,6]. Later on, a similar technique was employed by Walter Freeman and James Watts, whose lay term was "lobotomy". Widespread and often indiscriminate use of this neurosurgical intervention was conducted in the 1940s and 1950s [7,8].

The lessons from the "lobotomy years" had shown that widespread leucotomy lesions in the brain were often associated to severe adverse events. That led to new attempts of precisely refining the anatomic lesions made by the neurosurgeries using smaller targets. In 1947, the neurologist Spiegel and the neurosurgeon Wycis developed the first stereotactic apparatus, allowing neurosurgical lesions to become more precise and smaller [9]. Later on, in 1949, Talairach in France developed the first stereotactic radiofrequency thermocoagulation neurosurgery aiming at the internal capsules of psychiatric patients [10]. Leksell in Sweden had adopted a similar approach. In 1953, without trephination, Leksell also delivered sharply collimated x-ray beams to the internal capsule, in the first radiosurgical psychiatric surgery [11].

Only three years later, another stereotactic technique was developed in the United States, with lesions at the anterior cingulum, while in the following years other techniques, like the subcaudate tractotomy and a combined lesion (limbic leucotomy) were also developed for treating severe OCD cases [12,13,14]. In the following decades, radiofrequency lesions continued to be employed (especially with the capsulotomy and cingulotomy techniques), but other surgical modalities were incorporated, such as Gamma Knife® radiosurgery, deep brain stimulation, and the still experimental magnetic resonance guided focused ultrasound (Figure 21.1) [15,16].

The common feature among these different techniques is the injury of a neural network that later on was found to be associated to the pathophysiology of OCD. This pathway includes mainly the connections

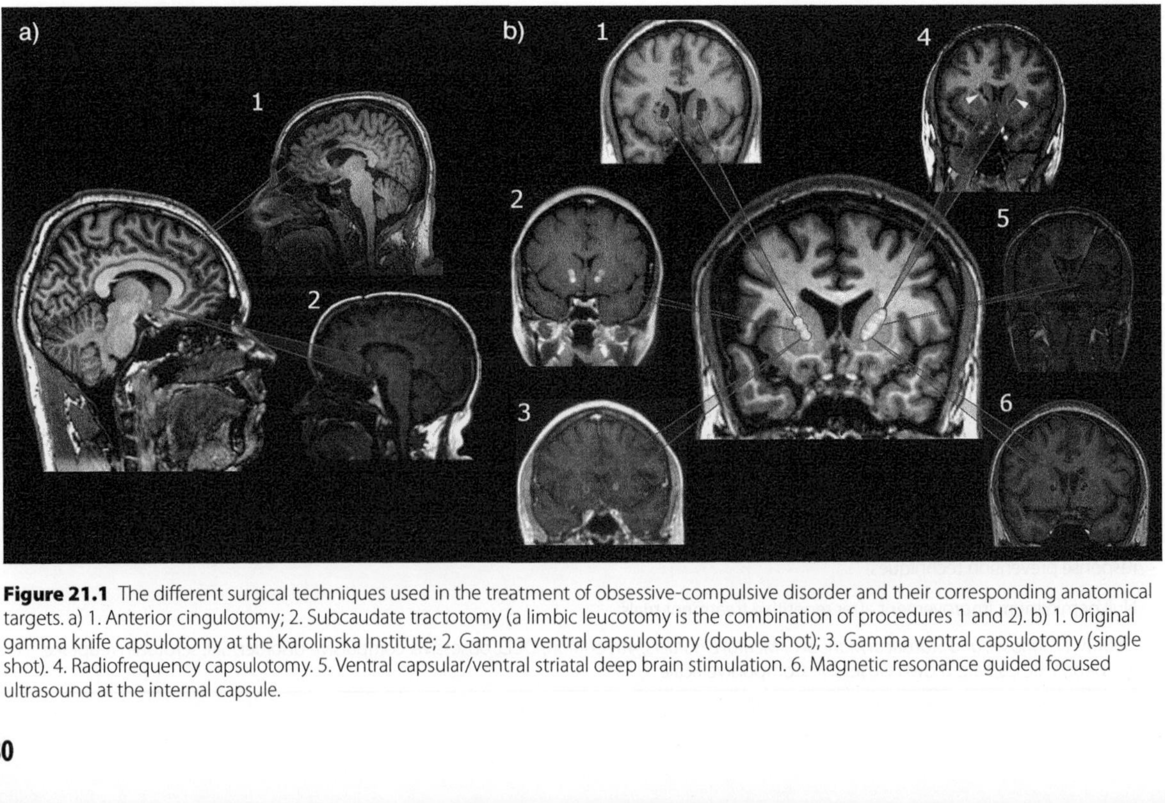

Figure 21.1 The different surgical techniques used in the treatment of obsessive-compulsive disorder and their corresponding anatomical targets. a) 1. Anterior cingulotomy; 2. Subcaudate tractotomy (a limbic leucotomy is the combination of procedures 1 and 2). b) 1. Original gamma knife capsulotomy at the Karolinska Institute; 2. Gamma ventral capsulotomy (double shot); 3. Gamma ventral capsulotomy (single shot). 4. Radiofrequency capsulotomy. 5. Ventral capsular/ventral striatal deep brain stimulation. 6. Magnetic resonance guided focused ultrasound at the internal capsule.

between cortical areas (such as the orbitofrontal cortex, ventromedial prefrontal cortex and anterior cingulate gyrus), ventral striatum areas and thalamic regions (e.g., the dorsomedial nucleus) [15,17]. A normalization of the metabolic activity of these interconnected areas has been associated to symptom improvement, both in drug therapy and neurosurgery studies [18].

The first descriptions of ablative neurosurgical interventions for OCD suggested that these procedures were possibly efficacious [19]. On the other hand, those were times when modern psychiatric diagnostic criteria and reliable psychometric assessments were not available yet, and thus precise measures of primary outcomes were not feasible. Moreover, adverse events were not systematically investigated in the follow-up of these patients.

The efficacy of radiofrequency or mechanical lesioning capsulotomy has ranged from 37% to 64% after one year of follow-up in contemporary studies (Table 21.1) [20,21,22,23,24,25]. Most adverse events were transient and did not lead to long-term complications [20,22,25]. However, uncommon and severe complications were sometimes described (such as hemorrhage, brain edema, frontal lobe syndrome, personality changes, urinary incontinence, episodic seizures or even hemiparesis) in radiofrequency, and especially with mechanical capsulotomy [20,21,23,25]. In this last procedure, the use of a leucotome has been implicated in a case series in a higher risk of hemorrhage and it was therefore abandoned [21].

As to the cingulotomy technique, a prospective, long-term follow-up study of 64 patients with refractory OCD at the Massachusetts General Hospital showed that 47% of the subjects reported a reduction of 35% or more in baseline Yale-Brown Obsessive Compulsive Scale (Y-BOCS) scores at their last follow-up assessment [26]. Note that this study comprised a mean follow-up of more than 5 years, and 30 patients who underwent more than one surgery (i.e., repeated cingulotomy or subcaudate tractotomy). Adverse events, such as seizures, subdural empyema and transient memory deficits were sometimes observed [26].

Recent Research Findings

Gamma Knife Radiosurgery for Obsessive-Compulsive Disorder

As already cited, the first radiosurgical intervention was done in 1953, using x-rays. Rather than opening the skull to deliver a thermal lesion inside the brain, this technique allowed focusing of ionizing radiation to create a lesion without trephination. However, it was ineffective for very small and precise lesions in the brain tissue [27]. Later on, in 1967, Lars Leksell developed a radiosurgery device that delivered gamma ray beams from a radioactive isotope of cobalt 60. Hundreds of these gamma ray beams could be focused in a single spot inside the brain, and in the small volume within the intersection of these beams, a high dose of radiation was produced, in such a way that it could lesion white-matter tracts.

Thus, in 1976, using hundreds of sharply collimated gamma ray beams, the first Gamma Knife radiosurgery was done in Sweden, aiming to treat psychiatric disorders [19,28]. In fact, the first patients treated with this technique included both OCD and various anxiety disorders, such as phobias, generalized anxiety and panic disorder. In the Karolinska Institute, using the first model of the Gamma Knife equipment, 36–56% of patients probably benefited from this intervention [19,29]. The most striking improvements were seen in the patients with OCD, but systematic assessments of symptoms by rating instruments were not available, and adverse events were not described in the initial studies.

In 1985 in Sweden, Per Mindus and Christer Lindquist began to use the second Gamma Knife model, which covered a smaller target volume than the first prototype, using 4-mm and 8-mm collimators. Even so, high doses of radiation were needed at the center of the shot (ranging from 160 Gy to 200 Gy) to produce a detectable lesion in the white-matter tracts. Three isocenters (round shots) were usually chosen in each hemisphere, aiming at the anterior limb of the internal capsules (Figure 21.1). The complete descriptions of their cohort of patients were available in 2008, when Christian Rück reported the results of the Swedish surgeries for OCD (Table 21.2) [23].

Radiofrequency and Gamma Knife capsulotomies were similarly efficacious, with response rates of 46.7% and 55.6%, respectively. However, they differed in terms of severe/permanent adverse events, with radiofrequency showing isolated cases of urinary incontinence, sexual disinhibition and substance abuse, while Gamma Knife capsulotomy showed additional cognitive changes, and signs of brain edema and radionecrosis. Note that radiosurgical complications were associated with very high doses of radiation (200 Gy) in larger volumes.

Table 21.2 Main ablative surgeries and deep brain stimulation studies in obsessive-compulsive disorder.

Study	Technique	Design	Site	Patients (*n*)	Diagnosis (*n*)	Mean Time of Follow-Up (months)	Responders, *n*/*N* (%)	Severe or Permanent Adverse Events (*n*)
Lippitz et al., 1997 [30]	Radiofrequency capsulotomy	Case series	ALIC	19	OCD (19)	n/a	9/19 (47.4)	n/a
Mindus et al., 1999 [31]	Radiofrequency capsulotomy	Case series	ALIC	19	OCD (19)	99.6?	8/19 (42.1)	Intraventricular hemorrhage (1)
Gascón et al., 2002 [32]	Radiofrequency capsulotomy	Case series	ALIC	15 (1C at completion)	OCD (15)	12	6/10 (60)	Brain edema, plus transient urinary incontinence and signs of frontal lobe syndrome (1); episodic convulsion (1)
Oliver et al., 2003 [20]	Radiofrequency capsulotomy	Case series	ALIC	18	OCD (18)	24	6/10 (60) at month 12	Brain edema with permanent "behavior disorder" (1)
Liu et al., 2008 [24]	Radiofrequency capsulotomy	Case series	ALIC	35	OCD (35)	36	Unclear	Cerebral hematoma with ventricular drainage (1), frontal lobe syndrome (2), weight loss (1)
Csigó et al., 2010 [25]	Radiofrequency capsulotomy	Case series	ALIC	5	OCD (5)	24	n/a	Increased appetite and weight gain (2)
D'Astous et al., 2013 [21]	Mechanical lesioning capsulotomy	Case series	ALIC	19	OCD (19)	84	7/19 (36.8)	Hemiplegia(1), cognitive deficits (1)
Zhan et al., 2014 [33]	Radiofrequency capsulotomy	Case series	ALIC	53	OCD (53)	67.5	33/53 (62.2)?	Apathy and lack of interest (3); impaired memory (1); urinary incontinence for up to 2 weeks (11)
Jung et al., 2015 [16]	Capsular magnetic resonance guided focused ultrasound	Case series	ALIC	4	OCD (4)	6	2/4 (50)	Weight gain (1)
Rylander et al., 1978 [19]	Gamma Knife® capsulotomy	Case series	ALIC	9	OCD (5); "chronic anxiety" (4)	5.4	5/9 (55.5)	n/a

Kihlström et al., 1995 [29]	Gamma Knife capsulotomy	Case series	ALIC	11	OCD (5); GAD or phobias (6)	n/a	4/11 (36.4)	Severe fatigue (3), signs of frontal lobe syndrome (apathy, fatigue, loss of initiative, occasional disinhibition) (2)
Lippitz et al., 1999 [22]	Gamma Knife capsulotomy	Case series	ALIC	9	OCD (9)	n/a	7/9 (77.7)	n/a
	Radiofrequency capsulotomy	Case series	ALIC	14	OCD (14)	n/a	9/14 (64.3)	n/a
Rasmussen et al., 2001 [34]	Gamma ventral capsulotomy, mainly double shot	Case series	VC/VS	15 (13 in the end)	OCD (15)	8	1/15 (6.7) single shot; 5/13 (38.5) with additional shot	Brain cyst (3), with neurological signs (headache, dizziness, visual changes) (1) requiring surgical cyst drainage; frontal syndrome (apathy, amotivation) (1)
Rück et al., 2008 [23]	Gamma Knife capsulotomy	Case series	ALIC	9	OCD (9)	139.6	5/9 (55.6)	Chronic brain edema (1), radiation necrosis with sequelae(1), cognitive changes (1), apathy (2), urinary incontinence (1), seizures (1), sexual disinhibition (1)
	Radiofrequency capsulotomy	Case series	ALIC	16	OCD (16)	126.4	7/15 (46.7)	Urinary incontinence (1), sexual disinhibition (1), substance abuse (1)
Lopes et al., 2009 [35]	Gamma ventral capsulotomy, double shot	Case series	VC/VS	5	OCD (5)	48	3/5 (60)	Weight changes (4)
Kondziolka et al., 2011 [36]	Gamma ventral capsulotomy, double shot	Case series	VC/VS	3	OCD (2); skin-picking disorder (1)	41.6 (13.5)	2/3 (66.7)	n/a
Sheehan et al., 2013 [37]	Gamma ventral capsulotomy, single shot	Case series	VC/VS	5	OCD (5)	22.2 (11.7)	4/5 (80)	None described

(continued)

Table 21.2 *(cont.)*

Study	Technique	Design	Site	Patients (*n*)	Diagnosis (*n*)	Mean Time of Follow-Up (months)	Responders, *n*/*N* (%)	Severe or Permanent Adverse Events (*n*)
Lopes et al., 2014 [38]	Gamma ventral capsulotomy, double shot	Sham-controlled, RCT, 12 months + case series	VC/VS	16	OCD (16)	55	0/8 (12 months) 2/8 (25) (12 months); 5/8 (62.5%) (last FU) 7/12 (58.3) (last FU, all operated patients)	Increased appetite and weight (4) (sham group) Manic episode (2), delirium + perseverations for 1 week (1), increased appetite and weight (6), memory deficits for 10 months (1), asymptomatic brain cyst (1), substance abuse (1) (all operated patients)
Sheth et al., 2013 [26]	Anterior cingulotomy	Case series	Anterior cingulum	64	OCD (64)	63.8 (7.7)	15/30 (50) for initial procedure; 12/38 (31.6%) for most recent FU	Temporary memory deficits (5), transient urinary retention (2), abulia (4), intraoperative convulsions (3), epilepsy (1), subdural empyema (1), pulmonary embolism (1), suicide (2)
Nuttin et al., 2003 [39]	DBS	RCT, 3 months on/off	ALIC/VC/VS	6	OCD (6)		4/6 (67) improved	Fatigue (1); subjective memory complaints (1); weight gain (2); transient disinhibition (2)
Abelson et al., 2005 [40]	DBS	RCT; 3 weeks on/off + case series	ALIC/VC/VS	4	OCD (4)		1/4 (25) improved in the randomized phase	Transient elevated mood (1), depressive symptoms (2) + suicide (1)
Goodman et al., 2010 [41]	DBS	RCT, 1 month on/off + case series	ALIC/VC/VS	6	OCD (6)		2/6 (33) after 1 month; 50% in 3 months; 67% in 12 months	Headache, nausea, sore throat, anxiety, panic, hypomania (4), insomnia, worse obsessive-compulsive symptoms (1)

Huff et al., 2010 [42]	DBS	RCT, 3 months on/off + case series	Unilateral NAcc	8	OCD (8)		1/10 (10) improved after 3 months ON; 1/10 (10) improved by month 12 of open phase	Subclavicular dysesthesia (1); transient agitation and anxiety (4); hypomania (2); concentration difficulties and failing memory (1); insomnia (1); weight gain (2); suicidal ideas (1)
Denys et al., 2010 [43]	DBS	RCT, 2 weeks on/off + case series	NAcc	6 on/off; 8 off/on	OCD (14)		8 /14 (57) during the RCT	Headache (3); transient paresthesias (3); forgetfulness (5); insomnia (3); hypomania (8); increased libido (7); micturition problems (2); taste reduction (3); stomach aches (4)
Mallet et al., 2008 [44]	DBS	RCT, 3 months on/off	Subthalamic nucleus	8 on/off; 8 off/on	OCD (16)		6/16 (40) during the RCT	CNS hemorrhage (1); CNS infection (2); transient diplopia (1); hypomania (3); transient dyskinesia (1); dysarthria/dysphagia transit (1)
Luyten et al., 2016 [45]	DBS	RCT, 3 months on/off + case series	ALIC/BNST	17	OCD (17)		11/17 (65) during the RCT	CNS hemorrhage (2); suicide attempts (4); epileptic seizures (5); morbid obesity (1); fatigue (18); memory complaints (16); disinhibition (12); logorrhea (10); hypomania (4); electrode misplacement (1)

ALIC, anterior limb of the internal capsule; BNST, bed nucleus of stria terminalis; CNS, central nervous system; DBS, deep brain stimulation; FU, follow-up; GAD, generalized anxiety disorder; n/a, not available; NAcc, nucleus accumbens; OCD, obsessive-compulsive disorder; OFF, stimulator off; ON, stimulator on; RCT, randomized controlled trial; VC/VS, ventral capsular/ventral striatal.

In the United States, Steven Rasmussen at Brown University made changes in the original Gamma Knife capsulotomy protocol. First, 15 patients received one bilateral midcapsular shot at the anterior limb of the internal capsule. Only one patient responded to treatment. Then, an additional lesion was made in the ventral portion of the internal capsule in 13 of these original patients. This time, 5 of 13 (38.5%) patients responded. This double-shot technique, aimed at the ventral portions of the anterior limb in the internal capsule, with 4-mm collimators and a total dose of 180 Gy, was then coined "gamma ventral capsulotomy" (GVC; Figure 21.1) [34].

Using the same technique as Rasmussen's group, we found that 3 of 5 (60%) patients were treatment responders after 24 months of follow-up, with 36% reduction of Y-BOCS scores [35]. Measures of anxiety and depression also improved in the sample. Later on, other patients received double-shot GVC in Pittsburgh, with the latest Gamma Knife model, using lower doses (140–150 Gy). Two of three (66.7%) patients were full responders [36].

The first double-blind, sham-controlled, randomized trial of an ablative surgical intervention in psychiatry was conducted with GVC for refractory OCD [46]. Sixteen patients were randomized between active and sham Gamma Knife. Two of eight (25%) patients were full responders at 12 months of blind follow-up, but none of the sham treatment group became responders. In spite of the small number of responders in the active group, changes in the Y-BOCS scores between the groups reached statistical significance. In the long-term follow-up, the most common adverse events were episodic headaches, nausea and weight changes. Two patients had hypomanic crises. One patient developed abnormal radionecrosis, with delirium and confabulation for a few days and, later on, an asymptomatic brain cyst.

Contrary to the findings of the Swedish group, no severe or permanent neuropsychological adverse changes were found in the GVC cohorts, possibly reflecting the lower induction of adverse events with smaller capsulotomy lesions and lower radiation doses [38,47]. Finally, a group from the University of Virginia proposed even smaller targets (single-shot lesions), at the most ventral border of the internal capsule, using 140 Gy and 160 Gy (Figure 21.1) [37]. Four of their five (80%) patients reached full response after a mean follow-up period of 22 months, with a mean 50% reduction on Y-BOCS scores. Adverse events were not described.

Deep Brain Stimulation for Obsessive-Compulsive Disorder

Deep brain stimulation is an alternative method for changing brain function without substantial injury of nervous tissue. It consists of the intracerebral installation of stimulation electrodes, connected to pulse generators, which are implanted in the subclavicular subcutaneous region. The subcutaneous neurostimulators continuously deliver electrical pulses to the tips of the intracerebral electrodes, and thus change the electrical activity of the targeted brain area and its related neural network. Since 1999, DBS has been studied in patients with refractory OCD, aimed at various brain targets [48,49]. Regardless of the study design, the global percentage of responders is estimated in 60% [50]. The main adverse events are anxiety, hypomanic symptoms and memory problems, in various techniques (Table 21.1), but occasional complications have been reported, such as wound infection (4.3%), intracerebral hemorrhage (2.6%), seizures (0.9%) and suicidal ideation (3.4%) [50]. The main advantage of this technique is its reversibility. Tissue damage is minimal and the effects on the stimulation site can be readily modified. Nevertheless, it is an expensive intervention, which requires expert neurosurgical and psychiatric teams throughout the procedure and in the follow-up. Detailed descriptions regarding the use of DBS in OCD are found in Chapter 20 of this book.

Cross-Diagnostic Approaches and Their Implications for Classification and Diagnosis

In the first decades after the advert of prefrontal leucotomy, a myriad of different mental disorders were subject to neurosurgical interventions, often in an indiscriminate way. In the 1950s and 1960s, as clinical experience accumulated, it was evident that severe OCD and depression were probably the best indications for surgery. In 1955, James Watts performed the first trans-orbital leucotomy for the treatment of patients with Tourette's disorder, but it was only in 1962 that Baker described the effects of neurosurgery (bi-medial leucotomy) in these patients [51]. Since then, various surgical techniques have been developed for treating refractory Tourette's disorder.

In 1970, Hassler and Dieckmann proposed to lesion the median and rostral intralaminar nuclei and the internal ventral oral nucleus of the thalamus selectively, which culminated in a response rate of 70% [52]. In spite of the smaller and refined target, adverse events secondary to this intervention were not negligible. In other case reports, ablative surgical techniques indicated for OCD were also employed in Tourette's disorder, such as limbic leucotomy and cingulotomy, especially when OCD or self-injurious behaviors were comorbid [53–56]. Positive results were reported in a few cases, generally associated with improvements in obsessive-compulsive symptoms and self-injury.

The first descriptions of deep brain stimulation surgery for OCD and Tourette's disorder were independently published in the same year, but with different targets: anterior limb of the internal capsule (ALIC) and thalamic nuclei, respectively [49,57]. Later, several targets have been chosen for deep brain stimulation in Tourette's disorder, especially in the thalamic nuclei, the globus pallidus pars interna or pars externa and the ALIC/anterior cingulate cortex. Today, probably more than 150 individuals with Tourette's disorder have received deep brain stimulation all around the world. When pooled together, all targets have shown similar efficacy, with an overall improvement of 53% in severity of tics [58].

Compared with no stimulation, 80% of patients with active stimulation of their electrodes had at least 25% reduction in symptom severity, or more than 50% improvements in 50% of patients. There were no significant correlations between obsessive-compulsive or depressive symptoms with the main outcome. The comorbidity between Tourette's disorder and OCD is high, and these diagnostic entities share some common pathophysiological neural pathways. However, Tourette's disorder has a large phenotypic variability, and comorbidity with attention deficit hyperactivity disorder and depression, which may partly explain why there are so many different target areas for deep brain stimulation in Tourette's disorder, when compared with OCD [59].

Another mental disorder that might benefit from a neurosurgical intervention is anorexia nervosa. Excessive preoccupation with body weight and "compulsive", compensatory behaviors (such as exaggerated physical activities) are some of the characteristic features of the disorder. In fact, anorexia nervosa can fit into the obsessive-compulsive spectrum disorders [60]. Moreover, functional neuroimaging studies suggest that some of the neural structures recruited in OCD can also take part in anorexia nervosa. For example, patients with anorexia nervosa, when exposed to food cues, can show signs of arousal, fear and avoidance, with activation of medial prefrontal cortex, anterior cingulate cortex, striatum and amygdala [61].

Regarding ablative neurosurgeries, there are only a few case reports with small numbers of patients with anorexia nervosa. There is one description in a patient with anorexia nervosa and OCD who received capsulotomy, with positive results [62]. Lesioning of the accumbens has also been described in six patients, with improved body mass index [63]. As to deep brain stimulation, some studies have targeted the subgenual cingulate cortex. One of these studies found that three of six (50%) patients with anorexia nervosa significantly gained weight at nine months of follow-up, accompanied by improvements in anorexia nervosa and mood symptoms [64]. Another study has assessed the effects of deep brain stimulation of the accumbens in four patients with anorexia nervosa. All patients improved over a long-term follow-up of three years [65]. Moreover, a patient with OCD with comorbid anorexia nervosa demonstrated normalization of the body mass index after ventral capsular/ventral striatal deep brain stimulation [66].

Clinical Implications of Cross-Diagnostic Approaches for Treatment and Prevention

In the fifth edition of the *Diagnostic and Statistical Manual of Mental Disorders* [67], OCD was included in a separate chapter, with a cluster of disorders that involve obsessional thoughts and/or compulsive behaviors. These include body dysmorphic disorder (BDD), hoarding disorder, trichotillomania (hair-pulling disorder) and excoriation (skin-picking) disorder. On the other hand, it is not clear whether grouping these different disorders in the same cluster would impact on the indication of neurosurgical procedures for these diagnostic entities. Literature on this issue is scarce.

A study by Gentil et al., in 2014 [68], assessed the influence of different obsessive-compulsive symptoms as a predictor of response to ablative neurosurgeries (cingulotomy, capsulotomy and GVC) in three different centers (Harvard University, the

Karolinska Institute and the University of São Paulo). The presence of symptoms of hoarding was the only dimension that was consistently associated with a worse prognosis in any type of surgery for OCD [69]. Note that many patients with OCD can have hoarding symptoms without fulfilling a diagnosis of hoarding disorder. To date, no studies have investigated the use of neurosurgical intervention for hoarding disorder.

In his series of three patients who received GVC, Kondziolka et al. [36] describes one patient who showed comorbid OCD and very severe skin-picking behaviors. After GVC, with a follow-up of 42 months, excoriation symptoms improved, together with OCD. This is the first description of neurosurgical treatment for excoriation disorder. In another study with a case series of five patients, one patient with refractory OCD had comorbid (and less severe) excoriation disorder. Her obsessive-compulsive symptoms improved in the long-term follow-up, but excoriation symptoms remained unaltered [35].

There are no reports of surgical interventions for BDD or trichotillomania. Of course, these two diagnoses may pose some extra challenges for a surgical indication, if patients become obsessed with minimal scar signs secondary to surgery on the face or the neck (like in some patients with BDD), or if patients maintain their compulsive urges to excoriate the skin that covers the deep brain stimulation electrodes or the pulse generator.

Conclusions and Future Directions

The indication of neurosurgical procedures for treating OCD is well established today. Clear criteria for refractoriness already exist and contraindications to such procedures have been investigated in different neurosurgical centers. However, there are many research questions in this area that are still underexplored. First, apart from OCD and Tourette's disorder, only a few small studies have investigated the role of neurosurgeries as a therapeutic option for some of the obsessive-compulsive spectrum disorders, such as anorexia nervosa or even post-traumatic stress disorder. To date, no studies have been published on surgical interventions for conditions such as hoarding disorder, BDD or trichotillomania.

In terms of surgical options, there are no studies comparing ablative techniques (like Gamma Knife or radiofrequency lesions) and deep brain stimulation with the same protocol, both in terms of efficacy/safety and cost effectiveness. Another key point is the choice for new targets or new surgical techniques. In deep brain stimulation for refractory depression, there is already a proposal to magnify the efficacy of this procedure by guiding the surgical targets according to the distribution of specific fiber tracts, as evidenced by diffusion tensor magnetic resonance imaging [68]. A similar approach will probably be employed in the following neurosurgical studies for OCD and related disorders.

In 2015, a proof-of-concept study on the use of magnetic resonance-guided focused ultrasound was published [16]. It is a new, therapeutic ultrasound surgery, which mimics the effects of Gamma Knife on brain tissue, but without the inconvenient exposure to radiation. A series of four patients with OCD indicates that 50% of the participants demonstrated more than 35% reductions in their Y-BOCS scores at six months of follow-up. The target was the anterior limb of the internal capsule. The only adverse events were mild headaches and vestibular symptoms, with no cognitive deficits so far. Larger studies using this surgical technique are certainly necessary.

In conclusion, neurosurgical techniques are part of the therapeutic options for the most severe patients with refractory OCD and Tourette's disorder. Other indications in the obsessive-compulsive spectrum are still under investigation. However, it has to be emphasized that only those patients with the most chronic, severe and refractory disorders should be referred for neurosurgery. Furthermore, all patients must be informed of potential benefits and risks secondary to these interventions and must always sign a consent form. Patients who are candidates for neurosurgery should be referred to experienced and specialized multidisciplinary teams consisting of psychiatrists, neurosurgeons, neuropsychologists, behavior therapists and so on. The neurosurgical facility must also guarantee that patients will receive long-term follow-up.

References

1. Ruscio AM, Stein DJ, Chiu WT, Kessler RC. The epidemiology of obsessive-compulsive disorder in the National Comorbidity Survey Replication. *Mol Psychiatry*. 2010;15(1):53–63.
2. Fernández de la Cruz L, Rydell M, Runeson B, et al. Suicide in obsessive-compulsive disorder: a population-based study of 36 788 Swedish patients. *Mol Psychiatry*. 2017;22(11):1626–1632.

3. McKay D, Sookman D, Neziroglu F, et al. Efficacy of cognitive-behavioral therapy for obsessive-compulsive disorder. *Psychiatry Res.* 2015;227(1):104–113.
4. Husted DS, Shapira NA. A review of the treatment for refractory obsessive-compulsive disorder: from medicine to deep brain stimulation. *CNS Spectr.* 2004;9(11):833–847.
5. Heller AC, Amar AP, Liu CY, Apuzzo MLJ. Surgery of the mind and mood: a mosaic of issues in time and evolution. *Neurosurgery.* 2006;59(4):720–739.
6. Feldman RP, Goodrich JT. Psychosurgery: a historical overview. *Neurosurgery.* 2001;48(3):647–659.
7. Mashour GA, Walker EE, Martuza RL. Psychosurgery: past, present, and future. *Brain Res Brain Res Rev.* 2005;48(3):409–419.
8. National Commission for the Protection of Human Subjects of Biomedical and Behavioral Research. *Appendix: Psychosurgery*. Publication no. 77-0002. Washington, DC: US Department of Health, Education and Welfare; 1977.
9. Spiegel EA, Wycis HT, Marks M, Lee AJ. Stereotaxic apparatus for operations on the human brain. *Science.* 1947;106(2754):349–350.
10. Talairach, Hecaen H, David M. Lobotomie préfrontal limitée par électro-coagulation des jikes thalamopontales à leur émergence du bras antérieur de la capoule interne. In: 4th International Congress of Neurology. Paris: ICN. Paris, France; 1949.
11. Leksell L, Herner T, Lidén K. Stereotaxic radiosurgery of the brain. Report of a case. *K Fysiogr Sällsk Lund Förhandl.* 1955;25(17):142–151.
12. Whitty CWM, Dufield JE, Tov' PM, Cairns H. Anterior cingulectomy in the treatment of mental disease. *Lancet.* 1952 Mar 8;1(6706):475–481.
13. Knight G. Stereotactic tractotomy in the surgical treatment of mental illness. *S J Neurol Neurosurg Psychiatry.* 1965 Aug;28:304–310.
14. Kelly D, Mitchell-Heggs N. Stereotactic limbic leucotomy--a follow-up study of thirty patients. *Postgrad Med J.* 1973 Dec;49(578):865–882.
15. Greenberg BD, Rauch SL, Haber SN. Invasive circuitry-based neurotherapeutics: stereotactic ablation and deep brain stimulation for OCD. *Neuropsychopharmacol Off Publ Am Coll Neuropsychopharmacol.* 2010 Jan;35(1):317–336.
16. Jung HH, Kim SJ, Roh D, et al. Bilateral thermal capsulotomy with MR-guided focused ultrasound for patients with treatment-refractory obsessive-compulsive disorder: a proof-of-concept study. *Mol Psychiatry.* 2015;20(10):1205–1211.
17. Haber SN, McFarland NR. The concept of the ventral striatum in nonhuman primates. *Ann N Y Acad Sci.* 1999;877:33–48.
18. Suetens K, Nuttin B, Gabriëls L, Van Laere K. Differences in metabolic network modulation between capsulotomy and deep-brain stimulation for refractory obsessive-compulsive disorder. *J Nucl Med Off Publ Soc Nucl Med.* 2014;55(6):951–959.
19. Rylander G. Försök med gammakapsulotomi vid ångest- och tvångsneuroser. *Läkartidningen.* 1978;75(7):547–549.
20. Oliver B, Gascón J, Aparicio A, et al. Bilateral anterior capsulotomy for refractory obsessive-compulsive disorders. *Stereotact Funct Neurosurg.* 2003;81(1–4):90–95.
21. D'Astous M, Cottin S, Roy M, Picard C, Cantin L. Bilateral stereotactic anterior capsulotomy for obsessive-compulsive disorder: long-term follow-up. *J Neurol Neurosurg Psychiatry.* 2013;84(11):1208–1213.
22. Lippitz BE, Mindus P, Meyerson BA, Kihlström L, Lindquist C. Lesion topography and outcome after thermocapsulotomy or gamma knife capsulotomy for obsessive-compulsive disorder: relevance of the right hemisphere. *Neurosurgery.* 1999;44(3):452–460.
23. Rück C, Karlsson A, Steele JD, et al. Capsulotomy for obsessive-compulsive disorder: long-term follow-up of 25 patients. *Arch Gen Psychiatry.* 2008;65(8):914–921.
24. Liu K, Zhang H, Liu C, et al. Stereotactic treatment of refractory obsessive compulsive disorder by bilateral capsulotomy with 3 years follow-up. *J Clin Neurosci Off J Neurosurg Soc Australas.* 2008;15(6):622–629.
25. Csigó K, Harsányi A, Demeter G, Rajkai C, Németh A, Racsmány M. Long-term follow-up of patients with obsessive-compulsive disorder treated by anterior capsulotomy: a neuropsychological study. *J Affect Disord.* 2010;126(1–2):198–205.
26. Sheth SA, Neal J, Tangherlini F, et al. Limbic system surgery for treatment-refractory obsessive-compulsive disorder: a prospective long-term follow-up of 64 patients. *J Neurosurg.* 2013;118(3):491–497.
27. Kondziolka D. Functional radiosurgery. *Neurosurgery.* 1999;44(1):12–22.
28. Leksell L. Stereotactic radiosurgery. *J Neurol Neurosurg Psychiatry.* 1983;46(9):797–803.
29. Kihlström L, Guo WY, Lindquist C, Mindus P. Radiobiology of radiosurgery for refractory anxiety disorders. *Neurosurgery.* 1995;36(2):294–302.
30. Lippitz B, Mindus P, Meyerson BA, Kihlström L, Lindquist C. Obsessive compulsive disorder and the right hemisphere: topographic analysis of lesions after anterior capsulotomy performed with thermocoagulation. *Acta Neurochir Suppl.* 1997;68:61–63.
31. Mindus P, Edman G, Andréewitch S. A prospective, long-term study of personality traits in patients with

intractable obsessional illness treated by capsulotomy. *Acta Psychiatr Scand.* 1999;99(1):40–50.

32. Gascón J, Martin MJ, Soler Insa PA, Alea E, Aparicio A, Oliver B. Efficacy of psychosurgery in obsessive-compulsive disorder. Preliminary results (September 2002). *Rev Psiquiatr Fac Med Barc.* 2002;29(6):398–409.
33. Zhan S, Liu W, Li D, et al. Long-term follow-up of bilateral anterior capsulotomy in patients with refractory obsessive-compulsive disorder. *Clin Neurol Neurosurg.* 2014;119:91–95.
34. Rasmussen SA. Anterior gamma capsulotomy for intractable OCD. In: Proceedings of the 5th International Obsessive Compulsive Disorder Conference. Sardinia, Italy; 2001.
35. Lopes AC, Greenberg BD, Norén G, et al. Treatment of resistant obsessive-compulsive disorder with ventral capsular/ventral striatal gamma capsulotomy: a pilot prospective study. *J Neuropsychiatry Clin Neurosci.* 2009;21(4):381–392.
36. Kondziolka D, Flickinger JC, Hudak R. Results following gamma knife radiosurgical anterior capsulotomies for obsessive compulsive disorder. *Neurosurgery.* 2011;68(1):28–32.
37. Sheehan JP, Patterson G, Schlesinger D, Xu Z. γ knife surgery anterior capsulotomy for severe and refractory obsessive-compulsive disorder. *J Neurosurg.* 2013;119(5):1112–1118.
38. Taub A, Lopes A, Fuentes D, et al. Neuropsychological outcome of ventral capsular/ventral striatal gamma capsulotomy for refractory obsessive-compulsive disorder: a pilot study. *J Neuropsychiatry Clin Neurosci.* 2009;21(4):393–397.
39. Nuttin BJ, Gabriëls LA, Cosyns PR, et al. Long-term electrical capsular stimulation in patients with obsessive-compulsive disorder. *Neurosurgery.* 2003;52(6):1263–1274.
40. Abelson JL, Curtis GC, Sagher O, et al. Deep brain stimulation for refractory obsessive-compulsive disorder. *Biol Psychiatry.* 2005;57(5):510–516.
41. Goodman WK, Foote KD, Greenberg BD, et al. Deep brain stimulation for intractable obsessive compulsive disorder: pilot study using a blinded, staggered-onset design. *Biol Psychiatry.* 2010;67(6):535–542.
42. Huff W, Lenartz D, Schormann M, et al. Unilateral deep brain stimulation of the nucleus accumbens in patients with treatment-resistant obsessive-compulsive disorder: outcomes after one year. *Clin Neurol Neurosurg.* 2010;112(2):137–143.
43. Denys D, Mantione M, Figee M, et al. Deep brain stimulation of the nucleus accumbens for treatment-refractory obsessive-compulsive disorder. *Arch Gen Psychiatry.* 2010;67(10):1061–1068.
44. Mallet L, Polosan M, Jaafari N, et al. Subthalamic nucleus stimulation in severe obsessive-compulsive disorder. *N Engl J Med.* 2008;359(20):2121–2134.
45. Luyten L, Hendrickx S, Raymaekers S, Gabriëls L, Nuttin B. Electrical stimulation in the bed nucleus of the stria terminalis alleviates severe obsessive-compulsive disorder. *Mol Psychiatry.* 2016;21(9):1272–1280.
46. Lopes AC, Greenberg BD, Canteras MM, et al. Gamma ventral capsulotomy for obsessive-compulsive disorder: a randomized clinical trial. *JAMA Psychiatry.* 2014;71(9):1066–1076.
47. Batistuzzo M Marcelo T, Anita G, et al. Visuospatial memory improvement after gamma ventral capsulotomy in treatment refractory obsessive-compulsive disorder patients. *Neuropsychopharmacology.* 2015;40(8):1837–1845.
48. Benabid AL, Pollak P, Louveau A, Henry S, de Rougemont J. Combined (thalamotomy and stimulation) stereotactic surgery of the VIM thalamic nucleus for bilateral Parkinson disease. *Appl Neurophysiol.* 1987;50(1–6):344–346.
49. Nuttin B, Cosyns P, Demeulemeester H, Gybels J, Meyerson B. Electrical stimulation in anterior limbs of internal capsules in patients with obsessive-compulsive disorder. *Lancet.* 1999;354(9189):1526.
50. Alonso P, Cuadras D, Gabriels L, et al. Deep brain stimulation for obsessive-compulsive disorder: a meta-analysis of treatment outcome and predictors of response. *PloS One.* 2015;10(7):e0133591.
51. Baker EF. Gilles de la Tourette syndrome treated by bimedial frontal leucotomy. *Can Med Assoc J.* 1962 Apr 21;86(16):746–747.
52. Hassler R, Dieckmann G. Stereotaxic treatment of tics and inarticulate cries or coprolalia considered as motor obsessional phenomena in Gilles de la Tourette's disease. *Rev Neurol (Paris).* 1970;123(2):89–100.
53. Robertson M, Doran M, Trimble M, Lees AJ. The treatment of Gilles de la Tourette syndrome by limbic leucotomy. *J Neurol Neurosurg Psychiatry.* 1990;53(8):691–694.
54. Sawle GV, Lees AJ, Hymas NF, Brooks DJ, Frackowiak RS. The metabolic effects of limbic leucotomy in Gilles de la Tourette syndrome. *J Neurol Neurosurg Psychiatry.* 1993;56(9):1016–1019.
55. Kurlan R, Kersun J, Ballantine HT Jr, Caine ED. Neurosurgical treatment of severe obsessive-compulsive disorder associated with Tourette's syndrome. *Mov Disord Off J Mov Disord Soc.* 1990;5(2):152–155.
56. Baer L, Rauch SL, Jenike MA, et al. Cingulotomy in a case of concomitant obsessive-compulsive disorder

and Tourette's syndrome. *Arch Gen Psychiatry.* 1994;51(1):73–74.

57. Vandewalle V, van der Linden C, Groenewegen HJ, Caemaert J. Stereotactic treatment of Gilles de la Tourette syndrome by high frequency stimulation of thalamus. *Lancet.* 1999;353(9154):724.

58. Baldermann JC, Schüller T, Huys D, et al. Deep brain stimulation for Tourette-syndrome: a systematic review and meta-analysis. *Brain Stimulat.* 2016;9(2):296–304.

59. Graat I, Figee M, Denys D. The application of deep brain stimulation in the treatment of psychiatric disorders. *Int Rev Psychiatry Abingdon Engl.* 2017;29(2):178–190.

60. Kachani AT, Barroso LP, Brasiliano S, Hochgraf PB, Cordás TA. Body checking and obsessive-compulsive symptoms in Brazilian outpatients with eating disorders. *Eat Weight Disord EWD.* 2014;19(2):177–182.

61. Giel KE, Friederich H-C, Teufel M, Hautzinger M, Enck P, Zipfel S. Attentional processing of food pictures in individuals with anorexia nervosa: an eye-tracking study. *Biol Psychiatry.* 2011;69(7):661–667.

62. Barbier J, Gabriëls L, van Laere K, Nuttin B. Successful anterior capsulotomy in comorbid anorexia nervosa and obsessive-compulsive disorder: case report. *Neurosurgery.* 2011;69(3):E745–E751.

63. Wang J, Chang C, Geng N, Wang X, Gao G. Treatment of intractable anorexia nervosa with inactivation of the nucleus accumbens using stereotactic surgery. *Stereotact Funct Neurosurg.* 2013;91(6):364–372.

64. Lipsman N, Woodside DB, Giacobbe P, et al. Subcallosal cingulate deep brain stimulation for treatment-refractory anorexia nervosa: a phase 1 pilot trial. *Lancet.* 2013;381(9875): 1361–1370.

65. Wu H, Van Dyck-Lippens PJ, Santegoeds R, et al. Deep-brain stimulation for anorexia nervosa. *World Neurosurg.* 2013;80(3–4):S29.e1–e10.

66. McLaughlin NCR, Didie ER, Machado AG, Haber SN, Eskandar EN, Greenberg BD. Improvements in anorexia symptoms after deep brain stimulation for intractable obsessive-compulsive disorder. *Biol Psychiatry.* 2013;73(9):e29–e31.

67. American Psychiatric Association. *Diagnostic and Statistical Manual of Mental Disorders,* 5th edition. Washington, DC: APA; 2013.

68. Gentil AF, Lopes AC, Dougherty DD, et al. Hoarding symptoms and prediction of poor response to limbic system surgery for treatment-refractory obsessive-compulsive disorder. *J Neurosurg.* 2014;121(1):123–130.

69. Riva-Posse P, Choi KS, Holtzheimer PE, et al. A connectomics approach for subcallosal cingulate deep brain stimulation surgery: prospective targeting in treatment-resistant depression. *Mol Psychiatry.* 2018;23(4):843–849.

Chapter 22

Alternative Treatments for Obsessive-Compulsive Disorder: Nutraceuticals and Lifestyle Interventions

Jerome Sarris and Georgina Oliver

Introduction

Advances have occurred in recent years in the study and appreciation of the role that adequate nutrition plays in general mental health [1], with certain nutrient deficiencies being correlated in sufferers of obsessive-compulsive disorder (OCD). Select nutraceuticals (standardized pharmaceutical-grade nutrients or plant medicines) may also have an application, especially in treating adjunctive depression [2]. Disorders such as OCD have been regarded as falling under the conceptual umbrella of "behavioral" addictions, that include gambling, sexual activity, eating, shopping, excoriation and trichotillomania [3]. This concept is posited as being due to an interrelated impairment of reward–punishment processing via the dopaminergic system (ventral striatum mediated), diminished prefrontal cortex mediated control, in combination with the limbic system being involved in negative reinforcement. While these particular neurobiological systems may only be modestly influenced by nutraceutical interventions, lifestyle interventions such as exercise and mindfulness meditation may have a role (in particular with regulation of the dopaminergic system and prefrontal cortex activity) [4]. Certain nutraceuticals may, however, have a beneficial effect on other pathways involved in impulsivity and compulsivity, by potentially enhancing GABA or serotonergic activity, or in the reduction of aberrant glutamate activity (detailed below). As a result of this beneficial effect, there is significant potential transdiagnostic application across a range of disorders, by mediating an array of underpinning and connected neurobiological processes.

This chapter first covers the data on nutrient deficiencies evident in OCD, and then discusses various nutraceuticals and lifestyle interventions with clinical trial evidence. It should be noted as an overall limitation in nutrient studies that none of the published research has included details of participants' dietary patterns. For some, it is plausible that nutrient deficiencies may be the result of restricted eating habits related to obsessions and compulsions of OCD, rather than being a causative factor in the manifestation of OCD.

Recent Research Findings

Nutrients for Obsessive-Compulsive Disorder (Deficiencies and Treatments)

Vitamin B12

Vitamin B12 (cobalamin) is a water-soluble micronutrient, predominately available in the diet through consumption of animal proteins such as meat, dairy and eggs [5]. It serves as a methyl donor to facilitate synthesis of the amino acid methionine from homocysteine in the cytoplasm, metabolites of which are required for DNA (demethylated tetrahydrofolate) and myelin synthesis (S-adenosylmethionine), the latter essential for maintaining neuronal integrity and neurotransmitter synthesis and activity [6]. Vitamin B12 deficiency (as detected in the blood) is common worldwide and is evident across the life span, however, its prevalence in psychiatric disorders is also of significance [7]. Given its involvement in methylation pathways, vitamin B12 influences the rate of serotonin and dopamine synthesis, prominent neurotransmitters implicated in the etiopathogenesis of OCD and other psychiatric disorders [8,9]. In addition, vitamin B12 deficiencies may contribute to impaired glutathione synthesis and activity, a tripeptide compound (comprised of the amino acids cysteine, glutamate and glycine), which possesses marked antioxidant activity [10]. Compromised glutathione and the presence of aberrant oxidative stress have been detected in individuals with OCD and in various other psychiatric disorders, which has prompted the investigation of various treatments to mitigate these occurrences [10,11,12,13].

Deficiencies in serum vitamin B12 levels have been highlighted in some individuals with OCD, however, only one published case study exists highlighting the therapeutic effects of B12 supplementation in deficiency states [14]. Intramuscular injections in a 39-year old male over a period of 10 weeks elicited a remission of obsessive-compulsive symptoms (Yale-Brown Obsessive Compulsive Scale, Y-BOCS, initial score of 24 reduced to 5) and these results were maintained for a seven-month period without the need for additional therapeutics. Another case report describes a 29-year-old female with OCD for over 11 years, who presented with a marked vitamin B12 deficiency (less than 30 pg/ml), which was reported to precede her psychiatric symptoms [15]. Oral nutritional therapies were started, however, the patient's response to these therapies were not detailed in the case report.

Case–control studies have also highlighted serum vitamin B12 deficiencies in patients with OCD. An early study comparing patients with OCD (n = 30), chronic schizophrenia (n = 30) and healthy controls (n = 30) revealed that six patients with OCD (20%) were B12 deficient (111–147 pg/ml), despite demonstrating no hematological or neurological abnormalities [16]. This was a significantly higher frequency than the other two groups combined. A more recent study revealed that mean vitamin B12 levels among patients with OCD (n = 35) were significantly lower than those in healthy controls (n = 22), and 31% of patients with OCD met criteria for vitamin B12 deficiency (less than 200 pg/ml) [17]. Higher levels of homocysteine, a metabolite often measured in the blood to provide a more sensitive indication of vitamin B12 deficiencies, have also been detected in individuals with OCD [17,18]. However, one study revealed that homocysteine levels were only significant in OCD when comorbid Major Depressive Disorder was present [17]. Collectively, these case reports and studies suggest vitamin B12 deficiency may be apparent in a sub-group of patients with OCD, however, evidence is lacking to indicate if supplementation of B12 will improve symptomatology in these individuals.

Zinc

Zinc is an essential trace mineral involved in a multitude and diverse range of biochemical processes including those involved in gene expression, DNA replication, transcription and protein synthesis; tissue and cell repair, hormone activity and cell-mediated immunity [19]. The activity of zinc in the central nervous system is widespread, being the most prevalent trace mineral in the amygdala, hippocampus and neocortex [20]. It is a modulator of inhibitory and excitatory neurotransmission with effects on glutamate and GABA, which may in part explain its role in the attenuation of excitotoxicity linked to some disorders [21,22]. A deficiency of dietary zinc has also been implicated in the excitability of glutamatergic neurons [23]. Further, zinc is involved in antioxidant and anti-inflammatory processes, including as a structural component of superoxide dismutase, maintaining metallothionein concentrations in tissues, sequestering the production of reactive oxygen species, inhibiting glutathione depletion and protecting against lipid peroxidation in the brain [19,24].

Serum zinc levels have been found to be significantly lower in individuals with OCD (n = 48) in comparison with healthy controls (n = 48) [25]. Interestingly, when stratified for severity, serum zinc levels were significantly lower in mild presentations of OCD (–69.2% difference between healthy controls), followed by non-significant differences in moderate (–29.4%) and severe presentations (–24.3%). To date, only one published randomized controlled trial (RCT) has investigated the effects of zinc supplementation in OCD [26]. Participants were randomized to take either fluoxetine (20 mg/day) and adjunctive oral zinc sulfate (220 mg twice a day) or fluoxetine plus placebo in an eight-week double-blind, placebo-controlled study. Zinc potentiated the therapeutic effects of fluoxetine, with mean Y-BOCS scores significantly lower in the adjunctive zinc group than fluoxetine alone after two weeks of treatment. Furthermore, after eight weeks of treatment, adjunctive zinc elicited significantly greater improvements in obsessive-compulsive symptoms.

Zinc status has also been implicated in other disorders sharing symptoms similar to that of OCD, with a recent meta-analysis identifying low plasma zinc levels in individuals with pica (five studies, with outliers included in the analysis), regardless of symptom dimensions (e.g., cravings for ice, dirt or purified starches) or life stage (pregnancy, adults or children) [27]. However, given that pica may reflect general significant nutritional deficiencies from disordered eating, the causal relationship of zinc to the disorder remains unknown.

Nutraceuticals for Obsessive-Compulsive Disorder and Related Disorders

N-acetylcysteine

N-acetylcysteine (NAC) is one of the most widely studied nutraceuticals for OCD and related disorders, as well as disorders possessing traits of compulsivity such as pathological gambling and drug addiction [28]. NAC is currently the most promising nutraceutical in addressing these conditions in a transdiagnostic context, due to its modulation of several overlapping neurological aberrations which underpin these disorders. NAC is an acetylated form of the essential amino acid cysteine, which has been used medicinally for over 50 years, initially in emergency departments for the treatment of paracetamol toxicity [29]. Cysteine is the rate-limiting amino acid required for endogenous glutathione production, and administration of NAC has been found to increase glutathione levels in the bloodstream and brain [30,31,32]. NAC also modulates glutamatergic neurotransmission, an attribute suggested to target core symptoms of compulsivity [33]. Animal models of addiction have highlighted NAC's ability to activate cystine-glutamate antiporters and restore glutamate transporter-1 activity in the nucleus accumbens, thereby regulating presynaptic glutamate release and extracellular glutamate clearance [34,35,36]. These mechanisms are postulated to be particularly beneficial for diminishing compulsive behaviors. Both preclinical and clinical studies have highlighted the ability of NAC to improve such behaviors [28,37,38]. Collectively, NAC's modulation of glutamate and involvement in the production of glutathione are believed to inhibit excessive N-methyl-D-aspartate receptor activation and subsequent excitotoxicity. Thus, NAC is also said to possess neuroprotective effects [39].

Various case reports have highlighted beneficial effects of NAC in OCD, trichotillomania and excoriation [40,41,42,43], whereas RCTs have revealed conflicting results (Table 22.1). The narrative emerging from these studies highlights that NAC may be beneficial for a sub-group of patients with obsessive and/or compulsive behaviors, perhaps those with glutathione and/or glutamate neurotransmitter abnormalities. In OCD, two Iranian RCTs have highlighted promising therapeutic effects of NAC, particularly in individuals with mild to moderate symptom severity [44,47]. Whereas one case series and two small RCTs highlighted minimal effect of NAC for ameliorating symptoms of OCD, particularly for those individuals considered to be treatment resistant, or having OCD of greater severity and chronicity [45,46,55]. NAC may, however, attenuate "compulsive" behaviors of the disorder, as evidenced from one RCT, where NAC was significant over placebo after 12 weeks of treatment for reducing Y-BOCS compulsive sub-score [45]. However, NAC may also alleviate repetitive, intrusive thoughts, evident in a recent excoriation study where NAC was effective for reducing reported urges to pick (as per Neurotic Excoriation-Y-BOCS sub-score) [52]. Further, it was found to be significantly effective for reducing the intrusive thought symptom domain of PTSD [56] and to decrease cravings for illicit substances in drug addiction [52,57,58]. Thus, while some clinical trials have failed to find a convincing effect for NAC on primary outcome measures, other studies highlight its benefits for improving certain features of psychiatric disorders. NAC has recently been suggested to be best employed alongside other pharmacotherapies to further improve symptomatology, specifically, that of intrusive thinking and subsequent compulsivity [58].

The therapeutic effects of NAC are typically seen after 8–12 weeks. Reported adverse effects include digestive complaints such as nausea, diarrhea and reflux, as well as a dry mouth, skin rashes, dizziness and headaches. The majority of these effects are reported to be of mild to moderate intensity and dissipate with continued use.

Myo-inositol

Myo-inositol (inositol) is an endogenous isomer of glucose, and the most biologically active form of the nine possible stereoisomer structures available. Inositol may be obtained through the diet in foods such as fruits, legumes, grains and nuts, as well as from *de novo* synthesis from glucose-6-phosphate [59]. Inositol is a structural component of phospholipid membranes and is a key metabolic precursor to phosphoinositide intracellular secondary messenger cycles [59]. These pathways are involved in neurotransmitter and receptor activity, as well as regulation of signaling proteins, mechanisms which may in turn improve serotonin reuptake and increase 5-HT_2 receptor density [60,61]. Inositol has also been found to increase striatal D_2 (dopamine) receptor density, and thus, may contribute to alleviating dopaminergic

Table 22.1 Clinical trials investigating the effects of N-acetylcysteine in compulsivity.

Study	Population			Study Design	NAC Max Dose (mg/day)	Results
	Patient type	Randomized (*n*)	Analyzed (*n*)			
Obsessive-Compulsive Disorder						
Paydary et al., 2016 [44]	Adult OCD	46	44	10-week parallel RCT	2000[a]	NAC potentiated the effects of fluvoxamine ($P = 0.012$). 12 of 22 patients taking NAC + fluvoxamine achieved symptom remission (Y-BOCS ≤ 16) vs. 5 of 22 patients taking fluvoxamine + placebo alone
Sarris et al., 2015 [45]	Adult OCD	44	35	16-week RCT	3000	NAC was not significant over placebo for improving OCD symptoms ($P = 0.15$). NAC beneficial for reducing compulsive behaviors at week 12 ($P = 0.013$); effect dissipated by week-16
Costa et al., 2015 [46]	Adult OCD	40	35	16-week RCT	3000	Both groups experienced a reduction in mean -Y-BOCS scores; NAC not significant over placebo in therapeutic effect ($P = 0.45$)
Afshar et al., 2012 [47]	Adult OCD	44	39	12-week RCT	2400	NAC significant over placebo for reducing OCD symptoms ($P = 0.003$), effect seen after 8 weeks; full clinical response experienced in 10 of 19 patients receiving NAC, vs. 3 of 20 taking placebo
Obsessive-Compulsive and Related Disorders						
Grant et al., 2009 [48]	Adult TTM	50	50	12-week RCT	2400	NAC significant over placebo for reducing TTM symptoms as per MGH-HPS ($P < 0.001$) and PITS ($P = 0.001$); therapeutic effect evident after 9 weeks of treatment
Bloch et al., 2013 [49]	Pediatric TTM	39	39	12-week RCT	2400	Modest decrease in symptoms detected in both placebo and NAC group (25% treatment responders in NAC group vs. 21% in placebo); NAC not significant over placebo ($P = 1$)
Ghanizadeh et al., 2013 [50]	Children and adolescents with chronic nail biting	42	25	8-week RCT	800	NAC showed significant effects over placebo for increasing nail length after first month ($P = 0.04$), but not by the second ($P = 0.59$)

(*continued*)

Table 22.1 *(cont.)*

Study	Population			Study Design	NAC Max Dose (mg/day)	Results
	Patient type	Randomized (*n*)	Analyzed (*n*)			
Miller & Angulo, 2014 [51]	Children and adults with excoriation in Prader Willi syndrome	35	35	12-week open label	1200	All participants experienced improvements in skin-picking behavior; 71% had complete resolution and 29% a significant reduction in the number of active lesions
Grant et al., 2016 [52]	Adult excoriation	66	66	12-week RCT	3000	NAC significant over placebo for reducing NE-Y-BOCS score at each time point (weeks 3, 6, 9, 12; $P = 0.048$ at week-12 end-point); 47% of participants receiving NAC were "much, or very much improved" vs. 19% in placebo group
				Pathological Gambling		
Grant et al., 2007 [53]	Adults with pathological gambling	29	27	8-week open label	1800	16 participants experienced clinical response to NAC (41.9% mean reduction in baseline PG-Y-BOCS, $P < 0.001$) and 40.2% mean reduction in G-SAS ($P < 0.001$)
Grant et al., 2007 [53]	Treatment responders from Grant et al.'s 2007 [53] open-label study	13	13	6-week RCT	1800	Of 6 patients randomized to continue on NAC therapy, 83.3% maintained clinical response criteria, vs. 28.6% in placebo group ($n = 7$; NAC not significant over placebo for reducing scores in either PG-Y-BOCS or G-SAS ($P = 0.095$ and 0.060, respectively)
Grant et al., 2014 [54]	Adults with pathological gambling and nicotine dependence	28	28	12-week RCT	3000[b]	Mean PG-Y-BOCS scores substantially decreased over 12 weeks in both groups; NAC not superior over placebo. Of 11 participants who completed week-24 follow-up (3 months after NAC/placebo cessation) those that had been treated with NAC ($n = 6$) demonstrated greater reduction in mean PG-Y-BOCS scores ($P = 0.043$) than those who were on placebo ($n = 5$)

G-SAS = Gambling Symptom Assessment Scale; MGH-HPS = Massachusetts General Hospital Hair Pulling Scale; NE-Y-BOCS; Neurotic Excoriation-Y-BOCS; OCD = Obsessive-Compulsive Disorder; PG-Y-BOCS; Pathological Gambling Y-BOCS; PITS = Psychiatric Institute TTM Scale; RCT = randomized controlled trial; SDS = Sheehan Disability Scale; TTM = trichotillomania; Y-BOCS = Yale-Brown Obsessive Compulsive Scale.

[a] Adjunctive to initiation of fluvoxamine treatment (200mg/day).

[b] Concurrent with initiation of psychological therapies.

hypofunction evident in some individuals with OCD and related disorders [3,62,63].

Inositol has been investigated for various psychiatric disorders including OCD, attention deficit and hyperactivity disorder, autism, schizophrenia, depression and panic disorder [60,64]. Several studies were published in the late 1990s exploring inositol's effects on OCD; the first was a double-blind, placebo-controlled crossover study where 18 g/day of inositol was found significant over placebo for reducing Y-BOCS scores in 13 patients who were not using selective serotonin reuptake inhibitors (SSRIs) at the time of the study [65]. In addition, an open-label study involving 14 patients with OCD (also medication free) revealed that 12 weeks of inositol therapy (18 g/day) induced a full clinical response in eight patients (Y-BOCS score reduction greater than 50% from baseline) [66]. Despite these positive results, inositol taken adjunctively to SSRIs appears a less promising strategy for OCD, highlighted in two seperate "negative" studies employing the same 18 g/day dose for six weeks [67,68]. Further, a double-blind placebo study published in 2017 failed to find a significant effect of inositol (6–18 g/day) over placebo in 38 individuals with trichotillomania after ten weeks of treatment [68]. These findings stand in contrast to a case series involving three individuals with excoriation, body dysmorphic disorder (BDD) and trichotillomania who experienced significant improvements in their symptoms on the same dose (18 g/day) [70].

Reported adverse effects with use of inositol primarily relate to gastrointestinal discomfort, including flatulence, diarrhea, abdominal cramps, nausea and bloating. Headaches and dizziness have also been reported. The majority of these effects are mild to moderate in severity and subside within one to two weeks of sustained use.

Glycine and Sarcosine

Glycine is an amino acid which possesses both inhibitory and excitatory neurotransmitter activity within the central nervous system [71]. Glycine has binding affinity for the strychnine-sensitive glycine-A site of ionotropic glycine receptors, and thus facilitates inhibitory neurotransmission. It is also a co-agonist (with L-glutamate) to strychnine-insensitive glycine-B sites located on the GluN1 sub-unit of NMDA receptors. Activation of this sub-unit inhibits glutamatergic activity in frontal regions of the brain, thus this amino acid has been a therapeutic target for schizophrenia, and more recently, OCD.

A case report has detailed the positive effects of high-dose glycine therapy (maximum dose 66 g/day, taken as a solution) over a five-year period in a male patient diagnosed with OCD and BDD [72]. He was treatment-resistant to three adequate trials of SSRIs, as well as atypical antipsychotics, and suffered severe impairment in his school and social life. Glycine treatment ameliorated both OCD and BDD symptoms, whereas cessation (which occurred at various times throughout the five-year period) resulted in a gradual relapse of symptoms and subsequent impairment in quality of life.

These positive results prompted an RCT investigating the therapeutic effects of glycine (30 g twice/daily), versus placebo, taken adjunctively to stable psychotropic medication for 12 weeks in 24 patients with OCD. [73]. Withdrawal rates in the study were high, with 9 of the 12 participants in the treatment group not completing the study because of reported adverse effects, including nausea and the disagreeable taste of the powder. Of the five who were evaluated in the treatment group, a mean decrease of six points in their Y-BOCS score occurred, in comparison with a one-point reduction in the placebo group (n = 9), an effect that reached clinical significance. No further studies have been published investigating glycine for OCD, or related disorders.

Sarcosine (N-methyl glycine) is a weak, but selective, inhibitor of the glycine transporter-1, and thereby increases the availability of synaptic glycine [71]. Thus far, it appears to have a superior tolerability profile to glycine [74,75]. To date, only one published study exists investigating the effects of sarcosine (500 mg/day, titrated to 2000 mg/day in the event of non-response) in patients with OCD (n = 26) [76]. The ten-week, open-label trial revealed that four of the eight participants who were medication naïve at time of entry into the study demonstrated a full clinical response to sarcosine (46.7–69.2% reduction in baseline Y-BOCS score). Five other participants who were taking psychotropic medication, or had previously trialed medication, also experienced positive effects (38.5–85.7% Y-BOCS score reduction). Adverse events were few; however, those that were reported led to withdrawal from the study (hypomanic symptoms and headache) and resolved with cessation of the treatment.

Herbal Medicine

Published clinical studies investigating the therapeutic effects of herbal medicines for OCD and related disorders are sparse, despite various preclinical studies highlighting a range of relevant pharmacological activity. Various herbal medicines have the potential to address some of the underlying pathophysiology in compulsive disorders, in part due to antioxidant, anti-inflammatory and monoamine modulatory effects [77]. It should be noted that, for many plant medicine products, there are potential quality issues regarding lack of standardization of active constituents, substitution and incorrect plant parts being used [78].

Withania Somnifera

Ashwagandha (*Withania somnifera*) is widely used in Ayurvedic plant medicine, and is renowned for its ability to improve adaptation to physical and psychological stress [79]. Various preclinical studies have highlighted its anti-inflammatory, antioxidant, neuroprotective, immunomodulatory, anxiolytic and antidepressant effects [79]. Isolated constituents, mainly from the roots (including withanolides and withanone), have been found to attenuate NMDA excitotoxicity *in vitro* [80,81], while extracts of the plant (leaf) have been found to restore glutathione levels and modulate superoxide dismutase and catalase activity in animals induced with neurological oxidative stress [82]. Extracts of the plant's roots enhance GABAergic signaling (potent agonist of $GABA\rho_1$ and activator of $GABA_A$ ionotropic channels), and increase GABA levels in the brain (more so than ethanol and with stronger anxiolytic effects) [83,84]. Furthermore, *W. somnifera* raises corticohippocampal serotonin levels and prevents stress-induced deficits of serotonin in this region [83,85]. In an animal model of addiction, *W. somnifera* prevented anxiety behaviors associated with ethanol withdrawal, and these effects were comparable to those of diazepam [82]. It also reduced drug-seeking and reinstatement behaviors for ethanol and inhibited tolerance and dependence on opioids [86,87]. In an animal model of OCD, extracts of *W. somnifera* root significantly reduced the number of marbles buried by mice in a dose-dependent manner, without affecting locomotor activity [88]. Further, the antidepressant effects of *W. somnifera* administrated to mice were comparable to those of fluoxetine [89].

Ashwagandha's various preclinical effects within the central nervous system suggest its utility for the treatment of anxiety, epilepsy, neurodegenerative disorders and addiction [79]. More recently, a small pilot study conducted in Iran investigated its therapeutic activity in OCD sufferers (Table 22.2). Although *W. somnifera* extract was significantly superior over placebo for reducing Y-BOCS scores after six weeks, baseline Y-BOCS scores were significantly higher in the treatment group, thereby limiting confidence in this finding. In addition, given the titration regimen used in this study, it is unclear which dose and for what duration may be beneficial for patients. No adverse effects were reported in either group during the study period.

Silybum Marianum

St Mary's thistle (*Silybum marianum*; milk thistle) is a plant medicine native to Mediterranean cultures used for over 2000 years to treat liver and biliary tract disorders [94]. Silymarin is considered one of the plant's most biologically active constituents. It has been widely studied to reveal potent antioxidant, anti-inflammatory and neuroprotective effects [95,96]. Preclinical studies have highlighted the ability of silymarin to directly sequester reactive oxygen species, increase cellular glutathione content and enhance superoxide dismutase activity in hepatocytes and neurons [97,98]. In addition, silymarin also influences monoamine activity, inhibiting its activity *in vitro* and increasing concentrations of serotonin in the cortex, as well as dopamine and norepinephrine levels in the cerebellum of mice [99]. One of silymarin's isolated constituents, the flavonolignan silibinin, was found to inhibit the reduction of serotonin in the hippocampus and dopamine in the prefrontal cortex in mice exposed to methamphetamine, and subsequently prevent cognitive impairment induced by the drug [100]. Anxiolytic and antidepressant activity has also been revealed in animal models, mediated in part by interactions with $5\text{-}HT_{1A}$ receptors and inhibiting elevations in serum corticosterone levels while restoring antioxidant enzymes (catalase and superoxide dismutase) following acute resistant stress [101,102].

Three case studies have highlighted positive effects of milk thistle supplementation for ameliorating hair-pulling behaviors (300 mg/day), OCD (600 mg/day) and chronic nail biting (300 mg/day) within four to eight weeks, and without reported adverse effects [103]. Further, a small pilot study, also conducted in Iran, revealed an extract of milk thistle (non-standardized) was as effective as fluoxetine for reducing

Table 22.2 Clinical trials of herbal medicines for Obsessive-Compulsive Disorder.

Study	Design	Dose of treatment	Baseline Y-BOCS score	End-point Y-BOCS
Jahanbakhsh et al., 2016 [90]	6-week RCT, pilot study ($n = 35$)	120 mg *Withania somnifera* root extract[a] adjunctive to SSRI mdx	26 *W. somnifera* (range 14–40); 18 placebo (range 11–33) ($P = 0.038$)	18 *W. somnifera* (range 4–40); 16 placebo (range 10–31) ($P < 0.001$)
Sayyah et al., 2010 [91]	8-week parallel study ($n = 35$)	Milk thistle leaf extract (600 mg/day) vs. fluoxetine (30 mg/day)	Mean Y-BOCS score reduction of 11 (± 4.15) in milk thistle group; 12.50 (± 4.54) in fluoxetine group; no significant difference between treatments at endpoint ($P = 0.43$)	
Taylor & Kobak, 2000 [92]	12-week open label ($n = 12$)	450 mg 0.3% hypericin taken twice daily	21.42 (± 4.10)	14 (± 7.54); mean decrease of 7.42 points ($P = 0.01$)
Kobak et al., 2005 [93]	12-week RCT, ($n = 60$)	St. John's wort L1 160 (0.3% hypericin) 600–1800 mg/day[b]	23.17 (± 3.81) SJW; 23.47 (± 5.54) placebo	17.77 (± 6.89) SJW; 18.62 (± 6.34) placebo; SJW not significant over placebo ($P = 0.899$)

RCT, randomized controlled trial; SJW, St. John's Wort; SSRI, selective serotonin reuptake inhibitor; Y-BOCS, Yale-Brown Obsessive Compulsive Scale.
[a] Dose of *W. somnifera* was titrated and then tapered down across the six weeks of the study.
[b] Titration dependent on clinical response.

severe obsessive-compulsive symptoms after eight weeks (Table 22.2). Clinical trials are currently being conducted investigating the effects of silymarin for trichotillomania and pathological gambling in the USA.

Hypericum Perforatum

St John's wort (*Hypericum perforatum*) is one of the most well-known herbal medicines, and is prescribed widely in Europe as an antidepressant agent [102]. Constituents found in the yellow, flowering tops of St John's wort, namely hypericin and hyperforin, exert a range of neurobiological effects demonstrated in preclinical studies, including nonselective inhibition of serotonin, dopamine and noradrenaline reuptake, increasing the amount of serotonin receptors in the brain, and weak inhibition of monoamine oxidase A and B enzymes [104]. Given its well-regarded antidepressant effects, and its superior tolerability profile to antidepressant medication [105], two clinical trials have investigated the potential of St John's wort in the treatment of OCD (Table 22.2). An open-label study revealed significant effects for reducing OCD symptoms within one week of use, suggesting a possible placebo response. Incongruent with the researcher's open-label study, an RCT of St John's wort for OCD failed to elicit a significant therapeutic effect over placebo [93,107].

Lifestyle Therapies

The importance of "lifestyle medicine", which includes modalities such as exercise, dietary modification/enhancement and stress management techniques including yoga and meditation practices, is becoming increasingly renowned in psychiatry. The inclusion of lifestyle medicine elements in the Royal Australian and New Zealand College of Psychiatrists clinical practice guidelines for mood disorders highlights their therapeutic potential [108]. However, at present, research studies exploring these modalities, particularly the influence of diet for OCD and related disorders are scarce. In a transdiagnostic context, the application of modifying several key lifestyle elements may not only provide benefits to mental health, these may potentially have a role in modulating compulsive behaviors.

Substantial evidence exists for the benefits of physical activity, and more in particular "prescriptive exercise" on depression, highlighted in a 2009 Cochrane review examining 23 trials with 907 participants collectively [109]. However, its effects for anxiety disorders, OCD and related disorders have been less rigorously studied. Engaging in exercise may provide acute relief for obsessive and compulsive symptoms as well as improvements in mood, and these benefits appear to be sustained with continued involvement [110,111].

A small pilot study published in 2015 examined the effects of a 12-week aerobic exercise program in combination with cognitive behavioral therapy (CBT) for 11 participants with OCD [4]. Each participant received an individualized exercise program which was advised to be completed on three days per week, with increasing intensity and duration (maximum 45-minute sessions). Participants also attended group CBT sessions for 15 weeks, which involved exposure and response prevention and other cognitive strategies specific for the treatment of OCD. All participants experienced significant improvements in their symptoms (self-reported and clinician-rated) as well as self-reported depressive symptoms, with effect sizes exceeding those typically evident with the use of psychological therapies alone [112]. No participant withdrew from the exercise component, and adherence rates to the exercise regimens was over 80%. Further, engaging in physical activity may be particularly important for individuals with OCD taking antipsychotic medications, given that the development of metabolic syndrome and other cardiovascular conditions are associated with their use [113].

Yoga practices may also provide benefits for alleviating compulsivity, however, many of the research studies which have investigated these effects possess various methodological flaws [114]. One study compared the practice of two forms of yoga: kundalini yoga, which employs various physical postures (asanas), dynamic movement and specific breathing techniques compared with a combination of mindfulness meditation and relaxation response in 21 participants with OCD [115]. After three months, results measured by Y-BOCS scores revealed a significantly greater reduction in favor of kundalini yoga (9.43 point reduction) over mindfulness meditation and relaxation response (2.86 point reduction). At 15-month follow-up, participants continuing with kundalini yoga had a mean score of 6.6 points on Y-BOCS. The authors reported, however, that only seven participants in each group completed the intervention, and that clinicians conducting the assessments were not blinded. Thus, the effect of yoga found over mindfulness and relaxation training is questionable. Another study evaluated the effects of a two-week yoga program (five sessions per week) in ten individuals with OCD [116]. Content of the program involved chanting, breathing exercises and various asanas that had been validated by ten yoga experts before they were demonstrated to the participants. Nine of the ten patients experienced a decrease in their Y-BOCS score after completion of the program, and the group's mean score reduction was significant at the endpoint (24.22 baseline, 14.77 endpoint).

Future Directions and Transdiagnostic Approaches

Current treatments for OCD are inadequate for many, and while pharmacotherapy and psychological interventions play an important role, to date no "silver bullet" has been discovered. Nutraceuticals offer a potential role in a transdiagnostic context via targeting an array of neurochemical pathways implicated in compulsive behaviors. One approach is the use of nutrient-based nutraceutical agents, which have been studied as effective adjuncts in a range of psychiatric disorders, including depression [2]. Further, the use of "combination" nutraceuticals may potentially exert greater effect than isolated nutrients via targeting a range of neurological pathways underlying the disorder, and potentially via synergism (as nutrients are often more effective in combination and may require certain cofactors for optimal nutrient metabolism) [117]. This principle may be applied across compulsive disorders and addictive behaviors, which may present with aberrations of glutamate neurotransmission, impairment of monoamine synthesis and function, disturbed inflammatory processes and the presence of atypical oxidative stress. Regardless, it should be noted that the future focus of research and clinical application should involve a more sophisticated targeting of neurochemical abnormalities and specific nutrients deficiencies based on the individual's psychophysiological presentation (i.e., beyond the "cookie-cutter" *Diagnostic and Statistical Manual of Mental Disorders* diagnoses). This will ideally be ascertained via our increased understanding of the underpinning differences in biomarkers and brain function (which can be in part analyzed via testing of nutrient blood level, and single nucleotide polymorphisms, gene expression, and neuroimaging studies). This also needs to be considered within context of the patient's environmental interaction.

In respect to the role of inflammation and oxidative stress (which have a role across many psychiatric disorders), although results are inconsistent, a series of studies have investigated the levels of circulating cytokines in patients with OCD in comparison with controls. A meta-analysis of studies measuring plasma cytokine levels reported that interleukin (IL) 1 beta

(IL-1β) is decreased in patients with OCD [118]. A key study revealed that significantly greater plasma levels of IL-2, IL-4, IL-6, IL-10, and tumor necrosis factor alpha in patients with OCD who were drug-naïve compared with sex- and age-matched healthy controls [119]. The role of the gut microbiota (an ecosystem consisting of tens of trillions of microorganisms residing primarily throughout the digestive tract) was highlighted in 2016 as having a key interface with immune system modulation and subsequent cytokine activity, as well as pivotal roles in neurotransmitter and hormone synthesis and activity [120].

Although studies for OCD and the use of probiotics (supplements containing specific compositions or singular strains of gut microorganisms) are lacking, one exists using *Lactobacillus rhamnosus* in mice induced with OCD-like behaviors via administration of RU24969 (a 5-$HT_{1A/1B}$ receptor agonist) [121]. Mice treated with *L. rhamnosus* demonstrated a decrease in marble burying and aberrant locomotor behavior compared with controls (saline). Further, the effects of the probiotic were comparable to those of fluoxetine, which was administered to a third group of mice. While there are no currently published human studies using a probiotic as a treatment intervention for OCD, Van Amerigen and colleagues are currently conducting a 12-week double-blind RCT using *Bifidobacterium longus* and *Lactobacillus helveticus* at McMaster University (results due in August 2019; [122]).

In summary, while evidence in this area is nascent, there is marked potential to explore a range of nutraceuticals for the treatment of various compulsive disorders. While this approach has almost wholly focused on specific disorders, for example OCD, trichotillomania and pathological gambling, there is much work needed to explore the effects of nutraceuticals on this symptomatology from a functional medicine perspective (treating the common underlying pathology). Lifestyle approaches, while not necessarily being considered standalone interventions for more serious compulsions and addictions, can be employed within an integrative context to attenuate rumination and compulsivity, improve management of stress and alleviate anxiety.

References

1. Sarris J, Logan AC, Akbaraly TN, et al. Nutritional medicine as mainstream in psychiatry. *Lancet Psychiatry*. 2015;2(3):271–274.
2. Sarris J, Murphy J, Mischoulon D, Fava M, Berk M, Ng C. Adjunctive nutrient nutraceuticals for depression: a systematic review and meta-analyses. *Am J Psychiatry*. 2016;173(6):575–587.
3. Figee M, Pattij T, Willuhn I, et al. Compulsivity in obsessive-compulsive disorder and addictions. *Eur Neuropsychopharmacol*. 2016;26(5):856–868.
4. Rector NA, Richter MA, Lerman B, Regev R. A pilot test of the additive benefits of physical exercise to CBT for OCD. *Cogn Behav Ther*. 2015;44(4):328–340.
5. Gille D, Schmid A. Vitamin B12 in meat and dairy products. *Nutr Rev*. 2015;73(2):106–115.
6. Gueant JL, Caillerez-Fofou M, Battaglia-Hsu S, et al. Molecular and cellular effects of vitamin B12 in brain, myocardium and liver through its role as co-factor of methionine synthase. *Biochimie*. 2013;95(5):1033–1040.
7. Hannibal L, Lysne V, Bjorke-Monsen AL, et al. Biomarkers and algorithms for the diagnosis of vitamin B12 deficiency. *Front Mol Biosci*. 2016;3:27.
8. Pauls DL, Abramovitch A, Rauch SL, Geller DA. Obsessive-compulsive disorder: an integrative genetic and neurobiological perspective. *Nat Rev Neurosci*. 2014;15(6):410–424.
9. Marazziti D. Understanding the role of serotonin in psychiatric diseases. *F1000Res*. 2017;6:180.
10. Zhang Y, Hodgson NW, Trivedi MS, et al. Decreased brain levels of vitamin B12 in aging, autism and schizophrenia. *PloS One*. 2016;11(1):e0146797.
11. Berk M, Ng F, Dean O, Dodd S, Bush AI. Glutathione: a novel treatment target in psychiatry. *Trends Pharmacol Sci*. 2008;29(7):346–351.
12. Brennan B, Jensen JE, Perriello C, et al. Lower posterior cingulate cortex glutathione levels in obsessive-compulsive disorder. *Neuropsychopharmacology*. 2015;40:S119–S120.
13. Kar S, Choudhury I. An empirical review on oxidative stress markers and their relevance in obsessive-compulsive disorder. *Int J Nutr Pharmacol Neurol Dis*. 2016;6(4):139–145.
14. Sharma V, Biswas D. Cobalamin deficiency presenting as obsessive compulsive disorder: case report. *Gen Hosp Psychiatry*. 2012;34(5):578 e7–e8.
15. Valizadeh M, Valizadeh N. Obsessive compulsive disorder as early manifestation of B12 deficiency. *Indian J Psychol Med*. 2011;33(2):203–204.
16. Hermesh H, Weizman A, Shahar A, Munitz H. Vitamin B12 and folic acid serum levels in obsessive compulsive disorder. *Acta Psychiatr Scand*. 1988;78(1):8–10.
17. Turksoy N, Bilici R, Yalciner A, et al. Vitamin B12, folate, and homocysteine levels in patients with

obsessive-compulsive disorder. *Neuropsychiatr Dis Treat*. 2014;10:1671–1675.

18. Atmaca M, Tezcan E, Kuloglu M, Kirtas O, Ustundag B. Serum folate and homocysteine levels in patients with obsessive-compulsive disorder. *Psychiatry Clin Neurosci*. 2005;59(5):616–620.
19. Gropper SA, Smith JA. *Advanced Nutrition and Human Metabolism*, 6th ed. Belmont, CA: Wadsworth Cengage Learning; 2013.
20. Szewczyk B, Kubera M, Nowak G. The role of zinc in neurodegenerative inflammatory pathways in depression. *Prog Neuropsychopharmacol Biol Psychiatry*. 2011;35(3):693–701.
21. Bancila V, Nikonenko I, Dunant Y, Bloc A. Zinc inhibits glutamate release via activation of pre-synaptic K channels and reduces ischaemic damage in rat hippocampus. *J Neurochem*. 2004;90(5):1243–1250.
22. Peters S, Koh J, Choi DW. Zinc selectively blocks the action of N-methyl-D-aspartate on cortical neurons. *Science*. 1987;236(4801):589–593.
23. Takeda A, Hirate M, Tamano H, Oku N. Release of glutamate and GABA in the hippocampus under zinc deficiency. *J Neurosci Res*. 2003;72(4):537–542.
24. Bagchi D, Vuchetich PJ, Bagchi M, et al. Protective effects of zinc salts on TPA-induced hepatic and brain lipid peroxidation, glutathione depletion, DNA damage and peritoneal macrophage activation in mice. *Gen Pharmacol*. 1998;30(1):43–50.
25. Shohag H, Ullah A, Qusar S, Rahman M, Hasnat A. Alterations of serum zinc, copper, manganese, iron, calcium, and magnesium concentrations and the complexity of interelement relations in patients with obsessive-compulsive disorder. *Biol Trace Elem Res*. 2012;148(3):275–280.
26. Sayyah M, Olapour A, Saeedabad Y, Yazdan Parast R, Malayeri A. Evaluation of oral zinc sulfate effect on obsessive-compulsive disorder: a randomized placebo-controlled clinical trial. *Nutrition*. 2012;28(9):892–895.
27. Miao D, Young SL, Golden CD. A meta-analysis of pica and micronutrient status. *Am J Hum Biol*. 2015;27(1):84–93.
28. Deepmala, Slattery J, Kumar N, et al. Clinical trials of N-acetylcysteine in psychiatry and neurology: a systematic review. *Neurosci Biobehav Rev*. 2015;55:294–321.
29. Prescott LF, Park J, Ballantyne A, Adriaenssens P, Proudfoot AT. Treatment of paracetamol (acetaminophen) poisoning with N-acetylcysteine. *Lancet*. 1977;2(8035):432–434.
30. Lavoie S, Murray MM, Deppen P, et al. Glutathione precursor, N-acetyl-cysteine, improves mismatch negativity in schizophrenia patients. *Neuropsychopharmacology*. 2008;33(9):2187–2199.
31. Dean OM, van den Buuse M, Berk M, Copolov DL, Mavros C, Bush AI. N-acetyl cysteine restores brain glutathione loss in combined 2-cyclohexene-1-one and d-amphetamine-treated rats: relevance to schizophrenia and bipolar disorder. *Neurosci Lett*. 2011;499(3):149–153.
32. Das P, Tanious M, Fritz K, et al. Metabolite profiles in the anterior cingulate cortex of depressed patients differentiate those taking N-acetyl-cysteine versus placebo. *Aust N Z J Psychiatry*. 2013;47(4):347–354.
33. Grados MA, Atkins EB, Kovacikova GI, McVicar E. A selective review of glutamate pharmacological therapy in obsessive-compulsive and related disorders. *Psychol Res Behav Manag*. 2015;8:115–131.
34. Baker DA, McFarland K, Lake RW, Shen H, Toda S, Kalivas PW. N-acetyl cysteine-induced blockade of cocaine-induced reinstatement. *Ann N Y Acad Sci*. 2003;1003:349–351.
35. Madayag A, Lobner D, Kau KS, et al. Repeated N-acetylcysteine administration alters plasticity-dependent effects of cocaine. *J Neurosci*. 2007;27(51):13968–13976.
36. Reissner KJ, Gipson CD, Tran PK, Knackstedt LA, Scofield MD, Kalivas PW. Glutamate transporter GLT-1 mediates N-acetylcysteine inhibition of cocaine reinstatement. *Addict Biol*. 2015;20(2):316–323.
37. Hurley MM, Resch JM, Maunze B, Frenkel MM, Baker DA, Choi S. N-acetylcysteine decreases binge eating in a rodent model. *Int J Obes (Lond)*. 2016;40(7):1183–1186.
38. Kupchik YM, Moussawi K, Tang XC, et al. The effect of N-acetylcysteine in the nucleus accumbens on neurotransmission and relapse to cocaine. *Biol Psychiatry*. 2012;71(11):978–986.
39. Samuni Y, Goldstein S, Dean OM, Berk M. The chemistry and biological activities of N-acetylcysteine. *Biochim Biophys Acta*. 2013;1830(8):4117–4129.
40. Lafleur DL, Pittenger C, Kelmendi B, et al. N-acetylcysteine augmentation in serotonin reuptake inhibitor refractory obsessive-compulsive disorder. *Psychopharmacology (Berl)*. 2006;184(2):254–256.
41. Rodrigues-Barata AR, Tosti A, Rodriguez-Pichardo A, Camacho-Martinez F. N-acetylcysteine in the treatment of trichotillomania. *Int J Trichol*. 2012;4(3):176–178.
42. Ozcan D, Seckin D. N-acetylcysteine in the treatment of trichotillomania: remarkable results in two patients. *J Eur Acad Dermatol Venereol*. 2016;30(9):1606–1608.
43. Yazici KU, Percinel I. N-acetylcysteine augmentation in children and adolescents diagnosed with

treatment-resistant obsessive-compulsive disorder case series. *J Clin Psychopharm*. 2015;35(4):486–489.

44. Paydary K, Akamaloo A, Ahmadipour A, Pishgar F, Emamzadehfard S, Akhondzadeh S. N-acetylcysteine augmentation therapy for moderate-to-severe obsessive-compulsive disorder: randomized, double-blind, placebo-controlled trial. *J Clin Pharm Ther*. 2016;41(2):214–219.
45. Sarris J, Oliver G, Camfield DA, et al. N-acetyl cysteine (nac) in the treatment of obsessive-compulsive disorder: a 16-week, double-blind, randomised, placebo-controlled study. *CNS Drugs*. 2015;29(9):801–809.
46. Costa DLC, Diniz JB, Joaquim M, et al. Poster sessions: P.4.d.006 Serotonin reuptake inhibitor augmentation with n-acetylcysteine in treatment resistant OCD: a double-blind randomized controlled trial. *Eur Neuropsychopharmacol*. 2015;25(Suppl 2):S570.
47. Afshar H, Roohafza H, Mohammad-Beigi H, et al. N-acetylcysteine add-on treatment in refractory obsessive-compulsive disorder: a randomized, double-blind, placebo-controlled trial. *J Clin Psychopharmacol*. 2012;32(6):797–803.
48. Grant JE, Odlaug BL, Kim SW. N-acetylcysteine, a glutamate modulator, in the treatment of trichotillomania: a double-blind, placebo-controlled study. *Arch Gen Psychiatry*. 2009;66(7):756–763.
49. Bloch MH, Panza KE, Grant JE, Pittenger C, Leckman JF. N-Acetylcysteine in the treatment of pediatric trichotillomania: a randomized, double-blind, placebo-controlled add-on trial. *J Am Acad Child Adolesc Psychiatry*. 2013;52(3):231–240.
50. Ghanizadeh A, Derakhshan N, Berk M. N-acetylcysteine versus placebo for treating nail biting, a double blind randomized placebo controlled clinical trial. *Antiinflamm Antiallergy Agents Med Chem*. 2013;12(3):223–228.
51. Miller JL, Angulo M. An open-label pilot study of N-acetylcysteine for skin-picking in Prader-Willi syndrome. *Am J Med Genet A*. 2014;164A(2):421–424.
52. Grant JE, Chamberlain SR, Redden SA, Leppink EW, Odlaug BL, Kim SW. N-acetylcysteine in the treatment of excoriation disorder: a randomized clinical trial. *JAMA Psychiatry*. 2016;73(5):490–496.
53. Grant JE, Kim SW, Odlaug BL. N-acetyl cysteine, a glutamate-modulating agent, in the treatment of pathological gambling: a pilot study. *Biol Psychiatry*. 2007;62(6):652–657.
54. Grant JE, Odlaug BL, Chamberlain SR, et al. A randomized, placebo-controlled trial of N-acetylcysteine plus imaginal desensitization for nicotine-dependent pathological gamblers. *J Clin Psychiatry*. 2014;75(1):39–45.
55. Sarris J, Oliver G, Camfield DA, Dean OM. Participant characteristics as modifiers of response to N-acetyl cysteine (NAC) in obsessive-compulsive disorder. *Clin Psychol Sci*. 2016;4(6):1104–1111.
56. Back SE, McCauley JL, Korte KJ, et al. A double-blind randomized controlled pilot trial of N-acetylcysteine in veterans with PTSD and substance use disorders. *J Clin Psychiatry*. 2016Nov;77(11):e1439.
57. LaRowe SD, Kalivas PW, Nicholas JS, Randall PK, Mardikian PN, Malcolm RJ. A double-blind placebo-controlled trial of N-acetylcysteine in the treatment of cocaine dependence. *Am J Addict*. 2013;22(5):443–452.
58. Kalivas BC, Kalivas PW. Corticostriatal circuitry in regulating diseases characterized by intrusive thinking. *Dialogues Clin Neuro*. 2016;18(1):65–76.
59. Kim H, McGrath BM, Silverstone PH. A review of the possible relevance of inositol and the phosphatidylinositol second messenger system (PI-cycle) to psychiatric disorders--focus on magnetic resonance spectroscopy (MRS) studies. *Hum Psychopharmacol*. 2005;20(5):309–326.
60. Harvey BH, Brink CB, Seedat S, Stein DJ. Defining the neuromolecular action of myo-inositol: application to obsessive-compulsive disorder. *Prog Neuropsychopharmacol Biol Psychiatry*. 2002;26(1):21–32.
61. Marazziti D, Masala I, Rossi A, et al. Increased inhibitory activity of protein kinase C on the serotonin transporter in OCD. *Neuropsychobiology*. 2000;41(4):171–177.
62. Harvey BH, Brink CB, Seedat S, Stein DJ. Defining the neuromolecular action of myo-inositol: application to obsessive-compulsive disorder. *Prog Neuro Psychopharmacol Biol Psychiatry*. 2002;26(1):21–32.
63. Vulink NC, Planting RS, Figee M, Booij J, Denys D. Reduced striatal dopamine D2/3 receptor availability in body dysmorphic disorder. *Eur Neuropsychopharmacol*. 2016;26(2):350–356.
64. Mukai T, Kishi T, Matsuda Y, Iwata N. A meta-analysis of inositol for depression and anxiety disorders. *Hum Psychopharmacol*. 2014;29(1):55–63.
65. Fux M, Levine J, Aviv A, Belmaker RH. Inositol treatment of obsessive-compulsive disorder. *Am J Psychiatry*. 1996;153(9):1219–1221.
66. Carey PD, Warwick J, Harvey BH, Stein DJ, Seedat S. Single photon emission computed tomography (SPECT) in obsessive-compulsive disorder before and after treatment with inositol. *Metab Brain Dis*. 2004;19(1–2):125–134.

67. Fux M, Benjamin J, Belmaker RH. Inositol versus placebo augmentation of serotonin reuptake inhibitors in the treatment of obsessive-compulsive disorder: a double-blind cross-over study. *Int J Neuropsychopharmacol.* 1999;2(3):193–195.
68. Seedat S, Stein DJ. Inositol augmentation of serotonin reuptake inhibitors in treatment-refractory obsessive-compulsive disorder: an open trial. *Int Clin Psychopharmacol.* 1999;14(6):353–356.
69. Leppink EW, Redden SA, Grant JE. A double-blind, placebo-controlled study of inositol in trichotillomania. *Int Clin Psychopharmacol.* 2017;32(2):107–114.
70. Seedat S, Stein DJ, Harvey BH. Inositol in the treatment of trichotillomania and compulsive skin picking. *J Clin Psychiatry.* 2001;62(1):60–61.
71. Cioffi CL, Guzzo PR. Inhibitors of glycine transporter-1: potential therapeutics for the treatment of CNS disorders. *Curr Top Med Chem.* 2016;16(29):3404–3437.
72. Cleveland WL, DeLaPaz RL, Fawwaz RA, Challop RS. High-dose glycine treatment of refractory obsessive-compulsive disorder and body dysmorphic disorder in a 5-year period. *Neural Plast.* 2009;2009:768398.
73. Greenberg WM, Benedict MM, Doerfer J, et al. Adjunctive glycine in the treatment of obsessive-compulsive disorder in adults. *J Psychiatr Res.* 2009;43(6):664–670.
74. Lane HY, Liu YC, Huang CL, et al. Sarcosine (N-methylglycine) treatment for acute schizophrenia: a randomized, double-blind study. *Biol Psychiatry.* 2008;63(1):9–12.
75. Tsai G, Lane HY, Yang P, Chong MY, Lange N. Glycine transporter I inhibitor, N-methylglycine (sarcosine), added to antipsychotics for the treatment of schizophrenia. *Biol Psychiatry.* 2004;55(5):452–456.
76. Wu PL, Tang HS, Lane HY, Tsai CA, Tsai GE. Sarcosine therapy for obsessive compulsive disorder a prospective, open-label study. *J Clin Psychopharm.* 2011;31(3):369–374.
77. Sarris J, Panossian A, Schweitzer I, Stough C, Scholey A. Herbal medicine for depression, anxiety and insomnia: a review of psychopharmacology and clinical evidence. *Eur Neuropsychopharmacol.* 2011;21(12):841–860.
78. Newmaster SG, Grguric M, Shanmughanandhan D, Ramalingam S, Ragupathy S. DNA barcoding detects contamination and substitution in North American herbal products. *BMC Med.* 2013;11:222.
79. Kulkarni SK, Dhir A. Withania somnifera: an Indian ginseng. *Prog Neuropsychopharmacol Biol Psychiatry.* 2008;32(5):1093–1105.
80. Dar NJ, Bhat JA, Satti NK, Sharma PR, Hamid A, Ahmad M. Withanone, an active constituent from *Withania somnifera*, affords protection against NMDA-induced excitotoxicity in neuron-like cells. *Mol Neurobiol.* 2017; 54(7):5061–5073.
81. Kumar G, Patnaik R. Exploring neuroprotective potential of *Withania somnifera* phytochemicals by inhibition of GluN2B-containing NMDA receptors: an in silico study. *Med Hypotheses.* 2016;92:35–43.
82. Rajasankar S, Manivasagam T, Surendran S. Ashwagandha leaf extract: a potential agent in treating oxidative damage and physiological abnormalities seen in a mouse model of Parkinson's disease. *Neurosci Lett.* 2009;454(1):11–15.
83. Bansal P, Banerjee S. Effect of *Withania somnifera* and shilajit on alcohol addiction in mice. *Pharmacogn Mag.* 2016;12(46):S121–S128.
84. Candelario M, Cuellar E, Reyes-Ruiz JM, et al. Direct evidence for GABAergic activity of *Withania somnifera* on mammalian ionotropic GABA(A) and GABAp receptors. *J Ethnopharmacol.* 2015;171:264–272.
85. Bhatnagar M, Sharma D, Salvi M. Neuroprotective effects of *Withania somnifera* dunal.: a possible mechanism. *Neurochem Res.* 2009;34(11):1975–1983.
86. Kulkarni SK, Ninan I. Inhibition of morphine tolerance and dependence by *Withania somnifera* in mice. *J Ethnopharmacol.* 1997;57(3):213–217.
87. Peana AT, Muggironi G, Spina L, et al. Effects of *Withania somnifera* on oral ethanol self-administration in rats. *Behav Pharmacol.* 2014;25(7):618–628.
88. Kaurav BP, Wanjari MM, Chandekar A, Chauhan NS, Upmanyu N. Influence of *Withania somnifera* on obsessive compulsive disorder in mice. *Asian Pac J Trop Med.* 2012;5(5):380–384.
89. Attari M, Jamaloo F, Shadvar S, Fakhraei N, Dehpour AR. Effect of *Withania somnifera* dunal root extract on behavioral despair model in mice: a possible role for nitric oxide. *Acta Med Iran.* 2016;54(3):165–172.
90. Jahanbakhsh SP, Manteghi AA, Emami SA, et al. Evaluation of the efficacy of *Withania somnifera* (ashwagandha) root extract in patients with obsessive-compulsive disorder: a randomized double-blind placebo-controlled trial. *Complement Ther Med.* 2016;27:25–29.
91. Sayyah M, Boostani H, Pakseresht S, Malayeri A. Comparison of *Silybum marianum* (L.) Gaertn. with fluoxetine in the treatment of obsessive-compulsive disorder. *Prog Neuropsychopharmacol Biol Psychiatry.* 2010;34(2):362–365.

92. Taylor LH, Kobak KA. An open-label trial of St. John's Wort (*Hypericum perforatum*) in obsessive-compulsive disorder. *J Clin Psychiatry.* 2000;61(8):575–578.

93. Kobak KA, Taylor LV, Bystritsky A, et al. St John's wort versus placebo in obsessive-compulsive disorder: results from a double-blind study. *Int Clin Psychopharmacol.* 2005;20(6):299–304.

94. Csupor D, Csorba A, Hohmann J. Recent advances in the analysis of flavonolignans of *Silybum marianum*. *J Pharm Biomed Anal.* 2016;130:301–317.

95. Hirayama K, Oshima H, Yamashita A, Sakatani K, Yoshino A, Katayama Y. Neuroprotective effects of silymarin on ischemia-induced delayed neuronal cell death in rat hippocampus. *Brain Res.* 2016;1646:297–303.

96. Shanmugam K, Holmquist L, Steele M, et al. Plant-derived polyphenols attenuate lipopolysaccharide-induced nitric oxide and tumour necrosis factor production in murine microglia and macrophages. *Mol Nutr Food Res.* 2008;52(4):427–438.

97. Valenzuela A, Aspillaga M, Vial S, Guerra R. Selectivity of silymarin on the increase of the glutathione content in different tissues of the rat. *Planta Med.* 1989;55(5):420–422.

98. Nencini C, Giorgi G, Micheli L. Protective effect of silymarin on oxidative stress in rat brain. *Phytomedicine.* 2007;14(2–3):129–135.

99. Osuchowski MF, Johnson VJ, He QR, Sharma RP. Alterations in regional brain neurotransmitters by silymarin, a natural antioxidant flavonoid mixture, in BALB/c mice. *Pharm Biol.* 2004;42(4–5):384–389.

100. Lu P, Mamiya T, Lu L, et al. Silibinin attenuates cognitive deficits and decreases of dopamine and serotonin induced by repeated methamphetamine treatment. *Behav Brain Res.* 2010;207(2):387–393.

101. Solati J, Yaghmaei P, Mohammdadi K. Role of the 5-HT1A serotonergic system in anxiolytic-like effects of silymarin. *Neurophysiology+.* 2012;44(1):49–55.

102. Thakare VN, Dhakane VD, Patel BM. Potential antidepressant-like activity of silymarin in the acute restraint stress in mice: modulation of corticosterone and oxidative stress response in cerebral cortex and hippocampus. *Pharmacol Rep.* 2016;68(5):1020–1027.

103. Grant JE, Odlaug BL. Silymarin treatment of obsessive-compulsive spectrum disorders. *J Clin Psychopharm.* 2015;35(3):340–342.

104. Jeschke E, Ostermann T, Vollmar HC, Tabali M, Matthes H. Depression, comorbidities, and prescriptions of antidepressants in a German network of GPs and specialists with subspecialisation in anthroposophic medicine: a longitudinal observational study. *Evid Based Complement Alternat Med.* 2012;2012:508623.

105. Klemow KM, Bartlow A, Crawford J, Kocher N, Shah J, Ritsick M. Medical attributes of St. John's wort (*Hypericum perforatum*). In: Benzie IFF, Wachtel-Galor S, eds. *Herbal Medicine: Biomolecular and Clinical Aspects*, 2nd ed. Boca Raton: CRC Press/Taylor and Francis; 2011.

106. Linde K, Berner MM, Kriston L. St John's wort for major depression. *Cochrane Database Syst Rev.* 2008(4):CD000448.

107. Kobak KA, Taylor LV, Warner G, Futterer R. St. John's wort versus placebo in social phobia: results from a placebo-controlled pilot study. *J Clin Psychopharmacol.* 2005;25(1):51–58.

108. Malhi GS, Bassett D, Boyce P, et al. Royal Australian and New Zealand College of Psychiatrists clinical practice guidelines for mood disorders. *Aust N Z J Psychiat.* 2015;49(12):1087–1206.

109. Mead GE, Morley W, Campbell P, Greig CA, McMurdo M, Lawlor DA. Exercise for depression. *Cochrane Database Syst Rev.* 2009(3):CD004366.

110. Abrantes AM, Strong DR, Cohn A, et al. Acute changes in obsessions and compulsions following moderate-intensity aerobic exercise among patients with obsessive-compulsive disorder. *J Anxiety Disord.* 2009;23(7):923–927.

111. Brown RA, Abrantes AM, Strong DR, et al. A pilot study of moderate-intensity aerobic exercise for obsessive compulsive disorder. *J Nerv Ment Dis.* 2007;195(6):514–520.

112. Olatunji BO, Davis ML, Powers MB, Smits JA. Cognitive-behavioral therapy for obsessive-compulsive disorder: a meta-analysis of treatment outcome and moderators. *J Psychiatr Res.* 2013;47(1):33–41.

113. Albert U, Aguglia A, Chiarle A, Bogetto F, Maina G. Metabolic syndrome and obsessive-compulsive disorder: a naturalistic Italian study. *Gen Hosp Psychiatry.* 2013;35(2):154–159.

114. Posadzki P, Choi J, Lee MS, Ernst E. Yoga for addictions: a systematic review of randomised clinical trials. *Focus Alt Complement Ther.* 2014;19(1):1–8.

115. Shannahoff-Khalsa DS, Ray LE, Levine S, Gallen CC, Schwartz BJ, Sidorowich JJ. Randomized controlled trial of yogic meditation techniques for patients with obsessive-compulsive disorder. *CNS Spectrums.* 1999;4(12):34–47.

116. Bhat S, Varambally S, Karmani S, Govindaraj R, Gangadhar BN. Designing and validation of a yoga-based intervention for obsessive compulsive disorder. *Int Rev Psychiatry.* 2016;28(3):327–333.

117. Sarris J, Kavanagh DJ, Byrne G. Adjuvant use of nutritional and herbal medicines with antidepressants, mood stabilizers and benzodiazepines. *J Psychiatr Res*. 2010;44(1): 32–41.

118. Gray SM, Bloch MH. Systematic review of proinflammatory cytokines in obsessive-compulsive disorder. *Curr Psychiatry Rep*. 2012;14(3):220–228.

119. Rao NP, Venkatasubramanian G, Ravi V, Kalmady S, Cherian A, Yc JR. Plasma cytokine abnormalities in drug-naive, comorbidity-free obsessive-compulsive disorder. *Psychiatry Res*. 2015;229(3):949–952.

120. Turna J, Grosman Kaplan K, Anglin R, Van Ameringen M. "What's Bugging the Gut in OCD?" A review of the gut microbiome in obsessive-compulsive disorder. *Depress Anxiety*. 2016;33(3):171–178.

121. Kantak PA, Bobrow DN, Nyby JG. Obsessive-compulsive-like behaviors in house mice are attenuated by a probiotic (*Lactobacillus rhamnosus* GG). *Behav Pharmacol*. 2014;25(1):71–79.

122. Van Ameringen M. Probiotic Treatment in Adult Obsessive-Compulsive Disorder. NCT02334644. ClinicalTrials.gov, 2017. Available from: https://clinicaltrials.gov/ct2/show/NCT02334644?term=probiotics&cond=%22Anxiety+Disorders%22&rank=7 (accessed July 19, 2018).

Chapter 23

Transdiagnostic and Unique Clinical and Treatment Factors of Dysmorphophobia: Body Dysmorphic Disorder and Olfactory Reference Disorder

Francesca Beilharz and Susan L. Rossell

VISUAL DYSMORPHOPHOBIA: BODY DYSMORPHIC DISORDER

Introduction

Diagnosis of Body Dysmorphic Disorder

Body dysmorphic disorder (BDD) is a psychiatric disorder characterized by a preoccupation with perceived flaws in appearance, which are considered "ugly" or "deformed", despite appearing minor or unnoticeable to others. This preoccupation causes clinically significant distress or functional impairment [1]. In response to these appearance concerns, people with BDD engage in repetitive behaviors, such as compulsive mirror checking, excessive grooming, cosmetic surgery and reassurance seeking [2,3]. Diagnostically, this preoccupation in appearance is not better explained by a focus on body weight or shape if symptoms also meet criteria for an eating disorder [1,4]. While any body part can be the focus of concern in BDD, specific facial features such as the nose, texture or color of one's hair or skin, or specific body parts such as thighs or breasts, are most commonly implicated [5].

BDD includes additional specifiers within the *Diagnostic and Statistical Manual of Mental Disorders*, fifth edition (DSM-5), including muscle dysmorphia, which is allocated if the patient's appearance preoccupation centers on the idea that their body build is insufficiently muscular [1]. This specifier can be given if there are both muscle build and other areas of appearance concern. Level of insight is also specified within the DSM-5 diagnosis, according to the strength of beliefs regarding one's appearance [1]. Insight ranges from good or fair (e.g., recognition that their appearance concerns may or may not be true), poor (e.g., appearance concerns are likely true) and absent or delusional (e.g., completely convinced that their appearance concerns are true) [1].

Within DSM-5, BDD has been reclassified as an obsessive-compulsive related disorder (OCRD), alongside obsessive-compulsive disorder (OCD), hoarding disorder, trichotillomania and excoriation disorder [1]. This reorganization was conducted with the following similarities of OCRDs in mind: "the cardinal symptoms of repetitive thoughts and behaviors with a failure of behavior inhibition, similar clinical profiles, shared brain circuitry and neurotransmitter abnormalities, and similar treatment response profiles" [6].

Recent Research Findings

Epidemiology and Demographic Features of Body Dysmorphic Disorder

Approximately 1.9% of the general population is diagnosed with BDD, with a slightly higher prevalence among women in the majority of settings [7]. The highest prevalence of BDD appears within general cosmetic surgery (13.2%), particularly rhinoplasty surgery (21.1%), as those with BDD often seek cosmetic procedures to try to "correct" their perceived defect in appearance [7]. Typically, those with BDD are less likely to have been married and are more likely to be divorced compared with the general population [8]. The typical onset of BDD is reported to be gradual, with a mean age range of 16–18.3 years [9,14]. If untreated, 92% of individuals endorsed a chronic and continuous progression, with 62% reporting their illness had worsened over time [10]. However, symptom severity and areas of concerns have been shown to wax and wane in intervals [9].

Comorbidities, Suicide and Quality of Life in Body Dysmorphic Disorder

BDD is associated with a high lifetime prevalence of comorbid psychological disorders, most commonly including depression (82%), substance use disorder (49%), social anxiety disorder (39%), eating disorders (32.5%) and OCD (27.5%) [11,12,13,14,15]. When these comorbid disorders occur alongside a primary diagnosis of BDD, individuals are at a higher risk of negative outcomes, including unemployment, being housebound, suicidal ideation and suicide attempts [11,13,16].

Approximately 78–81% of BDD participants have reported experiencing lifetime suicidal ideation, with 24–28% reporting prior suicide attempts [17,18,19,20,21]. These rates are particularly high among adolescents with BDD, with 80.6% reporting ideation and 44.4% having previously attempted suicide [20,22]. Compared with the general population, the rate of death by suicide among BDD sufferers is approximately 45 times higher [23].

As a consequence of the disorder, individuals with BDD often withdraw socially [23], and can have markedly and pervasively reduced quality of life compared with the general population. This includes a number of functioning domains, such as emotional wellbeing, occupation, education status, household functioning, leisure activities and all forms of social interaction and relationships [24,25,26].

Insight and Delusionality in Body Dysmorphic Disorder

As we have seen, insight in BDD involves the degree to which an individual holds their body image beliefs, and ranges from good to absent or delusional [27]. Using the well-validated Brown Assessment of Beliefs Scale, participants with BDD showed significantly poor insight into both their global insight and individual aspects of insight, such as conviction, perception of others' views and insight into the cause of belief [28,29]. Furthermore, low levels of insight have been associated with greater symptom severity and poor treatment response within BDD [28,29,30,31,32]. As insight involves the awareness and understanding of one's own mental health and perceptions, this can be instrumental in promoting change and engagement throughout treatment [27].

Visual Processing Abnormalities Within Body Dysmorphic Disorder

A major unique clinical feature of BDD involves abnormal visual processing. It has been suggested as a possible contributing or maintaining factor of the disorder. These abnormalities have been observed using a range of appearance and non-appearance-related visual stimuli, indicating that widespread differences in visual perception are present in individuals with BDD. A well-supported explanation for these differences in visual perception relates to changes in local and global visual processing. This theory states that individuals typically use two complementary systems to process incoming perceptual information: the first is the global system which is responsible for identifying overall shape and form, whereas the second, which is the local system, pieces together specific details to create a whole [33,34]. Healthy individuals can use either system, or a combination of the two, depending on the stimulus and environment in question; yet individuals with BDD appear to have a bias for processing information using the local system over the global system [35,36]. This bias reflects clinical characteristics of BDD as individuals report focusing on specific details, which most notably include areas of concern.

Visual tasks using face stimuli have provided the strongest evidence for this local bias, as patients with BDD demonstrate different strategies to recognize facial features and expressions compared with those without the disorder. It has been well documented in healthy individuals that a global template is used based on prior learning experiences, which comprises the eyes–nose–mouth triangle. This global process becomes automatic, as humans are required to recognize faces and emotional expressions quickly and effectively to socially interact with others. Eye-tracking technology has demonstrated that individuals with BDD use aberrant strategies to the global template, either by focusing on or avoiding facial areas of concern, which consequently impacts their ability to efficiently and accurately identify emotions and faces of individuals [37,38,39]. The scan paths of patients with BDD have also demonstrated significantly more blinks, fewer long fixations and less attention paid to salient facial features, with these abnormalities present in those with BDD whose predominant concerns were both head and body part related. This suggests that such differences in perception are present regardless of perceived "flaws" in BDD, and difficulties in processing emotional and social stimuli are a unique characteristic of the disorder [40]. Patients with BDD have additionally demonstrated superior recognition of neutral faces when the stimuli are inverted. While healthy individuals typically have disproportionate recognition delays and inaccuracies when recognizing an inverted compared with an upright face, patients with BDD were significantly faster [41,42] and more accurate [35]. It has been proposed individuals with BDD have an enhanced ability to efficiently and accurately process local visual information, which has negative effects when processing stimuli that are more efficiently processed globally, such as face stimuli [41,42].

These abnormalities in visual perception appear to extend to other visual stimuli such as houses, objects, gestalt shapes and negative disorder-related words [36,43]. Similarly, individuals with BDD have demonstrated differences to healthy controls with regard to attractiveness and symmetry ratings, which may reflect the aforementioned bias in local processing over global processing [44,45,46,47]. It is hypothesized that abnormal visual processes in BDD consequently influences behavioral components of the disorder, such as selective attention, mirror checking and avoidance and processing oneself as an "esthetic object". These perceptual abnormalities can then reinforce patterns of rumination, low mood and safety behaviors, creating maintaining mechanisms [48].

Brain Structure and Function in Body Dysmorphic Disorder

Neuroimaging studies have examined the brain structure, activation and connectivity of patients with BDD, with a focus on visual processing. Regarding volume, patients with BDD have shown abnormalities within the inferior frontal gyrus and the right amygdala, areas which are typically involved in processing faces [49,50]. These regions have been reported as smaller in volume compared with healthy controls, and are associated with increased symptom severity [49,51]. Functional imaging studies of BDD have typically focused on processing visual stimuli tasks, and have demonstrated abnormalities in regions associated with visual areas, such as reduced activity in primary and secondary visual cortices of the brain when recognizing face and house stimuli [36]. As these activation patterns have been replicated for a range of appearance and non-appearance-related stimuli among patients with BDD, this suggests more fundamental differences in visual processing.

Widespread structural connectivity issues have been noted across all four lobes of the brain, and both hemispheres in BDD [51,52]. Studies have demonstrated disrupted white matter connectivity across the whole of the brain in those with BDD. This has implications for how efficiently information is processed globally [53]. In addition connectivity abnormalities are significant when examining the cortical tracts that transfer visual information across the hemispheres, and between regions responsible for lower- and higher-order visual processing, as well as emotion and memory processing systems [53].

Treatment of Body Dysmorphic Disorder

Despite the aforementioned debilitating outcomes associated with a diagnosis of BDD, there has been relatively little research regarding the initiation and maintenance of symptoms, and consequently how to effectively treat the disorder. Current treatment guidelines for BDD were developed in tandem with OCD guidelines, owing to shared historical cognitive-behavioral models of the disorders. Depending on the level of functional impairment, these guidelines recommend an initial treatment of cognitive behavior therapy (CBT) including exposure and response prevention (ERP), selective serotonin reuptake inhibitors (SSRIs) such as escitalopram, fluvoxamine or citalopram or a combination of psychotherapy and medication [54].

CBT for BDD typically involves a combination of cognitive strategies to target maladaptive thoughts and behavioral techniques such as ERP to reduce appearance-related compulsions. ERP involves purposefully exposing, either in vivo or imaginary, individuals with BDD to a hierarchy of situations that provoke anxiety, without allowing the practice of safety behaviors [55]. This could include attending a public event without completing typical grooming techniques, so the perceived "flaw" is "exposed" to others [56,57]. Typical CBT components such as psychoeducation, formulation, modifying unhelpful cognitions, behavioral activation and altering avoidance behaviors, are also addressed in the treatment of BDD [57,58].

CBT for BDD also contains an optional component of perceptual mirror retraining, which teaches individuals to view themselves in a full-length mirror and scan from head to toe, while describing each body part nonjudgmentally and objectively [59]. The therapist guides clients through this retraining process, where they are simultaneously refraining from appearance-related rituals or other compulsive behaviors. While individuals with BDD have qualitatively reported mirror retraining to be among the most helpful aspects of treatment, no research is currently available which examines the use of this component outside of the CBT framework [60,61].

Recent systematic literature reviews have revealed that CBT for BDD appears to demonstrate moderate effect sizes, with symptoms generally reducing 50–78% on the BDD Yale-Brown Obsessive Compulsive Scale [5,60,61,62,63,64,65,66,67,68,69,70,71]. However, while reduced symptom severity has been maintained for up to four months, responding patients with BDD typically retain mild to moderate level symptoms at follow-up [64,72,73]. Pharmacologically, SSRIs such as fluoxetine and clomipramine have demonstrated some beneficial effects for BDD symptoms, although only a small number of randomized controlled trials are currently available [63]. Within these psychological and pharmacological treatment trials, it must be considered that a number of methodological factors limit comparison across studies.

Despite these moderate findings in symptom reduction, the most commonly pursued treatment by individuals with BDD concerns non-psychiatric medical treatments, such as cosmetic surgery. Research has identified up to 76.4% of patients with BDD sought such medical procedures, which were received by 66% of individuals, even though medical and surgical options often maintain or exacerbate the psychological condition [39,74]. Therefore, it appears as if current psychological, pharmacological and ill-advised surgical treatments may not be giving the best treatment outcome for individuals with BDD; perhaps as these methods do not address the visual abnormalities seen within BDD that appear to be a core component of the disorder.

Classification and Diagnostic Implications of Cross-Diagnostic Approaches for Body Dysmorphic Disorder

BDD was recently reclassified as an OCRD due to similarities regarding transdiagnostic factors, including obsessive thoughts, compulsive behaviors, CBT models, neurobiological abnormalities, epidemiology and similar treatment responses. Yet some concerns have been raised due to the lack of research supporting this restructure, and significant differences concerning insight and delusionality, suicide attempts and ideation, abnormal visual processing, neurobiology regarding brain volume, white matter integrity and functional activity [6,20,22,27,51,52,74,75,76]. Furthermore, treatment responses to psychotherapy including CBT and ERP appear to be less effective for BDD than originally thought, indicating reduced efficacy in comparison to OCD [63]. It is these clinical features which appear unique to BDD and differentiate BDD from other OCRDs.

To assist in differential diagnosis, a defining feature of BDD is the focus on body image distortions and concerns. It has been proposed that thoughts appear to be the primary feature of OCD. Alternatively, the disturbance of thoughts within BDD seems secondary to perceptual abnormalities with regard to body parts [77]. Indeed, it has been suggested that disorders such as BDD and eating disorders, including anorexia nervosa and bulimia nervosa, may be better classified within a "body image disorders" category, due to the intense focus on body image and shared perceptual disturbances [78]. Innovative methods to capture and assess this body image disturbance may be used clinically, such as drawing self-portraits, or change paradigms in which individuals are able to alter the form and dimensions of their facial and bodily features using a computer program [79,80]. Such methods can be especially valuable for the clinician to gain a shared understanding and conceptualization of the client's perceived "defects".

Clinical Treatment and Prevention Implications of Cross-Diagnostic Approaches for Body Dysmorphic Disorder

Although current treatment modalities for BDD such as CBT, ERP or SSRIs have demonstrated moderate efficacy in reducing symptoms and distress associated with the disorder, it is possible that because of the multifaceted nature of BDD, the established visual abnormalities present may not be addressed within these transdiagnostic methods [63,81]. As perceptual abnormalities appear to be a core feature of BDD, treatments that do not address this factor may result in higher rates of relapse as individuals can still "see" their areas of concern. Such studies generally demonstrate that while symptoms may reduce in severity through standard treatments, the majority of individuals with BDD remain symptomatic. For example, at four-year follow-up post-CBT, 37.8% of patients with BDD were in partial remission and 45.6% again met full diagnostic criteria [72,73,82]. As perceived "flaws" in appearance remain, it seems likely that individuals with BDD can easily resume previous obsessional thoughts and compulsive behaviors through sustained attention to visual details. Therefore, it is recommended that a greater understanding of such unique features within BDD, such as the perceptual abnormalities, is essential in developing more effective treatment methods.

Based on these findings, it is recommended that standard cross-diagnostic treatments are elaborated upon for BDD. This could involve ensuring that perceptual mirror retraining is a compulsory aspect of CBT, so that individuals are taught how to perceive their appearance in a global, non-judgmental and mindful manner. As reflective surfaces are used by individuals without BDD on a daily basis, it is important to ensure that patients with BDD are trained to use mirrors in a similar and healthy manner, reducing associated checking and avoidance behaviors. Additions could also be made to ERP techniques used in CBT for BDD, as it seems that the majority of current techniques involve participants being in a social situation where their areas of concern are "exposed" to *others*, for example, walking to the shops without wearing make-up [83,84,85]. This seems contrary to typical ERP practices for OCD, which involve direct exposure to the thoughts, images or situations that trigger obsessions and compulsions. Therefore, direct exposure to one's own appearance and perceived "flaws" may have the strongest effect for those with BDD. While only a few studies have specifically examined self-exposure in BDD, the majority of patients with BDD have benefited with significant reductions in symptom severity [85,86,87]. Similar exposure strategies could be used within an individual's mirror exposure hierarchy within perceptual mirror retraining, to ensure that self-perception is targeted as a core component of CBT for BDD.

Future Directions of Body Dysmorphic Disorder

While empirical studies have identified substantial visual abnormalities within BDD, current treatment methods do little to remedy this [62]. It is hypothesized that including perceptual mirror retraining and self-exposure as a compulsory module of CBT will modify how individuals with BDD perceive their appearance; however, the growing research literature supports visual abnormalities across a range of visual stimuli and levels of processing in BDD. Therefore, it may be beneficial to implement a separate visual training program to target broader perception skills outside of self-perception. Such a training program may be delivered independently alongside typical CBT for BDD to strengthen current treatment outcomes [88,89].

Despite overwhelming support for the implementation of a specific visual intervention for BDD [37,38,43,47,90,91,92,93], this has been examined only briefly in the literature, but with promising outcomes [94]. To date, only one published study has introduced a visual training program as a treatment method with BDD, where the well-documented deficit in processing emotional faces was targeted by Buhlmann et al. [94]. This program provided correctional feedback after each trial, and found that patients with BDD who participated in the training had significantly improved in identifying "neutral" and "scared" facial expressions compared with patients with BDD who did not receive the training. This study demonstrated that patients with BDD showed improved facial recognition after a single training session, which supports the potential for further visual training programs to be trialed with BDD, although the impact on symptoms is unknown.

Based on these findings, it seems logical to develop and implement a visual training program that addresses broader aspects of visual perception, as guided by research identifying visual abnormalities within BDD. For example, this could involve a bottom-up training process of developing general visual skills (such as processing speed, scanning, attention, motion and details), face and emotion recognition skills and mirror retraining for self-perception. Further investigation is required as specifically targeting visual deficits has only been attempted in a healthy sample with sub-clinical body image concerns [94,95].

Although the utility and efficacy of such visual training used to treat BDD are still within the experimental stage, research supports the efficacy of similar visual programs within cognitive remediation treatments for alternative populations. For example, patients with schizophrenia who demonstrate similar visual abnormalities to those with BDD have shown significant improvements after using a cognitive remediation and social cognition computer intervention, including superior emotion recognition, faster processing speed and increased attention, vigilance and working memory [96,97]. Such emotion training programs have remediated atypical scan paths within schizophrenia to reflect those seen in healthy controls, such as greater fixations on relevant features [98]. Based on these findings, visual training and social cognition programs demonstrate good feasibility and promising outcomes, and may be generalizable to other disorders with shared phenomenology [97,99,100].

Future research may also implement eye-tracking technology to create a personalized visual training program based on each individual's specific processing patterns. Patients with BDD can demonstrate different patterns of atypical scanning, including avoidance, over-focusing and a combination of both disproportionate focus and intermittent scanning, so different visual training techniques may be required, according to the pattern displayed by the individual [40].

Advances in our understanding of neuroplasticity have highlighted the brain's ability to refine or modify existing neural pathways through repeated learning, and have shown the positive impact this can have on mental health [101]. For example, visual plasticity has been demonstrated by strengthening neural connections between the visual areas of the brain, resulting in improvements in spatial field, local and global processing, attention and visual discrimination [102]. Such findings indicate that both functional and structural brain changes can be induced in individuals with impaired and healthy visual processing systems [101]. Therefore, such visual training programs may remediate perceptual abnormalities within BDD at a neural level for longer-lasting effects. These novel interventions are not designed to supersede traditional psychotherapies for BDD, but to complement and enhance existing modalities. CBT for BDD demonstrates moderate improvements within the majority of clients, but owing to the multifaceted nature of BDD, with a unique clinical feature involving abnormal visual processing, it is recommended that this be an additional target of treatment.

OLFACTORY DYSMORPHOPHOBIA: OLFACTORY REFERENCE DISORDER

Introduction

Diagnosis of Olfactory Reference Disorder

Compared with a perceived "defect" in one's visual appearance as in BDD, olfactory reference disorder (ORD; or olfactory reference syndrome) is characterized by a concern and preoccupation with emitting an unpleasant or offensive body odor. While the individual may or may not be able to "smell" the odor in question, it cannot be perceived by others. A number of body odors can be of concern, including those originating from the mouth, anus, genitals, feet or underarms, and can also include non-bodily odors, such as rotten food. Individuals with ORD experience significant distress and impairment, particularly relating to a fear of rejection or humiliation from others. Similar obsessive and compulsive behaviors can be seen in ORD, such as reassurance seeking, camouflaging the perceived odor, frequent bathing and grooming rituals [103]. While ORD is not considered an official diagnosis within DMS-5, it is now referenced as an example of an "otherwise specified OCRD". Diagnostically, an OCRD requires symptoms characteristic of an OCRD that do not meet full criteria for any specific OCRDs, but involve significant distress and impairment to functioning [1].

Recent Research Findings

Epidemiology and Demographics of Olfactory Reference Disorder

Owing to limited research data on ORD, community prevalence rates are estimated to range from 0.5% to 2.1% based on body odor concern self-report data [104]. However, it is likely that the prevalence of ORD is underreported within the general population because of the embarrassment associated with symptoms, and the lack of awareness within the community and medical professions. Demographically, slightly more females (60%) appear to experience ORD than males, with mean age of onset at 15.6 years [105]. If left untreated, ORD appears to be chronic in the majority of cases (84.2%), with the potential for deterioration, such as new odor concerns emerging over time [105].

Comorbidities, Suicide and Quality of Life in Olfactory Reference Disorder

ORD is associated with a high lifetime prevalence of comorbid psychological disorders, with the most common including depression (95%), anxiety (80%), social anxiety disorder (65%), substance use disorder (50%) and OCD (30%) [105,106]. Primary ORD, and associated comorbid conditions, have significant impacts on stress and impairment across a range of functioning modalities. A high percentage (50%) often avoid occupational, academic and family roles, often resulting in individuals becoming completely housebound [104,107]. Individuals with ORD typically have high service use, seeking specialists in medical, surgery and specialist fields, often pursuing on average 2.5 specialist opinions to treat their perceived odor.

Suicide is also common within ORD, with lifetime prevalence up to 68.4% for suicidal ideation and 31.6% reported past suicidal behaviors [108,109]. It has additionally been reported that 5.6% of a study with 36 participants with ORD had completed suicide by the time of the 17-year follow-up [103,110].

Insight and Delusionality in Olfactory Reference Disorder

While ORD was previously considered to be a delusional disorder, research now demonstrates that patients can experience varying degrees of insight regarding the validity of their beliefs and olfactory sensations [103]. It appears the majority of those with ORD can experience delusional beliefs where they can actually "smell" their perceived odor (57–85%), while others demonstrate fair insight and can express doubts regarding their odor concerns (15–43%) [103,105,108].

Often associated with delusional levels of insight, individuals with ORD can experience ideas of reference, where coincidental or random events are interpreted with a high level of personal significance. Within ORD, this typically involves misattributing and misinterpreting the actions of others to one's perceived odor, such as scratching their nose, facing away or opening windows [103,104]. The lifetime prevalence of ideas of reference is estimated to occur in up to 88% of those with ORD [105].

Treatment of Olfactory Reference Disorder

Owing to the widely misunderstood nature of ORD, and limited assessment and diagnosis options, research supporting treatment options is fairly lacking. Similar to those with BDD, individuals with ORD often seek non-psychiatric medical or surgical treatments, including specialists such as dentists, gynecologists, gastroenterologists, dermatologists and nose, ear and mouth specialists, in an attempt to reduce or eliminate their perceived odor. However, medical treatments for ORD have been ineffective in all studied cases [105].

Throughout case studies and anecdotal evidence, CBT appears to garner the most support of psychotherapy for ORD, for example improvements were found in 14 of 18 patients (78%), with reduced core ORD symptoms and associated anxiety and mood concerns [108,111]. Most commonly used techniques appear to include those similar to OCD treatment, such as ERP, shared conceptualizations, identifying and modifying unhelpful beliefs, relaxation techniques and behavioral activation [103]. These techniques appear very similar to those used in CBT for BDD, except that the clinical focus explores appraisal of olfactory experience and perceived reactions of others [111,112].

Additional case studies support the combination of CBT alongside pharmacological treatments [113,114]. Historically, medication for ORD has involved antipsychotics, yet more recent evidence supports the use of SSRIs and tricyclic antidepressants, including clomipramine, paroxetine, sertraline and citalopram [115,116,117]. These improvements in medication have predominantly resulted in a significant reduction of ORD symptoms, which have been maintained up to two years of follow-up with continued use [115]. Despite these promising case studies, the current available literature is insufficient to provide treatment recommendations. This is complicated by the lack of randomized controlled trials, and additional methodological differences which limit comparison [103].

Classification, Diagnosis and Treatment Implications of Cross-Diagnostic Approaches for Olfactory Reference Disorder

While ORD currently is not recognized in DSM-5 as a distinct disorder, there is some support for this introduction to be classified as an OCRD. This argument is based on perceived similarities between ORD and OCRDs, such as preoccupations and compulsive behaviors, high comorbidity with OCD and superior treatment outcomes of SSRIs over antipsychotics [118]. Because of the significant shame and embarrassment regarding symptoms, it has also been theorized that individuals with ORD may instead present with more transdiagnostic and "acceptable" symptoms such as in OCD or social anxiety [107]. However, similarly to BDD, ORD appears to involve unique factors around insight and delusionality, the focus of preoccupations being upon one's odor and increased use of non-psychiatric services [118]. It has been hypothesized that ORD could be an olfactory variant of BDD, due to parallel negative interpretations of oneself, which are believed to be shared by others [109,119], although research specifically comparing these disorders is not currently available.

As the current literature relies upon case studies to identify effective treatments for ORD, limited implications of cross-diagnostic approaches can be considered. Although positive outcomes have been noted in case studies using CBT and SSRIs to reduce symptoms of ORD, it seems possible that the unique factors as discussed above may have some impact on treatment efficacy. Similarly to BDD, it is possible that through transdiagnostic treatments, the unique disturbance in olfaction is not addressed, however further research is required.

Future Directions of Olfactory Reference Disorder

There are many areas of ORD which require both research and clinical attention to better understand and treat the disorder. As the current research literature on ORD is solely composed of case reports and case series, larger group studies are required to limit researcher bias and provide group data on epidemiology, classification, demographics and symptom severity [118]. Additionally, neuroimaging studies into the structure, function and connectivity status of the brain in ORD would provide important knowledge regarding the development of the disorder. Of particular interest would be whether similar abnormalities exist in ORD in the primary olfactory cortex which is responsible for the sensation of smell, parallel to abnormalities in the visual cortex as seen in BDD.

Once a greater understanding of the diagnosis, maintaining factors, neurobiological underpinnings and unique clinical factors are gained, the literature on ORD would benefit from evidence-based controlled treatment trials [118]. Such treatment trials could examine the efficacy of psychotherapy compared with pharmacotherapy, and benefits of specific therapeutic modalities. Future comparisons of treatment outcomes to conceptually similar disorders like OCD and BDD would also be beneficial, to help elucidate transdiagnostic or unique treatment factors.

Conclusion

In conclusion, while BDD, ORD and OCD share some commonalities in regard to clinical, epidemiological and functional factors, there are distinct differences within these domains which question the clinical utility of placing these disorders within the same conceptual framework. Furthermore, the amount of research on BDD and ORD is severely lacking compared with OCD, and so the support for this decision is simply not available. Particularly, there is a need for direct comparisons of BDD and ORD with OCD, as only a few studies have been conducted. However, the available research indicates that individuals with BDD and ORD may differ significantly from those with OCD in terms of insight and delusionality, suicide attempts and ideation, visual processing of faces and other stimuli, neurobiology and response to psychological treatments including CBT. As classification systems are vital in understanding and treating psychological conditions, it is essential to clarify the similarities and differences among these disorders, so that appropriate treatment recommendations can be implemented to provide the best possible outcomes for clients.

Acknowledgments

The authors would like to acknowledge the support of the Australian Government Research Training Program Scholarship in preparing this chapter.

References

1. American Psychiatric Association. *Diagnostic and Statistical Manual of Mental Disorders*, 5th ed. Washington, DC: APA; 2013.
2. Buhlmann U, Glaesmer H, Mewes R, et al. Updates on the prevalence of body dysmorphic disorder: a population-based survey. *Psychiatry Res.* 2010;178(1):171–175.
3. Veale D, Riley S. Mirror, mirror on the wall, who is the ugliest of them all? The psychopathology of mirror

gazing in body dysmorphic disorder. *Behav Res Ther.* 2001;39(12):1381–1393.

4. Cororve MB, Gleaves DH. Body dysmorphic disorder: a review of conceptualizations, assessment, and treatment strategies. *Clin Psychol Rev.* 2001;21(6):949–970.
5. Veale D, Boocock A, Gournay K, et al. Body dysmorphic disorder. A survey of fifty cases. *Br J Psychiatry.* 1996;169(2):196–201.
6. Van Ameringen M, Patterson B, Simpson W. DSM-5 obsessive-compulsive and related disorders: clinical implications of new criteria. Review: DSM-5 OCD and Related Disorders. *Depress Anxiety.* 2014;31(6):487–493.
7. Veale D, Gledhill LJ, Christodoulou P, Hodsoll J. Body dysmorphic disorder in different settings: a systematic review and estimated weighted prevalence. *Body Image.* 2016;18:168–186.
8. Koran LMA, Abujaoude E; Large, MD, Serpe, RT. The prevalence of body dysmorphic disorder in the United States adult population. *CNS Spectr.* 2008;13(4):316–322.
9. Phillips KA, Pagano ME, Menard W, Stout RL. A 12-month follow-up study of the course of body dysmorphic disorder. *Am J Psychiatry.* 2006;163(5):907–912.
10. Phillips KA. "I look like a monster": pharmacotherapy and cognitive-behavioral therapy for body dysmorphic disorder. In: Spitzer RL, ed. *DSM-IV-TR Casebook Experts Tell How They Treated Their Own Patients.* Washington, DC: American Psychiatric Association; 2006:263–276.
11. Gunstad J, Phillips KA. Axis I comorbidity in body dysmorphic disorder. *Compr Psychiatry.* 2003;44(4):270–276.
12. Grant JE, Menard W, Pagano ME, Fay C, Phillips KA. Substance use disorders in individuals with body dysmorphic disorder. *J Clin Psychiatry.* 2005;66(3):309–316.
13. Coles ME, Phillips KA, Menard W, et al. Body dysmorphic disorder and social phobia: cross-sectional and prospective data. *Depress Anxiety.* 2006;23(1):26–33.
14. Ruffolo JS, Phillips KA, Menard W, Fay C, Weisberg RB. Comorbidity of body dysmorphic disorder and eating disorders: severity of psychopathology and body image disturbance. *Int J Eat Disord.* 2006;39(1):11–19.
15. Frias A, Palma C, Farriols N, Gonzalez L. Comorbidity between obsessive-compulsive disorder and body dysmorphic disorder: prevalence, explanatory theories, and clinical characterization. *Neuropsychiatr Dis Treat.* 2015;11:2233–2244.
16. Fang A, Hofmann SG. Relationship between social anxiety disorder and body dysmorphic disorder. *Clin Psychol Rev.* 2010;30(8):1040–1048.
17. Didie E, Kelly MM, Phillips K. Clinical features of body dysmorphic disorder. *Psychiatr Ann.* 2010;40(7):310–316.
18. Angelakis I, Gooding PA, Panagioti M. Suicidality in body dysmorphic disorder (BDD): a systematic review with meta-analysis. *Clin Psychol Rev.* 2016;49:55–66.
19. Perugi G, Giannotti D, Frare F, et al. Prevalence, phenomenology and comorbidity of body dysmorphic disorder (dysmorphophobia) in a clinical population. *Int J Psychiatry Clin Pract.* 1997;1(2):77.
20. Phillips KA. Suicidality in body dysmorphic disorder. *Prim Psychiatry.* 2007;14(12):58–66.
21. Phillips KA, Coles ME, Menard W, Yen S, Fay C, Weisberg RB. Suicidal ideation and suicide attempts in body dysmorphic disorder. *J Clin Psychiatry.* 2005;66(6):717–725.
22. Phillips K, Didie E, Menard W, Pagano ME, Fay C, Weisberg R. Clinical features of body dysmorphic disorder in adolescents and adults. *Psychiatry Res.* 2006;141(3):305–314.
23. Phillips K, Menard W. Suicidality in body dysmorphic disorder: a prospective study. *Am J Psychiatry.* 2006;163(7):1280-U2.
24. IsHak WW, Bolton MA, Bensoussan JC, et al. Quality of life in body dysmorphic disorder. *CNS Spectr.* 2012;17(4):167–175.
25. Phillips KA, Menard W, Fay C, Pagano ME. Psychosocial functioning and quality of life in body dysmorphic disorder. *Compr Psychiatry.* 2005;46(4):254–260.
26. Didie ER, Pinto A, Mancebo M, et al. A comparison of quality of life and psychosocial functioning in obsessive-compulsive disorder and body dysmorphic disorder. *Ann Clin Psychiatry.* 2007;19(3):181–186.
27. Phillips KA, Hart AS, Simpson HB, Stein DJ. Delusional versus nondelusional body dysmorphic disorder: recommendations for DSM-5. *CNS Spectr.* 2014;19(1):10–20.
28. Phillips K, Pinto A, Hart A, et al. A comparison of insight in body dysmorphic disorder and obsessive-compulsive disorder. *J Psychiatr Res.* 2012;46(10):1293–1299.
29. Eisen J, Phillips K, Coles ME, Rasmussen SA. Insight in obsessive compulsive disorder and body dysmorphic disorder. *Compr Psychiatry.* 2004;45(1):10–15.
30. Mancuso SG, Knoesen N, Castle D. Delusional versus nondelusional body dysmorphic disorder. *Compr Psychiatry.* 2010;51(2):177–182.

31. Jacob ML, Larson MJ, Storch EA. Insight in adults with obsessive–compulsive disorder. *Compr Psychiatry.* 2014;55(4):896–903.
32. Neziroglu F, Stevens K, McKay D, Yaryura-Tobias J. Predictive validity of the overvalued ideas scale: outcome in obsessive-compulsive and body dysmorphic disorders. *Behav Res Ther.* 2001;39(6):745–756.
33. Kimchi R. Primacy of wholistic processing and global/local paradigm: a critical review. *Psychol Bull.* 1992;112(1):24–38.
34. Love B, Rouder J, Wisniewski E. A structural account of global and local processing. *Cognit Psychol.* 1999;38(2):291–316.
35. Feusner JD, Moller H, Altstein L, et al. Inverted face processing in body dysmorphic disorder. *J Psychiatr Res.* 2010;44(15):1088–1094.
36. Feusner JD, Hembacher E, Moller H, Moody TD. Abnormalities of object visual processing in body dysmorphic disorder. *Psychol Med.* 2011;41(11):2385–2397.
37. Greenberg JL, Reuman L, Hartmann AS, Kasarskis I, Wilhelm S. Visual hot spots: an eye tracking study of attention bias in body dysmorphic disorder. *J Psychiatr Res.* 2014;57:125–132.
38. Grocholewski A, Kliem S, Heinrichs N. Selective attention to imagined facial ugliness is specific to body dysmorphic disorder. *Body Image.* 2012;9(2):261–269.
39. Crerand CE, Menard W, Phillips KA. Surgical and minimally invasive cosmetic procedures among persons with body dysmorphic disorder. *Ann Plast Surg.* 2010;65(1):11–16.
40. Toh WL, Castle DJ, Rossell SL. How individuals with body dysmorphic disorder (BDD) process their own face: a quantitative and qualitative investigation based on an eye-tracking paradigm. *Cogn Neuropsychiatry.* 2017;22(3):213–232.
41. Jefferies K, Laws K, Hranov G, Fineberg NA. P.1.g.003 Cognitive and perceptual processing in body dysmorphic disorder. *Eur Neuropsychopharmacol.* 2010;20(Supplement 3):S309–S310.
42. Jefferies K, Laws KR, Fineberg NA. Superior face recognition in body dysmorphic disorder. *J Obsessive Compuls Relat Disord.* 2012;1(3):175–179.
43. Li W, Lai TM, Bohon C, et al. Anorexia nervosa and body dysmorphic disorder are associated with abnormalities in processing visual information. *Psychol Med.* 2015;45(10):2111–2122.
44. Buhlmann U, Etcoff NL, Wilhelm S. Facial attractiveness ratings and perfectionism in body dysmorphic disorder and obsessive-compulsive disorder. *J Anxiety Disord.* 2008;22(3):540–547.
45. Moody TD, Shen VW, Hutcheson NL, et al. Appearance evaluation of others' faces and bodies in anorexia nervosa and body dysmorphic disorder. *Int J Eat Disord.* 2017;50(2):127–138.
46. Lambrou C, Veale D, Wilson G. The role of aesthetic sensitivity in body dysmorphic disorder. *J Abnorm Psychol.* 2011;120(2):443–453.
47. Stangier U, Adam-Schwebe S, Muller T, Wolter M. Discrimination of facial appearance stimuli in body dysmorphic disorder. *J Abnorm Psychol.* 2008;117(2):435–443.
48. Veale D. Cognitive behaviour therapy for body dysmorphic disorder. In: Phillips DJCKA, ed. *Disorders of Body Image.* Petersfield: Wrightson Biomedical; 2002:121–138.
49. Feusner JD, Townsend J, Bystritsky A, McKinley M, Moller H, Bookheimer S. Regional brain volumes and symptom severity in body dysmorphic disorder. *Psychiatry Res Neuroimag.* 2009;172(2):161–167.
50. Feusner JD, Townsend J, Bystritsky A, Bookheimer S. Visual information processing of faces in body dysmorphic disorder. *Arch Gen Psychiatry.* 2007;64(12):1417–1426.
51. Buchanan B, Rossell S, Maller JJ, Toh WL, Brennan S, Castle D. Regional brain volumes in body dysmorphic disorder compared to controls. *Aust N Z J Psychiatry.* 2014;48(7):654–662.
52. Buchanan BG, Rossell SL, Maller JJ, Toh WL, Brennan S, Castle DJ. Brain connectivity in body dysmorphic disorder compared with controls: a diffusion tensor imaging study. *Psychol Med.* 2013;43(12):2513–2521.
53. Arienzo D, Leow A, Brown JA, et al. Abnormal brain network organization in body dysmorphic disorder. *Neuropsychopharmacology.* 2013;38(6):1130–1139.
54. National Institute for Health and Care Excellence. *Obsessive-Compulsive Disorder and Body Dysmorphic Disorder: Treatment.* Clinical Guideline CG31. London: NICE; 2005.
55. Foa EB, Yadin E, Lichner TK, eds. *Exposure and Response (Ritual) Prevention for Obsessive-Compulsive Disorder Therapist Guide*, 2nd ed. Oxford University Press; 2012.
56. Folke F, Von Bahr M, Assadi-Talaremi V, Ramnerö J. Exposure and response prevention in the treatment of body dysmorphic disorder: a case series. *PCSP.* 2012;8(4):255–287.
57. Wilhelm S, Phillips KA, Steketee G. *Cognitive-Behavioral Therapy for Body Dysmorphic Disorder: A Treatment Manual.* New York, NY: Guilford Press; 2012.
58. Veale D. Cognitive behavioural therapy for body dysmorphic disorder. *Adv Psychiatr Treat.* 2001;7:125–132.

59. Wilhelm S, Phillips KA, Fama JM, Greenberg JL, Steketee G. Modular cognitive–behavioral therapy for body dysmorphic disorder. *Behav Ther.* 2011;42(4):624–633.

60. Greenberg JL, Markowitz S, Petronko MR, Taylor CE, Wilhelm S, Wilson GT. Cognitive-behavioral therapy for adolescent body dysmorphic disorder. *Cogn Behav Pract.* 2010;17(3):248–258.

61. Veale D, Anson M, Miles S, Pieta M, Costa A, Ellison N. Efficacy of cognitive behaviour therapy versus anxiety management for body dysmorphic disorder: a randomised controlled trial. *Psychother Psychosom.* 2014;83(6):341–353.

62. Beilharz F, Castle DJ, Grace S, Rossell SL. A systematic review of visual processing and associated treatments in body dysmorphic disorder. *Acta Psychiatr Scand.* 2017;36(1):16–36.

63. Phillipou A, Rossell SL, Wilding HE, Castle DJ. Randomised controlled trials of psychological and pharmacological treatments for body dysmorphic disorder: a systematic review. *Psychiatry Res.* 2016;245:179–185.

64. Harrison A, Fernandez de la Cruz L, Enander J, Radua J, Mataix-Cols D. Cognitive-behavioral therapy for body dysmorphic disorder: a systematic review and meta-analysis of randomized controlled trials. *Clin Psychol Rev.* 2016;48:43–51.

65. Fang A, Schwartz RA, Wilhelm S. Treatment of an adult with body dysmorphic disorder. In: Storch EA, Lewin AB, eds. *Clinical Handbook of Obsessive-Compulsive and Related Disorders: A Case-Based Approach to Treating Pediatric and Adult Populations.* Cham, Switzerland: Springer International; 2016:259–271.

66. Greenberg JL, Mothi SS, Wilhelm S. Cognitive-behavioral therapy for body dysmorphic disorder by proxy. *Behav Ther.* 2016;47(4):515–526.

67. Mataix-Cols D, de la Cruz LF, Isomura K, et al. A pilot randomized controlled trial of cognitive-behavioral therapy for adolescents with body dysmorphic disorder. *J Am Acad Child Adolesc Psychiatry.* 2015;54(11):895–904.

68. Weingarden H, Marques L, Fang A, et al. Culturally adapted cognitive behavioral therapy for body dysmorphic disorder: case examples. *Int J Cogn Ther.* 2011;4(4):381–396.

69. Wilhelm S, Buhlmann U, Hayward LC, Greenberg JL, Dimaite R. A cognitive-behavioral treatment approach for body dysmorphic disorder. *Cogn Behav Pract.* 2010;17(3):241–247.

70. Wilhelm S, Otto MW, Lohr B, Deckersbach T. Cognitive behavior group therapy for body dysmorphic disorder: a case series. *Behav Res Ther.* 1999;37(1):71–75.

71. Wilhelm S, Phillips KA, Didie E, et al. Modular cognitive-behavioral therapy for body dysmorphic disorder: a randomized controlled trial. *Behav Ther.* 2014;45(3):314–327.

72. Veale D, Miles S, Anson M. Long-term outcome of cognitive behavior therapy for body dysmorphic disorder: a naturalistic case series of 1 to 4 years after a controlled trial. *Behav Ther.* 2015;46(6):775–785.

73. Krebs G, Turner C, Heyman I, Mataix-Cols D. Cognitive behaviour therapy for adolescents with body dysmorphic disorder: a case series. *Behav Cogn Psychother.* 2012;40(4):452–461.

74. Phillips KA, Grant J, Siniscalchi J, Albertini RS. Surgical and nonpsychiatric medical treatment of patients with body dysmorphic disorder. *Psychosomatics.* 2001;42(6):504–510.

75. Toh WL, Castle DJ, Rossell SL. Facial affect recognition in body dysmorphic disorder versus obsessive-compulsive disorder: an eye-tracking study. *J Anxiety Disord.* 2015;35:49–59.

76. Feusner JD, Moody T, Hembacher E, et al. Abnormalities of visual processing and frontostriatal systems in body dysmorphic disorder. *Arch Gen Psychiatry.* 2010;67(2):197–205.

77. Rossell SL, Labuschagne I, Dunai J, Kyrios M, Castle DJ. Using theories of delusion formation to explain abnormal beliefs in Body Dysmorphic Disorder (BDD). *Psychiatry Res.* 2014;215(3): 599–605.

78. Phillipou A, Castle DJ, Rossell SL. Anorexia nervosa: eating disorder or body image disorder? *Aust N Z J Psychiatry.* 2018;52(1):13–14.

79. Silver J, Reavey P, Anne Fineberg N. How do people with body dysmorphic disorder view themselves? A thematic analysis. *Int J Psychiatry Clin Pract.* 2010;14(3):190–197.

80. Yaryura-Tobias JA, Neziroglu F, Chang R, Lee S, Pinto A, Donohue L. Computerized perceptual analysis of patients with body dysmorphic disorder: a pilot study. *CNS Spectr.* 2002;7(6):444–446.

81. Neziroglu FA, Yaryura-Tobias JA. Body dysmorphic disorder: phenomenology and case descriptions. *Behav Psychother.* 1993;21(1):27–36.

82. Phillips KA, Grant JE, Siniscalchi JM, Stout R, Price LH. A retrospective follow-up study of body dysmorphic disorder. *Compr Psychiatry.* 2005;46(5):315–321.

83. McKay D, Todaro J, Neziroglu F, Campisi T. Body dysmorphic disorder: a preliminary evaluation of treatment and maintenance using exposure with response prevention. *Behav Res Ther.* 1997;35(1):67–70.

84. McKay D. Two-year follow-up of behavioral treatment and maintenance for body dysmorphic disorder. *Behav Modif.* 1999;23(4):620–629.

85. Neziroglu F, McKay D, Todaro J, Yaryura-Tobias JA. Effect of cognitive behavior therapy on persons with body dysmorphic disorder and comorbid axis II diagnoses. *Behav Ther.* 1996;27(1):67–77.

86. Rosen JC, Reiter J, Orosan P. Cognitive-behavioral body image therapy for body dysmorphic disorder. *J Consult Clin Psychol.* 1995;63(2):263–269.

87. Gorbis E. Crooked mirrors: the externalization of self-image in body dysmorphic disorder. *Behav Ther.* 2004;27(4):74–76.

88. Baldock E, Anson M, Veale D. The stopping criteria for mirror-gazing in body dysmorphic disorder. *Br J Clin Psychol.* 2012;51(3):323–344.

89. Windheim K, Veale D, Anson M. Mirror gazing in body dysmorphic disorder and healthy controls: effects of duration of gazing. *Behav Res Ther.* 2011;49(9):555–564.

90. Buhlmann U, Etcoff NL, Wilhelm S. Emotion recognition bias for contempt and anger in body dysmorphic disorder. *J Psychiatr Res.* 2006;40(2):105–111.

91. Kerwin L, Hovav S, Hellemann G, Feusner JD. Impairment in local and global processing and set-shifting in body dysmorphic disorder. *J Psychiatr Res.* 2014;57:41–50.

92. Li W, Lai TM, Loo SK, et al. Aberrant early visual neural activity and brain-behavior relationships in anorexia nervosa and body dysmorphic disorder. *Front Hum Neurosci.* 2015;9:301.

93. Marks IM, Mishan J. Dysmorphophobic avoidance with disturbed bodily perception: a pilot study of exposure therapy. *Br J Psychiatry.* 1988;152:674–678.

94. Buhlmann U, Gleiss MJ, Rupf L, Zschenderlein K, Kathmann N. Modifying emotion recognition deficits in body dysmorphic disorder: an experimental investigation. *Depress Anxiety.* 2011;28(10):924–931.

95. Beilharz FL, Atkins KJ, Duncum AJ, Mundy ME. Altering visual perception abnormalities: a marker for body image concern. *PloS One.* 2016;11(3): e0151933.

96. Silver H, Bilker WB. Social cognition in schizophrenia and healthy aging: differences and similarities. *Schizophr Res.* 2014;160(1–3):157–162.

97. Lindenmayer J-P, McGurk SR, Khan A, et al. Improving social cognition in schizophrenia: a pilot intervention combining computerized social cognition training with cognitive remediation. *Schizophr Bull.* 2013;39(3):507–517.

98. Drusch K, Stroth S, Kamp D, Frommann N, Wölwer W. Effects of training of affect recognition on the recognition and visual exploration of emotional faces in schizophrenia. *Schizophr Res.* 2014;159(2–3):485–490.

99. Darmedru C, Demily C, Franck N. Cognitive remediation and social cognitive training for violence in schizophrenia: a systematic review. *Psychiatry Res.* 2017;251:266–274.

100. Frommann N, Streit M, Wölwer W. Remediation of facial affect recognition impairments in patients with schizophrenia: a new training program. *Psychiatry Res.* 2003;117(3):281–284.

101. Kays JL, Hurley RA, Taber KH. The dynamic brain: neuroplasticity and mental health. *J Neuropsychiatry Clin Neurosci.* 2012;24(2):118–124.

102. Martins Rosa AM, Silva MF, Ferreira S, Murta J, Castelo-Branco M. Plasticity in the human visual cortex: an ophthalmology-based perspective. *BioMed Res Int.* 2013;2013:568354.

103. Thomas E, Plessis S, Chiliza B, Lochner C, Stein D. Olfactory reference disorder: diagnosis, epidemiology and management. *CNS Drugs.* 2015;29(12):999–1007.

104. Feusner JD, Phillips KA, Stein DJ. Olfactory reference syndrome: issues for DSM-V. *Depress Anxiety.* 2010;27(6):592–599.

105. Phillips KA, Menard W. Olfactory reference syndrome: demographic and clinical features of imagined body odor. *Gen Hosp Psychiatry.* 2011;33(4):398.

106. Lochner C, Stein DJ. Prevalence of olfactory reference syndrome in obsessive-compulsive disorder and social anxiety disorder. *J Clin Psychiatry.* 2014;75(11):1266.

107. Veale D, Matsunaga H. Body dysmorphic disorder and olfactory reference disorder: proposals for ICD-11. *Rev Bras Psiquiatr.* 2014;36:14–20.

108. Begum M, McKenna PJ. Olfactory reference syndrome: a systematic review of the world literature. *Psychol Med.* 2011;41(3):453–461.

109. Prazeres AM, Fontenelle LF, Mendlowicz MV, et al. Olfactory reference syndrome as a subtype of body dysmorphic disorder. *J Clin Psychiatry.* 2010;71(1):87–89.

110. Pryse-Phillips W. An olfactory reference syndrome. *Acta Psychiatr Scand.* 1971;47(4):484–509.

111. Allen-Crooks R, Challacombe F. Cognitive behaviour therapy for olfactory reference disorder (ORD): a case study. *J Obsessive Compuls Rel Disord.* 2017;13:7–13.

112. Martin-Pichora AL, Antony MM. Successful treatment of olfactory reference syndrome with cognitive behavioral therapy: a case study. *Cogn Behav Pract.* 2011;18(4):545–554.

113. Thomas E, Voges J, Chiliza B, Stein DJ, Lochner C. Sniffing out olfactory reference syndrome. *SAJP.* 2017;23:5.

114. Bizamcer AN, Dubin WR, Hayburn B. Olfactory reference syndrome. *Psychosomatics*. 2008;49(1): 77–81.

115. Teraishi T, Takahashi T, Suda T, et al. Successful treatment of olfactory reference syndrome with paroxetine. *J Neuropsychiatry Clin Neurosci*. 2012;24(1):E24.

116. Michael S, Boulton M, Andrews G. Two cases of olfactory reference syndrome responding to an atypical antipsychotic and SSRI. *Aust N Z J Psychiatry*. 2014;48(9):878–879.

117. Stein DJ, Le Roux L, Bouwer C, Van Heerden B. Is olfactory reference syndrome an obsessive-compulsive spectrum disorder? *J Neuropsychiatry Clin Neurosci*. 1998;10(1):96–99.

118. Ferreira JA, Dallaqua RP, Fontenelle LF, Torres AR. Olfactory reference syndrome: a still open nosological and treatment debate. *Gen Hosp Psychiatry*. 2014;36(6):760.e1-3.

119. Gebara CM, de Barros Neto TP. Considerações sobre a clínica e o tratamento de uma manifestação incomum do transtorno dismórfico corporal: A síndrome de referência olfatória. [Considerations on the clinical picture and treatment of an unusual manifestation of body dysmorphic disorder the olfactory reference syndrome.] *J Bras Psiquiatr*. 2011;60(4):347–349.

Chapter 24

Hypochondriasis

Vladan Starcevic

Introduction

Hypochondriasis has a fascinating history that spans the centuries. Despite its early description as a disorder, there have always been controversies about what hypochondriasis encompasses, whether it is better understood as a part of another condition and how it should be conceptualized and classified. In light of these conundrums, it is not surprising that treatment of hypochondriasis has also been a challenging endeavor. The aim of this chapter is to reexamine hypochondriasis and its relationship with obsessive-compulsive disorder (OCD).

Clinical Picture

The two components of hypochondriasis that have been identified consistently are: (i) fear of already being ill with a serious or life-threatening disease (disease fear, also referred to as disease phobia) and (ii) suspicion that one is already ill or preoccupation with a belief that one is ill (disease belief, also referred to as disease conviction) [1,2,3]. The prototypical cases of hypochondriasis are characterized by both of these components, but in clinical practice some individuals present with the predominance of disease fear or disease belief. If there is only a prominent disease fear without the corresponding belief, such a clinical presentation resembles other anxiety disorders and is also known as "health anxiety". If there is a prominent disease belief with or without prominent disease fear, this presentation may be phenomenologically closer to OCD or even a delusional disorder.

Individuals with hypochondriasis present with or without physical symptoms. Such symptoms tend to be misinterpreted as an ominous sign, suggesting that the person is seriously ill. The usual way of coping with disease fear is through reassurance seeking and checking whether one is actually ill; the former is typically sought from a physician or a family member. In recent times, an increasing number of people with hypochondriasis seek reassurance via the Internet; if their health anxiety increases after online health-related searches, this is referred to as cyberchondria [4,5].

A common but puzzling feature of hypochondriasis is an apparent unwillingness to accept routine medical reassurance. Individuals with the condition thus both seek reassurance and seem to reject it. This usually complicates the relationship with primary care physicians and other healthcare providers. A physician's interpretation of this paradoxical resistance to reassurance often determines how patients with hypochondriasis are regarded and dealt with. If the apparent resistance to reassurance is interpreted as deliberate, patients with hypochondriasis are likely to be treated with suspicion and perceived as being manipulative, not "wanting" to get better, indulging in "doctor shopping", exaggerating complaints or even fabricating symptoms. If the apparent resistance to reassurance is interpreted as a consequence of an underlying psychiatric disorder, patients may be referred to a psychiatrist with psychotic disorder or severe depression as the usual provisional diagnosis.

Conceptualization and Diagnosis

In the *Diagnostic and Statistical Manual of Mental Disorders* (DSM) system, hypochondriasis was an official diagnosis until the publication of its fifth edition (DSM-5) [6]. Thus, in the DSM-IV [7], hypochondriasis was defined as a chronic preoccupation with fears of having, or the idea that one has, a serious disease, which is based on misinterpretation of bodily symptoms and persists despite appropriate medical evaluation and reassurance. Hypochondriasis was excluded from the DSM-5 mainly because of its conceptual heterogeneity in the DSM-IV and pejorative connotations of the term. Instead of hypochondriasis, two diagnostic concepts were introduced in the DSM-5: illness anxiety disorder (IAD) and somatic symptom disorder (SSD).

Both IAD and SSD are conceptualized as chronic conditions, with the key difference being that SSD is characterized by at least one "distressing" or "disruptive" somatic symptom, whereas in IAD such symptoms are absent or only mild. According to the DSM-5, about 25% of individuals meeting the DSM-IV criteria for hypochondriasis would qualify for the diagnosis of IAD and the remaining 75% would be diagnosed with SSD. The construct of IAD refers to a pattern of high level of health anxiety *and* excessive or disproportionate preoccupation with having or acquiring a serious illness, which *must* be accompanied by repeated checking of one's body for signs of illness or health-related avoidance (e.g., avoidance of medical appointments and facilities). In contrast, features of SSD are intense health anxiety *or* "excessive" thoughts about the seriousness of symptoms *or* "excessive time and energy" spent on somatic symptoms or health concerns.

The constructs of IAD and SSD have been criticized as being distinguished on the basis of the presence of intense somatic symptoms without any empirical support [8,9]. SSD appears to be too broad and vague conceptually [8,9,10] and has a very low diagnostic threshold, thereby unnecessarily allowing too many diagnostic "false positives", and its diagnostic criteria to be easily met by people with serious medical conditions [11]. Moreover, the constructs of IAD and SSD fail to capture the disease belief component of hypochondriasis [12,13]. Finally, IAD includes a concern about becoming ill in the future and avoidance of health- and disease-related cues and situations, which prior to DSM-5 characterized a type of specific phobia referred to as disease/illness phobia; it is questionable whether concerns about being already ill and concerns about becoming ill in the future should be treated interchangeably as the same diagnostic criterion [9].

The DSM-5 approach to hypochondriasis has not been espoused by the architects of the 11th revision of the International Classification of Disease (ICD-11), which is currently being developed. According to the available information and literature [14,15], the term "hypochondriasis" will be retained in ICD-11 and its diagnostic criteria will be very similar to those found in the DSM-IV. The proposal for ICD-11 emphasizes the overlap between hypochondriasis on one hand and OCD and anxiety disorders on the other, stipulating that hypochondriasis is also characterized either by "repetitive and excessive health-related behaviors" or "maladaptive avoidance behaviors related to health". Consequently, hypochondriasis is proposed to be classified both among "obsessive-compulsive and related disorders" (OCRDs) and the "anxiety and fear-related disorders". In line with the other OCRDs in ICD-11 and on the basis of the degree of insight, two subtypes of hypochondriasis have been proposed for ICD-11: one is with "fair to good insight" and the other is with "poor to absent insight". The presence of physical symptoms is not required for the diagnosis of hypochondriasis in ICD-11, but the diagnosis is not incompatible with the presence of such symptoms. Consequently, hypochondriasis in ICD-11 is not proposed to be conceptualized and classified as a "disorder of bodily distress or bodily experience". This is in contrast to the classification of hypochondriasis in DSM-IV as a somatoform disorder and the classification of IAD and SSD in DSM-5 among somatic symptom disorders.

The current conceptual and nosological situation with hypochondriasis is complicated, confusing and controversial. While the condition does not exist in the DSM system, it is present in the ICD classification. The disorders that have replaced hypochondriasis in DSM-5 have not been fully embraced by clinicians and researchers, and it is uncertain to what extent they will be used in the future. It is unknown whether the proposed changes in ICD-11 will adequately address the deficiencies of the DSM-IV concept of hypochondriasis. A need for more research cannot be overemphasized if we are to better understand this intriguing condition.

Differential Diagnosis

Differential diagnosis of hypochondriasis includes conditions that can be mistaken for hypochondriasis or vice versa, due to symptom overlap (i.e., shared symptoms). Determining whether a diagnosis of hypochondriasis is appropriate requires a good understanding of both the similarities and differences between hypochondriasis and these conditions. Disorders that should be considered in this regard are medical diseases, psychotic disorders, major depressive disorder, panic disorder, generalized anxiety disorder (GAD), a disorder characterized by physical symptoms that do not have an adequate medical explanation (somatization disorder in DSM-IV, somatic symptom disorder in DSM-5 and bodily distress disorder proposed for ICD-11), certain types of personality disturbance and OCD. These conditions preempt the diagnosis of hypochondriasis if they better explain clinical features that are shared with hypochondriasis; in other cases when features of hypochondriasis co-occur with those of other disorders, hypochondriasis may be used as an additional diagnosis, but this needs to be ascertained on a case-by-case basis. Establishing the correct diagnosis has important treatment implications.

An underlying medical disease may need to be considered when patients present with prominent or persistent physical symptoms. Any further investigation of such a disease should be done very carefully and tactfully because patients are already preoccupied with this possibility and have often consulted many doctors or undergone numerous diagnostic procedures. This usually means that additional medical investigations may be in order only if new symptoms appear or if clinicians have other reasons to suspect a medical condition.

Distinguishing between hypochondriasis and psychotic disorder such as delusional disorder can be difficult. It involves examining the characteristics of disease beliefs and distinguishing between overvalued ideas that characterize hypochondriasis and delusions that are a hallmark of psychotic disorders. The key criteria for making this distinction are a greater conviction (extent to which the person is convinced that his or her belief is true) and greater fixity (tendency for the belief to remain despite the person being presented with contrary evidence) of delusions [16]. In addition, the content of delusions may be bizarre or less plausible than that of overvalued ideas and patients with delusions may provide delusional evidence in support of their beliefs.

Disease fears and beliefs may occur in individuals suffering from major depressive disorder. Therefore, it is important to ascertain whether features of hypochondriasis can be attributed to depression. Enquiring about other symptoms of depression (e.g., anhedonia, guilt feelings, sleep disturbance and poor appetite) is usually helpful in this regard. The onset of a hypochondriasis-like disorder later in life may be due to depression [17], calling for a careful assessment of possible depression in such cases.

Typical features of hypochondriasis are often secondary to panic disorder. Many panic patients report disease fear and may be convinced that they are dying during panic attacks, usually from a heart attack, suffocation or stroke. Patients with hypochondriasis and panic disorder have a similar cognitive style characterized by prominent anxiety sensitivity, catastrophic misinterpretation of innocuous bodily sensations, body-focused vigilance and somatosensory amplification. Still, hypochondriasis and panic disorder can be distinguished on the basis of a greater variety of physical symptoms (i.e., not just symptoms of autonomic hyperarousal) being experienced and feared in hypochondriasis, with these symptoms being more persistent in hypochondriasis and limited to panic attacks in panic disorder. A sense of an impending doom is typically reported during panic attacks, leading to urgent help seeking; in contrast, the threat from disease and death in hypochondriasis is not necessarily experienced as immediate, with help-seeking patterns showing less urgency. However, help-seeking behavior in hypochondriasis tends to be more persistent than in panic disorder.

Hypochondriasis may resemble GAD because both conditions are characterized by excessive and uncontrollable worries. However, these concerns pertain to health- and disease-related matters in hypochondriasis, whereas worries in GAD relate to a variety of topics besides health (e.g., work, relationships and finances).

The relationship between hypochondriasis and disorders characterized by prominent physical symptoms that do not have an adequate medical explanation remains obscure because of the ever-changing conceptualizations of both disorders. Still, they can be distinguished clinically in terms of what patients experience as most distressing: in hypochondriasis, it is the frightening meaning and implications of the symptoms, whereas in somatization disorder/ somatic symptom disorder/bodily distress disorder, it is the symptoms themselves and the associated disability.

Certain aspects of hypochondriasis may overlap with features of personality disturbance, most notably obsessive-compulsive personality disorder. This pertains to an excessive need for control, rigidity and perfectionist tendencies. In such cases, the usual task is to ascertain whether obsessive-compulsive personality disorder exists in addition to hypochondriasis because this may affect the choice of treatment and its outcome.

The relationship between hypochondriasis and OCD is discussed in detail in the section entitled

"Cross-diagnostic approaches and their implications for classification and diagnosis".

Recent Research Findings

Epidemiology

Epidemiological data about hypochondriasis are discrepant, depending on the diagnostic criteria and assessment instruments used, timeframe and the population and setting in which the studies were conducted. The point prevalence rate of the DSM-IV hypochondriasis in the general population ranged from 0.05% to 0.4% [18,19,20]. For diagnostically subthreshold DSM-IV hypochondriasis (without the requirement to meet the diagnostic criterion of preoccupation that persists despite reassurance), prevalence rates in the general population were 0.58% [19] and 1.3% [18]. The prevalence rates of various components or aspects of hypochondriasis and constructs related to hypochondriasis (e.g., illness worry, prominent health anxiety and conviction of having a serious illness) in the general population ranged between 2.12% and 10% [18,19,20,21,22].

The prevalence rates of the DSM-III-R, DSM-IV or ICD-10 hypochondriasis were higher in primary care settings (0.8–3.4%) [23,24] and specialized medical settings (3.5–6.3%) [25,26] than in the general population. Likewise, the prevalence rates of prominent health anxiety and hypochondriacal concerns were quite high in primary care samples (7.7–10.3%) [27,28] and samples from the specialized medical settings (8.6–24.9%) [29,30]. Some studies reported the rates outside of these ranges, which highlights inconsistencies in establishing diagnostic thresholds and cut-offs on measures of dimensional constructs. Demographic and social variables such as age, sex, marital and employment status and level of education have not been consistently associated with hypochondriasis or constructs related to hypochondriasis.

Treatment

The key general aspects of the treatment approach to hypochondriasis are taking patients' symptoms and concerns seriously, refraining from arguing with patients about the origin of the symptoms and making an effort to understand the circumstances in which the specific disease concerns occur. In addition, it is important to foster effective communication and nurture trust because patients with hypochondriasis are prone to misunderstanding or misinterpreting health-related information and because they tend to harbor intense interpersonal mistrust. Scheduling regular visits and emphasizing therapist's availability, accessibility, reliability and predictability are the means of engaging patients and fostering consistency and continuity of the therapeutic relationship. The goal of the treatment should be realistic and clear (e.g., "care rather than cure"), focusing on the alleviation of distress and improvement in coping and functioning. This goal should be communicated to patients early on to avoid their unrealistic expectations (e.g., that treatment will result in symptom disappearance).

Psychological Treatments

Various psychological treatments have been used in hypochondriasis and health anxiety: cognitive-behavior therapy (CBT), interpersonal therapy, psychodynamic therapy and supportive therapy. Of these, CBT has the strongest empirical support for efficacy, as demonstrated by numerous randomized controlled trials [31,32,33,34,35,36,37,38,39]. CBT was also found to produce better outcomes than pharmacotherapy [36]. This treatment is based on the cognitive, behavioral and information-processing models of hypochondriasis [40,41], which postulate that assumptions or beliefs that amplify health anxiety are the key etiological factor in hypochondriasis. For example, people who believe that good health means an absence of any symptoms become easily alarmed when experiencing innocuous physical symptoms. Cognitive factors that maintain hypochondriasis have been identified as follows: selective attention and selective perception of health- and illness-related information and stimuli (including bodily symptoms), and their catastrophic misinterpretation, memory bias for illness-related information and exaggerated estimation of threat posed by bodily symptoms. Typical behavioral factors that maintain hypochondriasis include health anxiety-driven checking and reassurance seeking; these behaviors may alleviate health anxiety temporarily, but usually keep anxiety levels high in the long run.

Cognitive therapy techniques aim to remove the specific health anxiety-amplifying assumptions and beliefs, as well as cognitive factors that maintain hypochondriasis, usually by identifying, challenging and modifying them. Attentional training targets selective attention to bodily symptoms and external sources of health- and illness-related information. Behavior therapy techniques such as exposure and response prevention aim to eliminate behaviors that are presumed to maintain hypochondriasis. They have been derived from the techniques used in phobic disorders and OCD, and entail controlled exposure to cues that elicit health anxiety, combined with modified response prevention (i.e., refraining from checking one's health status and seeking reassurance about health).

Psychoeducation is an important component of every variant of CBT. Cognitive and behavior therapy techniques are usually combined, but some techniques are more represented than others in certain treatment "packages". Studies did not find significant differences in efficacy between more or less "pure" cognitive therapy on one hand and "pure" behavior therapy (exposure and response prevention) on the other [32,34]. CBT can be delivered in an individual or group format. Individual CBT and CBT-based group therapy can also be used sequentially. Internet-based CBT was found to be efficacious in randomized controlled trials in patients with "severe health anxiety" [42] and in those with IAD and SSD, the DSM-5 successors of hypochondriasis [43]. There is also evidence to support the efficacy of mindfulness-based cognitive therapy for hypochondriasis [44].

The disadvantages of CBT for hypochondriasis include its limited availability and perception as difficult or demanding. The latter explains the finding of one study that only 30% of patients with hypochondriasis found CBT "attractive", with a dropout rate of 25% [35]. This suggests that there is much room for refining CBT.

Pharmacological Treatment

Evidence of the efficacy of pharmacotherapy in hypochondriasis is scant and medications are rarely used as the only treatment modality. Pharmacological agents may be more useful against fear of disease and obsession-like preoccupation with disease than for treating somatic symptoms and somatization.

Four open-label pharmacotherapy studies were conducted in patients with hypochondriasis. They involved very small samples (less than 20 patients) and used selective serotonin reuptake inhibitors (SSRIs; fluoxetine, paroxetine, fluvoxamine) [45,46,47] or imipramine, a tricyclic antidepressant [48]. The results suggested that these medications might be useful for hypochondriasis.

Three randomized controlled trials were subsequently conducted, one with paroxetine [36], the other two with fluoxetine [49,50]. The findings of these studies, conducted in larger, but still modestly sized samples, did not unequivocally favor medication over placebo. For example, in one study, paroxetine was superior to placebo only in completer analysis, but not in the intention-to-treat analysis [36]. In another trial, fluoxetine was significantly more efficacious than placebo only in secondary analyses, using a continuous measure of hypochondriasis as an outcome variable [50]. One study examining 45 individuals who had participated in hypochondriasis treatment studies with SSRIs 4–16 years prior to assessment reported greater remission rates for those who had used SSRIs for at least 1 month and concluded that long-term use of SSRIs in hypochondriasis was correlated with extended symptom remission [51].

Pharmacological treatment may be justified or necessary in the presence of severe anxiety or depressive symptoms and disorders that co-occur with hypochondriasis. Hypochondriacal manifestations that are a part of another primary disorder, such as panic disorder and major depressive disorder ("secondary hypochondriasis"), may subside with successful pharmacological treatment of the primary condition.

Combined Treatment

Limited evidence exists for the role of combined treatment (CBT plus pharmacotherapy) in hypochondriasis. Only one study that compared combined treatment with CBT alone, treatment with fluoxetine alone and placebo showed that combined treatment had only a small incremental advantage over fluoxetine alone [50]. Although this finding suggests little benefit of combining CBT with pharmacotherapy, this may be due to problems with the delivery of CBT that resulted in generally poorer performance of CBT compared with other studies. Combined treatment approach to hypochondriasis may still be useful and appears to be common in clinical practice. As in other situations when psychological and pharmacological treatments are combined, this should be done in a complementary way that is likely to maximize positive outcomes.

Cross-Diagnostic Approaches and Their Implications for Classification and Diagnosis

As already noted, the strength of the relationships between hypochondriasis on one hand and OCD and anxiety disorders on the other has been recognized in the proposal for ICD-11, with a suggestion that hypochondriasis should be classified in ICD-11 among both OCRDs and anxiety and fear-related disorders. However, IAD and SSD, the DSM-5 successors of hypochondriasis, are classified as somatic symptom disorders. While reflecting a rampant disagreement about the conceptualization and classification of hypochondriasis, this also points to a need to reexamine its relationships with OCD and anxiety disorders. This section focuses on the links with OCD.

A notion that hypochondriasis is related to OCD dates back to the conceptualization of obsessive-compulsive spectrum disorders, based on the assumption that these disorders share a difficulty in delaying or inhibiting repetitive behaviors such as compulsions, reassurance seeking, impulsive acts, drug use, self-harm, tics and so on [52]. Another criterion for membership of the spectrum was a similar, favorable response to the same treatment (e.g., serotonin reuptake inhibitors, exposure and response prevention or habit reversal) [53]. The group of obsessive-compulsive spectrum disorders initially included very diverse conditions that were placed on a compulsive-impulsive continuum; hypochondriasis was posited to be closer to the compulsive, risk-avoiding, harm-overestimating end of this continuum [53,54].

A recent reconsideration of the concepts of compulsivity and impulsivity has led to a notion that they are not mutually exclusive and should not necessarily be placed at the extreme ends of a continuum; this is supported by findings of a neurobiological overlap between compulsivity and impulsivity [55,56]. With this in mind, the conceptualization of hypochondriasis as a disorder primarily characterized by compulsivity (i.e., a repetitive health-related checking and reassurance seeking performed to prevent or avoid perceived negative consequences of not doing so) appears somewhat simplistic. In other words, hypochondriasis also seems to be characterized by some elements of impulsivity, such as inability to resist urges to engage in health-related checking and reassurance seeking, and the apparent importance attached to an immediate relief or reward obtained from these behaviors. Persistence of health-related checking and reassurance seeking, despite their negative consequences, can be interpreted as a manifestation of both compulsivity and impulsivity.

The idea of classifying hypochondriasis in the obsessive-compulsive spectrum disorders has received some support [57], based on a number of clinical similarities between hypochondriasis and OCD. Preoccupations with being ill in hypochondriasis resemble somatic and doubting obsessions in OCD because both are persistent or recurrent, very difficult or impossible to control, distressing or eliciting anxiety and compelling a person to find a way of coping with them. Also, individuals with hypochondriasis may worry about germs and infection in a way that is usually seen in the context of contamination obsessions in OCD.

High levels of intolerance of uncertainty characterize both hypochondriasis and OCD [58]. Furthermore, in both conditions there is a prominent need to engage in behaviors that aim to alleviate anxiety or distress. This need may be resisted, but usually without success. As a result, individuals with hypochondriasis resort to repeated and excessive health-related checking, similar to checking compulsions in OCD. Another feature common to hypochondriasis and OCD is reassurance seeking. This behavior is related to checking and often occurs along with it or instead of it. Checking and reassurance seeking usually lead to a short-term alleviation of anxiety in both hypochondriasis and OCD, but a need to repeat checking or reassurance seeking generally follows.

Many differences between features of hypochondriasis and OCD appear to be quantitative. Thus, preoccupation with being ill in hypochondriasis is usually experienced as less intrusive and more ego-syntonic than obsessions in OCD [59]. Disease beliefs in hypochondriasis may be held with more strength compared with obsession-related beliefs in OCD, and one study reported that patients with hypochondriasis exhibited more prominent overvalued ideas than those with OCD [57]. Although the level of insight varies in both conditions, it may be generally lower in individuals with hypochondriasis.

As a result, urges to check or seek reassurance are generally met with less resistance in hypochondriasis than in OCD [59]. Individuals with hypochondriasis and OCD have also been found to differ in terms of the former exhibiting less prominent OCD symptoms [60], more somatic symptoms [59], higher levels of health anxiety [58,60,61], greater body vigilance [58], more catastrophic beliefs about disease [61] and greater avoidance [57]. One study reported that while hypochondriasis and OCD did not differ significantly in terms of the levels of "obsessionality", OCD was associated with higher levels of "compulsivity" than hypochondriasis, as measured by the obsessions and compulsions subscales of the Yale-Brown Obsessive-Compulsive Scale [57].

From a neurobiological perspective, hypochondriasis and OCD share some characteristics and differ with respect to others. Thus, differences between hypochondriasis and panic disorder on one hand and OCD on the other were reported in terms of the neuroanatomical correlates of attentional bias in response to threat [62]. A more widespread cortical activation pattern and generalized emotional interference effects while completing a cognitive and emotional Stroop task were found in patients with hypochondriasis and panic disorder, compared with those with OCD [62]. In another imaging study, however, patients with hypochondriasis, panic disorder, and OCD did not differ significantly in terms of alterations in frontostriatal and limbic activation during a planning task [63].

Lifetime rates of OCD among patients with hypochondriasis were up to 9.5% [64], whereas lifetime rates of hypochondriasis in patients with OCD were reported to range from 8.2% to 15% [65,66,67]. These co-occurrence rates are higher than the lifetime rates of either hypochondriasis or OCD in the general population, but lower than the likelihood of most depressive and anxiety disorders occurring in hypochondriasis [60,64] or in OCD [60,67]. This suggests that hypochondriasis and OCD may not be related in a specific or unique way.

Should hypochondriasis be conceptualized and classified as a disorder related to OCD? While there are both similarities and differences between the two conditions, studies suggest that they can be distinguished on the basis of disorder-specific symptoms [58,60,68]. Literature reviews provide generally little support for inclusion of hypochondriasis into the group of OCRDs [69,70]. Some studies suggest that the relationships between hypochondriasis and the anxiety disorders (especially panic disorder) are more important than the links between hypochondriasis and OCD [62]. However, most authors are inconclusive with respect to the issue of whether hypochondriasis is closer to OCD or to panic disorder [57,58,63,71,72]. This helps to explain the rationale for the proposal to classify hypochondriasis in ICD-11 among both OCRDs and anxiety and fear-related disorders.

The fact that it is still uncertain whether the similarities are sufficient to classify hypochondriasis and OCD together despite their differences highlights the lack of clear criteria that would stipulate the minimal degree of relatedness between disorders required for them to be classified together and the minimal degree of distinctness necessitating their separate classification [73]. Consequently, the question of the membership of hypochondriasis in the group of OCRDs remains open.

Implications of Cross-Diagnostic Approaches for Treatment and Prevention

There is some evidence referred to in the previous sections of this chapter that certain psychological and pharmacological treatments for OCD (i.e., exposure and response prevention and SSRIs) may also be effective for hypochondriasis. The evidence is more convincing for psychological than pharmacological treatments and raises an important practical question of the extent to which these treatments for OCD can be used for hypochondriasis and whether and how they need to be adapted. There is very little research addressing this question.

In one study, exposure and response prevention that was used to treat OCD patients, also decreased levels of health anxiety without the latter being a direct target of treatment [74]. In another study, exposure and response prevention that was modified for "severe health anxiety" had a moderate to large therapeutic effect on OCD symptoms in patients with a co-occurring OCD, although OCD was not targeted directly [60]. Such effects of treatments developed and used for one disorder on a related, co-occurring disorder may be a consequence of therapeutic targeting of the common mechanisms (e.g., certain metacognitions) underpinning both OCD and hypochondriasis/health anxiety [74]. Alternatively, these therapeutic effects may be attributed to the application of the same therapeutic principles and techniques across a variety of OCD-specific and hypochondriasis/health anxiety-specific cues and triggering situations [60].

Findings of these studies strongly support "transdiagnostic" (i.e., not diagnosis-focused) psychological treatment approaches because certain therapy ingredients seem to be broadly effective for related co-occurring disorders, regardless of the primary disorder. Considering the high frequency of co-occurrence of mental disorders, including

OCD and hypochondriasis/health anxiety, the value of diagnosis-specific psychological treatment "packages" should be reconsidered and compared with transdiagnostic approaches. With regard to transdiagnostic treatments for hypochondriasis, the optimal proportion of "generic" components (i.e., those that are applicable to hypochondriasis, OCD and related disorders, as well as anxiety and depressive disorders) and components relatively specific for hypochondriasis remains to be determined.

In the realm of psychopharmacotherapy, SSRIs are a good example of transdiagnostic treatment because their effectiveness is not confined to a certain type of psychopathology or even to a group of disorders. However, SSRIs are not unique among psychopharmacological agents in this regard. The reasons for the effectiveness of SSRIs across various disorders are still elusive, but it is possible that despite being superficially distinct, these disorders share the characteristics at a neurobiological level that are targeted by SSRIs. It would be important to investigate whether individuals with diverse SSRI-responsive disorders who actually fail to respond to SSRIs also have some neurobiological similarities.

The fact that some research supports the role of SSRIs in the treatment of hypochondriasis does not by itself suggest that hypochondriasis is specifically related to any of the various SSRI-responsive disorders, including OCD. In pharmacotherapy studies conducted so far, SSRIs tended to be used in higher doses for hypochondriasis [36,45,46,47,49,50], just as they are often used for OCD. Although higher doses of fluoxetine appear more effective for hypochondriasis than lower doses [50], there is no evidence that higher doses of SSRIs are necessarily associated with better outcomes in hypochondriasis. In addition to dosing, further research should aim to establish whether there are any other aspects of the treatment of hypochondriasis with SSRIs that resemble the treatment of OCD with SSRIs (e.g., a delayed response). This will also help an effort to better understand what may be specific in the relationship between hypochondriasis and OCD.

Future Directions

The key obstacle to progress in our understanding of the relationship between hypochondriasis, OCD, and other psychopathology is the lack of agreement about the optimal conceptualization of hypochondriasis and related constructs. It would be irresponsible to wait for these conceptual dilemmas to be resolved before proceeding with research. For now, studies need to take into account diagnostic approaches espoused by both DSM-5 and ICD-11/DSM-IV and use the corresponding sets of diagnostic criteria simultaneously. Undoubtedly, this will be complicated and time consuming, but it seems to be the only way to clarify the relationships between the ICD-11/DSM-IV hypochondriasis and the DSM-5 constructs of IAD and SSD. Such research will be crucial for reaching a conceptual consensus on hypochondriasis.

Studies of the relationships between hypochondriasis and OCD should acknowledge the heterogeneity within both psychopathological entities as it is likely that this accounts for at least some of the equivocal findings of the research conducted so far. The specificity of the links between hypochondriasis and OCD needs to be investigated by comparing them with the relationships with other forms of psychopathology, especially other disorders in the obsessive-compulsive spectrum and anxiety and depressive disorders. Symptom-level comparisons will not be sufficient and should be supplemented by genetic and neurobiological comparisons. As already noted, a more sophisticated understanding of hypochondriasis will be based on measuring the extent to which it is associated with both compulsivity and impulsivity. All this will ultimately lead to a more precise positioning of hypochondriasis in the realm of psychopathology, with a clearer delineation of its relatedness to OCD, anxiety disorders and other conditions. Such endeavor should also clarify what components of hypochondriasis, OCD and other disorders are shared and which aspects appear to be specific or even unique for each disorder.

There is a great potential for novel approaches to both expand our knowledge of psychopathology and improve treatment efforts. For example, the network model of psychopathology [75,76] posits that mental disorders represent complex networks of interacting symptoms, a few of which are central, while most are peripheral to the disorders. This model may explain why some disorders co-occur with others and is able to suggest key targets for therapeutic intervention by identifying a degree of symptom centrality. Owing to the network model's ability to accommodate both nomothetic and idiographic designs, it also holds promise to further develop personalized medicine in psychiatry [77]. Application of this model to hypochondriasis and OCD may lead to new insights and possible breakthroughs in both the theoretical realm and clinical practice.

A better understanding of hypochondriasis and its relationships with OCD and other disorders has clear treatment implications. Future studies should directly compare psychological and pharmacological treatment modalities between patients with hypochondriasis, those with OCD and patients who suffer from both conditions. A greater variety of treatments (e.g., cognitive therapy strategies and pharmacological agents other than SSRIs) may need to be used in these studies. Also, transdiagnostic therapy approaches merit further scrutiny, refinement and testing of efficacy. Treatment studies should ideally be driven by hypotheses generated from new insights into the interactions between hypochondriasis and all other psychopathological entities.

References

1. Pilowsky I. Dimensions of hypochondriasis. *Br J Psychiatry.* 1967;113:89–93.
2. Kellner R. *Somatization and Hypochondriasis.* New York, NY: Praeger Publishers; 1986.
3. Fergus TA, Valentiner DP. Disease phobia and disease conviction are separate dimensions underlying hypochondriasis. *J Behav Ther Exp Psychiatry.* 2010;41:438–444.
4. Starcevic V, Berle D. Cyberchondria: towards a better understanding of excessive health-related Internet use. *Exp Rev Neurother.* 2013;13:205–213.
5. Starcevic V. Cyberchondria: challenges of problematic online searches for health-related information. *Psychother Psychosom.* 2017;86:129–133.
6. American Psychiatric Association. *Diagnostic and Statistical Manual of Mental Disorders*, 5th ed. Washington, DC: APA; 2013.
7. American Psychiatric Association. *Diagnostic and Statistical Manual of Mental Disorders*, 4th ed. Washington, DC: APA; 1994.
8. Rief W, Isaac M. The future of somatoform disorders: somatic symptom disorder, bodily distress disorder or functional syndromes? *Curr Opin Psychiatry.* 2014;27:315–319.
9. Starcevic V. Should we deplore the disappearance of hypochondriasis from DSM-5? *Aust N Z J Psychiatry.* 2014;48:373–374.
10. Rief W, Martin A. How to use the new DSM-5 somatic symptom disorder diagnosis in research and practice: a critical evaluation and a proposal for modifications. *Annu Rev Clin Psychol.* 2014;10:339–367.
11. Frances A, Chapman S. DSM-5 somatic symptom disorder mislabels medical illness as mental disorder. *Aust N Z J Psychiatry.* 2013;47:483–484.
12. Sirri L, Fava GA. Diagnostic criteria for psychosomatic research and somatic symptom disorders. *Int Rev Psychiatry.* 2013;25:19–30.
13. Starcevic V. Hypochondriasis and health anxiety: conceptual challenges. *Br J Psychiatry.* 2013;202:7–8.
14. van den Heuvel OA, Veale D, Stein DJ. Hypochondriasis: considerations for ICD-11. *Rev Bras Psiquiatria.* 2014;36:S21–S27.
15. World Health Organization. *ICD-11 Beta Draft.* 2017. Available from: www.who.int/classifications/icd/revision/en/ (accessed July 19, 2018).
16. Brakoulias V, Starcevic V. The characterization of beliefs in obsessive-compulsive disorder. *Psychiatr Q.* 2011;82:151–161.
17. Hegeman JM, Kok RM, van der Mast RC, Giltay EJ. Phenomenology of depression in older compared with younger adults: meta-analysis. *Br J Psychiatry.* 2012;200:275–281.
18. Looper KJ, Kirmayer LJ. Hypochondriacal concerns in a community population. *Psychol Med.* 2001;31:577–584.
19. Martin A, Jacobi F. Features of hypochondriasis and illness worry in the general population in Germany. *Psychosom Med.* 2006;68:770–777.
20. Bleichhardt G, Hiller W. Hypochondriasis and health anxiety in the German population. *Br J Health Psychol.* 2007;12:511–523.
21. Rief W, Hessel A, Braehler E. Somatization symptoms and hypochondriacal features in the general population. *Psychosom Med.* 2001;63:595–602.
22. Sunderland M, Newby JM, Andrews G. Health anxiety in Australia: prevalence, comorbidity, disability and service use. *Br J Psychiatry.* 2013;202:56–61.
23. Gureje O, Ustun TB, Simon GE. The syndrome of hypochondriasis: a cross-national study in primary care. *Psychol Med.* 1997;27:1001–1010.
24. Escobar JI, Gara M, Waitzkin H, et al. DSM-IV hypochondriasis in primary care. *Gen Hosp Psychiatry.* 1998;20:155–159.
25. Barsky AJ, Wyshak G, Klerman GL, et al. The prevalence of hypochondriasis in medical outpatients. *Soc Psychiatry Psychiatr Epidemiol.* 1990;25:89–94.
26. Fink P, Hansen MS, Oxhoj ML. The prevalence of somatoform disorders among internal medical inpatients. *J Psychosom Res.* 2004;56:413–418.

27. Palsson N. Functional somatic symptoms and hypochondriasis among general practice patients: a pilot study. *Acta Psychiatr Scand.* 1988;78:191–197.

28. Kirmayer LJ, Robbins JM. Three forms of somatization in primary care: prevalence, co-occurrence, and sociodemographic characteristics. *J Nerv Ment Dis.* 1991;179:647–655.

29. Seivewright H, Salkovskis P, Green J, et al. Prevalence and service implications of health anxiety in genitourinary medicine clinics. *Int J STD AIDS.* 2004;15:519–522.

30. Kehler MD, Hadjistavropoulos HD. Is health anxiety a significant problem for individuals with multiple sclerosis? *J Behav Med.* 2009;32:150–161.

31. Warwick HMC, Clark DM, Cobb A, et al. A controlled trial of cognitive-behavioural treatment of hypochondriasis. *Br J Psychiatry.* 1996;169:189–195.

32. Bouman TK, Visser S. Cognitive and behavioural treatments of hypochondriasis. *Psychother Psychosom.* 1998;67:214–221.

33. Clark DM, Salkovskis PM, Hackman A, et al. Two psychological treatments for hypochondriasis: a randomized controlled trial. *Br J Psychiatry.* 1998;173:218–225.

34. Visser S, Bouman TK. The treatment of hypochondriasis: exposure and response prevention vs. cognitive therapy. *Behav Res Ther.* 2001;39:423–442.

35. Barsky AJ, Ahern DK. Cognitive behavior therapy for hypochondriasis: a randomized controlled trial. *JAMA.* 2004;291:1464–1470.

36. Greeven A, van Balkom AJ, Visser S, et al. Cognitive behavior therapy and paroxetine in the treatment of hypochondriasis: a randomized controlled trial. *Am J Psychiatry.* 2007;164:91–99.

37. Seivewright H, Green J, Salkovskis PM, et al. Cognitive-behavioural therapy for health anxiety in a genitourinary medicine clinic: randomized controlled trial. *Br J Psychiatry.* 2008;198:332–337.

38. Sørensen P, Birket-Smith M, Wattar U, et al. A randomized clinical trial of cognitive behavioural therapy versus short-term psychodynamic psychotherapy versus no intervention for patients with hypochondriasis. *Psychol Med.* 2011;41:431–441.

39. Tyrer P, Cooper S, Salkovskis P, et al. Clinical and cost-effectiveness of cognitive behaviour therapy for health anxiety in medical patients: a multicentre randomised controlled trial. *Lancet.* 2014;383:219–225.

40. Warwick HMC, Salkovskis PM. Hypochondriasis. *Behav Res Ther.* 1990;24:597–602.

41. Rachman S. Health anxiety disorders: a cognitive construal. *Behav Res Ther.* 2012;50:502–512.

42. Hedman E, Andersson G, Andersson E, et al. Internet-based cognitive-behavioural therapy for severe health anxiety: randomised controlled trial. *Br J Psychiatry.* 2011;198:230–236.

43. Hedman E, Axelsson E, Andersson E, et al. Exposure-based cognitive-behavioural therapy via the internet and as bibliotherapy for somatic symptom disorder and illness anxiety disorder: randomised controlled trial. *Br J Psychiatry.* 2016;209:407–413.

44. McManus F, Surawy C, Muse K, Vazques-Montes M, Williams JMG. A randomized clinical trial of mindfulness-based cognitive therapy versus unrestricted services for health anxiety (hypochondriasis). *J Consult Clin Psychol.* 2012;80:817–828.

45. Fallon BA, Liebowitz MR, Salmán E, et al. Fluoxetine for hypochondriacal patients without major depression. *J Clin Psychopharmacol.* 1993;13:438–441.

46. Oosterbaan DB, van Balkom AJ, van Boeijen CA, et al. An open study of paroxetine in hypochondriasis. *Prog Neuro-Psychopharmacol Biol Psychiatry.* 2001;25:1023–1033.

47. Fallon BA, Qureshi AI, Schneier FR, et al. An open trial of fluvoxamine for hypochondriasis. *Psychosomatics.* 2003;44:298–303.

48. Wesner RB, Noyes R. Imipramine an effective treatment for illness phobia. *J Affect Disord.* 1991;22:43–48.

49. Fallon BA, Petkova E, Skritskaya N, et al. A double-masked, placebo-controlled study of fluoxetine for hypochondriasis. *J Clin Psychopharmacol.* 2008;28:638–645.

50. Fallon BA, Ahern DK, Pavlicova M, et al. A randomized controlled trial of medication and cognitive-behavioral therapy for hypochondriasis. *Am J Psychiatry.* 2017;174(8):756–764.

51. Schweitzer PJ, Zafar U, Pavlicova M, et al. Long-term follow-up of hypochondriasis after selective serotonin reuptake inhibitor treatment. *J Clin Psychopharmacol.* 2011;31:365–368.

52. Hollander E, Benzaquen S. The obsessive-compulsive spectrum disorders. *Int Rev Psychiatry.* 1997;9:99–109.

53. Hollander E, Braun A, Simeon D. Should OCD leave the anxiety disorders in DSM-V? The case for obsessive compulsive-related disorders. *Depress Anxiety.* 2008;25:317–329.

54. Hollander E. *Obsessive-Compulsive Related Disorders.* Washington, DC: American Psychiatric Press; 1993.

55. Fineberg NA, Chamberlain SR, Goudriaan AE, et al. New developments in human neurocognition: clinical, genetic, and brain imaging

correlates of impulsivity and compulsivity. *CNS Spectr.* 2014;19:69–89.

56. Grant JE, Kim SW. Brain circuitry of compulsivity and impulsivity. *CNS Spectr.* 2014;19:21–27.

57. Neziroglu F, McKay D, Yaryura-Tobias JA. Overlapping and distinctive features of hypochondriasis and obsessive-compulsive disorder. *J Anxiety Disord.* 2000;14:603–614.

58. Deacon B, Abramowitz JS. Is hypochondriasis related to obsessive-compulsive disorder, panic disorder, or both? An empirical evaluation. *J Cogn Psychoter.* 2008;22:115–127.

59. Barsky AJ. Hypochondriasis and obsessive compulsive disorder. *Psychiatr Clin North Am.* 1992;15:791–801.

60. Hedman E, Ljótsson B, Axelsson E, et al. Health anxiety in obsessive compulsive disorder and obsessive compulsive symptoms in severe health anxiety: an investigation of symptom profiles. *J Anxiety Disord.* 2017;45:80–86.

61. Abramowitz JS, Olatunji BO, Deacon BJ. Health anxiety, hypochondriasis, and the anxiety disorders. *Behav Ther.* 2007;38:86–94.

62. van den Heuvel OA, Veltman DJ, Groenewegen HJ, et al. Disorder-specific neuroanatomical correlates of attentional bias in obsessive-compulsive disorder, panic disorder, and hypochondriasis. *Arch Gen Psychiatry.* 2005;62:922–933.

63. van den Heuvel OA, Mataix-Cols D, Zwitser G, et al. Common limbic and frontal-striatal disturbances in patients with obsessive-compulsive disorder, panic disorder and hypochondriasis. *Psychol Med.* 2011;41:2399–2410.

64. Barsky AJ, Wyshak G, Klerman GL. Psychiatric comorbidity in DSM-III-R hypochondriasis. *Arch Gen Psychiatry.* 1992;49:101–108.

65. Bienvenu OJ, Samuels JF, Riddle MA, et al. The relationship of obsessive-compulsive disorder to possible spectrum disorders: results from a family study. *Biol Psychiatry.* 2000;48:287–293.

66. du Toit P, van Kradenburg J, Niehaus D, et al. Comparison of obsessive-compulsive disorder patients with and without comorbid putative obsessive-compulsive spectrum disorders using a structured clinical interview. *Compr Psychiatry.* 2001;42:291–300.

67. Bienvenu OJ, Samuels JF, Wuyek LA, et al. Is obsessive-compulsive disorder an anxiety disorder, and what, if any, are spectrum conditions? A family study perspective. *Psychol Med.* 2012;42:1–13.

68. Greeven A, van Balkom AJLM, van Rood YR, et al. The boundary between hypochondriasis and obsessive-compulsive disorder: a cross-sectional study from the Netherlands. *J Clin Psychiatry.* 2006;67:1682–1689.

69. Phillips KA, Stein DJ, Rauch SL, et al. Should an obsessive-compulsive spectrum grouping of disorders be included in DSM-V? *Depress Anxiety.* 2010;27:528–555.

70. Starcevic V, Janca A. Obsessive-compulsive spectrum disorders: still in search of the concept-affirming boundaries. *Curr Opin Psychiatry.* 2011;24:55–60.

71. Fallon BA, Qureshi AI, Laje G, Klein B. Hypochondriasis and its relationship to obsessive-compulsive disorder. *Psychiatr Clin North Am.* 2000;23:605–616.

72. Olatunji BO, Deacon BJ, Abramowitz JS. Is hypochondriasis an anxiety disorder? *Br J Psychiatry.* 2009;194:481–482.

73. Starcevic V. Classification of anxiety disorders: changes, conundrums and consequences. *Aust N Z J Psychiatry.* 2014;48:1164–1165.

74. Solem S, Borgejordet S, Haseth S, Hansen B, Håland Å, Bailey R. Symptoms of health anxiety in obsessive-compulsive disorder: relationship with treatment outcome and metacognition. *J Obsessive Compuls Relat Disord.* 2015;5:76–81.

75. Cramer AOJ, Waldorp LJ, van der Maas HLJ, Borsboom D. Comorbidity: a network perspective. *Behav Brain Sci.* 2010;33:137–150.

76. Borsboom D, Cramer AOJ. Network analysis: an integrative approach to the structure of psychopathology. *Annu Rev Clin Psychol.* 2013;9:91–121.

77. Fried EI, van Borkulo CD, Cramer AOJ, Boschloo L, Schoevers RA, Borsboom D. Mental disorders as networks of problems: a review of recent insights. *Soc Psychiatry Psychiatr Epidemiol.* 2017;52:1–10.

Chapter 25

Hoarding Disorder

Lorena Fernández de la Cruz and David Mataix-Cols

Introduction

Hoarding disorder is a mental disorder that was newly introduced in the *Diagnostic and Statistical Manual of Mental Disorders*, fifth edition (DSM-5) [1]. It is also planned for inclusion in the forthcoming 11th revision of the International Classification of Diseases (ICD-11) [2]. In DSM-5, hoarding disorder is included under the broad umbrella of obsessive-compulsive and related disorders (OCRDs), which, in addition to obsessive-compulsive disorder (OCD), also includes body dysmorphic disorder, hair pulling disorder (trichotillomania) and excoriation (skin picking) disorder. ICD-11 will adopt a similar approach and will be even more inclusive (e.g., hypochondriasis and olfactory reference disorder are suggested for inclusion in the OCRDs section) [2].

The reasons for classifying hoarding disorder alongside OCD and related disorders are primarily historical, given the previous conceptualization of problematic hoarding as being a criterion of obsessive-compulsive personality disorder (OCPD) and/or a symptom of OCD [3]. While there are similarities and overlapping etiological factors between hoarding disorder and other OCRDs [4], it is also apparent that it shares features with other emotional, impulse control and neurodevelopmental disorders, such as attention deficit and hyperactivity disorder (ADHD) [5].

This chapter first summarizes the main clinical features and diagnostic criteria for hoarding disorder. It then reviews the most recent data on its epidemiology, etiology, assessment and treatment. Finally, it offers an overview of the cross-diagnostic aspects of hoarding disorder and their implications for psychiatric classification, diagnosis and treatment. Future directions of research in the field are also outlined.

Clinical Features, Diagnostic Criteria and Specifiers

Diagnostic Criteria

The DSM-5 diagnostic criteria for hoarding disorder [1] are based on an earlier operational definition of "compulsive" hoarding [6]. The landmark feature is a persistent difficulty with discarding or parting with possessions (criterion A). The most commonly saved items include newspapers, old clothing, bags, books and paperwork, but any item can be saved. The nature of items is not limited to worthless possessions because many individuals collect and save valuable things too (e.g., gifts in their original wrapping).

These discarding difficulties are generally motivated by the perceived utility of the items (e.g., toilet paper rolls that are saved because they might be useful for art projects), their esthetic value (e.g., Christmas decorations that are never used but are kept for years because they are nice), the strong sentimental attachment to the possessions (e.g., objects that have emotional value because they are linked with important people or events in their life, such as memorabilia from trips done in the past), the fear of losing important information (e.g., newspapers that are accumulated to be read at some point in case there is something relevant in them), a desire to avoid being wasteful (e.g., keeping a large amount of glass jars because there is no recycling point near the house), or, typically, a combination of these factors [6]. The prospect of discarding or parting with possessions causes substantial distress to the individual (criterion B).

These difficulties result in the disorganized accumulation of possessions that congest and clutter active living areas and substantially compromise their intended use (criterion C). Affected individuals may not be able to sleep in their beds, cook in the kitchen or sit on the sofas in their living rooms. Frequently, the clutter extends beyond the person's actual home, with accumulation of possessions taking place in garages, gardens, vehicles and even workplaces. Some individuals may pay for private storage spaces or ask family members or friends to keep items in their homes.

Criterion C can still be met if the living areas are uncluttered only because of the intervention of third parties (e.g., family members, cleaners or authorities). Because children and adolescents typically do not control their living environment and have limited acquisitive power, the possible intervention of third parties (e.g., parents keeping the spaces usable and thus reducing interference) should be considered when making the diagnosis. Young individuals with hoarding disorder who live at their parent's home may not have unduly cluttered bedrooms but still fulfill all other diagnostic criteria.

Criterion D requires that the difficulties with discarding and/or clutter cause clinically significant distress or impairment in social, occupational or other important areas of functioning, including maintaining a safe environment for self and others. In severe cases, hoarding can put individuals at risk for fire, falling, poor sanitation and other health risks. Some individuals, particularly those with poor insight, may not report distress, and the impairment may only be apparent to those around the individual. However, any attempts to discard or clear the possessions by third parties result in high levels of distress. Quality of life is often severely impaired and family relationships are frequently strained [7]. Legal proceedings ranging from forced clearings to evictions and, where relevant, the removal of dependents from the home (e.g., children, elderly) are relatively common [8]. A diagnosis of hoarding disorder can only be given once other general medical conditions (criterion E) and mental disorders (criterion F) have been ruled out (see Differential diagnosis section below). For a diagnosis of hoarding disorder, all six criteria (A–F) must be met.

Specifiers

For individuals fulfilling diagnostic criteria for hoarding disorder, clinicians may also assess the presence of two specifiers: excessive acquisition and insight. The *excessive acquisition* specifier is endorsed when the individual engages in excessive acquisition of free items, excessive buying, or, less frequently, stealing items that are not needed or for which there is no space available. In approximately 63–90% of people with hoarding disorder, the difficulty discarding is accompanied by concurrent excessive acquisition [9,10,11,12]; these individuals typically experience distress if they are unable to acquire items or are prevented from acquiring items. Reducing excessive acquisition is one of the main goals in the treatment of hoarding disorder.

The *insight* specifier has three categories (good/fair, poor and absent/delusional) and refers to the degree to which the individual recognizes that hoarding-related beliefs and behaviors are problematic. A substantial proportion of sufferers lack insight into their difficulties and are reluctant to seek help for their problems [13]. Increasing motivation for change is an integral part of the current psychological treatment for hoarding disorder, particularly in cases with reduced insight.

Other Clinical Features, Squalor and Animal Hoarding

Other common features of hoarding disorder include indecisiveness, perfectionism, avoidance, procrastination, difficulty with planning and organizing tasks and distractibility [6]. Some individuals with hoarding disorder live in various degrees of unsanitary conditions (*squalor*) that may be a logical consequence of severely cluttered spaces and/or related to planning and organizing difficulties [14]. However, the majority of individuals living in severe domestic squalor do not meet criteria for hoarding disorder; rather, squalid homes are typically seen in other medical or neurocognitive conditions (see Differential diagnosis section below).

Some individuals are known to accumulate large numbers of animals. In *animal hoarding*, there is generally a failure to provide minimal standards of nutrition, sanitation and veterinary care for the animals; and a failure to act on the deteriorating condition of the animals and the environment. It is unclear if animal hoarding is a special manifestation of hoarding disorder, but most individuals who hoard animals also hoard inanimate objects [15].

Differential Diagnosis

A diagnosis of hoarding disorder can be made only after other medical conditions and mental disorders that can lead to the excessive accumulation of possessions have been ruled out. A careful psychopathological interview is necessary to establish the differential diagnosis. The presence of cluttered living spaces alone does not necessarily signal the presence of hoarding disorder because cluttered (and sometimes unhygienic) living spaces may be the consequence of multiple conditions.

Other Medical Conditions

Hoarding disorder is not diagnosed if the symptoms are judged to be a direct consequence of another medical condition (criterion E), such as traumatic brain injury, surgical resection for the treatment of a tumor or seizure control, cerebrovascular disease, infections of the central nervous system (e.g., herpes simplex encephalitis) or neurogenetic conditions such as Prader-Willi syndrome [3,16].

Damage to the anterior ventromedial prefrontal and cingulate cortices has been particularly associated with the excessive accumulation of objects [17,18]. In these individuals, the hoarding behavior is not present prior to the onset of the brain damage and appears shortly after the brain damage occurs [17]. Some of these individuals appear to have little interest in the accumulated items and are able to discard them easily or do not care if others discard them, whereas others appear to be very reluctant to discard anything [18].

Neurodevelopmental Disorders

Hoarding disorder is not diagnosed if the accumulation of objects is judged to be a direct consequence of a neurodevelopmental disorder, such as autism spectrum disorders (ASD) or intellectual disability. Individuals with ASD may, for example, excessively acquire or retain possessions that correspond to a particular sensory preoccupation (e.g., intense fascination with visual stimuli such as shiny objects or tactile stimuli such as smooth surfaces – different from a fondness for the aesthetic value of an item) or "special interest" (i.e., a circumscribed area of intense interest in a specific, narrow and often unusual topic). This contrasts with the much broader range of diverse objects that are typically accumulated by individuals with hoarding disorder. Another distinguishing feature is that in ASD, significant periods of time are spent in the continued use of or interaction with objects as part of current special interest, whereas in hoarding disorder time may be spent seeking out items, but there is little apparent use or interaction with objects already owned.

Schizophrenia Spectrum and other Psychotic Disorders

Hoarding disorder is not diagnosed if the accumulation of objects is judged to be a direct consequence of positive or negative symptoms in schizophrenia spectrum and other psychotic disorders [3,19]. When the hoarding behavior is secondary to positive symptoms (delusions or hallucinations), the clinical picture tends to be idiosyncratic and there is normally a delusional explanation for the hoarding behavior [16]. When the hoarding behavior is secondary to negative symptoms, the accumulation of possessions is typically a passive phenomenon and is more accurately described as failure to discard waste. Furthermore, these individuals do not feel emotionally attached to the hoarded items, nor do they attribute an intrinsic or practical value to them. For this reason, helping these individuals clear out the waste items does not tend to be challenging [16]. Many of the homes of these individuals present high levels of unsanitary conditions (severe domestic squalor), a rare phenomenon in hoarding disorder [14].

Major Depressive Episode

Hoarding disorder is not diagnosed if the accumulation of objects is judged to be a direct consequence of psychomotor retardation, fatigue or loss of energy during a major depressive episode. Individuals suffering from depression may fail to tend to the household and may fail to discard items received in the mail, waste items and rubbish. This may lead to the accumulation of clutter. Carefully investigating the onset of symptoms may be the main differentiator. If the symptoms of depression precede the hoarding behavior, the diagnosis is more likely to be one of depressive disorder rather than hoarding disorder. Additionally, an individual with depression will most likely be unconcerned with the items and clearing them will not usually be met with opposition [16].

Obsessive-Compulsive Disorder

Although approximately 5–10% of patients with OCD display hoarding symptoms, the majority of individuals (more than 80%) with hoarding difficulties do not display other OCD symptoms [9,10,20,21]. Hoarding disorder is not diagnosed if the symptoms are judged to be a direct consequence of typical obsessions or compulsions, such as fears of contamination, harm or feelings of incompleteness. In such cases, OCD should be diagnosed instead [22]. Symmetry obsessions and compulsions are the most commonly associated with this form of hoarding. The accumulation of objects can also be the result of persistently avoiding onerous rituals (e.g., not discarding to avoid endless washing or checking rituals) [3,19].

Some additional clinical features are helpful in differentiating hoarding disorder from OCD. In OCD, the behavior is generally unwanted and highly distressing, and the individual experiences no pleasure or reward from it. Excessive acquisition is usually not present; if excessive acquisition is present, items are acquired because of a specific obsession (e.g., the need to buy items that have been accidentally touched to avoid contaminating other people), not because of a genuine desire to possess the items. These individuals are also more likely to accumulate bizarre items, such as trash, feces, urine, nails, hair, used diapers or rotten food [20]. Accumulation of such items is very unusual in hoarding disorder. Both disorders may be diagnosed when severe hoarding appears concurrently with other typical symptoms of OCD, but is judged to be independent of these symptoms [3].

Neurocognitive Disorders

Hoarding disorder is not diagnosed if the accumulation of objects is judged to be a direct consequence of a degenerative disorder, such as neurocognitive disorder associated with frontotemporal lobar degeneration or Alzheimer's disease. Typically, onset of the accumulating behavior is gradual and follows onset of the neurocognitive disorder. The accumulating behavior may be accompanied with self-neglect and severe domestic squalor (where there is trash, rotten food or excrement), alongside other neuropsychiatric symptoms, such as disinhibition, gambling, rituals/stereotypies, tics and self-injurious behaviors [14].

Normal Collecting

While technically not a differential diagnosis, it is worth delineating the differences between normative or healthy collecting and pathological hoarding [23]. This is particularly relevant because quite a few individuals meeting criteria for hoarding disorder define themselves as "collectors," as they perceive this term as being somewhat less pejorative [23]. Normative collecting is a common activity that is both benign and pleasurable. Most children and up to 30% of adults collect items at some time in their lives [24].

Collectors report the acquisition of, attachment to and reluctance to discard objects, but they do not have the disorganized clutter, distress and impairment that is characteristic of hoarding disorder. In contrast to hoarding, the process of collecting is highly structured and planned, very selective (i.e., confined to a narrow range of items), pleasurable and often a social activity. Most collectors, even those who might be considered eccentric, are unlikely to meet the diagnostic criteria for hoarding disorder [23,24].

Comorbidities

The most common psychiatric comorbidities among hoarding cases are generalized anxiety disorder (31–37%), major depressive disorder (26–31%), OCD (15–20%), panic disorder (17%), social anxiety disorder (14%) and post-traumatic stress disorder (PTSD; 14%) [9,10,12,19,25]. Symptoms typical of ADHD, particularly inattention, are also commonly reported [5,10]. These comorbidities, rather than the hoarding, may often be the main reason for clinical consultation [26]. General medical conditions may also be highly frequent in patients with hoarding disorder. Its presence has been associated with both poorer perceived physical health and higher rates of disability [12]. These limitations may be particularly evident in elderly individuals, who appear to have a disproportionally high rate of medical complications in association with hoarding disorder, compared with age-matched controls [27].

Recent Research Findings

Epidemiology

Initial prevalence estimates, primarily from questionnaire studies conducted in Europe and the United States, estimated the point prevalence of clinically significant hoarding to be approximately 2–6% among adults [19] and 2% among adolescents [28]. However, in the only epidemiological study to date to employ the current DSM-5 criteria, conducted in the United Kingdom, the prevalence was estimated to be approximately 1.5% in both adult men and women [12]. This estimate, which was obtained principally through diagnostic interviews conducted face to face in the participants' homes, contrasts with some prior work in its suggestion that rates of hoarding disorder are balanced across the genders. Help-seeking clinical samples are predominantly female, perhaps reflecting better insight and motivation for change.

Epidemiological studies are more consistent in their finding that the prevalence of hoarding disorder seems to increase with advancing age [12,19]. Individuals with hoarding disorder are more frequently unemployed, and more often unmarried, separated or divorced than individuals from the general community [12,23,29]. Additionally, they are more likely to feel that their hoarding difficulties impair their social and occupational functioning [7,12].

The functional impairments caused by the disorder typically extend to the relatives or carers of the person who hoards [7]. Retrospective reports indicate that hoarding difficulties begin early and span well into the late stages of life. Hoarding symptoms may first emerge around ages 11–15 years, start interfering with the individual's everyday functioning by the mid-20s, and cause clinically significant impairment by the mid-30s [30,31,32]. Problems with acquisition, when they do emerge, appear to do so (or become more evident) earlier than problems with discarding [30].

Participants in clinical research studies are usually in their 50s [9,20]. A steady worsening of symptoms is typically reported over each decade of life [33]. Once symptoms begin, the course of hoarding is often chronic, with few individuals reporting a waxing and waning course [32]. Given the absence of treatment studies with long follow-up periods, the long-term prognosis for treated hoarding disorder is currently unknown. Most research into hoarding disorder has been carried out in Western contexts, but there is growing evidence to indicate that it occurs and has largely similar phenomenology across cultures [34,35].

Etiology

Genetic and Environmental Factors

Although controlled family studies have not yet been carried out, patient self-report suggests that hoarding runs in families [20]. Consistently, a number of twin studies conducted in large, population-based adolescent and adult twin samples suggest that this familiality is largely attributable to additive genetic factors (heritabilities ranging between 36% and 50%), with the remaining variance attributable to non-shared environmental factors and measurement error [36,37,38].

The mechanisms by which either genetic or environmental factors, or their interaction, confer risk to the development of hoarding disorder remain unknown. Specific genes implicated in the condition have not yet been identified. Although research has suggested some unique environmental risk factors (e.g., traumatic life events), small samples and retrospective self-report methods leave the role of such exposures in the onset or exacerbation of hoarding disorder unclear [31,36]. Anecdotal links between material deprivation (e.g., childhood poverty) and hoarding have received no support in the literature [31].

Future work is warranted to understand how specific genetic and environmental risk factors interact to confer risk to individuals carefully diagnosed as having hoarding disorder. It is likely that these genetic and environmental risk factors will be, at least in part, shared with related conditions such as OCD and other related disorders [39]. The potential etiological overlaps between hoarding disorder and other neuropsychiatric conditions (e.g., anxiety and mood disorders, ADHD) remain to be explored.

Neurocognitive Correlates

The neural substrates of hoarding behavior have been well studied in animals that naturally display hoarding behaviors as part of their behavioral repertoire (e.g., rodents, birds), as well as primates. These studies clearly implicate subcortical limbic structures (nucleus accumbens, ventral tegmental area, amygdala, hippocampus, thalamus, hypothalamus) and the ventromedial prefrontal cortex in the mediation of hoarding behavior [18]. Research with animals also suggests that the dopaminergic system plays a crucial role in hoarding behavior (for a review see Mataix-Cols et al. [18]).

Much less is known about normal and abnormal hoarding behavior in humans. Useful clues come from case studies of patients with brain damage and of individuals with dementia, particularly of the frontotemporal type. This research suggests that the ventromedial prefrontal and anterior cingulate cortices, as well as medial temporal regions, may be implicated in hoarding behavior [18]. One theory is that the former cortical regions modulate or suppress subcortically driven predispositions to acquire and collect and adjust these predispositions to environmental context [17]. Damage to these cortical regions may result in dysregulated collecting and hoarding behavior.

The neuroimaging literature of "non-organic" hoarding has also implicated the ventromedial prefrontal and anterior cingulate cortices, and subcortical limbic structures (e.g., amygdala/hippocampus) in patients who hoard [40,41,42]. However, the evidence is preliminary, obtained from small samples, and confounded in many cases by the presence of comorbid obsessive-compulsive symptoms [18]. A small number of functional neuroimaging and electrophysiological studies have compared the patterns of brain activation in hoarding disorder compared with OCD, using a variety of neurocognitive tasks [42,43,44,45]. Overall, these studies converge to highlight potential differences in the neural substrates of the two disorders, but these results should be considered preliminary until the findings are consistently replicated.

Similarly, it is difficult to draw firm conclusions from early reports on the neurocognitive profile of hoarding disorder [18]. Many of the initial neuropsychological studies recruited patients with OCD who showed hoarding symptoms (with different degrees of severity), whereas others recruited individuals with severe hoarding but predominantly without OCD. The neuropsychological tests employed have been heterogeneous and have tapped into different domains, and few employed psychiatric control groups. Findings to date suggest possible impairments in spatial planning, visuospatial learning and memory, sustained attention/working memory organization, response inhibition, set shifting, probabilistic learning and reversal [18,46,47]. Future work in this area should include carefully characterized samples of individuals meeting strict criteria for hoarding disorder.

Assessment

The Clinical Interview and Risk Assessment

The diagnosis of hoarding disorder is usually made on the basis of a direct interview with the person being evaluated to establish whether the diagnostic criteria are met. The Structured Interview for Hoarding Disorder [48] is available for this purpose and has been translated to several languages, including Spanish, Portuguese and Japanese [35]. Because hoarding may not always be the initial reason for consultation [26], clinicians often need to ask direct questions, such as "Do you find it difficult to discard or part with possessions?" or "Do you have a large number of possessions that congest and clutter the main rooms in your home?". An affirmative answer to these questions can initiate a dialog that may lead to diagnosis.

A home visit is recommended for the assessment of clutter, impairment and associated risks. If a home visit is not feasible, the clinician should try to gather additional information from reliable informants, such as a spouse or relative (with the patient's consent). This is particularly important for affected persons with limited insight, because they may underestimate the extent and consequences of their difficulties. Informants may also help establish whether the current presentation is long-standing or transient, whether third parties have intervened to clear away some of the clutter and whether there are potential risks that require attention.

Photographs of the patient's home can also be very useful in helping to document the presence of clinically significant clutter and to track treatment outcomes [49,50], particularly when home visits are not possible or are impractical. However, photographs should not be a substitute for a thorough psychopathological interview. The diagnostic interview provides an opportunity to carry out a thorough risk assessment. Attention should be paid to potential fire hazards, the risk of clutter avalanches, the presence of rodent or insect infestation and unsanitary living conditions that pose a risk to health. In addition, it is important to establish whether other vulnerable persons (e.g., children and elderly people) cohabit with the person who is hoarding.

Clinician and Self-Administered Rating Scales

Numerous clinician and self-administered measures of hoarding severity exist and can be used to quantify the severity of various aspects of hoarding such as difficulties discarding, clutter, distress, etc. While useful, these measures do not allow a diagnosis of hoarding disorder, primarily because it is not possible to rule out other disorders that may cause hoarding. Therefore, they should be restricted to quantify the severity of hoarding in already diagnosed individuals or to screen individuals in population-based studies.

The most widely used clinician administered measures are the Hoarding Rating Scale-Interview [51] and the Clutter Image Rating [49]. Among the most widely used self-administered measures are the Hoarding Rating Scale-Self Report [52], the Saving Inventory-Revised (SI-R) [53], the University of California, Los Angeles, Hoarding Severity Scale (UHSS) [54] and the Hoarding Disorder Dimensional Scale [55]. Typically, these measures have empirically derived cut-off points, which give an indication of whether the person is likely to have clinically significant hoarding problems.

Supplementary measures that assess saving cognitions (e.g., the Saving Cognitions Inventory)

[56], problematic acquisition (e.g., the Compulsive Acquisition Scale [57]), self-reported squalor (e.g., the Environmental Cleanliness and Clutter Scale [58,59] and the Home Environment Index [60]) and caregiver burden and accommodation (e.g., the Family Impact Scale for Hoarding [61]) are available and may prove useful for clarifying the clinical picture and monitoring treatment outcomes.

Treatment

Few treatment studies have specifically included individuals fulfilling DSM-5 criteria for hoarding disorder and therefore the evidence to guide treatment choice is currently weak. Additionally, the available treatment studies for hoarding disorder have a significant number of methodological shortcomings. In a systematic review assessing the quality of the available evidence regarding interventions for hoarding disorder [62], none of the 20 evaluated studies scored above the cut-off in the Clinical Trials Assessment Measure, a scale created to judge the methodological quality of clinical trials. Characteristics that contributed to lower scores were, among others, the small sample sizes and the lack of control groups [62]. To date, only five randomized controlled trials (RCTs) have evaluated the efficacy of treatments for hoarding disorder (including four cognitive behavioral therapy-based interventions and one cognitive remediation trial [63,64,65,66,67]). Of these, only three have included active control conditions [63,64,65].

Psychological Treatment

Currently, the intervention that has the strongest evidence base for hoarding disorder is a multicomponent psychological treatment that is based on a cognitive behavioral model of "compulsive hoarding" [6]. The intervention includes office and in-home sessions; motivational interviewing methods to address ambivalence about therapy; education about hoarding; goal-setting; organizing, decision making and problem-solving skills training; exposure to sorting, discarding and not acquiring; and cognitive strategies to facilitate this work [68].

Tolin and colleagues [69] conducted a meta-analysis of all open-label trials or RCTs of CBT or behavioral therapy for hoarding in adults. The eligible studies used hoarding-specific outcome measures and hoarding disorder was the primary condition being studied, as opposed to hoarding measured in the context of another psychiatric disorder (e.g., OCD). Ten relevant studies comprising 12 samples were identified, of which three were RCTs including a total of 103 patients. Four samples used individual CBT, whereas the remaining eight used a group format. Three samples employed a peer-directed, bibliotherapy-based program of CBT with no professional therapist present.

The number of CBT sessions ranged from 13 to 35 (mean 20.2 sessions), and the number of visits conducted in patients' homes ranged from 0 to 33 (mean 5.6 sessions). Overall hoarding symptom severity decreased significantly across studies with a large effect size (Hedges' g 0.82 for the overall hoarding disorder severity score). Significant effects were evident on all outcome domains. The strongest effects were seen for difficulty discarding (Hedges' g 0.89). Clutter and acquiring showed effects in the moderate range (Hedges' g 0.70 and 0.72, respectively). Functional impairment (which was not used in the calculation of overall hoarding disorder symptom severity) showed the smallest effect, in the moderate range (Hedges' g 0.52) [69].

More recently, a novel CBT-based treatment enhanced with cognitive rehabilitation techniques has been evaluated in elderly patients with hoarding disorder. Fifty-eight elderly patients meeting DSM-5 criteria for hoarding disorder were randomized to cognitive rehabilitation and exposure/sorting therapy (CREST) or to geriatric case management [65]. Participants in the CREST group achieved a significantly higher decrease in hoarding symptoms as measured by the SI-R. Participants in CREST averaged a 38% decrease on the SI-R and participants who completed case management averaged a 25% decrease (Cohens' d for completers = 0.63).

Thus, although encouraging, the clinical outcomes of CBT interventions for hoarding are relatively modest (many individuals still require additional treatment) and there is still significant room for improvement. The long-term benefit of such interventions is unclear but data from a single trial suggests that the treatment gains of CBT for hoarding disorder were largely maintained at 12-month follow-up [70]. Studies with even longer follow-up times are needed.

While the current psychological treatments emphasize the importance of motivational interviewing techniques, the patients that generally participate in the treatment trials have sufficient insight to at least seek help. It is currently unclear how to best approach individuals with absent or delusional insight and who may only come to the attention of mental health services against their will. The clinical management of these cases may require an unprecedented level of interagency coordination. Several countries have set up local or federal, multi-agency task forces (often including mental health, fire, pest control, housing, legal and social services) to tackle the most severe cases of hoarding who do not voluntarily seek or want help [71].

Pharmacological Treatment

Pharmacotherapy has also been suggested as a treatment for hoarding disorder. However, data regarding the use of such treatment are extremely limited and derived from small, uncontrolled studies. While no randomized controlled trials of medication for hoarding disorder have been conducted, some data are available from studies in patients with OCD who also have hoarding symptoms. In patients diagnosed with OCD, the presence of hoarding symptoms is consistently associated with a worse response to serotonin reuptake inhibitors, alone or in combination with CBT [72]. Specifically, patients with OCD who have hoarding symptoms are, on average, 50% less likely to respond to serotonin reuptake inhibitors than patients with OCD who do not hoard [72].

In an open-label study of paroxetine that included 79 patients with OCD (32 patients meeting criteria for "compulsive hoarding syndrome" [6] and 47 patients with non-hoarding OCD), hoarding symptoms improved as much as other obsessive-compulsive symptoms. However, paroxetine was not well tolerated (adverse effects included sedation, fatigue, constipation, akathisia, headache and sexual dysfunction), and the overall response was moderate in both groups.

To date, only three studies (two open-label trials and one case series) have included samples of individuals diagnosed with hoarding disorder according to the DSM-5 criteria. An open study evaluated the efficacy of a 12-week trial of venlafaxine and classed 16 of 24 participants as responders (defined as at least 30% reduction in UHSS and SI-R scores, as well as a rating of at least "much improved" on the Clinical Global Impression–Improvement scale) [73]. Two other studies have used ADHD treatments to treat hoarding symptoms. The first of these studies was a case series of four patients treated with methylphenidate extended release treated for four weeks. Of the four patients, two had a modest reduction in hoarding symptoms (25% and 32% decrease in the SI-R) but the drug was not well tolerated and all patients discontinued treatment [74]. More recently, another uncontrolled trial reported that 9 of 12 participants with hoarding disorder showed some degree of reduction in their hoarding symptoms in a 12-week trial of atomoxetine [75]. Eleven patients completed the trial and, of these, six were classified as full responders based on the UHSS (mean reduction of 57%); three other patients were classified as partial responders (mean reduction of 27%).

Cross-Diagnostic Approaches and Their Implication for Classification and Diagnosis

As noted in the introduction, hoarding disorder is currently classified in DSM-5 in the OCRDs chapter and ICD-11 will adopt a similar approach. The reasons for classifying hoarding disorder alongside OCD and related disorders are primarily historical, given the previous conceptualization of problematic hoarding as being a criterion of OCPD and/or a symptom of OCD [3]. While there are similarities and overlapping etiological factors between hoarding disorder and other OCRDs [4], it is also apparent that it shares features with other disorders.

There are phenomenological links between hoarding and impulse control disorders, in particular, compulsive buying, which in DSM-5 is considered under "other specified disruptive, impulse control, and conduct disorder" [3,76,77]. The ego-syntonic and sometimes pleasurable nature of excessive acquisition in hoarding resembles the phenomenology in compulsive buying [76]. Many hoarders feel compelled to collect or acquire free items, and to buy excessively and, conversely, many compulsive buyers hoard [10,76]. Some authors have suggested that hoarding and buying could represent manifestation of a broader psychopathological construct [11,78]. However, not everyone with hoarding problems reports excessive acquisition (see Diagnosis and clinical picture section, above) and, similarly, not all compulsive buyers report hoarding symptoms. Furthermore, as opposed to hoarding, compulsive buyers find excitement in the buying process itself, not in the bought items [79].

Preliminary data also suggest a link with other impulse control disorders. For example, Samuels et al. [80] reported a greater frequency of trichotillomania and skin picking among patients with OCD and hoarding symptoms, compared with those without hoarding symptoms. Frost and colleagues [81] reported high levels of hoarding symptoms in a sample of pathological gamblers. An association between kleptomania and compulsive buying has also been proposed [82], and anecdotal experience gathered by Steketee and Frost [76] suggests a link between kleptomania and hoarding, but clearly more research is needed.

A link has also been established between ADHD and hoarding [5,83]. Individuals who hoard usually present with attention difficulties [5,84] and other executive functioning deficits such as difficulties in strategic planning, feedback response, impulsivity, concept formation and decision making [5,47,85,86]. ADHD may even play a more important role in hoarding than OCD [87], with comorbid ADHD [88] occurring more frequently than comorbid OCD [9]. Further, epidemiological studies have shown that symptoms of inattention in childhood are specifically associated with hoarding symptoms in adulthood over and above the presence of obsessive-compulsive symptoms, suggesting that inattention symptoms in childhood might be a precursor of hoarding difficulties later in life [89]. It has also been suggested that executive functioning may provide a marker for genetic vulnerability toward hoarding symptoms in individuals with ADHD [83].

There is also a strong correlation between hoarding and depressive and anxiety symptoms [90,91], which suggests a non-specific link with emotional disorders in general. In fact, hoarding has been associated with a number of anxiety-related transdiagnostic dispositional tendencies such as anxiety sensitivity, experiential avoidance and emotion regulation difficulties.

Anxiety sensitivity is a well-known general risk factor for psychopathology. Also known as "fear of fear", anxiety sensitivity refers to beliefs that experiences of anxiety, such as bodily sensations, have negative implications [92]. Higher levels of anxiety sensitivity are thought to amplify anxious reactions and fear-related responses, which subsequently lead to greater levels of avoidance [92,93]. This construct has been particularly associated with panic disorder and agoraphobia, but also with a range of other psychiatric disorders including a number of anxiety disorders, OCD, PTSD, substance use disorders, depression and increased suicidality [94].

Similarly, a robust association between anxiety sensitivity and hoarding has been established in a number of studies using both clinical [95] and non-clinical samples [94,96,97].These results add to the idea that anxiety sensitivity acts as a general diathesis for the development of psychopathology, including hoarding, which may play a role in the development and maintenance of these conditions [94].

Experiential avoidance, defined as the tendency to avoid contact with particular unwanted internal experiences, such as bodily sensations, emotions, thoughts and memories [98], is hypothesized to underlie much psychopathology, and has been investigated in a number of psychological disorders such as OCD, generalized anxiety disorder, PTSD, trichotillomania and skin picking [99]. Existing conceptualizations of pathological hoarding disorder [6,76] appear broadly consistent with an experiential avoidance model. For example, they suggest that saving possessions (as opposed to discarding them) enables individuals to avoid distressing feelings associated with the action – or thought – of discarding, such as loss, guilt or fear of having made a mistake [99]. Indeed, a number of studies have found high levels of experiential avoidance in individuals with hoarding symptoms [100] and in individuals diagnosed with hoarding disorder [99,101].

Emotion regulation is defined as the ability to monitor, evaluate and modulate emotional reactions, especially in the context of goal-related behavior [102]. Difficulties in emotion regulation have been mentioned as a vulnerability factor for the development of a number of emotional problems [103]. Further, significant difficulties in emotion regulation have been found in people who hoard [99]. It has been suggested that hoarding symptoms may rely on items for emotion regulation, leading to stronger beliefs that items are integral to emotional wellbeing [104]. Additionally, some research suggests that people who hoard may attempt to regulate their emotions by using maladaptive behaviors such as using alcohol [105] or eating excessively [106].

Cross-Diagnostic Approaches and Their Implication for Treatment

The emergent literature reviewed in the previous section, together with data from the psychopathology, behavior genetics, neuroimaging and neurocognition literature, suggests that a number of transdiagnostic processes may be relevant across several psychiatric disorders, including hoarding disorder, and which are not limited to those included in the OCD and related disorders grouping. Indeed, hoarding disorder appears to share psychopathological features with OCRDs, emotional disorders in general, ADHD, impulse control disorders and even behavioral addictions. Whether this knowledge will eventually result in the development of better treatments, by targeting some of these transdiagnostic risk factors, compared with traditional disorder-focused treatments, is currently unknown.

A step in this direction involves the development and evaluation of cognitive rehabilitation or cognitive remediation protocols that target some of the information processing deficits that are typical of the disorder. This approach has been evaluated in two RCTs [64,65] with promising results (see Psychological treatment section, above). Similarly, trials of ADHD medication (evaluated in two open trials of methylphenidate and atomoxetine, totaling 16 patients) have resulted in modest reductions in hoarding symptoms, although methylphenidate was not well tolerated. Further controlled trials are needed to establish the efficacy and tolerability of such pharmacological approaches, and whether these are particularly suited for patients with a certain profile (e.g., prominent information processing difficulties). It is possible that these drugs may improve some of the cognitive difficulties associated with hoarding disorder, which may in turn facilitate compliance with additional behavioral interventions. In the authors' view, pharmacological approaches alone are unlikely to suffice in such a complex disorder, which has a natural history of several decades.

The resemblance between hoarding disorder and impulse control disorders or behavioral addictions, has also been noted above. Motivational interviewing techniques are generally included in treatment protocols of both hoarding and impulse control problems, such as gambling or compulsive buying, given the lack of insight and low motivation for change that usually characterize these disorders. While these techniques are not meant to be used alone, they are helpful when patients present with ambivalence about change that interferes with the treatment progress [68]. These techniques were first developed to treat addiction problems such as alcoholism [107]. Whether current treatments for impulse control disorders or addictions – beyond motivational interviewing techniques – may be of help to address hoarding difficulties is still unknown. An RCT of augmentation with naltrexone (a drug generally used to treat addiction to opioids) for OCD, where two of ten patients presented with hoarding symptoms, did not show any advantage for the naltrexone in the improvement of OCD symptoms, compared with placebo [108]. Further treatment studies are needed to explore the relation between hoarding disorder and impulse disorders and addictions.

Future Directions

Hoarding disorder was included in the DSM-5 and is also planned for inclusion as an independent disorder in the forthcoming ICD-11. The consideration of hoarding disorder as a discrete diagnostic entity has definitely been a major achievement for the field. Many previously undiagnosed persons are now entitled to receive appropriate care for their condition. Because hoarding disorder is a newly recognized disorder, most of the current knowledge is preliminary. Virtually all areas require investigation. Particularly, efforts to identify genetic and environmental risk factors for the disorder as well as the development and dissemination of more efficacious and cost-effective treatments should be regarded as a priority. Like most mental disorders, hoarding disorder almost certainty shares etiological risk factors and mechanisms with other disorders not limited to those in the OCRDs chapter. Identification of disorder-specific risk factors, as well as those shared with other disorders, will aid future research into the etiology, nosology and management of this disabling condition.

References

1. American Psychiatric Association. *The Diagnostic and Statistical Manual of Mental Disorders, Fifth Edition (DSM-5)*. Washington, DC: APA; 2013.
2. Stein DJ, Kogan CS, Atmaca M, et al. The classification of obsessive-compulsive and related disorders in the ICD-11. *J Affect Disord*. 2016;190:663–674.
3. Mataix-Cols D, Frost RO, Pertusa A, et al. Hoarding disorder: a new diagnosis for DSM-V? *Depress Anxiety*. 2010;27:556–572.
4. Phillips KA, Stein DJ, Rauch SL, et al. Should an obsessive-compulsive spectrum grouping of disorders be included in DSM-V? *Depress Anxiety*. 2010;27:528–555.
5. Tolin DF, Villavicencio A. Inattention, but not OCD, predicts the core features of hoarding disorder. *Behav Res Ther*. 2011;49:120–125.
6. Frost RO, Hartl TL. A cognitive-behavioral model of compulsive hoarding. *Behav Res Ther*. 1996;34:341–350.

7. Drury H, Ajmi S, Fernández de la Cruz L, Nordsletten AE, Mataix-Cols D. Caregiver burden, family accommodation, health, and well-being in relatives of individuals with hoarding disorder. *J Affect Disord.* 2014;159:7–14.

8. Frost RO, Steketee G, Williams L. Hoarding: a community health problem. *Health Soc Care Commun.* 2000;8:229–234.

9. Frost RO, Steketee G, Tolin DF. Comorbidity in hoarding disorder. *Depress Anxiety.* 2011;28:876–884.

10. Mataix-Cols D, Billotti D, Fernández de la Cruz L, Nordsletten AE. The London field trial for hoarding disorder. *Psychol Med.* 2013;43:837–847.

11. Frost RO, Tolin DF, Steketee G, Fitch KE, Selbo-Bruns A. Excessive acquisition in hoarding. *J Anxiety Disord.* 2009;23:632–639.

12. Nordsletten AE, Reichenberg A, Hatch SL, et al. Epidemiology of hoarding disorder. *Br J Psychiatry.* 2013;203:445–452.

13. Tolin DF, Fitch KE, Frost RO, Steketee G. Family informants' perceptions of insight in compulsive hoarding. *Cogn Ther Res.* 2010;34:69–81.

14. Snowdon J, Pertusa A, Mataix-Cols D. On hoarding and squalor: a few considerations for DSM-5. *Depress Anxiety.* 2012;29:417–424.

15. Frost RO, Patronek G, Rosenfield E. Comparison of object and animal hoarding. *Depress Anxiety.* 2011;28:885–891.

16. Pertusa A, Fonseca A. Hoarding behavior in other disorders. In: Frost RO, Steketee G, eds. *The Oxford Handbook of Hoarding and Acquiring.* New York, NY: Oxford University Press; 2014:59–74.

17. Anderson SW, Damasio H, Damasio AR. A neural basis for collecting behaviour in humans. *Brain.* 2005;128:201–212.

18. Mataix-Cols D, Pertusa A, Snowdon J. Neuropsychological and neural correlates of hoarding: a practice-friendly review. *J Clin Psychol.* 2011;67:467–476.

19. Pertusa A, Frost RO, Fullana MA, et al. Refining the diagnostic boundaries of compulsive hoarding: a critical review. *Clin Psychol Rev.* 2010;30:371–386.

20. Pertusa A, Fullana MA, Singh S, Alonso P, Menchon JM, Mataix-Cols D. Compulsive hoarding: OCD symptom, distinct clinical syndrome, or both? *Am J Psychiatry.* 2008;165:1289–1298.

21. Samuels J, Bienvenu OJ, Grados MA, et al. Prevalence and correlates of hoarding behavior in a community-based sample. *Behav Res Ther.* 2008;46:836–844.

22. Pertusa A, Frost RO, Mataix-Cols D. When hoarding is a symptom of OCD: a case series and implications for DSM-V. *Behav Res Ther.* 2010;48:1012–1020.

23. Nordsletten AE, Fernández de la Cruz L, Billotti D, Mataix-Cols D. Finders keepers: the features differentiating hoarding disorder from normative collecting. *Compr Psychiatry.* 2013;54:229–237.

24. Nordsletten AE, Mataix-Cols D. Hoarding versus collecting: where does pathology diverge from play? *Clin Psychol Rev.* 2012;32:165–176.

25. Fullana MA, Vilagut G, Rojas-Farreras S, et al. Obsessive-compulsive symptom dimensions in the general population: results from an epidemiological study in six European countries. *J Affect Disord.* 2010;124:291–299.

26. Tolin DF, Meunier SA, Frost RO, Steketee G. Hoarding among patients seeking treatment for anxiety disorders. *J Anxiety Disord.* 2011;25:43–48.

27. Ayers CR, Iqbal Y, Strickland K. Medical conditions in geriatric hoarding disorder patients. *Aging Ment Health.* 2014;18:148–151.

28. Ivanov VZ, Mataix-Cols D, Serlachius E, et al. Prevalence, comorbidity and heritability of hoarding symptoms in adolescence: a population based twin study in 15-year olds. *PloS One.* 2013;8:e69140.

29. Timpano KR, Exner C, Glaesmer H, et al. The epidemiology of the proposed DSM-5 hoarding disorder: exploration of the acquisition specifier, associated features, and distress. *J Clin Psychiatry.* 2011;72:780–789.

30. Grisham JR, Frost RO, Steketee G, Kim HJ, Hood S. Age of onset of compulsive hoarding. *J Anxiety Disord.* 2006;20:675–686.

31. Landau D, Iervolino AC, Pertusa A, Santo S, Singh S, Mataix-Cols D. Stressful life events and material deprivation in hoarding disorder. *J Anxiety Disord.* 2011;25:192–202.

32. Tolin DF, Meunier SA, Frost RO, Steketee G. Course of compulsive hoarding and its relationship to life events. *Depress Anxiety.* 2010;27:829–838.

33. Ayers CR, Saxena S, Golshan S, Wetherell JL. Age at onset and clinical features of late life compulsive hoarding. *Int J Geriatr Psychiatry.* 2010;25:142–149.

34. Fernández de la Cruz L, Nordsletten AE, Mataix-Cols D. Ethnocultural aspects of hoarding disorder. *Curr Psychiatry Rev.* 2016;12:115–123.

35. Nordsletten AE, Fernández de la Cruz L, Aluco E, et al. A transcultural study of hoarding disorder: insights from the United Kingdom, Spain, Japan, and Brazil. *Transcult Psychiatry.* 2018;55:261–285.

36. Iervolino AC, Perroud N, Fullana MA, et al. Prevalence and heritability of compulsive hoarding: a twin study. *Am J Psychiatry.* 2009;166:1156–1161.

37. López-Solà C, Fontenelle LF, Alonso P, et al. Prevalence and heritability of obsessive-compulsive spectrum and

anxiety disorder symptoms: a survey of the Australian Twin Registry. *Am J Med Genet B*. 2014;165:314–325.

38. Mathews CA, Delucchi K, Cath DC, Willemsen G, Boomsma DI. Partitioning the etiology of hoarding and obsessive-compulsive symptoms. *Psychol Med*. 2014;44:2867–2876.
39. Monzani B, Rijsdijk F, Harris J, Mataix-Cols D. The structure of genetic and environmental risk factors for dimensional representations of DSM-5 obsessive-compulsive spectrum disorders. *JAMA Psychiatry*. 2014;71:182–189.
40. Saxena S, Brody AL, Maidment KM, et al. Cerebral glucose metabolism in obsessive-compulsive hoarding. *Am J Psychiat*. 2004;161:1038–1048.
41. An SK, Mataix-Cols D, Lawrence NS, et al. To discard or not to discard: the neural basis of hoarding symptoms in obsessive-compulsive disorder. *Mol Psychiatry*. 2009;14:318–331.
42. Tolin DF, Stevens MC, Villavicencio AL, et al. Neural mechanisms of decision making in hoarding disorder. *Arch Gen Psychiatry*. 2012;69:832–841.
43. Hough CM, Luks TL, Lai K, et al. Comparison of brain activation patterns during executive function tasks in hoarding disorder and non-hoarding OCD. *Psychiatry Res*. 2016;255:50–59.
44. Tolin DF, Witt ST, Stevens MC. Hoarding disorder and obsessive-compulsive disorder show different patterns of neural activity during response inhibition. *Psychiat Res*. 2014;221:142–148.
45. Mathews CA, Perez VB, Roach BJ, et al. Error-related brain activity dissociates hoarding disorder from obsessive-compulsive disorder. *Psychol Med*. 2016;46:367–379.
46. Woody SR, Kellman-McFarlane K, Welsted A. Review of cognitive performance in hoarding disorder. *Clin Psychol Rev*. 2014;34:324–336.
47. Morein-Zamir S, Papmeyer M, Pertusa A, et al. The profile of executive function in OCD hoarders and hoarding disorder. *Psychiatry Res*. 2014;215:659–667.
48. Nordsletten AE, Fernández de la Cruz L, Pertusa A, Reichenberg A, Hatch SL, Mataix-Cols D. The Structured Interview for Hoarding Disorder (SIHD): development, usage and further validation. *J Obsess Compuls Relat Disord*. 2013;2:346–350.
49. Frost RO, Steketee G, Tolin DF, Renaud S. Development and validation of the clutter image rating. *J Psychopathol Behav Assess*. 2008;30:193–203.
50. Fernández de la Cruz L, Nordsletten AE, Billotti D, Mataix-Cols D. Photograph-aided assessment of clutter in hoarding disorder: is a picture worth a thousand words? *Depress Anxiety*. 2013;30:61–66.
51. Tolin DF, Fitch KE, Frost RO, Steketee G. Family informants' perceptions of insight in compulsive hoarding. *Cogn Ther Res*. 2010;34:69–81.
52. Tolin DF, Frost RO, Steketee G. A brief interview for assessing compulsive hoarding: the Hoarding Rating Scale-Interview. *Psychiatry Res*. 2010;178:147–152.
53. Frost RO, Steketee G, Grisham J. Measurement of compulsive hoarding: saving inventory-revised. *Behav Res Ther*. 2004;42:1163–1182.
54. Saxena S, Ayers CR, Dozier ME, Maidment KM. The UCLA hoarding severity scale: development and validation. *J Affect Disord*. 2015;175:488–493.
55. LeBeau RT, Mischel ER, Simpson HB, et al. Preliminary assessment of obsessive-compulsive spectrum disorder scales for DSM-5. *J Obsess Compuls Relat Disord*. 2013;2:114–118.
56. Steketee G, Frost RO, Kyrios M. Cognitive aspects of compulsive hoarding. *Cogn Ther Res*. 2003;27:463–479.
57. Frost RO, Steketee G, Williams L. Compulsive buying, compulsive hoarding, and obsessive-compulsive disorder. *Behav Therapy*. 2002;33:201–214.
58. Halliday G, Snowdon J. The Environmental Cleanliness and Clutter Scale (ECCS). *Int Psychogeriatr*. 2009;21:1041–1050.
59. Snowdon J, Halliday G, Hunt GE. Two types of squalor: findings from a factor analysis of the Environmental Cleanliness and Clutter Scale (ECCS). *Int Psychogeriatr*. 2013;25: 1191–1198.
60. Rasmussen JL, Steketee G, Frost RO, Tolin DF, Brown TA. Assessing squalor in hoarding: the home environment index. *Community Ment Health J*. 2014;50:591–596.
61. Nordsletten AE, Fernández de la Cruz L, Drury H, Ajmi S, Saleem S, Mataix-Cols D. The Family Impact Scale for Hoarding (FISH): measure development and initial validation. *J Obsess Compuls Relat Disord*. 2014;3:29–34.
62. Thompson C, Fernández de la Cruz L, Mataix-Cols D, Onwumere J. A systematic review and quality assessment of psychological, pharmacological, and family-based interventions for hoarding disorder. *Asian J Psychiatr*. 2017;27:53–66.
63. Muroff J, Steketee G, Bratiotis C, Ross A. Group cognitive and behavioral therapy and bibliotherapy for hoarding: a pilot trial. *Depress Anxiety*. 2012;29:597–604.
64. DiMauro J, Genova M, Tolin DF, Kurtz MM. Cognitive remediation for neuropsychological impairment in hoarding disorder: a pilot study. *J Obsess Compuls Relat Disord*. 2014;3:132–138.
65. Ayers CR, Dozier ME, Twamley EW, et al. Cognitive Rehabilitation and Exposure/Sorting Therapy (CREST)

for hoarding disorder in older adults: a randomized clinical trial. *J Clin Psychiatry*. 2018;79:ii. doi: 10.4088/JCP.16m11072.

66. Steketee G, Frost RO, Tolin DF, Rasmussen J, Brown TA. Waitlist-controlled trial of cognitive behavior therapy for hoarding disorder. *Depress Anxiety*. 2010;27:476–484.
67. Frost RO, Ruby D, Shuer LJ. The buried in treasures workshop: waitlist control trial of facilitated support groups for hoarding. *Behav Res Ther*. 2012;50:661–667.
68. Steketee G, Frost RO. *Compulsive Hoarding and Acquiring: Therapist Guide (Treatments That Work)*. New York, NY: Oxford University Press; 2007.
69. Tolin DF, Frost RO, Steketee G, Muroff J. Cognitive behavioral therapy for hoarding disorder: a meta-analysis. *Depress Anxiety*. 2015;32:158–166.
70. Muroff J, Steketee G, Frost RO, Tolin DF. Cognitive behavior therapy for hoarding disorder: follow-up findings and predictors of outcome. *Depress Anxiety*. 2014;31:964–971.
71. Bratiotis C. Community hoarding task forces: a comparative case study of five task forces in the United States. *Health Soc Care Community*. 2013;21:245–253.
72. Bloch MH, Bartley CA, Zipperer L, et al. Meta-analysis: hoarding symptoms associated with poor treatment outcome in obsessive-compulsive disorder. *Mol Psychiatry*. 2014;19:1025–1030.
73. Saxena S, Sumner J. Venlafaxine extended-release treatment of hoarding disorder. *Int Clin Psychopharm*. 2014;29:266–273.
74. Rodriguez CI, Bender J, Jr., Morrison S, Mehendru R, Tolin D, Simpson HB. Does extended release methylphenidate help adults with hoarding disorder?: a case series. *J Clin Psychopharmacol*. 2013;33:444–447.
75. Grassi G, Micheli L, Di Cesare Mannelli L, et al. Atomoxetine for hoarding disorder: a pre-clinical and clinical investigation. *J Psychiatr Res*. 2016;83:240–248.
76. Steketee G, Frost R. Compulsive hoarding: current status of the research. *Clin Psychol Rev*. 2003;23:905–927.
77. Mueller A, Mueller U, Alberta P, et al. Hoarding in a compulsive buying sample. *Behav Res Ther*. 2007;45:2754–2763.
78. Mollenkamp M, de Zwaan M, Muller A. Hoarding with and without excessive buying: results of a pilot study. *Psychopathology*. 2015;48:56–59.
79. Muller A, Mitchell JE, de Zwaan M. Compulsive buying. *Am J Addiction*. 2015;24:132–137.
80. Samuels J, Bienvenu OJ, Riddle MA, et al. Hoarding in obsessive compulsive disorder: results from a case-control study. *Behav Res Ther*. 2002;40:517–528.
81. Frost RO, Meagher BM, Riskind JH. Obsessive-compulsive features in pathological lottery and scratch-ticket gamblers. *J Gambl Stud*. 2001;17:5–19.
82. Fishbain DA. Do compulsive buyers and kleptomaniacs share identical characteristics? *J Clin Psychiatry*. 1994;55:545–546.
83. Lynch FA, McGillivray JA, Moulding R, Byrne LK. Hoarding in attention deficit hyperactivity disorder: understanding the comorbidity. *J Obsess Compuls Relat Disord*. 2015;4:37–46.
84. Hacker LE, Park JM, Timpano KR, et al. Hoarding in children with ADHD. *J Atten Disord*. 2016;20:617–626.
85. Grisham JR, Brown TA, Savage CR, Steketee G, Barlow DH. Neuropsychological impairment associated with compulsive hoarding. *Behav Res Ther*. 2007;45:1471–1483.
86. McMillan SG, Rees CS, Pestell C. An investigation of executive functioning, attention and working memory in compulsive hoarding. *Behav Cogn Psychother*. 2013;41:610–625.
87. Woerner M, Selles RR, De Nadai AS, Salloum A, Storch EA. Hoarding in college students: exploring compulsive spectrum and ADHD. *J Obsess Compuls Relat Disord*. 2017;12:95–101.
88. Sheppard B, Chavira D, Azzam A, et al. ADHD Prevalence and association with hoarding behaviors in childhood-onset OCD. *Depress Anxiety*. 2010;27:667–674.
89. Fullana MA, Vilagut G, Mataix-Cols D, et al. Is ADHD in childhood associated with lifetime hoarding symptoms? An epidemiological study. *Depress Anxiety*. 2013; 30:741–748.
90. Wu KD, Watson D. Hoarding and its relation to obsessive-compulsive disorder. *Behav Res Ther*. 2005;43:897–921.
91. Abramowitz JS, Wheaton MG, Storch EA. The status of hoarding as a symptom of obsessive-compulsive disorder. *Behav Res Ther*. 2008;46:1026–1033.
92. Reiss S, Peterson RA, Gursky DM, McNally RJ. Anxiety sensitivity, anxiety frequency and the prediction of fearfulness. *Behav Res Ther*. 1986;24:1–8.
93. Taylor S, Koch WJ, Mcnally RJ. How does anxiety sensitivity vary across the anxiety disorders. *J Anxiety Disord*. 1992;6:249–259.
94. Raines AM, Oglesby ME, Allan NP, Short NA, Schmidt NB. Understanding DSM-5 hoarding disorder: a triple vulnerability model. *Psychiatry*. 2016;79:120–129.
95. Medley AN, Capron DW, Korte KJ, Schmidt NB. Anxiety sensitivity: a potential vulnerability factor for compulsive hoarding. *Cogn Behav Therapy*. 2013;42:45–55.

96. Timpano KR, Buckner JD, Richey JA, Murphy DL, Schmidt NB. Exploration of anxiety sensitivity and distress tolerance as vulnerability factors for hoarding behaviors. *Depress Anxiety.* 2009;26:343–353.

97. Coles ME, Frost RO, Heimberg RG, Steketee G. Hoarding behaviors in a large college sample. *Behav Res Ther.* 2003;41:179–194.

98. Hayes SC, Strosahl KD, Wilson KG. *Acceptance and Commitment Therapy: An Experiential Approach to Behavior Change.* New York, NY: Guilford Press; 1999.

99. Fernández de la Cruz L, Landau D, Iervolino AC, et al. Experiential avoidance and emotion regulation difficulties in hoarding disorder. *J Anxiety Disord.* 2013;27:204–209.

100. Wheaton MG, Abramowitz JS, Franklin JC, Berman NC, Fabricant LE. Experiential avoidance and saving cognitions in the prediction of hoarding symptoms. *Cogn Ther Res.* 2011;35:511–516.

101. Ayers CR, Castriotta N, Dozier ME, Espejo EP, Porter B. Behavioral and experiential avoidance in patients with hoarding disorder. *J Behav Ther Exp Psychiatry.* 2014;45:408–414.

102. Gratz KL, Roemer L. Multidimensional assessment of emotion regulation and dysregulation: development, factor structure, and initial validation of the difficulties in emotion regulation scale. *J Psychopathol Behav Assess.* 2004;26:41–54.

103. Berking M, Wupperman P. Emotion regulation and mental health: recent findings, current challenges, and future directions. *Curr Opin Psychiatry.* 2012;25:128–134.

104. Phung PJ, Moulding R, Taylor JK, Nedeljkovic M. Emotional regulation, attachment to possessions and hoarding symptoms. *Scand J Psychol.* 2015;56:573–581.

105. Raines AM, Chavarria J, Allan NP, Short NA, Schmidt NB. Hoarding behaviors and alcohol use: the mediating role of emotion dysregulation. *Subst Use Misuse.* 2017:1–8.

106. Raines AM, Boffa JW, Allan NP, Short NA, Schmidt NB. Hoarding and eating pathology: the mediating role of emotion regulation. *Compr Psychiatry.* 2015;57:29–35.

107. Miller W, Rollnick S. *Motivational Interviewing: Preparing People for Change.* New York, NY: Guilford Press; 2002.

108. Amiaz R, Fostick L, Gershon A, Zohar J. Naltrexone augmentation in OCD: a double-blind placebo-controlled cross-over study. *Eur Neuropsychopharmacol.* 2008;18:455–461.

Chapter 26

Transdiagnostic Factors in Obsessive-Compulsive Personality Disorder

Michael G. Wheaton and Anthony Pinto

Introduction

Clinical Picture and Diagnosis

Obsessive-compulsive personality disorder (OCPD) is a chronic and impairing condition characterized by maladaptive perfectionism, preoccupation with orderliness and detail and an excessive need to exert control over one's environment [1]. Individuals with OCPD are often described as being rigid and inflexible interpersonally, resulting in impaired social functioning. They frequently experience high levels of internal distress, causing high rates of treatment, both in medical and mental health settings.

Although the central features of OCPD were noted in the literature more than 100 years ago, OCPD remains an understudied phenomenon, with several important questions outstanding. In fact, the current diagnostic system includes two separate conceptualizations of OCPD, suggesting that some elements of OCPD remain in flux. The first section of this chapter reviews the essential features of OCPD according to the current model, as well as recent data on the prevalence, associated features and available treatments for OCPD.

The fifth edition of the *Diagnostic and Statistical Manual of Mental Disorders* (DSM-5) [1] provides two sets of diagnostic criteria for OCPD. The first of these is based on the existing model of OCPD as a categorical entity as defined in previous editions of the DSM. The first edition of the DSM [2] included a description of "compulsive personality" based on the Freudian concept of the "anal character" (characterized by excessive orderliness and obstinacy). Subsequent editions of the DSM expanded and refined this notion to define OCPD based on the presence of a set of polythetic criteria.

The current set of criteria employed in DSM-5 are the same as in DSM-IV [3] and define OCPD as a pervasive pattern of preoccupation with orderliness, perfectionism, and mental and interpersonal control as indicated by at least four of the following criteria: (1) preoccupation with details, (2) self-limiting perfectionism, (3) excessive devotion to work/productivity, (4) excessive conscientiousness with regard to morals/ethics, (5) difficulty discarding worn-out or useless items, (6) difficulty delegating, (7) miserliness and (8) rigidity and stubbornness. Notably, to meet diagnostic criteria for OCPD, the patient can endorse any combination of four of these eight criteria, leading to heterogeneity in symptom presentation across patients with OCPD.

The second diagnostic conceptualization of OCPD in DSM-5 is contained in the appendix (Section III), among the emerging measures and models for future study. This section is intended as an alternative model for research, which proposes a reconceptualization of personality disorders broadly based on a hybrid dimensional–categorical model. This model aims to account for the variation in personality traits present in the population (which may be distributed along a continuum), while also retaining diagnostic categories to identify individuals with personality disorders. In this model, a personality disorder is present when there is a significant disruption in personality functioning as demonstrated in at least two life domains (including identity, self-direction, empathy and intimacy). Personality pathology can then be divided into personality disorder types based on characteristic pathological personality traits.

The cardinal feature of OCPD according to this model is *rigid perfectionism* (pursuit of perfection at the expense of task completion). In addition, patients must also meet criteria for at least one other characteristic OCPD trait: perseveration (a pattern of persisting in nonfunctional behaviors), intimacy avoidance (problems manifest in close relationships and attachments) and restricted affectivity (reduced ability to experience inner

Table 26.1 DSM-5 criteria for obsessive-compulsive personality disorder.

Model	DSM-5 Criteria
Official criteria for diagnosis and treatment	A. A pervasive pattern of preoccupation with orderliness, perfectionism and mental and interpersonal control as indicated by four or more of the following: 1. Preoccupation with details 2. Perfectionism 3. Excessive devotion to work 4. Overconscientiousness/ hypermorality 5. Inability to discard worthless objects 6. Reluctance to delegate tasks 7. Miserliness 8. Rigidity
Alternative model for OCPD for research	A. At least moderate impairment in personality functioning, defined as difficulty in two or more domains: 1. Identity (e.g., sense of self with undue emphasis on work productivity) 2. Self-direction (e.g., difficulty completing tasks due to unrealistic goals and standards) 3. Empathy (e.g., difficulty appreciating the viewpoints of others) 4. Intimacy (e.g., relationship conflict caused by rigidity and stubbornness) B. Three or more pathological personality traits, one of which must be [1]: 1. Rigid perfectionism (e.g., pursuit of perfection that interferes with task completion) 2. Perseveration (e.g., persistence in tasks beyond what would be considered functional) 3. Intimacy avoidance (e.g., impairment in interpersonal attachments) 4. Restricted affectivity (e.g., limited emotional experience, with little reaction to emotional events)

emotions or ability to express only a limited range of emotions). Table 26.1 presents the criteria for both the official and alternative diagnostic conceptualizations for OCPD in DSM-5 for comparison.

The alternative OCPD criteria set represents an important change from the previous conceptualization. By including perfectionism as a necessary feature, this alternative model may be more narrow because the group defined as having OCPD by this criteria set may be less heterogeneous [4]. In addition, the alternative model adds new criteria (perseveration, intimacy avoidance and restricted affectivity) and deletes several of the current DSM criteria (e.g., miserliness, difficulty discarding worn-out/worthless items, difficulty delegating tasks). These changes suggest that some individuals who would meet existing DSM-IV/5 criteria would no longer be diagnosed under the alternative model and vice versa.

These differences also have important implications for estimating community prevalence rates as well as developing treatments. Unfortunately, research investigating the alternative model remains in its early stages and therefore the majority of this section reviews studies that have employed the official DSM-IV/5 criteria set in terms of prevalence and treatment. However we return to the alternative model of OCPD later in this chapter in relation to transdiagnostic approaches to obsessions and compulsions.

Recent Research Findings

Prevalence

According to DSM-5, OCPD is one of the most common personality disorders in the general population, with an estimated lifetime prevalence of 2.1% to 7.9% [1]. This estimate represents a marked increase from the previous estimate in DSM-IV of approximately 1% prevalence in the community [3]. However, the more recent estimate reported in DSM-5 is in line with epidemiological studies, which suggest a 7.7–7.8% prevalence rate [5,6].

The DSM-5 suggests a distinct gender imbalance in OCPD prevalence, estimating that OCPD is approximately twice as common in men compared with women. Of note however, research reports from the community have provided mixed findings regarding this gender imbalance. For example, while some studies have indeed reported OCPD to be more common in males [7], two large community-based studies reported equal prevalence in OCPD for men and women [6,8]. Some clinical samples of treatment-seeking patients have also reported no difference in OCPD rates by gender [9,10].

Similarly, results are inconsistent as to whether OCPD is more common in some communities. Whereas some studies suggest that OCPD has equal prevalence among ethnic/racial groups [10,11], two nationally representative studies reported significantly lower rates of OCPD in Asian-American and Hispanic participants compared with white and African-American participants [6,8]. Other data suggest that OCPD may be relatively common in outpatient samples from the Hispanic population, with one study estimating that up to 26% of this population had OCPD [12].

Importantly, all of the prevalence estimates reported above have only employed existing DSM-IV/5 criteria. As of now, no study has formally estimated the prevalence of OCPD when diagnosed with the alternative DSM-5 criteria set, although it has been suggested that the prevalence rate using the new criteria may be somewhat lower due to their "stricter" nature [4].

Course

As with all personality disorders, OCPD is typically diagnosed in adulthood. Rates of OCPD diagnosis may increase with age, as an epidemiological study found that OCPD was less prevalent in younger individuals (aged 20–29 years) than in individuals older than 30 years [8]. However, some studies suggest that OCPD traits may begin in childhood [13]. Although personality disorders are typically considered to be chronic conditions, evidence that OCPD diagnoses are stable across time has been somewhat mixed. For example Nestadt et al. [14] found OCPD to be less temporally stable than certain other personality disorders (antisocial, avoidant, borderline, histrionic and schizotypal), though this study employed DSM-III criteria. A study employing DSM-IV/5 criteria found OCPD diagnoses to be somewhat more stable, with half of individuals diagnosed with OCPD continuing to meet diagnostic criteria two years later [15]. It is possible that the use of polythetic criteria and associated heterogeneity of symptom profiles may have contributed to some of the temporal inconsistencies reported in these studies. It is therefore possible that the alternative DSM-5 criteria set will evidence better temporal stability.

Impairment and Treatment Take-Up

In spite of the commonly held misconception that perfectionism is an adaptive trait, individuals with OCPD suffer from marked impairment in their functioning. The great majority of OCPD sufferers (nearly 90% in the Collaborative Longitudinal Personality Disorders Study sample [16]) are estimated to have at least moderate impairment in one or more life domains. In addition, individuals with OCPD report significantly lower levels of quality of life compared with the general community [17]. In fact, a 2014 study estimated equivalent impairment in quality of life and psychosocial functioning comparing individuals with OCPD to patients with obsessive-compulsive disorder (OCD) [18].

Of all life domains, OCPD is typically most associated with impaired interpersonal functioning. Sufferers with OCPD often become involved in social conflicts, frequently relating to their impossibly high standards for the behavior of others and need for control [19]. Individuals with OCPD are known to have difficulty delegating tasks and often come across as being uncompromising and demanding of others [20]. As a potential explanation for these interpersonal difficulties, a 2014 study of interpersonal functioning reported that individuals with OCPD had more hostile-dominant interpersonal problems and less empathic perspective taking relative to healthy controls [21].

Not surprisingly, individuals with OCPD frequently present for treatment and have high rates of treatment take-up, including both primary care [22] and psychotherapy [23]. In fact, some data suggest that individuals with OCPD are up to three times more likely than patients with depression to seek and receive psychotherapy [23].

Etiology

Several models have been postulated to account for the etiology of OCPD, including both biological and psychological conceptualizations.

Biological Models

Biological models have focused on genetic and neurochemical influences on OCPD traits. In terms of genetic contributions, an early twin study using DSM-III-R criteria found substantial heritability for OCPD diagnoses (0.8 [24]). However research on specific vulnerability genes has been inconclusive as yet. In a community study, Blom et al. [25] found a single nucleotide polymorphism in the promoter region of the serotonin transporter gene (*SLC64A*, designated 5HTTPLPR) to be linked to OCPD traits, albeit with a specific gender moderation; whereas men with the short form of the gene have fewer OCPD traits, the relationship was the opposite in women [25].

However, this specific gene has been commonly linked to both anxiety and depression [26] suggesting that it is not specific to OCPD. Another study found no difference in serotonin transporter promoter genes comparing individuals with OCPD with healthy controls [27]. In terms of neurochemistry, some data suggest a role for altered serotonergic functioning in OCPD. For example, one report found males with OCPD had blunted fenfluramine-mediated prolactin responses (indicating serotonergic dysfunction) compared with healthy controls and patients with other personality disorders [28].

Neurocognitive models

Some have suggested that OCPD traits (e.g., preoccupation with rules and organization, inflexibility) may represent attempts to compensate for executive functioning deficits [29]. In line with this approach, some studies have reported impaired functioning on neuropsychological assessments in individuals with OCPD. For example, a 2015 comprehensive study [30] administered the Cambridge Neuropsychological Test Automated Battery (CANTAB) to individuals high and low in OCPD traits.

Results showed that the high OCPD trait group had performance deficits in spatial working memory and attentional set shifting. Similarly, in another 2015 study using the CANTAB, Fineberg et al. [31] reported impaired performance indicating cognitive inflexibility and executive planning deficits among 21 adults meeting DSM-IV criteria for OCPD compared with 15 healthy controls.

Psychological Models

Psychological conceptualizations of OCPD have evolved over time. Early models derived from the psychoanalytic tradition formulated OCPD as involving fixation at the anal stage of development [32]. According to this account, struggles with parental figures (e.g., over issues such as toilet training) result in an overdeveloped and punitive superego, although notably these approaches were not empirically investigated [33].

Subsequently, behavioral models emphasized the role of early learning that reinforces strict behavioral control and punishes novelty and affection, leading to patterns of rigid behavior and overcontrol of emotions [20,34]. Cognitive models then expanded upon these perspectives by incorporating the role of beliefs and schemas, including dichotomous thinking ("anything less than perfection is failure") and the need for control ("other people will make mistakes"). The current cognitive-behavioral conceptualization is supported by a growing body of research [35].

Dimensional Models

Dimensional approaches to personality disorders suggest that all personality traits exist along a continuum in the population, and that individuals with personality disorders (including OCPD) may simply represent the extreme end of the distribution of a combination of traits. The most widely used dimensional model of personality traits is the five-factor model [36], which identifies the following five basic traits: openness, neuroticism, agreeableness, extraversion and conscientiousness. Of these five traits, OCPD has consistently been linked to elevated levels of conscientiousness [37,38], which includes concerns related to order, dutifulness, self-discipline, competence and deliberation.

The hybrid model of personality disorders offered as an alternative model in DSM-5 incorporates a dimensional approach. This model is based on the idea that personality disorders result from a combination of stable personality traits and less stable symptomatic behaviors [39]. Whereas traits are thought to be dimensional in nature (ranging from adaptive to pathological), symptomatic behaviors (dysfunctional adaptations used to compensate for pathological traits) are considered categorical (present or absent). Dimensional conceptualizations of OCPD are in line with transdiagnostic approaches, as discussed in more detail below.

Treatment

Despite the high rate at which individuals with OCPD seek health care, there is remarkably little research on treatments for primary OCPD. Although there is no empirically supported "gold standard" treatment for OCPD, limited data support both medication and psychotherapeutic approaches.

Pharmacotherapy

Perhaps surprisingly, there has been only one published controlled trial evaluating the efficacy of psychiatric medication as a treatment for OCPD [40]. In this small trial (24 patients), individuals with DSM-IV OCPD without comorbid depression were randomized to receive fluvoxamine (a selective serotonin reuptake inhibitor, SSRI) or pill placebo for up to 12 weeks.

Results showed that those treated with fluvoxamine (n = 12) had significantly greater improvement in OCPD trait severity compared with individuals in the placebo group (n = 12). However, OCPD is noted to co-occur with mood and anxiety disorders typically treated with serotonin reuptake inhibitors (SRIs) and trials for these conditions present some additional evidence suggesting that OCPD symptoms may respond to these medications. For example, in an early trial of SRI treatment (clomipramine and imipramine) for OCD, Volavka et al. [41] reported that 12 weeks of treatment was associated with significant reduction in co-occurring OCPD symptoms as measured using the Self-Rating Obsessive-Compulsive Personality Inventory. Similarly, in a large trial of patients with depression (n = 308), treatment with 24 weeks of an SSRI (citalopram or sertraline) was associated with a significant reduction in OCPD symptoms [42]. In light of the relative lack of controlled medication trials, treatment recommendations for OCPD typically focus on psychotherapy [33], or recommend a combination of SSRI pharmacotherapy and psychotherapy [35]. However, as discussed below, empirical work validating psychotherapy for OCPD also suffers from several limitations, such as relying on open studies with mixed samples, or comparing two active treatments.

Psychodynamic Psychotherapy

Psychodynamic treatment employs an insight-oriented approach to examine how OCPD trait behaviors may function to protect the individual against internal feelings of insecurity and distress. The rationale for this approach is that with increased insight, patients with OCPD would then be empowered to improve their interpersonal functioning by relinquishing inflexible patterns and demands for perfection. Some empirical work supports the use of this form of therapy as a treatment for OCPD. For example, Barber et al. [43] conducted an uncontrolled trial of supportive-expressive psychodynamic therapy for a mixed personality disorder sample and reported significant improvement among 14 individuals with OCPD after 52 treatment sessions.

Two subsequent psychodynamic trials that also employed mixed personality disorder samples (including some with OCPD) also reported improvement in general functioning relative to waitlist control groups [44,45], though neither of these two studies specifically investigated improvement among those with OCPD. In the first trial, Winston [45] randomized 81 patients with personality disorders to short-term psychodynamic psychotherapy (n = 25), brief adaptive psychotherapy (n = 30) or waitlist (n = 26). Both psychotherapies led to improved scores on the Symptom Checklist-90 and Social Adjustment Scale relative to waitlist (there were no significant differences between therapies). Although 36 patients (44% of the sample) were diagnosed with a cluster C personality disorder, the authors did not report how many specifically had OCPD, limiting the ability of this study to provide evidence for OCPD specifically.

In the second trial, Abbass et al. [44] randomized 27 patients to intensive short-term dynamic psychotherapy or minimal contact waitlist control. Ten patients (37% of the sample) met criteria for OCPD, making it the second most common personality disorder in the sample after borderline personality disorder (44.4%). Results revealed that the treatment group experienced significantly greater improvement in scores on the Brief Symptom Inventory and the Inventory of Interpersonal Problems. Importantly these trials evaluated outcomes in terms of global functioning and improvement and have not assessed changes in OCPD symptoms specifically. Thus, additional work is needed to support the effectiveness of psychodynamic psychotherapy for OCPD.

Cognitive-Behavioral Therapy

CBT typically involves a combination of both cognitive and behavioral techniques. The general cognitive therapy approach involves identifying and restructuring the maladaptive cognitions and dysfunctional beliefs associated with pathological emotions [46,47]. In the case of OCPD, cognitive approaches have focused on restructuring cognitive distortions such as "all or nothing" thinking to lessen the individual's tendencies to be rigid, overestimate negative consequences and catastrophize minor imperfections [46,47,48]. CBT often also includes behavioral elements, such as exposure to feared situations and stimuli (e.g., purposefully making small mistakes) [33]. Although several approaches to treating OCPD with CBT have been described [49], relatively little empirical research has been conducted as of yet.

In the largest ever trial of CBT for OCPD, Enero et al. [50] enrolled 116 outpatients who met DSM-IV criteria for OCPD in an open trial of ten weeks of group therapy for OCPD consisting of psychoeducation, cognitive restructuring, behavioral experiments and relapse prevention planning. They reported significant reductions in OCPD severity following treatment and that pretreatment distress predicted OCPD response rate such that patients with lower levels of trait anxiety and depression were more likely to show a response in OCPD symptoms following treatment. However, a notable limitation of this trial is that it did not include a control group. These results are in line with previous studies of cognitive therapy for OCPD, which have also showed positive effects but are limited by small sample sizes and lack of control groups. For example, an open trial of cognitive therapy focusing on OCPD conducted in Hong Kong [51], demonstrated significant improvement in anxiety and depression symptoms in a small sample ($n = 10$) of individuals with co-occurring OCPD and major depression. Moreover, at post-treatment, nine of ten patients no longer met diagnostic criteria for OCPD. However, as mentioned, sample size was small and there was no control group.

Similarly, Strauss et al. [52] conducted an open trial of cognitive therapy for a mixed personality disorder sample, and reported positive effects in a sub-group of patients with OCPD ($n = 16$), among whom 83% had clinically significant reductions in OCPD trait severity and 53% had clinically significant improvement in depression. However, this trial did not include a comparison condition.

There are few data to suggest which form of psychotherapy (psychodynamics or CBT) is superior in the treatment of OCPD, as very few studies have directly compared these two modalities. In one study, Svartberg et al. [53] randomized a mixed personality disorder group (including OCPD, avoidant and dependent personality disorders) to 40 sessions of either cognitive ($n = 25$) or short-term psychodynamic therapy ($n = 25$). Avoidant was the most frequent personality disorder in the sample, though OCPD was also relatively common, comprising 32% of the cognitive therapy group and 36% of the psychodynamic group. Results showed that both treatment groups demonstrated significant improvement in distress, interpersonal problems and core personality pathology (at post-treatment and at two-year follow-up). There was no significant difference in improvement comparing CBT and psychodynamic treatments across the full sample. However, the authors did not specifically compare treatment effects for the patients with OCPD in particular. Thus, it is unclear whether CBT and psychodynamic treatments are equally effective and more work is needed in this area.

It is noteworthy that all of the extant OCPD treatment literature has used the categorical approach to conceptualizing OCPD (as codified in DSM-III and DSM-IV). To date, no trials have specifically enrolled patients diagnosed with the hybrid dimensional-categorical approach to OCPD proposed in DSM-5.

Transdiagnostic Approaches and Their Implications for Classification and Diagnosis

Transdiagnostic approaches to OCPD have often focused on the relationship between OCPD and OCD. These two conditions share a longstanding yet frequently misunderstood relationship. Historical clinical opinion closely linked the two conditions, as early psychoanalysts often referred to the features of both OCD and OCPD as obsessive-compulsive neurosis [54]. Indeed, there is some overlap in the symptoms of the two conditions as individuals with OCPD often make lists as a function of being preoccupied with details; at the same time, excessive list-making is considered an OCD compulsion as listed on the Yale-Brown Obsessive Compulsive Scale [55,56] symptom checklist.

However, on a functional level, the symptoms of OCD and OCPD appear qualitatively distinct. OCD symptoms (intrusive, distressing, time-consuming obsessions and compulsions aimed at relieving obsessional anxiety) are considered to be *ego-dystonic* because they are experienced as unwanted and upsetting. In contrast, OCPD symptoms are often considered *ego-syntonic*, as they are viewed to be rational and appropriate by the individual. Further, while OCD and OCPD are both impairing disorders marked by repetitive time-consuming behaviors (e.g., list-making, rereading and rewriting to improve work, checking for mistakes), they can be differentiated by the presence of obsessions in OCD [18]. Thus, despite apparent similarities, consensus opinion conceptualizes OCD and OCPD as distinct entities.

Yet despite the differences between OCD and OCPD, these conditions can and do co-occur. Recent estimates using DSM-IV criteria have found high rates of OCPD in OCD patients, ranging from 23% to 32% [9,57,58]. The comorbidity rate was even higher among some treatment-seeking OCD samples (47.3%) [59]. Transdiagnostic approaches suggest that the substantial rates of co-occurrence may be driven by overlap in transdiagnostic processes that could contribute to the development of both conditions. For example, in a recent theoretical review paper, Fineberg et al. [60] propose that OCPD and OCD share common features of "compulsivity", defined as repetitive urges to perform a narrow repertoire of behaviors designed to relieve distress. In OCD, this compulsivity is seen to manifest as repetitive compulsive behaviors, while in OCPD, individuals are highly bound by rules and routines. In addition, the new alternative model of OCPD proposed in DSM-5 suggests that perseveration (persistence in tasks beyond what would be considered functional) be considered as a specific OCPD characteristic trait, which would seem to overlap substantially with the concept of compulsivity. The DSM-5 does not offer specific guidelines for differentiating perseverative behaviors from compulsive behaviors. The description of perseverative behaviors would appear to apply to a broad class of repetitive behaviors (marked by continuance of the same behavior despite repeated failures or clear reasons for stopping), and perseveration is often noted in diverse conditions including traumatic brain injury, attention deficit and hyperactivity disorder and autism spectrum disorders. Compulsive behaviors are often described in terms of attempts to escape a negative internal emotional state (e.g., anxiety or distress) or to prevent feared consequences, suggesting that compulsive behaviors are often experienced as being unwanted (ego-dystonic). In contrast, perseverative behaviors may be experienced in a more ego-syntonic way, and the DSM-5 alternative model considers perseveration to be a facet of the broad personality trait domain negative affectivity.

Fineberg et al. [60] further discuss the possibility that based on shared features of compulsivity, OCPD perhaps could be considered for inclusion within the module of OCD-related disorders (including body dysmorphic disorder, hoarding disorder, trichotillomania and excoriation disorder). As the authors discuss, it is possible that classifying OCPD as an OCD-related disorder might revitalize neuropsychological investigation of the disorder, reduce stigma, and facilitate comparative study with other disorders that share compulsivity as a key mechanism. However, in DSM-5, OCPD was maintained in the personality disorders module. In our opinion, increased research from a transdiagnostic viewpoint might allow researchers to transcend these classification boundaries.

In their proposed dimensional psychiatry model, Robbins et al. [61] differentiate between conditions defined by impulsivity (characterized by poorly planned maladaptive behaviors that result in negative consequences) and compulsivity (in which individuals persist in actions that are no longer appropriate to the situation or result in undesirable consequences). To the extent that compulsivity and impulsivity populate opposite ends of a spectrum of behaviors, tasks of self-control might be conceptualized to distinguish between the two (i.e., impulsive individuals would seek immediate rewards whereas compulsive individuals would prioritize delayed rewards).

In a 2014 investigation, Pinto et al. [18] employed a neuropsychological test of the capacity to delay reward to study self-control in relation to OCPD. Specifically, the authors compared patients diagnosed with DSM-IV OCPD (n = 25) to patients with OCD (n = 25), as well as those with comorbid OCD and OCPD (n = 25) and healthy controls (n = 25), on an intertemporal choice task in which participants were asked whether they would prefer a smaller amount of money immediately or a larger amount offered later.

Results showed that the participants with OCPD (including those with comorbid OCD) showed less temporal discounting, indicating an increased capacity to delay reward, relative to individuals with OCD and healthy controls. The excessive self-control demonstrated by those with OCPD could be conceptualized as excessive compulsivity (as opposed to impulsivity). Moreover, the conceptualization of compulsivity is congruent with the behavioral phenotype of perfectionism, rigidity and a desire to control one's environment.

Another transdiagnostic process associated with both OCPD and OCD is perfectionism. In the alternative model of OCPD proposed in DSM-5, maladaptive perfectionism is hierarchically linked to OCPD in that it is required for the diagnosis as a characteristic OCPD trait. Yet perfectionism is also frequently noted in OCD, as many studies have found that patients with OCD display significantly higher levels of perfectionism than controls [62,63]. Perfectionism has also been described as a contributing factor to OCD, as beliefs about the need for perfection are included among those postulated to relate to the etiology and maintenance of OCD (so-called "obsessive beliefs" [64]). Thus perfectionism may drive some of the association between OCD and OCPD.

Perfectionism has also been linked to many other psychiatric conditions and conceptualized as a transdiagnostic process. For example, a 2011 review [65] found elevated rates of perfectionism among participants with eating disorders, anxiety disorders and mood disorders. In addition, perfectionism has also been implicated across personality disorders [66], offering further evidence for the transdiagnostic role of perfectionism.

The idea that perfectionism may contribute to multiple conditions might explain some of the high rates of comorbidity between OCPD and other disorders. For example depressive disorders are very commonly observed in OCPD patients. In the Collaborative Longitudinal Personality Disorders Study dataset, more than 75% of individuals with OCPD met lifetime criteria for major depression [67]. Of note, perfectionism has been linked to the development of depression [68].

Finally, a third transdiagnostic factor recently associated with OCPD is experiential avoidance, a construct from the field of acceptance and commitment therapy (ACT) [69]. Experiential avoidance has been conceptualized as an unwillingness to experience or remain in contact with unpleasant emotions, thoughts and sensations, coupled with deliberate attempts to escape from and avoid these experiences [69]. Heightened experiential avoidance has been suggested to be a contributing factor to several forms of psychopathology, including mood and anxiety disorders as well as substance use disorders and borderline personality disorder [69,70].

A 2016 study reported that individuals with self-identified OCPD ($n = 53$) endorsed heightened levels of experiential avoidance relative to community controls ($n = 571$), even after accounting for group differences in distress symptoms [17]. Moreover, experiential avoidance mediated the relationship between higher OCPD trait severity and worse quality of life. Although it requires replication, this study suggests that experiential avoidance may be another transdiagnostic factor contributing to OCPD features. In line with the clinical phenotype of OCPD, difficulty experiencing unpleasant inner experiences (i.e., negative thoughts and emotions) could relate to the restricted affectivity noted in OCPD as well as the attempt to exert control over one's inner emotional state.

Recent advances in transdiagnostic approaches to psychopathology offer several potential benefits to how OCPD is diagnosed and categorized. Elucidation of distinct processes that contribute to OCPD, including but not necessarily limited to those discussed here, offer a potential lens to understand the heterogeneity that has been described in the OCPD phenotype. Specifically, if one were to imagine these contributing factors as related and yet distinct factors, the manifest differences observed in OCPD presentations could be understood in terms of varying degrees of underlying transdiagnostic factors. In addition, consistent with dimensional models of OCPD traits reviewed above, transdiagnostic approaches suggest an alternative model in which OCPD severity may be distributed continuously in the population, rather than solely present as an all or none category.

Clinical Implications of Transdiagnostic Approaches for Treatment and Prevention

Recent advances in transdiagnostic approaches to OCPD may also offer avenues to improve OCPD treatments. Specifically, to the extent that these transdiagnostic features contribute to the development and maintenance of OCPD, they also represent potential treatment targets. For example, some empirical and theoretical work has already been done to develop a treatment protocol for transdiagnostic perfectionism.

Fairburn et al. [71] developed a protocol for perfectionism targeting four elements: (i) identifying perfectionism as a problem and establishing what maintains it (e.g., avoidance, checking and, cognitive biases); (ii) conducting behavioral experiments to challenge beliefs and interpretations (e.g., reducing rewriting rituals, exposure to small mistakes); (iii) psychoeducation and cognitive techniques to modify personal standards, rigidity and self-criticism; (iv) encouraging a broader and more flexible self-evaluation system so that self-esteem is not wholly dependent on not making errors. CBT for clinical perfectionism (CBT-P) has been found to reduce perfectionistic thinking and behaviors in several trials [72,73,74].

Although this exact manual has not been tested in a clinical trial of individuals meeting full diagnostic criteria for OCPD, Pinto [75] describes positive results from using elements of CBT-P with an individual patient with OCPD. Although CBT-P is quite similar in some respects to the existing CBT for OCPD, its focus on perfectionism broadly may help to focus the treatment on a particularly important aspect of OCPD. Specifically, a treatment focused on perfectionism may be clinically important, as perfectionism has been identified as a risk factor for suicidal ideation [76].

Transdiagnostic models of compulsivity have associated compulsive behaviors with abnormalities in frontostriatal brain circuits, suggesting that pharmacological interventions acting on these targets might help in a range of conditions characterized by compulsivity [61]. This raises the possibility of testing novel medication treatments for OCPD, which given the paucity of pharmacotherapy trials conducted to date, would be important. Targeting compulsivity might also involve novel psychotherapeutic ideas for OCPD.

For example, Gillan et al. [77] published in 2017 a transdiagnostic model of OCD that emphasizes compulsivity as a key factor in the disorder, as manifest by the excessive tendency toward habitual behaviors. They proposed that OCD treatment might be improved by supplementing standard exposure and response prevention treatment with habit reversal training. It could also be the case that psychotherapy for OCPD could be improved with added techniques to help break habitual routines as a way of decreasing compulsivity. However, this possibility requires empirical testing.

The transdiagnostic process of experiential avoidance is one of the primary therapeutic targets of ACT [69]. ACT targets experiential avoidance by encouraging patients to accept and endure negative inner experiences (e.g., emotions, thoughts and memories) through the use of metaphors, mindfulness training and behavioral therapy techniques. Some evidence suggests that directly targeting experiential avoidance in treatment leads to symptom improvement for disorders such as depression and post-traumatic stress disorder [70].

When applied to OCPD, ACT might involve educating individuals with OCPD about the paradoxical consequences of emotional avoidance (i.e., attempts to control or eliminate unpleasant emotional states often amplify emotions and drive problematic coping strategies). Treatment would instead encourage individuals with OCPD to accept and tolerate negative emotional experiences rather than reacting in a controlling way.

For example, patients could work to mindfully tolerate distressing emotions caused by imperfection and sudden changes in plans without immediately attempting to control the environment or situation. However, to date, there have been no trials of ACT for OCPD, though a single case study describes the use of emotion regulation skills (which also may target experiential avoidance) in the successful treatment of an individual with OCPD [75]. Thus, future work testing interventions targeting experiential avoidance as OCPD treatments is needed.

Future Directions

OCPD is an impairing condition characterized by maladaptive perfectionism, rigidity and excessive need for control. Although OCPD has been the subject of clinical and research attention for more than a century, much remains unknown about how to best conceptualize and treat individuals with this disorder. Existing biological and psychological models have failed to fully account for the OCPD phenotype, and the current state of research on OCPD has been described as being "in flux", as exemplified by the current diagnostic system including two separate conceptualizations of OCPD.

Transdiagnostic approaches to psychopathology may help to improve our understanding of OCPD, including its complicated patterns of psychiatric comorbidity. In particular, a transdiagnostic approach might help to understand the often misunderstood relationship between OCPD and OCD. Whereas obsessions may predominate in OCD, both OCPD and OCD may be characterized by compulsivity and perfectionism. Moreover, OCPD may also involve heightened experiential avoidance, a transdiagnostic factor in many forms of psychopathology. Future work is needed to determine whether consideration of these factors provides any incremental utility relative to the existing categorical model.

Importantly, investigation of transdiagnostic factors has the potential to catalyze new research on OCPD, which has been described as "dying" [78]. This is an important endeavor, as OCPD remains an understudied yet common phenomenon. Strikingly, although individuals with OCPD frequently present for treatment, as yet there is no "gold standard" treatment for OCPD. Thus, treatments focusing on transdiagnostic factors may provide novel treatment options for OCPD. However, as yet, these treatments have not been systematically tested in this population. Thus, much more research is needed in this area.

References

1. American Psychiatric Association. *Diagnostic and Statistical Manual of Mental Disorders*, 5th ed. Washington, DC: APA; 2013.

2. American Psychiatric Association. *Diagnostic and Statistical Manual of Mental Disorders*, 2nd ed. Washington, DC: APA; 1968.

3. American Psychiatric Association. *Diagnostic and Statistical Manual of Mental Disorders*, 4th ed. Washington, DC: APA; 1994.

4. Starcevic V, Brakoulias V. New diagnostic perspectives on obsessive-compulsive personality disorder and its links with other conditions. *Curr Opin Psychiatry.* 2014;27(1):62–67.
5. Ekselius L, Tillfors M, Furmark T, Fredrikson M. Personality disorders in the general population: DSM-IV and ICD-10 defined prevalence as related to sociodemographic profile. *Personal Indiv Diff.* 2001;30:311–320.
6. Grant BF, Hasin DS, Stinson FS, et al. Prevalence, correlates, and disability of personality disorders in the United States: results from the national epidemiologic survey on alcohol and related conditions. *J Clin Psychiatry.* 2004;65(7):948–958.
7. Torgersen S, Kringlen E, Cramer V. The prevalence of personality disorders in a community sample. *Arch Gen Psychiatry.* 2001;58:590–596.
8. Grant JE, Mooney ME, Kushner MG. Prevalence, correlates, and comorbidity of DSM-IV obsessive-compulsive personality disorder: results from the National Epidemiologic Survey on Alcohol and Related Conditions. *J Psychiatr Res.* 2012;46(4):469–475.
9. Albert U, Maina G, Forner F, Bogetto F. DSM-IV obsessive-compulsive personality disorder: prevalence in patients with anxiety disorders and in healthy comparison subjects. *Compr Psychiatry.* 2004;45(5):325–332.
10. Chavira DA, Grilo CM, Shea MT, et al. Ethnicity and four personality disorders. *Compr Psychiatry.* 2003;44(6):483–491.
11. Karno M, Golding I, Sorenson S, Burnam M. The epidemiology of obsessive-compulsive disorder in five US communities. *Arch Gen Psychiatry.* 1988;45:1094–1099.
12. Ansell EB, Pinto A, Crosby RD, et al. The prevalence and structure of obsessive-compulsive personality disorder in Hispanic psychiatric outpatients. *J Behav Ther Exp Psychiatry.* 2010;41(3):275–281.
13. Bernstein DP, Cohen P, Velez CN, Schwab-Stone M, Siever LJ, Shinsato L. Prevalence and stability of the DSM-III-R personality disorders in a community-based survey of adolescents. *Am J Psychiatry.* 1993;150(8):1237–1243.
14. Nestadt G, Di C, Samuels J, et al. The stability of DSM personality disorders over twelve to eighteen years. *J Psychiatr Res.* 2010;44(1):1–7.
15. Grilo CM, Skodol AE, Gunderson JG, et al. Longitudinal diagnostic efficiency of DSM-IV criteria for obsessive-compulsive personality disorder: a 2-year prospective study. *Acta Psychiatr Scand.* 2004;110:64–68.
16. Skodol AE, Gunderson JG, McGlashan TH, et al. Functional impairment in patients with schizotypal, borderline, avoidant, or obsessive-compulsive personality disorder. *Am J Psychiatry.* 2002;159(2):276–283.
17. Wheaton MG, Pinto A. The role of experiential avoidance in obsessive–compulsive personality disorder traits. *Personal Disord.* 2017;8(4):383–388.
18. Pinto A, Steinglass JE, Greene AL, Weber EU, Simpson HB. Capacity to delay reward differentiates obsessive-compulsive disorder and obsessive-compulsive personality disorder. *Biol Psychiatry.* 2014;75(8):653–659.
19. Pollak JM. Obsessive-compulsive personality: theoretical and clinical perspectives and recent research findings. *J Personal Disord.* 1987; 1(3):248–262.
20. Millon T. *Disorders of Personality: DSM-III, Axis II.* New York, NY: Wiley; 1981.
21. Cain NM, Ansell EB, Simpson HB, Pinto A. Interpersonal functioning in obsessive-compulsive personality disorder. *J Personal Assess.* 2015;97(1):90–9.
22. Sansone RA, Hendricks CM, Gaither GA, Reddington A. Prevalence of anxiety symptoms among a sample of outpatients in an internal medicine clinic: a pilot study. *Depress Anxiety.* 2004;19(2):133–136.
23. Bender DS, Skodol AE, Pagano ME, et al. Prospective assessment of treatment use by patients with personality disorders. *Psychiatr Serv.* 2006;57(2):254–257.
24. Torgersen S, Lygren S, Oien PA, et al. A twin study of personality disorders. *Compr Psychiatry.* 2000;41(6):416–425.
25. Blom RM, Samuels JF, Riddle MA, et al. Association between a serotonin transporter promoter polymorphism (5HTTLPR) and personality disorder traits in a community sample. *J Psychiatr Res.* 2011;45(9):1153–1159.
26. Caspi A, Hariri AR, Holmes A, Uher R, Moffitt TE. Genetic sensitivity to the environment: the case of the serotonin transporter gene and its implications for studying complex diseases and traits. *Focus.* 2010;8(3):398–416.
27. Perez M, Brown JS, Vrshek-Schallhorn S, Johnson F, Joiner TE, Jr. Differentiation of obsessive-compulsive-, panic-, obsessive-compulsive personality-, and non-disordered individuals by variation in the promoter region of the serotonin transporter gene. *J Anxiety Disord.* 2006;20(6):794–806.
28. Stein DJ, Trestman RL, Mitropoulou V, Coccaro EF, Hollander E, Siever LJ. Impulsivity and serotonergic function in compulsive personality disorder. *J Neuropsychiatry Clin Neurosci.* 1996;8(4):393–398.

29. Dinn WM, Harris CL, Aycicegi A, Greene P, Andover MS. Positive and negative schizotypy in a student sample: neurocognitive and clinical correlates. *Schizophr Res.* 2002;56(1–2):171–185.

30. García-Villamisar D, Dattilo J. Executive functioning in people with obsessive-compulsive personality traits: evidence of modest impairment. *J Personal Disord.* 2015;29(3):418–430.

31. Fineberg NA, Day GA, de Koenigswarter N, et al. The neuropsychology of obsessive-compulsive personality disorder: a new analysis. *CNS Spectr.* 2015;20(5):490–499.

32. Kline P. Obsessional traits, obsessional symptoms and anal eroticism. *Br J Med Psychol.* 1968;41:299–305.

33. Sperry L. *Handbook of Diagnosis and Treatment of DSM-IV-TR Personality Disorders*, 2nd ed. New York, NY: Brunner-Routledge; 2003.

34. Millon T, Everly G. *Personality and Its Disorders.* New York, NY: Wiley; 1985.

35. Diedrich A, Voderholzer U. Obsessive–compulsive personality disorder: a current review. *Curr Psychiatry Rep.* 2015;17(2):1–10.

36. Costa PT, Jr., McCrae RR. *Revised NEO Personality Inventory (NEO-PI-R) and NEO Five-Factor Inventory (NEO-FFI) professional manual.* Odessa, FL: Psychological Assessment Resources; 1992.

37. Lynam DR, Widiger TA. Using the five-factor model to represent the DSM-IV personality disorders: an expert consensus approach. *J Abnorm Psychol.* 2001;110(3):401–412.

38. Samuel DB, Widiger TA. Conscientiousness and obsessive-compulsive personality disorder. *Personal Disord.* 2011;2(3):161–174.

39. McGlashan TH, Grilo CM, Sanislow CA, et al. Two-year prevalence and stability of individual DSM-IV criteria for schizotypal, borderline, avoidant, and obsessive-compulsive personality disorders: toward a hybrid model of axis II disorders. *Am J Psychiatry.* 2005;162(5):883–889.

40. Ansseau M. Serotonergic antidepressants in obsessive personality. *L'Encephale.* 1996;22:309–310.

41. Volavka J, Neziroglu F, Yaryura-Tobias JA. Clomipramine and imipramine in obsessive-compulsive disorder. *Psychiatry Res.* 1985;14(1):85–93.

42. Ekselius L, Von Knorring L. Changes in personality traits during treatment with sertraline or citalopram. *Br J Psychiatry.* 1999;174:444–448.

43. Barber JP, Morse JQ, Krakauer I, Chittams J, Crits-Christoph K. Change in obsessive-compulsive and avoidant personality disorders following time-limited supportive-expressive therapy. *Psychotherapy.* 1997;34:133–143.

44. Abbass A, Sheldon A, Gyra J, Kalpin A. Intensive short-term dynamic psychotherapy for DSM-IV personality disorders: a randomized controlled trial. *J Nerv Ment Dis.* 2008;196(3):211–216.

45. Winston A, Laikin M, Pollack J, Samstag LW, McCullough L, Muran JC. Short-term psychotherapy of personality disorders. *Am J Psychiatry.* 1994;151(2):190–194.

46. Beck AT, Freeman A. *Cognitive Therapy of Personality Disorders.* New York, NY: Guilford Press; 1990.

47. Beck JS. Cognitive approaches to personality disorders. In: Wright JH, Thase ME, eds. *Cognitive Therapy: 16 (American Psychiatric Press Review of Psychiatry).* Washington, DC: American Psychiatric Press; 1997:173–1106.

48. Bailey GR, Jr. Cognitive-behavioral treatment of obsessive-compulsive personality disorder. *J Psychol Pract.* 1998;4(1):51–59.

49. Kyrios M. A cognitive-behavioural approach to the understanding and management of obsessive-compulsive personality disorder. In: Perris C, McGorry PD, eds. *Cognitive Psychotherapy of Psychotic and Personality Disorders: Handbook of Theory and Practice.* New York, NY: Wiley; 1998:351–378.

50. Enero C, Soler A, Ramos I, Cardona S, Guillamat R, Valles V. 2783–Distress level and treatment outcome in obsessive-compulsive personality disorder (OCPD). *Eur Psychiatry.* 2013;28:1.

51. Ng RM. Cognitive therapy for obsessive-compulsive personality disorder-a pilot study in Hong Kong Chinese patients. *Hong Kong J Psychiatry.* 2005;15(2):50.

52. Strauss JL, Hayes AM, Johnson SL, et al. Early alliance, alliance ruptures, and symptom change in a nonrandomized trial of cognitive therapy for avoidant and obsessive-compulsive personality disorders. *J Consult Clin Psychol.* 2006;74(2):337–345.

53. Svartberg M, Stiles TC, Seltzer MH. Randomized, controlled trial of the effectiveness of short-term dynamic psychotherapy and cognitive therapy for cluster C personality disorders. *Am J Psychiatry.* 2004;161(5):810–817.

54. Angyal A. *Neurosis and Treatment: A Holistic Theory.* New York, NY: Wiley; 1965.

55. Goodman WK, Price LH, Rasmussen SA, et al. The Yale-Brown Obsessive Compulsive Scale. II. Validity. *Arch Gen Psychiatry.* 1989;46(11):1012–1016.

56. Goodman WK, Price LH, Rasmussen SA, et al. The Yale-Brown Obsessive Compulsive Scale. I. Development, use, and reliability. *Arch Gen Psychiatry.* 1989;46(11):1006–1011.

57. Pinto A, Mancebo MC, Eisen JL, Pagano ME, Rasmussen SA. The Brown Longitudinal

Obsessive Compulsive Study: clinical features and symptoms of the sample at intake. *J Clin Psychiatry.* 2006;67:703–711.

58. Samuels J, Nestadt G, Bienvenu OJ, et al. Personality disorders and normal personality dimensions in obsessive-compulsive disorder. *Br J Psychiatry.* 2000;177:457–462.
59. Starcevic V, Berle D, Brakoulias V, et al. Obsessive-compulsive personality disorder co-occurring with obsessive-compulsive disorder: conceptual and clinical implications. *Aust N Z J Psychiatry.* 2013;47(1):65–73.
60. Fineberg NA, Reghunandanan S, Kolli S, Atmaca M. Obsessive-compulsive (anankastic) personality disorder: toward the ICD-11 classification. *Revista Brasil Psiquiatria.* 2014;36:40–50.
61. Robbins TW, Gillan CM, Smith DG, de Wit S, Ersche KD. Neurocognitive endophenotypes of impulsivity and compulsivity: towards dimensional psychiatry. *Trends Cogn Sci.* 2012;16(1):81–91.
62. Antony M, Downie F, Swinson R. Diagnostic issues and epidemiology in obsessive-compulsive disorder. In: Swinson R, Antony M, Rachman S, Richter M, eds. *Obsessive-Compulsive Disorder: Theory, Research, and Treatment.* New York, NY: Guilford Press; 1998:3–32.
63. Antony MM, Purdon CL, Huta V, Swinson RP. Dimensions of perfectionism across the anxiety disorders. *Behav Res Ther.* 1998;36(12):1143–1154.
64. OCCW. Cognitive assessment of obsessive-compulsive disorder. *Behav Res Ther.* 1997;35(7):667–681.
65. Egan SJ, Wade TD, Shafran R. Perfectionism as a transdiagnostic process: a clinical review. *Clin Psychol Rev.* 2011;31(2):203–212.
66. Stoeber J. Multidimensional perfectionism and the DSM-5 personality traits. *Personal Indiv Diff.* 2014;64:115–120.
67. McGlashan TH, Grilo CM, Skodol AE, et al. The Collaborative Longitudinal Personality Disorders Study: baseline Axis I/II and II/II diagnostic co-occurrence. *Acta Psychiatr Scand.* 2000;102(4):256–264.
68. Rice KG, Aldea MA. State dependence and trait stability of perfectionism: a short-term longitudinal study. *J Counsel Psychol.* 2006;53:205–212.
69. Hayes SC. Acceptance and commitment therapy, relational frame theory, and the third wave of behavioral and cognitive therapies. *Behav Ther.* 2004;35(4):639–665.
70. Chawla N, Ostafin B. Experiential avoidance as a functional dimensional approach to psychopathology: an empirical review. *J Clin Psychol.* 2007;63(9):871–890.
71. Fairburn CG, Cooper Z, Shafran R. Cognitive behaviour therapy for eating disorders: a "transdiagnostic" theory and treatment. *Behav Res Ther.* 2003;41(5):509–528.
72. Egan SJ, Hine P. Cognitive behavioural treatment of perfectionism: a single case experimental design series. *Behav Change.* 2008;25(4):245–258.
73. Riley C, Lee M, Cooper Z, Fairburn CG, Shafran R. A randomised controlled trial of cognitive-behaviour therapy for clinical perfectionism: a preliminary study. *Behav Res Ther.* 2007;45(9):2221–2231.
74. Shafran R, Egan SJ, Wade TD. *Overcoming Perfectionism: A Self-Help Guide Using Cognitive-Behavioural Techniques.* London: Constable and Robinson; 2010.
75. Pinto A. Treatment of obsessive-compulsive personality disorder. In: Storch EA, Lewin AB, eds. *Clinical Handbook of Obsessive-Compulsive and Related Disorders*: Berlin: Springer; 2016:415–429.
76. Hewitt PL, Newton J, Flett GL, Callander L. Perfectionism and suicide ideation in adolescent psychiatric patients. *J Abnorm Child Psychol.* 1997;25(2):95–101.
77. Gillan C, Fineberg N, Robbins T. A trans-diagnostic perspective on obsessive-compulsive disorder. *Psychol Med.* 2017:1–21.
78. Villemarette-Pittman NR, Stanford MS, Greve KW, Houston RJ, Mathias CW. Obsessive-compulsive personality disorder and behavioral disinhibition. *J Psychol.* 2004;138(1):5–22.

Chapter 27

Tourette's and Other Tic Disorders

Andrea E. Cavanna

Introduction

Tics are defined as involuntary, sudden, rapid, recurrent, non-rhythmic movements (motor tics) or vocalizations (vocal tics) [1]. Tic disorders are among the most common hyperkinetic movement disorders and Tourette's disorder (also known as Tourette syndrome) is the most complex and challenging tic disorder, as it is characterized by the presence of multiple motor and vocal tics with onset in early life, and is frequently accompanied by behavioral problems [2,3,4]. The exact etiology and pathophysiology associated with tic development and tic expression are still largely unknown. Converging evidence points toward dopaminergic neurotransmission alterations within corticostriatocorticofrontal circuitries as a key pathophysiological pathway [5,6]. The role of other central nervous system components in tic generation and modulation is currently being investigated [7]. Genetic predisposition has been shown by early family studies and confirmed by subsequent genetic studies. The complexity of possible heritability pathways indicates that Tourette's disorder is a genetically heterogeneous disorder [8,9]. As in most neuropsychiatric disorders, environmental factors (streptococcal infections and autoimmune dysfunction, as well as pre- and perinatal problems) have been proposed to play a contributory role to the etiopathogenesis of Tourette's disorder [10,11,12].

The first description of Tourette's disorder in the medical literature dates back to the case series published in 1885 by French physician Georges Gilles de la Tourette (Figure 27.1), who famously published a case series of nine patients affected by this syndrome in 1885 [13,14], following a previous report on the *tic non douloureux* by another French physician, Armand Trousseau [15].

Recent Research Findings

Epidemiology

For a long time, Tourette's disorder was considered a rare, bizarre medical curiosity, with scattered early reports of patients presenting with the clinical triad of symptoms initially portrayed by Gilles de la Tourette (tics, urges to repeat other people's sounds/words or echolalia, involuntary swearing or coprolalia). The development of standardized diagnostic criteria marked a paradigm shift in the epidemiology of the syndrome. Crucially, complex symptoms such as coprolalia and echolalia, which were originally reported by Georges Gilles de la Tourette as core features of the condition he described, do not feature among the current diagnostic criteria. Since the new millennium, Tourette's disorder has no longer been considered a rare medical condition, as large epidemiological studies and meta-analyses have shown that 0.3–1% of school-age children fulfill established diagnostic criteria, with different degrees of severity [16,17]. Tic symptoms are thought to be even more common, potentially affecting around 5% of the general population at any point in life [18], although prevalence figures show a wide variability, ranging from 1% to 29%, depending on the different study designs, methodologies and sampled populations [19]. For example, the prevalence of tics is known to be higher in children than in adults, in boys than in girls, and in special education settings than in the general community [20].

Clinical Picture

Tic disorders are neurodevelopmental conditions. The average age at tic onset is around six years, with eye blinking as the most common initial tic [21], followed by other simple tics, such as eye rolling,

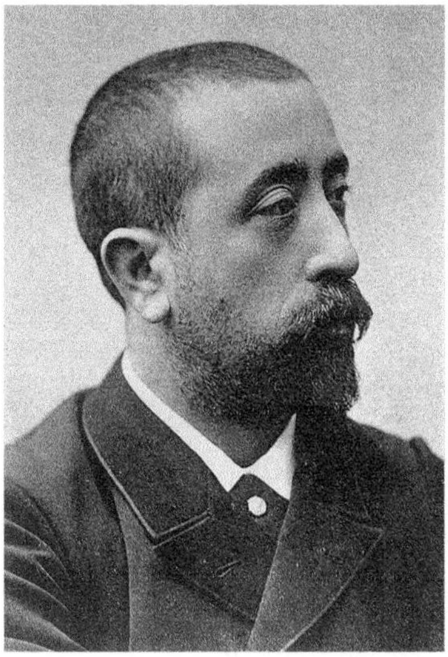

Figure 27.1 Georges Gilles de la Tourette (1857–1904).

mouth opening, jaw movements, facial grimacing, neck stretching, shoulder shrugging, abdominal crunching, arm stretching and kicking. Complex motor tics can subsequently develop. These involve multiple muscular segments, resulting in whole body movements, abnormal gait, forced touching, repeating actions a certain number of times or until they "feel right" (palipraxia), copying other people's movements (echopraxia), involuntary production of rude gestures (copropraxia). With regard to vocal tics, the most frequent are sniffing, grunting, throat clearing, coughing, snorting, squeaking, humming, as well as simple vocalizations ("ah", "ooh"). In addition to echolalia and coprolalia (originally described by Gilles de la Tourette), a proportion of patients can present with other complex vocal tics (e.g., uttering entire words; palilalia or repeating one's own words, usually for a set number of times or until they "sound right"). Of note, despite extensive media coverage especially in recent years, socially inappropriate complex tics such as coprophenomena are relatively rare, as coprolalia has been documented in about 10% of patients with Tourette's disorder in the community and in up to 30% of patients referred to specialist clinics, where more complex or severe cases tend to be seen [22].

Tics present with a male to female ratio of four to one [1,2,3] and characteristically follow a waxing and waning course, with significant variations in frequency, severity and body distribution throughout life. Prospective studies involving large cohorts of patients with tic disorders are needed to confirm the clinical impression that tics peak in severity during early teenage years and in the majority of cases improve or stabilize after puberty [23]. Importantly, tics persist into adulthood in approximately 90% of cases, often with milder severity. Environmental factors are known to modulate tic expression in day-to-day life. Tiredness, excitement, psychological stress, anxiety, boredom and self-consciousness, have all been reported as aggravating factors. Alleviating factors typically include relaxation and engagement in non-stressful mental and physical tasks requiring active concentration (e.g. sports, music). Social interactions are also known to affect tic expression [24,25,26], including the production of context-specific socially inappropriate behaviors [27].

Tic symptoms show both interindividual and intraindividual variability, ranging from mild twitches that do not cause significant impairment and tend to go unnoticed, to forceful movements and loud noises that can sometimes cause injury and call other people's attention. Interestingly, the results of clinical studies using principal component factor analysis and hierarchical cluster analysis have confirmed the existence of multiple phenotypes within the so-called "Tourette's disorder spectrum" [28]. Moreover, converging evidence shows that about 90% of patients with Tourette's disorder present with co-associated behavioral problems [28,29,30,31], most commonly obsessive-compulsive disorder (OCD) or sub-threshold obsessive-compulsive behaviors (approximate comorbidity rate 30% each) [32,33] and attention deficit and hyperactivity disorder (ADHD; 60%) [33,34]. Other frequently co-occurring conditions include autism spectrum disorders [35,36], affective disorders [37,38] and impulse control disorders [39,40]. The recent development of disease-specific instruments to measure health-related quality of life in patients with Tourette's disorder [41,42,43] has allowed a more accurate assessment of the differential impact of tics and behavioral co-morbidities on patients' wellbeing [44].

Diagnosis

The fifth edition of the *Diagnostic and Statistical Manual for Mental Disorders* (DSM-5), published in 2013, classifies tic disorders as movement disorders within the "Neurodevelopmental disorders" section [45,46]. Specifically, the DSM-5 lists four criteria for Tourette's disorder (DSM-5 code 307.23): the presence of both motor and vocal tics at some time during the illness (not necessarily concurrently); the

Table 27.1 Key features of chronic tic disorders.

Tics	Tourette's Disorder	Persistent Motor Tic Disorder	Persistent Vocal Tic Disorder
Motor	2+	1+	0
Vocal	1+	0	1+

persistence of tics for more than one year since onset (irrespective of the duration of tic-free periods); the onset age before 18 years; the absence of underlying organic causes. Up until the text revision of the DSM-IV (published in 2000), a further criterion based on the level of impairment caused by the symptoms was required to diagnose tic disorders, similarly to most psychiatric disorders. In addition to Tourette's disorder, the current classification system lists other types of tic disorders, coded according to the presence of motor and/or vocal tics and their temporal trajectories. "Persistent (chronic) motor or vocal tic disorder" (DSM-5 code 307.22) is diagnosed when single or multiple motor or vocal tics (but not both motor and vocal tics) are present, and criteria for Tourette's disorder are not fully met (Table 27.1).

The category of "provisional tic disorder" (DSM-5 code 307.21) can be applied to diagnose patients with single or multiple motor and/or vocal tics that have been present for less than one year since onset. The "other specified tic disorder" category (DSM-5 code 307.20) should be used when there is strong evidence from the history, physical examination, and/or laboratory results to suggest a plausible underlying cause for the tic symptoms (e.g., Huntington disease, post-viral encephalitis, cocaine use), when the age at tic onset is above 18 years, and whenever tics are present, but full criteria for a tic/neurodevelopmental disorder are not met. Finally, the "Unspecified tic disorder" category (DSM-5 code 307.20) covers situations where there is insufficient information to make a more specific diagnosis in patients with tics who do not meet the criteria for a tic/neurodevelopmental disorder. The diagnostic criteria proposed by the World Health Organization International Classification of Diseases [47] and by the Tourette Syndrome Classification Study Group [48] show a considerable overlap with the outlined DSM criteria, with minor differences (for example, age at tic onset before 21 years rather than 18, according to the Study Group criteria).

The diagnosis of Tourette's disorder is based on clinical grounds and requires expert observation and in-depth history taking to document the chronic presence of at least two motor tics and one vocal tic since childhood. Patients characteristically report that their tics are preceded by a subjective feeling of mounting inner tension, that is only temporarily relieved by actual tic expression [49,50,51,52]. The presence of these sensory symptoms or "premonitory urges" to tic is taken into consideration by clinicians for the differential diagnosis between tics and other repetitive behaviors, such as stereotypies and mannerisms. Assessing the degree of tic suppressibility (described as a distressing feeling like when "holding back a sneeze", at the expense of mounting inner tension and subsequent rebound in tic severity) is also helpful in the differential diagnosis with a range of other hyperkinetic movement disorders [53]. Specific investigations, including laboratory tests and neuroimaging, are only indicated in particular cases to rule out possible underlying causes for tics in patients with atypical presentations, such as acute onset, onset in adulthood or sustained/dystonic tics (possibly resembling motor symptoms of Wilson disease). While the absence of rhythmicity makes it relatively easy to differentiate tics from tremor, some patients present with dystonic tics (slow and sustained muscle contractions) or catatonic features as part of their tic repertoire, which can pose considerable diagnostic challenges [54]. Electroencephalography can sometimes be useful to rule out absence seizures in young patients presenting with staring tics or other symptoms resulting in transient motor arrest.

In consideration of the young age of patients first presenting with tics, and the high rate of comorbidity with attention deficit and hyperactivity symptoms in this age group, particular care has to be taken in the differential diagnosis between motor tics and hyperactivity. As the diagnosis of children and adolescents with Tourette's disorder can be complicated by the co-occurrence of attention deficit and hyperactivity symptoms, child specialists' input is often helpful [34]. Not surprisingly, young patients with tics are restless and hyperactive; furthermore, the constant efforts they have to produce to actively suppress their tics can interfere with their ability to sustain concentration in school settings, thus mimicking primary attention deficit problems. It is therefore recommended that the diagnosis of comorbid ADHD is established by experienced child and adolescent psychiatrists, pediatricians or adult psychiatrists/neuropsychiatrists after a comprehensive clinical assessment, which can involve collecting information from third parties (especially parents and teachers) [3,34,55].

Treatment

In patients with more severe and persistent forms of Tourette's disorder, tics and/or behavioral symptoms can affect health-related quality of life in different ways throughout life [56]. Although the majority of children with mild symptoms might only require psychoeducation, patients with uncertain diagnosis, more severe symptoms or complex presentations should be referred to a specialist clinic, where an in-depth assessment from the behavioral neurology point of view can help establishing the diagnosis and formulating an individualized treatment plan. In 2011, the European Society for the Study of Tourette Syndrome published the first internationally agreed set of guidelines for the assessment and management of Tourette's disorder [57,58,59,60]. These recommendations were followed by the publication in 2012 of the Canadian guidelines for the evidence-based treatment of tic disorders [61,62]. The main treatment strategies include psychoeducation, behavioral interventions, pharmacotherapy and, for severe and refractory cases, deep brain stimulation.

According to current evidence, habit reversal training and exposure and response prevention are the most effective behavioral strategies targeting tic symptoms [63]. The results of two large randomized controlled trials conducted in the last few years in children/adolescents [64] and adults [65] with Tourette's disorder or other chronic tic disorders have shown that a comprehensive behavioral intervention for tics incorporating the habit reversal training component contributed to significant reduction in tic severity in about half of the patients. Further trials conducted in other centers actively involved in clinical research on tic disorders are needed to replicate these promising results. A range of cognitive-behavioral approaches can be useful in the clinical management of comorbid behavioral problems [59].

Pharmacotherapy is often required, based on a comprehensive assessment of the nature and severity of individual tics, combined with evaluation of tic-related behavioral problems and overall impact on health-related quality of life. The recommendations of the European Society for the Study of Tourette Syndrome on the indications to pharmacotherapy in patients with Tourette's disorder are based on expert consensus: presence of tics causing subjective discomfort, sustained problems in social life, emotional problems or functional interference in school or at work should prompt consideration of pharmacological interventions for tic management [58,66]. Agents belonging to a range of pharmacological classes have proven useful in patients with Tourette's disorder, depending on their clinical presentation and most prominent symptoms.

Since adequate numbers of double-blind randomized controlled trials are available only for older agents, practical recommendations often have to take into account the results of more recent open-label studies and large case series [67,68]. Both newer (risperidone) and newest (aripiprazole) atypical antipsychotics have replaced older neuroleptics, mainly because of their better tolerability profile, especially in terms of extrapyramidal adverse effects. The better tolerability profile of aripiprazole is particularly significant in terms of cardiological effects, which have been associated with neuroleptics (e.g. pimozide) and, to a lesser extent, other atypical antipsychotics [69]. In addition to haloperidol and pimozide, the monoamine presynaptic depletor tetrabenazine and the substituted benzamide sulpiride have licensed indications for tic disorders, although their use is usually restricted to second- or third-line pharmacological options, as these anti-tic medications can be associated with significant adverse effects, including extrapyramidal and metabolic problems (e.g., hyperprolactinemia and weight gain), as well as sedation and depression. Alpha-2 agonists, such as clonidine and guanfacine, are often offered as first-line pharmacological options to young patients with chronic disorders, based on a good level of evidence for efficacy and, importantly, tolerability (apart from dose-dependent hypotensive effects and mild sedation). Alpha-2 agonists can be particularly useful in young patients with Tourette's disorder and comorbid ADHD, since their anti-noradrenergic action has been shown to be potentially effective also for attentional problems and hyperactivity [70]. It should be noted that there is no evidence that stimulants necessarily exacerbate tics when used to treat comorbid attention deficit and hyperactivity symptoms in patients with Tourette's disorder, especially if administered in lower doses and with gradual titration [71,72]. In terms of different pharmacological classes, antiepileptic drugs with GABA-ergic properties (especially topiramate) have proven beneficial for tic control in small open-label and double-blind controlled trials, although further research is needed to confirm these initial findings.

Finally, in the medical literature there is a growing number of reports of patients with severe and treatment-refractory Tourette's disorder who have undergone deep brain stimulation, a functional procedure which is less invasive than ablative neurosurgery [73,74,75]. There is uncertainty about the optimal target for the stimulation; however, the most commonly targeted subcortical structures are the pars interna of the globus pallidus and the ventromedian–parafascicular nucleus of the thalamus, which are thought to be involved in the modulation of the pathophysiological pathways underlying tic disorders. In recent years, different sets of guidelines have been developed in the effort to move toward an agreement on optimal brain targets and suitable candidates [76,77]. Overall, the use of this procedure for the treatment of tic disorders is still in its infancy and can only be recommended as a last resort option, also in consideration of the many unanswered questions.

Cross-Diagnostic Approaches and Their Implications for Classification and Diagnosis

Complex tics and compulsions share similarities, primarily in that they can both be described as repetitive behaviors and have high familial loading. Treating clinicians are familiar with the observation that the symptoms of both OCD and Tourette's disorder can be exacerbated by stress or anxiety [78]. However, in-depth assessment reveals a number of key differences, which are important aspects of the differential diagnosis [79]. Unlike tics, the compulsions reported by patients with OCD are often purposeful, ritualistic and routine-like in nature. Moreover, compulsive behaviors are typically performed as a method to reduce psychological anxiety caused by intrusive (obsessional) thoughts, whereas tics are driven by premonitory urges that are described as physical sensations of somatic discomfort, incompleteness, pain or tension. It has been noted that both sub-threshold obsessive-compulsive symptoms and OCD diagnosed in patients with Tourette's disorder have earlier onset than symptoms in patients with "pure" forms of OCD [80]. Finally, the gender ratio in the two conditions is different, with tics being more prevalent in males and obsessive-compulsive symptoms in females.

The high prevalence of comorbid obsessive-compulsive symptoms in patients with Tourette's disorder can pose considerable diagnostic challenges [32]. Interestingly, patients with tics often report the presence of urge-driven obsessive-compulsive behaviors which are phenomenologically different from the symptoms reported by patients with a primary diagnosis of OCD [81]. Specifically, in patients with Tourette's disorder there is a significantly higher prevalence of concerns for symmetry, evening-up behaviors, obsessional counting (arithmomania), ordering and "just-right" perceptions, whereas patients with pure OCD tend to report a higher rate of concerns for contamination and cleaning/washing rituals. Tic-related OCD, in contrast to non-tic-related OCD, is characterized by a higher percentage of forced touching, tapping and rubbing, as well as higher frequencies of violent and aggressive intrusive thoughts and images [80]. Moreover, the majority of patients with Tourette's disorder do not report mental obsessions or symptoms of autonomic anxiety (e.g., tachycardia, shortness of breath, sweating, pallor) preceding their repetitive behaviors [82].These phenomenological differences are likely to reflect separate underlying pathophysiological mechanisms and have important implications in terms of both classification and diagnosis [32]. It is important to note, however, that clinical presentations are often multifaceted and exceptions to the abovementioned differences have been reported [83].

Clinical Implications of Cross-Diagnostic Approaches for Treatment and Prevention

A better understanding of the phenomenological continuum between OCD and Tourette's disorder can inform targeted management pathways and ultimately improve treatment approaches. For instance, specific behavioral approaches could prove useful for patients with tic-related OCD who report sensory phenomena, rather than obsessional thoughts, preceding their repetitive behaviors. In such cases, instead of looking for obsessions, clinicians should focus on helping patients to recognize their subjective experiences. In fact, both habit reversal training and exposure and response prevention are therapeutic techniques based on patients' awareness of their premonitory urges to facilitate tic suppression. The most extensively investigated approach is habit reversal training, according to which patients are encouraged to resist their urges for a specific tic by using a tailored competing response (a more comfortable or acceptable movement/sound) in place of the actual tic [84]. Conversely, cognitive-behavioral therapy strategies, which are used as first-line treatment interventions for patients with primary OCD, tend to focus primarily on changing cognitions [78]. Overall, a thorough evaluation of symptoms in terms of cognitive, emotional and physiological factors is important in informing behavioral treatment selection for patients with repetitive behaviors on the tic–compulsion spectrum.

Likewise, antidopaminergic agents can be a useful additional intervention as augmentation therapy in patients with tic disorders and comorbid OCD treated with serotonergic agents (selective serotonin reuptake inhibitors or the tricyclic clomipramine) [85,86]. The possible role of the presence of tics in modulating the clinical response to augmentation strategies in OCD treatment is to some extent controversial. Initial findings of significantly increased response rate to antipsychotic augmentation in patients with OCD and comorbid tics were not replicated in subsequent studies, possibly due to small sample sizes [80,87]. Likewise, the findings of initial studies looking for treatment response in patients with OCD showed that the presence of tics in patients with OCD was associated with a worse response to monotherapy with a selective serotonin reuptake inhibitor. Again, these findings did not find confirmation in subsequent studies, suggesting that the treatment of OCD in patients with tics should start with first-line serotonergic therapies for OCD, plus first-line antidopaminergic treatment for tics when necessary [80]. The few studies conducted in this field have relevant limitations, including variations in the measurement and categorization of symptoms as tics or OCD-related compulsions [78]. Overall, it seems premature to draw firm conclusions about whether repetitive behaviors in Tourette's disorder and tic-related OCD exhibit a different response to serotonin reuptake inhibitors from tic-free OCD.

Future Directions

Although advances in clinical research on Tourette's disorder and OCD have allowed us to find more homogeneous phenotypes of both disorders, there is need for further studies at the interface between tic disorders and obsessive-compulsive spectrum disorders. Questions for future research encompass a wide range of themes on the nature and implications of the differences between Tourette's disorder and OCD, with high relevance for the cases in which the two conditions are present in comorbidity. The environmental, genetic, neurobiological and neurophysiological mechanisms contributing to phenotypical differences between the two conditions are still largely unknown. Therefore, future research lines should include the characterization of patients by using a variety of multidimensional clinical and neurobiological measures: different genotypes, response to neurophysiological paradigms, findings from neuroimaging techniques and neuropsychological measures with endophenotypic value). Key differences in subjective reports associated with tics in patients with Tourette's disorder (hyperawareness of sensory/physical experiences) and with repetitive behaviors in patients with OCD (mental obsessions including imagined scenarios) is likely to reflect the different neurobiological changes thought to underpin each disorder. Findings from neuroimaging studies have provided consistent evidence of orbitofrontal involvement in OCD, and more sensorimotor areas involvement in Tourette's disorder. This could reflect predominant involvement of corticostriatothalamocortical networks dysfunction in Tourette's disorder compared with greater involvement of lateral–orbitofrontal networks in OCD [78].

Despite the close relationship between tic disorders and OCD, no clinical trials have specifically evaluated the treatment of obsessive-compulsive symptoms in patients with Tourette's disorder. For example, the efficacy of currently available treatment approaches for childhood-onset OCD in patients with coexisting OCD and Tourette's disorder is still unknown. Further studies are necessary to understand and predict the effect of the presence of tics on OCD treatment response. Since most clinical trials for OCD did not include patients with comorbid Tourette's disorder, the available data are scarce. Specifically, it would be useful to know whether antipsychotic augmentation can be exploited for the treatment of co-morbid OCD in patients with Tourette's disorder. Clinicians would be particularly interested to know which antipsychotic agents (or behavioral interventions) are most likely to help in this context. The better characterization of a specific tic-related OCD group can increase our knowledge of phenotypic expressions and help patients to understand their symptoms, as well as fostering the development of specific behavioral and pharmacological treatments.

Conversely, it is still not possible to predict the exact role of the presence of OCD or other common comorbidities in Tourette's disorder treatment response. In particular, future studies should elucidate whether OCD or other common comorbidities worsen or improve Tourette's disorder treatment response.

Acknowledgments

The author is a former member of the Medical Advisory Board of the USA Tourette Syndrome Association and has received board membership fees and research grants from Eisai Pharmaceuticals and lectureship grants from Eisai Pharmaceuticals, UCB Pharma and Janssen-Cilag.

References

1. Ganos C, Martino D. Tics and Tourette syndrome. *Neurol Clin.* 2015;33:115–136.
2. Cavanna AE, Termine C. Tourette syndrome. *Adv Exp Med Biol.* 2012;724:375–383.
3. Cavanna AE, Seri S. Tourette's syndrome. *Br Med J.* 2013;347:f4964.
4. Hallett M. Tourette syndrome: update. *Brain Dev.* 2015;37:651–655.
5. Felling RJ, Singer HS. Neurobiology of Tourette syndrome: current status and need for further investigation. *J Neurosci.* 2011;31:12387–12395.
6. Yael D, Vinner E, Bar-Gad I. Pathophysiology of tic disorders. *Mov Disord.* 2015;30:1171–1178.
7. Nagai Y, Cavanna AE, Critchley HD. Influence of sympathetic arousal on tics: implications for a therapeutic behavioral intervention for Tourette syndrome. *J Psychosom Res.* 2009;67:599–605.
8. Deng H, Gao K, Jankovic J. The genetics of Tourette syndrome. *Nature Rev Neurol.* 2012;8:203–213.
9. Ali F, Morrison KE, Cavanna AE. The complex genetics of Gilles de la Tourette syndrome: implications for clinical practice. *Neuropsychiatry.* 2013;3:321–330.
10. Martino D, Draganski B, Cavanna AE, et al. Anti-basal ganglia antibodies and Tourette's syndrome: a voxel based morphometry and diffusion tensor imaging study in an adult population. *J Neurol Neurosurg Psychiatry.* 2008;79:820–822.
11. Madhusudan N, Cavanna AE. The role of immune dysfunction in the development of tics and susceptibility to infections in Tourette syndrome: a systematic review. *Basal Ganglia.* 2013;3:77–84.
12. Martino D, Zis P, Buttiglione M. The role of immune mechanisms in Tourette syndrome. *Brain Res.* 2015;1617:126–143.
13. Gilles de la Tourette G. Etude sur une affection nerveuse caracterisée par de l'incoordination motrice accompagnée d'écholalie et de coprolalie. *Archives de Neurologie (Paris).* 1885;9:19–42, 158–200.
14. Rickards H, Cavanna AE. Gilles de la Tourette: the man behind the syndrome. *J Psychosom Res.* 2009;67:469–474.
15. Rickards H, Woolf I, Cavanna AE. Trousseau's disease: a description of Gilles de la Tourette syndrome 12 years before 1885. *Mov Disord.* 2010;25:2285–2289.
16. Robertson MM, Eapen V, Cavanna AE. The international prevalence, epidemiology and clinical phenomenology of Tourette syndrome: a cross-cultural perspective. *J Psychosom Res.* 2009;67:475–483.
17. Scharf JM, Miller LL, Gauvin CA, et al. Population prevalence of Tourette syndrome: a systematic review and meta-analysis. *Mov Disord.* 2015;30:221–228.
18. Ong MT, Mordekar SR, Seal A. 15 minute consultation: tics and Tourette syndrome. *Arch Dis Child Educ Pract Ed.* 2016;101:87–94.
19. Robertson MM. The prevalence and epidemiology of Gilles de la Tourette syndrome. Part 1: the epidemiological and prevalence studies. *J Psychosom Res.* 2008;65:461–472.
20. Knight T, Steeves T, Day L, et al. Prevalence of tic disorders: a systematic review and meta-analysis. *Pediatr Neurol.* 2012;47:77–90.
21. Martino D, Cavanna AE, Robertson MM, Orth M. Prevalence and phenomenology of eye tics in Gilles de la Tourette syndrome. *J Neurol.* 2012;259:2137–2140.
22. Eddy CM, Cavanna AE. "It's a curse!": coprolalia in Tourette syndrome. *Eur J Neurol.* 2013;20:1467–1470.
23. Hassan N, Cavanna AE. The prognosis of Tourette syndrome: implications for clinical practice. *Funct Neurol.* 2012;27:23–27.
24. Eddy C, Mitchell IJ, Beck SR, et al. Altered attribution of intention in Tourette's syndrome. *J Neuropsychiatry Clin Neurosci.* 2010;22:348–351.
25. Eddy CM, Mitchell IJ, Beck SR, et al. Social reasoning in Tourette syndrome. *Cogn Neuropsychiatry.* 2011;16:326–347.
26. Eddy CM, Cavanna AE. Altered social cognition in Tourette syndrome: nature and implications. *Behav Neurol.* 2013;27:15–22.

27. Eddy CM, Cavanna AE. On being your worst enemy: an investigation of socially inappropriate symptoms in Tourette syndrome. *J Psychiatr Res.* 2013;47:1259–1263.

28. Cavanna AE, Rickards H. The psychopathological spectrum of Gilles de la Tourette syndrome. *Neurosci Biobehav Rev.* 2013;37:1008–1015.

29. Freeman RD, Fast DK, Burd L, et al. An international perspective on Tourette syndrome: selected findings from 3500 individuals in 22 countries. *Dev Med Child Neurol.* 2000;42:436–447.

30. Khalifa N, Von Knorring A-L. Tourette syndrome and other tic disorders in a total population of children: clinical assessment and background. *Acta Paediatrica.* 2005;94:1608–1614.

31. Cavanna AE, Critchley HD, Orth M, et al. Dissecting the Gilles de la Tourette spectrum: a factor analytic study on 639 patients. *J Neurol Neurosurg Psychiatry.* 2011;82:1320–1323.

32. Lombroso PJ, Scahill L. Tourette syndrome and obsessive-compulsive disorder. *Brain Dev.* 2008;30:231–237.

33. Eddy CM, Cavanna AE, Gulisano M, et al. The effects of comorbid obsessive-compulsive disorders and attention-deficit hyperactivity disorder on quality of life in Tourette syndrome. *J Neuropsychiatry Clin Neurosci.* 2012;24:458–462.

34. Simpson HA, Jung L, Murphy TK. Update on attention-deficit/hyperactivity disorder and tic disorders: a review of the current literature. *Curr Psychiatry Rep.* 2011;13:351–356.

35. Baron-Cohen S, Scahill VL, Izaguirre J, et al. The prevalence of Gilles de la Tourette syndrome in children and adolescents with autism: a large scale study. *Psychol Med.* 1999;29:1151–1159.

36. Canitano R, Vivanti G. Tics and Tourette syndrome in autism spectrum disorders. *Autism.* 2007;11:19–28.

37. Robertson MM. Mood disorders and Gilles de la Tourette's syndrome: an update on prevalence, etiology, comorbidity, clinical associations, and implications. *J Psychosom Res.* 2006;61:349–358.

38. Eddy CM, Rickards H, Critchley HD, Cavanna AE. A controlled study of personality and affect in Tourette syndrome. *Compr Psychiatry.* 2013;54:105–110.

39. Frank MC, Piedad J, Rickards H, Cavanna AE. The role of impulse control disorders in Tourette syndrome: an exploratory study. *J Neurol Sci.* 2011;310:276–278.

40. Wright A, Rickards H, Cavanna AE. Impulse control disorders in Gilles de la Tourette syndrome. *J Neuropsychiatry Clin Neurosci.* 2012;24:16–27.

41. Cavanna AE, Schrag A, Morley D, et al. The Gilles de la Tourette Syndrome-Quality of Life scale (GTS-QOL): development and validation. *Neurology.* 2008;71:1410–1416.

42. Cavanna AE, Luoni C, Selvini C, et al. The Gilles de la Tourette Syndrome-Quality of Life Scale for Children and Adolescents (GTS-QOL-C&A): development and validation of the Italian version. *Behav Neurol.* 2013;27:95–103.

43. Cavanna AE, Luoni C, Selvini C, et al. Disease-specific quality of life in young patients with Tourette syndrome. *Pediatr Neurol.* 2013;48:111–114.

44. Cavanna AE, David K, Bandera V, et al. Health-related quality of life in Gilles de la Tourette syndrome: a decade of research. *Behav Neurol.* 2013;27:83–93.

45. American Psychiatric Association. *Diagnostic and Statistical Manual of Mental Disorders*, 5th ed. Washington, DC: APA; 2013.

46. Cavanna AE. Improved criteria for the diagnosis of tic disorders in DSM-5. *Future Neurol.* 2014;9:251–253.

47. Woods DW, Thomsen PH. Tourette and tic disorders in ICD-11: standing at the diagnostic crossroads. *Rev Bras Psiquiatria.* 2014;36(Suppl 1):51–58.

48. Tourette Syndrome Classification Study Group. Definitions and classification of tic disorders. *Arch Neurol.* 1993;50:1013–1016.

49. Crossley E, Cavanna AE. Sensory phenomena: clinical correlates and impact on quality of life in adult patients with Tourette syndrome. *Psychiatry Res.* 2013;209:705–710.

50. Rajagopal S, Seri S, Cavanna AE. Premonitory urges and sensorimotor processing in Tourette syndrome. *Behav Neurol.* 2013;27:65–73.

51. Crossley E, Seri S, Stern JS, et al. Premonitory urges for tics in adult patients with Tourette syndrome. *Brain Dev.* 2014;36:45–50.

52. Eddy CM, Cavanna AE. Premonitory urges in adults with complicated and uncomplicated Tourette syndrome. *Behav Modif.* 2014;38:264–275.

53. Van der Salm SMA, de Haan RJ, Cath DC, et al. The eye of the beholder: inter-rater agreement among experts on psychogenic jerky movement disorders. *J Neurol Neurosurg Psychiatry.* 2013;84:742–747.

54. Cavanna AE, Robertson MM, Critchley HD. Catatonic signs in Gilles de la Tourette syndrome. *Cogn Behav Neurol.* 2008;21:34–37.

55. Termine C, Selvini C, Balottin U, et al. Self-, parent-, and teacher-reported behavioural symptoms in young people with Tourette syndrome: a case–control study. *Eur J Paediatr Neurol.* 2011;15:95–100.

56. Cavanna AE, David K, Robertson MM, Orth M. Predictors during childhood of future health-related

quality of life in adults with Gilles de la Tourette syndrome. *Eur J Paediatr Neurol.* 2012;16:605–612.

57. Cath DC, Hedderly T, Ludolph AG, et al. European clinical guidelines for Tourette syndrome and other tic disorders. Part I: assessment. *Eur Child Adolesc Psychiatry.* 2011;20:155–171.
58. Roessner V, Plessen KJ, Rothenberger A, et al. European clinical guidelines for Tourette syndrome and other tic disorders. Part II: pharmacological treatment. *Eur Child Adolesc Psychiatry.* 2011;20:173–196.
59. Verdellen C, van de Griendt J, Hartmann A, et al. European clinical guidelines for Tourette syndrome and other tic disorders. Part III: behavioural and psychosocial interventions. *Eur Child Adolesc Psychiatry.* 2011;20:197–207.
60. Muller-Vahl KR, Cath DC, Cavanna AE, et al. European clinical guidelines for Tourette syndrome and other tic disorders. Part IV: deep brain stimulation. *Eur Child Adolesc Psychiatry.* 2011;20:209–217.
61. Pringsheim T, Doja A, Gorman D, et al. Canadian guidelines for the evidence-based treatment of tic disorders: pharmacotherapy. *Can J Psychiatry.* 2012;57:133–143.
62. Steeves T, McKinlay D, Gorman D, et al. Canadian guidelines for the evidence-based treatment of tic disorders: behavioural therapy, deep brain stimulation and transcranial magnetic stimulation. *Can J Psychiatry.* 2012;57:144–151.
63. Frank M, Cavanna AE. Behavioural treatments for Tourette syndrome: an evidence-based review. *Behav Neurol.* 2013;27:105–117.
64. Piacentini J, Woods DW, Scahill L, et al. Behavior therapy for children with Tourette disorder: a randomized controlled trial. *J Am Med Assoc.* 2010;303:1929–1937.
65. Wilhelm S, Peterson AL, Piacentini J, et al. Randomized trial of behavior therapy for adults with Tourette syndrome. *Arch Gen Psychiatry.* 2012;69:795–803.
66. Rickards H, Cavanna AE, Worrall R. Treatment practices in Tourette syndrome: the European perspective. *Eur J Paediatr Neurol.* 2012;16:361–364.
67. Waldon K, Hill S, Termine C, et al. Trials of pharmacological interventions for Tourette syndrome: a systematic review. *Behav Neurol.* 2013;26:265–273.
68. Thomas R, Cavanna AE. The pharmacology of Tourette syndrome. *J Neural Transm.* 2013;120:689–694.
69. Gulisano M, Calì PV, Cavanna AE, et al. Cardiovascular safety of aripiprazole and pimozide in young patients with Tourette syndrome. *Neurol Sci.* 2011;32:1213–1217.
70. Bloch MH, Panza KE, Landeros-Weisenberger A, Leckman JF. Meta-analysis: treatment of attention-deficit hyperactivity disorder in children with comorbid tic disorders. *J Am Acad Child Adolesc Psychiatry.* 2009;48:884–893.
71. Erenberg G. The relationship between Tourette syndrome, attention deficit hyperactivity disorder, and stimulant medication: a critical review. *Semin Pediatr Neurol.* 2005;12:217–221.
72. Robertson MM. Attention deficit hyperactivity disorder, tics and Tourette's syndrome: the relationship and treatment implications. *Eur Child Adolesc Psychiatry.* 2006;15:1–11.
73. Rickards H, Wood C, Cavanna AE. Hassler and Dieckmann's seminal paper on stereotaxic thalamotomy for Gilles de la Tourette syndrome: translation and critical reappraisal. *Mov Disord.* 2008;23:1966–1972.
74. Vandewalle V, van der Linden C, Groenewegen HJ, Caemaert J. Stereotactic treatment of Gilles de la Tourette syndrome by high frequency stimulation of thalamus. *Lancet.* 1999;353:724.
75. Piedad JCP, Rickards HE, Cavanna AE. What patients with Gilles de la Tourette syndrome should be treated with deep brain stimulation and what is the best target? *Neurosurgery.* 2012;71:173–192.
76. Cavanna AE, Eddy CM, Mitchell R, et al. An approach to Deep Brain Stimulation for severe treatment-refractory Tourette syndrome: the UK perspective. *Br J Neurosurg.* 2011;25:38–44.
77. Porta M, Sassi M, Ali F, et al. Neurosurgical treatment for Gilles da la Tourette syndrome: the Italian perspective. *J Psychosom Res.* 2009;67:585–590.
78. Eddy CM, Cavanna AE. Tourette syndrome and obsessive compulsive disorder: compulsivity along the continuum. *J Obs Compuls Relat Dis.* 2014;3:363–371.
79. Worbe Y, Mallet L, Golmard JL, et al. Repetitive behaviours in patients with Gilles de la Tourette syndrome: tics, compulsions, or both? *PLoS One.* 2010;5:e12959.
80. Ferrao YA, Gomes de Alvarenga P, Hounie AG, et al. The phenomenology of obsessive-compulsive symptoms in Tourette syndrome. In: Martino D, Leckman JP, eds. *Tourette Syndrome.* Oxford University Press; 2013:50–73.
81. Robertson MM. A personal 35 year perspective on Gilles de la Tourette syndrome: prevalence, phenomenology, comorbidities, and coexistent psychopathologies. *Lancet Psychiatry.* 2015;2:68–87.

82. Miguel EC, Coffey BJ, Baer L, et al. Phenomenology of intentional repetitive behaviors in obsessive-compulsive disorder and Tourette's disorder. *J Clin Psychiatry.* 1995;56:246–255.

83. Robertson MM, Cavanna AE. The disaster was my fault! *Neurocase.* 2007;13:446–451.

84. Dutta N, Cavanna AE. Effectiveness of habit reversal therapy in the treatment of Tourette syndrome and other chronic tic disorders: a systematic review. *Funct Neurol.* 2013;28:7–12.

85. Bloch MH, Landeros-Weisenberger A, Kelmendi B, et al. A systematic review: antipsychotic augmentation with treatment refractory obsessive-compulsive disorder. *Mol Psychiatry.* 2006;11:622–632.

86. Masi G, Pfanner C, Brovedani P. Antipsychotic augmentation of selective serotonin reuptake inhibitors in resistant tic-related obsessive-compulsive disorder in children and adolescents: a naturalistic comparative study. *J Psychiatr Res.* 2013;47:1007–1012.

87. Cardona F, Rizzo R. Treatment of psychiatric comorbidities of Tourette syndrome. In: Martino D, Leckman JP, eds. *Tourette Syndrome.* Oxford University Press; 2013:553–582.

Chapter 28

Body-Focused Repetitive Behaviors

Jon E. Grant and Samuel R. Chamberlain

Introduction

The term body-focused repetitive behavior (BFRB) refers to a group of psychiatric disorders characterized by recurrent hair pulling and picking one's own body, resulting in physical damage. Trichotillomania and excoriation (skin picking) disorder (SPD) are the BFRBs currently classified in the *Diagnostic and Statistical Manual of Mental Disorders*, fifth edition (DSM-5) [1] and are discussed in detail in this chapter.

The act of pulling one's own hair in response to an intense emotional reaction or distress has long been described through history. In fact, there is a common idiom used by English speakers that says "I could pull my hair out". This sentence usually applies to designate strong feelings and frustration. In literature and art, hair pulling is frequently a portrayal of mental illnesses. Nonetheless, it was only in 1889 that hair pulling was identified as a medical problem. In that year, Francois Hallopeau suggested the name trichotillomania to describe a patient that had pulled out all his body hair [2]. However, trichotillomania was only officially established as a psychiatric diagnosis in 1987 when it became part of the DSM-III-R. At that time it was classified as an impulse control disorder not elsewhere classified. Later research suggested that trichotillomania's psychopathology resembles the compulsive behavior seen in obsessive-compulsive related disorders [3]. As a consequence, in 2013 the DSM-5 reclassified trichotillomania as an obsessive-compulsive and related disorder.

The following are the DSM-5 diagnostic criteria for trichotillomania (hair-pulling disorder): (i) recurrent pulling out of one's hair, resulting in hair loss; (ii) repeated attempts to decrease or stop hair pulling; (iii) the hair pulling causes clinically significant distress or impairment in social, occupational or other important areas of functioning; (iv) the hair pulling or hair loss is not attributable to another medical condition (e.g., a dermatological condition); and (v) the hair pulling is not better explained by the symptoms of another mental disorder (e.g., attempts to improve a perceived defect or flaw in appearance in body dysmorphic disorder) [1].

SPD, also referred to as pathological skin picking, neurotic excoriation, dermatillomania or psychogenic excoriation, is characterized by the repetitive and compulsive picking of skin, leading to tissue damage [1]. The medical literature has long noted compulsive picking as a health problem. Erasmus Wilson, in 1875, first coined the term "neurotic excoriation" to describe excessive picking behaviors in neurotic patients that were extremely difficult, if not impossible, to control [4].

Even with a long history in the medical literature, SPD was not explicitly listed in the DSM until the fifth edition. The following are the diagnostic criteria for SPD: (i) recurrent skin-picking resulting in skin lesions; (ii) repeated attempts to decrease or stop skin-picking; (iii) the skin picking causes clinically significant distress or impairment in social, occupational or other important areas of functioning; (iv) the skin picking is not due to the direct physiological effects of a substance (e.g., cocaine) or a general medical condition (e.g., scabies; Prader-Willi syndrome); and (v) the skin picking is not restricted to the symptoms of another mental disorder (e.g., skin picking due to fixed beliefs about skin infestation in delusional disorder, preoccupation with appearance in body dysmorphic disorder) [1].

Recent Research Findings

Epidemiology

Trichotillomania

Although long thought to be a rare disorder, recent research has shown that trichotillomania is in fact more common than previously thought. Nationwide epidemiological studies of trichotillomania are not yet available, but some small studies have examined the prevalence of trichotillomania, mostly in college student settings. In the United States, individual studies conducted using questionnaires in college students have estimated the lifetime prevalence of trichotillomania to be around of 0.6%; and point prevalence to be up to 3.9% [5]. The sample size of these studies, considered individually, ranged from 200 to 2579 participants. One study examined 832 people who were visiting retail stores in a US college city, and identified trichotillomania in five individuals (0.6%) [6]. There are a handful of studies from non-US settings. King and colleagues explored hair pulling using questionnaires and interviews, in 794 Israeli 17-year-olds who were undertaking preinduction for military service [7]. The lifetime prevalence of hair pulling was estimated at 1%, but none of the subjects met DSM-III-R criteria for trichotillomania. In a cross-sectional study conducted in 210 students at medical colleges in Karachi (Pakistan), probable trichotillomania (measured using a "habit" questionnaire) was found in 13.3% of the sample [8]. Collectively, prevalence estimates appear higher when using more recently formulated diagnostic criteria according to DSM, which are less strict. It should also be considered that people with trichotillomania are often ashamed and embarrassed about their condition, and so the above may be underestimates of the true population prevalence.

Trichotillomania in adults appears to be more common in females. Some data suggest a female to male ratio being as high as ten to one [9]. These numbers may possibly be overestimates, and findings have agreed that the female preponderance of trichotillomania is particularly high [5]. Interestingly, in children, both genders appear to be equally affected [10].

The onset of trichotillomania most commonly occurs in late childhood/early teenage years, with an average age at onset of 13 years. Thus, the onset of trichotillomania frequently coincides with the beginning of puberty, which may hint at neurodevelopmental or hormonal influences [6].

Skin-Picking Disorder

Two community prevalence studies have found that SPD is fairly commonplace. In a study of 354 subjects, 19 (5.4%) reported significant picking with associated distress/impact and thereby met criteria for SPD [11]. This study demonstrated that although 63% of the subjects engaged in some form of picking, only a small percentage met criteria for SPD. A second study, comprising 2513 telephone interviews, found that 10% picked to the point of having noticeable skin damage which was not secondary to a medical condition [12]. When distress or impairment was required to establish the diagnosis, 1.4% of the sample met criteria for SPD. These studies demonstrate that as a behavior, skin picking appears to be quite common, and often presents along a continuum from mild to severe. Mild cases of picking presumably rarely require interventions. When picking meets the criteria for SPD, however, interventions are needed.

Clinical Findings

Trichotillomania

The main characteristic of trichotillomania is the pulling out of one's hair. Although any body part with hair can be affected, the most common is the scalp, followed by eyelashes and eyebrows. Other sites, such as pubic area, may be involved and multiple areas can be implicated in the same patient. Approximately half of individuals with trichotillomania pull exclusively from one body part [4]. The hair pulling can present with an "automatic" quality, when the patient is not fully aware of the behavior. More frequently, this type of pulling is triggered by emotional components; for example, boredom, anxiety, anger and frustration. In contrast, when the pulling happens with a "focused" characteristic, meaning that the patient is entirely conscious of the behavior, it can be triggered by cognitions and tactile sensations. In these cases, patients might pull thicker or more irregular hairs, or the ones they believe are in wrong places or are impairing an esthetical pattern they are pursuing. Patients usually present with both styles of behavior to varying degrees. Pulling the hair may be followed by other acts like manipulating or even swallowing it.

Trichotillomania is associated with many negative consequences. By analyzing quality of life scores, a recent study found that almost 30% of adults with trichotillomania reported a low or very low quality of life [13]. Individuals frequently report feeling ashamed of their behavior and avoiding social situations either due to the alopecia (hair loss) or fear that they might have the urge to pull in public. Additionally, they may isolate themselves and even avoid working so as not to have contact with other people. In addition, individuals might spend considerable amounts of time each day hiding the alopecia by the use of wigs or hats.

Besides the social and emotional distress, trichotillomania can also result in medical problems. Lesions in different degrees of severity can happen to the skin, especially when instruments such as scissors and tweezers are used to pull the hair. Additionally, more than 20% of the patients with trichotillomania ingest their hair after pulling it (trichophagia). This fact usually is a source of great embarrassment, and patients frequently omit this information when talking with their physician. Clinicians need to ask about this behavior because the ingestion of hair may result in a trichobezoar which could eventually obstruct the gastrointestinal system, resulting in a serious medical complication [14]. There are still some discrepancies in the literature regarding the prevalence of trichobezoars. Nonetheless, it is an important condition because of its potential severity.

Skin-Picking Disorder

Research suggests that the age of onset for SPD varies substantially and may occur during childhood (less than 10 years old), adolescence (mean age approximately 13–15 years) or at a later age (between the ages of 30 and 45) [15,16,17,18]. The clinical characteristics of SPD appear the same across age cohorts and across cultures – Europe, Africa, North America, South America and the Middle East [18].

Individuals with SPD spend a significant amount of time each day picking their skin, with many reporting that the picking behavior constitutes several hours each day [19]. Due to the amount of time spent picking, individuals report missing or being late for work, school or social activities.

Triggers to pick vary greatly between individuals and multiple triggers are the norm, not the exception. Stress, anxiety, time away from scheduled activities (e.g., sitting on the couch, watching television, reading), boredom and feeling tired or angry, have all been reported as triggers [18,19]. Emotion regulation difficulties and emotion reactivity have been shown to predict picking behavior after controlling for depression, anxiety and worry [20]. Picking can also be triggered by the feel (e.g., a bump or unevenness) or look (e.g., blemish or discoloration) of the skin. Picking often begins unconsciously but becomes conscious after a period of time. This is similar to the characteristics of other repetitive behaviors such as trichotillomania, where the act of pulling has been described as automatic (i.e., unconscious) or focused (i.e., conscious). The percentage of time patients with SPD report being aware of their picking behavior ranges from 68.9% to 78.1%. In many cases, however, the picking behavior only becomes conscious when someone else brings it to their attention or the site begins to bleed.

Diagnostic Considerations

Trichotillomania

Patients with trichotillomania are unlikely to seek mental health treatment for their condition. In fact, one study found that only 27.3% of individuals with trichotillomania had ever sought psychiatric treatment [5]. Thus, many patients will instead seek dermatological help due to the cosmetic damage. Out of embarrassment, some patients might not admit to pulling their hair.

Co-occurring psychiatric conditions are common among those with trichotillomania. Proper diagnosis of these comorbid conditions can be crucial for successful treatment of the hair pulling.

The most common associated conditions in trichotillomania are anxiety, mood and substance use disorders. The available literature suggests the following rates: major depressive disorder (39–65%), anxiety disorder (27–32%) and substance use disorders (15–19%) [5].

Skin-Picking Disorder

Although the course of illness may vary, when untreated, SPD is most often considered a chronic disorder with fluctuations in intensity over time. A study of 29 patients with SPD found a mean illness duration of 20.1 years [21], which is similar to the 18.9 year duration found in a sample of 24 patients [22]. Individuals report that the symptoms of their picking, although waxing and waning in intensity over many years, are essentially unchanged with time. Seeking medical help from a physician is uncommon among individuals who pick their skin. In fact, some studies have indicated that less than 20% of subjects seek treatment for their picking [19]. Individuals with SPD often report being unaware that viable treatments are available.

Psychiatric comorbidity is common in excoriation disorder, with rates of co-occurring disorders ranging from 54.5% to 100% [15,16,23]. SPD is often misdiagnosed as either obsessive-compulsive disorder (OCD) or body dysmorphic disorder (BDD). Rates of co-occurring OCD are significantly higher in individuals with SPD (6–52%) than those found in the community (1–3%), and rates of SPD among individuals with OCD have ranged from 8.9% to 24.0%, which is greater than the rate of 1.4–5.4% found in the community. The repetitive motor symptoms of SPD share some similarity with the repetitive compulsive rituals in OCD. These findings raise the possibility of an underlying common neurobiological pathway, but several lines of evidence suggest that SPD is distinct from OCD. Individuals with SPD are more likely to be female, report higher rates of co-occurring BFRBs, and are more likely to have first-degree relatives with BFRBs. Neurocognitive data also demonstrate a distinction between individuals with SPD (i.e., demonstrating poor motor inhibition) and individuals with OCD (problems with cognitive flexibility) [18].

Treatment

Studies regarding pharmacological treatment for BFRBs have produced mixed results and therefore have complicated treatment recommendations. Antidepressants seem to have limited value in treating BFRBs although they may be beneficial for the co-occurring anxiety or mood disorders. More recent studies with N-acetyl cysteine (NAC, dose ranging from 1200 mg to 3000 mg/day) have shown promising results and might point to a new direction for BFRB treatment guidelines [5]. Additionally, treating key psychiatric comorbidities is important to help maximize treatment outcomes for patients with BFRBs.

Trichotillomania

Individuals with trichotillomania rarely seek psychological or psychiatric treatment for their condition. Patients avoid seeking treatment because of social embarrassment or due to a belief that their condition is just a "bad habit" or that it is untreatable. Without treatment, response rates in adults are low (approximately 14%). When diagnosed early and appropriately treated, however, up to 50% of individuals may experience symptom reduction at least for the short term.

The evidence base for psychotherapy for trichotillomania is small but supports the use of behavioral therapy. Behavioral therapy for trichotillomania has generally used habit-reversal therapy and has sometimes included components of acceptance and commitment therapy and dialectical behavior therapy too [24]. There are seven controlled studies of behavioral therapy, using habit-reversal therapy alone or with other components, for trichotillomania.

Habit-reversal therapy was first developed approximately 40 years ago by Azrin and Nunn for the treatment of nervous habits and tics. Typically, habit-reversal therapy is conducted on a weekly basis, although higher severity of the disorder may necessitate more frequent sessions. It has shown benefit in many different frequency formats and anywhere from 4 to 22 sessions (usually 60-minute sessions) may be helpful. The core aspects of habit-reversal therapy include self-monitoring (i.e., asking the patient to track his/her hair pulling, picking), awareness training, competing response training and stimulus control procedures (i.e., modifying the environment to reduce cues for hair pulling or skin-picking). Habit-reversal therapy appears to be superior to waitlist and minimal attention control based on controlled studies. In addition, habit-reversal therapy has shown benefit with the addition of components of acceptance and commitment therapy and dialectical behavior therapy [24,25]. Habit-reversal therapy can be delivered in person, online using a self-help method or in a group format [26]. Acute treatment gains obtained from habit-reversal therapy have been generally maintained from three to six months. Although in practice many clinicians use a combination of habit-reversal therapy and more traditional cognitive therapy, the empirical data support habit-reversal therapy as the first-line psychotherapy treatment for these disorders. In a systematic review of available randomized controlled clinical trials, quality scores of psychotherapy studies were in the moderate to good range [27].

In terms of medication options, there are currently no pharmacotherapies that would be universally accepted as first-line treatments for trichotillomania. A Cochrane review of randomized controlled trials concluded that although clomipramine has demonstrated some benefit for trichotillomania, there is no strong evidence of a treatment effect for the selective serotonin reuptake inhibitors (SSRIs) [28]. The quality of studies was not quantified numerically, but the authors noted there to be a limited number of studies in a limited number of participants, with high attrition rates and lack of intent-to-treat analyses in several of the trials [28].

Other medications that might be beneficial for trichotillomania include glutamatergic agents, antipsychotic medications and cannabinoid agonists. In terms of glutamate agents, NAC has demonstrated benefit in a double-blind placebo-controlled study for trichotillomania using a dose of 1200 mg twice a day and giving it approximately nine weeks to work [29]. Adverse effects with NAC are generally mild and usually only involve some bloated feelings and flatulence. Theoretically, NAC may worsen asthma and therefore should be used only cautiously in individuals with respiratory disorders. The antipsychotic medication, olanzapine, has also been studied in one small (n = 23) double-blind, placebo-controlled trial. After 12 weeks using a mean dose of 10.8 mg/day, olanzapine significantly reduced symptoms of trichotillomania [30]. Olanzapine has been associated with metabolic syndrome and so the decision to use it in the treatment of trichotillomania needs to be tempered by its adverse-effect profile. In the aforementioned Cochrane review [28], the authors noted that these two trials for NAC and olanzapine were of high quality and that they merit replication.

Finally, an open-label study of dronabinol, a cannabinoid agonist, demonstrated marked reductions in trichotillomania symptoms during a 12-week trial using a mean dose of 11.6 mg/day [31]. Dronabinol, a generally well-tolerated medication at these low doses with only slight sedation, may be a promising option, but without a controlled trial the results must be viewed cautiously.

Skin-Picking Disorder

As for trichotillomania, people with SPD rarely seek dermatological or psychiatric treatment for their condition. Treatment for SPD has largely focused on cognitive-behavioral interventions and pharmacology. Early psychosocial treatment studies provided preliminary evidence for skin-picking reduction with habit-reversal or acceptance-enhanced behavior therapy [32]. Teng and colleagues [33] conducted a waitlist controlled study of habit-reversal therapy and demonstrated significantly greater reductions in skin picking at post-treatment and follow-up with active treatment. Similarly, Schuck and colleagues demonstrated the efficacy of a brief, four-session CBT protocol for SPD in comparison with a waitlist control, with treatment effects maintained at a two-month follow-up [34].

Double-blind, placebo-controlled clinical trials in patients with SPD have been conducted over the past decade [35]. Data regarding the efficacy of serotonin reuptake inhibitors have been mixed, with some demonstrating improvement on certain measures of picking behavior [35]. One study of fluoxetine in 21 patients with SPD found that, among the 17 completers (6 fluoxetine, 11 placebo), the fluoxetine group improved significantly more than the placebo group at a mean dosage of 55 mg/day after ten weeks of treatment, but patients responded on only one of the three measures and full remission was not observed [36]. In a second fluoxetine study, 15 subjects were given six weeks of open-label fluoxetine followed by a six-week double-blind discontinuation phase for responders. At the end of the six-week open-label treatment phase, eight subjects (53.3%) were considered responders. The four patients randomized to fluoxetine maintained their improvement during the double-blind discontinuation phase while the placebo group returned to baseline levels of picking severity [37]. In a double-blind study of 45 patients with SPD treated with citalopram (20 mg/day) for four weeks, scores on the Yale-Brown Obsessive Compulsive Scale modified for SPD decreased significantly for the citalopram group but not for the placebo group [38]. However, there was no significant medication effect on the primary outcome measure, a visual analog scale of picking behavior [38].

Lamotrigine, an antiepileptic medication, was examined in 24 patients with SPD [22]. Although an open-label study demonstrated some benefit, a follow-up double-blind, placebo-controlled study failed to demonstrate greater benefit than placebo [39].

Opioid antagonists reduce self-licking or self-chewing in 63–91% of dogs with acral lick dermatitis, a possible animal model of SPD [34]. In humans with SPD, the efficacy of opioid antagonists is supported only by case reports.

Glutamatergic agents have shown early promise for the treatment of SPD. One example is NAC, which has demonstrated benefit for SPD in a recent double-blind, placebo-controlled study. In that study, 66 participants (31 randomized to placebo and 35 to NAC) were compared and NAC treatment was associated with significant improvements in reducing urges and behavior. At the study's end point, of the 53 participants who completed the study, 15 of the 32 participants (47%) receiving NAC were much or very much improved compared with 4 of the 21 participants (19%) receiving placebo [40].

Cross-Diagnostic Approaches and Their Implications for Classification and Diagnosis

Cross-diagnostic approaches to BFRBs will rely on an understanding of the underlying pathophysiology of these disorders and their similarities and differences to other disorders.

Family History and Genetics

Data regarding the pathophysiology of trichotillomania are limited, but there is a familial component. Several family studies have reported elevated rates of trichotillomania in first-degree relatives of probands with trichotillomania, along with elevated rates of mood and anxiety disorders [41]. In a 2014 study, Keuthen and colleagues found that the relatives of probands with trichotillomania had higher recurrence risk estimates for hair pulling [42].

Existing family history data suggests that SPD is familial. In a study of 60 patients with SPD, 28.3% of their first-degree family members had SPD [43]. Another study of 40 patients with SPD found that 43% had a first-degree relative with SPD [23]. Although family studies of OCD have found that SPD occurs more frequently in case relatives [44], a comparison between probands with SPD and those with OCD found that individuals with SPD were significantly more likely to have at least one first-degree relative with SPD or compulsive nail biting compared with patients with OCD [45].

Monzani and colleagues (personal communication) examined the prevalence and heritability of skin-picking in a sample of 2518 twins from the Twins UK adult twin registry. Clinically significant skin picking was endorsed by 1.2% of twins. Significantly higher concordance rates for the monozygotic versus dizygotic twin pairs indicated a strong genetic influence on skin picking. Additive and non-additive genetics factors accounted for slightly over 40% of the variance in skin picking, with the remaining variance attributable to non-shared environmental factors (with shared environmental factors negligible and non-significant).

Neuroimaging

Several brain structures and functions have been implicated in both trichotillomania and SPD. Excess gray-matter density has been found in patients with trichotillomania compared with controls, in the striatum, amygdalohippocampal formation, frontal and cingulate cortices and supplementary motor cortex [46]. In a 2013 functional neuroimaging study, patients with trichotillomania exhibited dampening of nucleus accumbens responses to reward anticipation (but relative hypersensitivity to gain and loss outcomes) as compared with controls [47]. Other neuroimaging studies have found disorganization of white-matter tracts involved in motor generation and suppression (i.e. bilateral anterior cingulate and right orbitofrontal and inferior frontal cortices) in both disorders [48,49]. Neuropsychological studies have also shown that patients with trichotillomania and SPD exhibit deficits in cognitive abilities that are linked to the functioning of the frontal lobe and its related frontosubcortical structures, such as executive functioning deficits, motor impulsivity and insufficient cognitive-behavioral flexibility [50,51].

Psychological Theories of Body-Focused Repetitive Behavior Etiology

Because negative emotions such as anxiety, tension and sadness often precede pulling and picking episodes, the question arises as to the role of these behaviors in regulating emotional states or stressful events [20,52]. Picking and pulling may therefore function as a means for the person to escape from or avoid aversive experiences and the temporary reduction in these negative emotions maintains the behavior through a negative reinforcement cycle [52]. Studies that have measured emotional regulation in individuals with and without pulling and picking found that individuals have greater difficulty regulating negative affective states than controls [53]. In a related fashion, boredom may also trigger picking and pulling in some individuals [23,54]. This has led some to hypothesize that pulling and picking may similarly help to adjust negative emotions brought on by a feeling of perfectionism characterized by unwillingness to relax [54]. This theory suggests that the perfectionism leads to feelings of frustration, impatience and dissatisfaction when standards are not met and to boredom when productivity is impossible. Picking and pulling may therefore function as a means of releasing tension generated by these emotions. Pulling and picking are perhaps positively reinforced by a feeling of "taking action" [5].

Animal Models

Animal models represent useful tools for investigating the pathophysiology of BFRBs. One possible candidate model is the *hoxb8* gene knockout mouse. Greer and Capecchi [55] reported that, compared with their control counterparts, mice with mutations of *Hoxb8* gene groomed excessively to the point of skin lesions. Mutant mice demonstrated normal cutaneous sensation and there was no evidence of an inflammatory response suggesting that this behavior was not due to skin or other abnormalities of the peripheral nervous system. This transgenic model is promising because the excessive grooming of *Hoxb8* mutants is similar to the excessive grooming seen in BFRBs, thus offering face similarity to symptoms observed in BFRBs. Moreover, the *Hoxb8* gene is expressed in the orbital cortex, the anterior cingulate, the striatum and the limbic system.

A possible genetic model for BFRBs can be found in the animal research on the gene encoding SAPAP3, a scaffolding protein found in excitatory glutamate-responsive synapses largely in the striatum. Mice which were deficient in SAPAP3 demonstrated extreme excessive grooming [56]. This research was later reinforced in a human genetic association study which found that a variation in the *SAPAP3* gene is associated with human grooming disorders, such as SPD [44]. A study of 383 families phenotyped for OCD genetics studies (1618 participants) used a family-based association analysis and found that 32% of the participants met criteria for a grooming disorder (20% for SPD). The study found that SPD was associated with a variant of the *SAPAP3* gene which was not associated with OCD.

Future Directions

Clinical treatment trials for BFRBs have been largely short term and have predominantly involved young or middle-aged adults. Data are lacking on the long-term benefit and risks among both children and the elderly. More research is also needed to identify predictors of poor outcomes.

Habit-reversal therapy has demonstrated some benefit for BFRBs, but there are no data regarding how well it is performed in the community and how effective the treatment is when performed by non-specialists. It has shown some promise but there are few, if any, data on whether more traditional therapies such as cognitive therapy or supportive therapy might also be beneficial for trichotillomania and SPD.

The genetic features of BFRBs remain incompletely understood. Genes that confer susceptibility to these disorders have not yet been identified. Studies are needed to identify childhood and adolescent risk factors, and on how these variables interact with genetic factors. This may allow for the identification of children at risk and the development of early-intervention strategies.

Although a range of etiological theories have been proposed, there is still a paucity of data examining this important area.

Declaration of Interest

Dr. Grant has received research grants from National Institute of Mental Health, National Center for Responsible Gaming, the American Foundation for Suicide Prevention, the Trichotillomania Learning Center, Brainsway, Forest, Roche, Takeda and Psyadon Pharmaceuticals. He receives yearly compensation from Springer Publishing for acting as Editor-in-Chief of the *Journal of Gambling Studies* and has received royalties from Oxford University Press, American Psychiatric Publishing, Inc., Norton Press and McGraw Hill. Dr. Chamberlain's research is supported by a Clinical Fellowship from the Wellcome Trust (110049/Z/15/Z).

References

1. American Psychiatric Association. *Diagnostic and Statistical Manual of Mental Disorders*, 5th ed. Washington, DC: APA; 2013.
2. Stein DJ, Chtistenson GA, Hollander E, eds. *Trichotillomania*. Washington, DC: American Psychiatric Association Publishing; 1999.
3. Stein DJ, Grant JE, Franklin ME, et al. Trichotillomania (hair pulling disorder), skin picking disorder, and stereotypic movement disorder: toward DSM-V. *Depress Anxiety*. 2010;27(6):611–626.
4. Grant JE, Stein DJ, Woods DW, Keuthen NJ. *Trichotillomania, Skin Picking, and Other Body-Focused Repetitive Behaviors*. Washington, DC:American Psychiatric Association Publishing; 2012.
5. Grant JE, Chamberlain SR. Trichotillomania. *Am J Psychiatry*. 2016;173(9):868–874.
6. Duke DC, Keeley ML, Geffken GR, Storch EA. Trichotillomania: a current review. *Clin Psychol Rev*. 2010;30(2):181–193.
7. King RA, Zohar AH, Ratzoni G, et al. An epidemiological study of trichotillomania in Israeli adolescents. *J Am Acad Child Adolesc Psychiatry*. 1995;34(9):1212–1215.
8. Siddiqui EU, Naeem SS, Naqvi H, Ahmed B. Prevalence of body-focused repetitive behaviors

in three large medical colleges of Karachi: a cross-sectional study. *BMC Res Notes*. 2012;5:614.

9. Grant JE, Redden SA, Leppink EW, et al. Sex differences in trichotillomania. *Ann Clin Psychiatry*. 2016;28(2):118–124.
10. Lewin AB, Piacentini J, Flessner CA, et al. Depression, anxiety, and functional impairment in children with trichotillomania. *Depress Anxiety*. 2009;26(6):521–527.
11. Hayes SL, Storch EA, Berlanga L. Skin picking behaviors: an examination of the prevalence and severity in a community sample. *J Anxiety Disord*. 2009;23:314–319.
12. Keuthen NJ, Koran LM, Aboujaoude E, Large MD, Serpe RT. The prevalence of pathological skin picking in US adults. *Compr Psychiatry*. 2010;51:183–186.
13. Odlaug BL, Kim SW, Grant JE. Quality of life and clinical severity in pathological skin picking and trichotillomania. *J Anxiety Disord*. 2010;24(8):823–829.
14. Grant JE, Odlaug BL. Clinical characteristics of trichotillomania with trichophagia. *Compr Psychiatry*. 2008;49(6):579–584.
15. Arnold LM, McElroy SL, Mutasim DF, Dwight MM, Lamerson CL, Morris EM. Characteristics of 34 adults with psychogenic excoriation. *J Clin Psychiatry*. 1998;59:509–514.
16. Bohne A, Wilhelm S, Keuchen NJ, Baer L, Jenike MA. Skin picking in German students: prevalence, phenomenology, and associated characteristics. *Behav Modif*. 2002;26:320–339.
17. Calikusu C, Yucel B, Polat A, Baykal C. The relation of psychogenic excoriation with psychiatric disorders: a comparative study. *Compr Psychiatry*. 2003;44:256–361.
18. Grant JE, Odlaug BL, Chamberlain SR, Keuthen NJ, Lochner C, Stein DJ. Skin picking disorder. *Am J Psychiatry*. 2012;169(11):1143–1149.
19. Tucker BT, Woods DW, Flessner CA, Franklin SA, Franklin ME. The Skin Picking Impact Project: phenomenology, interference, and treatment utilization of pathological skin picking in a population-based sample. *J Anxiety Disord*. 2011;25:88–95.
20. Snorrason I, Smari J, Olafsson RP. Emotion regulation in pathological skin picking: findings from a non-treatment seeking sample. *J Behav Ther Exp Psychiatry*. 2010;41:238–245.
21. Keuthen NJ, Jameson M, Loh R, Deckersbach T, Wilhelm S, Dougherty SS. Open-label escitalopram treatment for pathological skin picking. *Int Clin Psychopharmacol*. 2007;22:268–274.
22. Grant JE, Odlaug BL, Kim SW. Lamotrigine treatment of pathologic skin picking: an open-label study. *J Clin Psychiatry*. 2007;68:1384–1391.
23. Neziroglu F, Rabinowitz D, Breytman A, Jacofsky M. Skin picking phenomenology and severity comparison. *Prim Care Companion J Clin Psychiatry*. 2008;10:306–312.
24. Rehm I, Moulding R, Nedelijkovic M. Psychological treatments for trichotillomania: update and future directions. *Australas Psychiatry*. 2015;23(4):365–368.
25. Keuthen NJ, Rothbaum BO, Fama J, et al. DBT-enhanced cognitive-behavioral treatment for trichotillomanai: a randomized controlled trial. *J Behav Addict*. 2012;1(3):106–114.
26. Rogers K, Banis M, Falkenstein MJ, et al. Stepped care in treatment of trichotillomania. *J Consult Clin Psychol*. 2014;82(2):361–367.
27. Bloch MH, Landeros-Weisenberger A, Dombrowski P, et al. Systematic review: pharmacological and behavioral treatment for trichotillomania. *Biol Psychiatry*. 2007;62(8):839–846.
28. Rothbart R, Amos T, Siegfried N, et al. Pharmacotherapy for trichotillomania. *Cochrane Database Syst Rev*. 2013;11:CD007662.
29. Odlaug BL, Grant JE. N-acetyl cysteine in the treatment of grooming disorders. *J Clin Psychopharmacol*. 2007;27:227–229.
30. Van Ameringen M, Mancini C, Patterson B, Bennett M, Oakman J. A randomized, double-blind, placebo-controlled trial of olanzapine in the treatment of trichotillomania. *J Clin Psychiatry*. 2010;71(10):1336–1343.
31. Grant JE, Odlaug BL, Chamberlain SR, Kim SW. Dronabinol, a cannabinoid agonist, reduces hair pulling in trichotillomania: a pilot study. *Psychopharmacology (Berl)*. 2011;218(3):493–502.
32. Siev J, Reese HE, Timpano K, Wilhelm S. Assessment and treatment of pathological skin picking. In: Grant JE, Potenza MN, eds., *The Oxford Handbook of Impulse Control Disorder*. Oxford University Press; 2012:360–374.
33. Teng EJ, Woods DW, Twohig M. Habit reversal as a treatment for chronic skin picking: a pilot investigation. *Behav Modif*. 2006;30:411–422.
34. Schuck L, Keijsers G, Rinck M. The effects of brief cognitive-behavioral therapy for pathological skin picking: a randomized comparison to wait-list control. *Behav Res Ther*. 2011;49:11–17.
35. Grant JE, Stein DJ, Woods DW, Keuthen NJ. *Pharmacotherapy, in Trichotillomania, Skin Picking and Other Body-Focused Repetitive Behaviors*. Washington, DC: American Psychiatric Association Publishing; 2012:205–221.
36. Simeon D, Stein DJ, Gross S, Islam N, Schmeidler J, Hollander E. A double-blind trial of fluoxetine

in pathologic skin picking. *J Clin Psychiatry.* 1997;58:341–347.

37. Bloch MR, Elliot M, Thompson H, Koran LM. Fluoxetine in pathologic skin picking: open-label and double-blind results. *Psychosomatics.* 2001;42:314–319.

38. Arbabi M, Farina V, Balighi K, et al. Efficacy of citalopram in treatment of pathological skin picking: a randomized double blind placebo controlled trial. *Acta Med Iran.* 2008;46:367–372.

39. Grant JE, Odlaug BL, Chamberlain SR, Kim SW. A double-blind, placebo-controlled trial of lamotrigine for pathologic skin picking: treatment efficacy and neurocognitive predictors of response. *J Clin Psychopharmacol.* 2010;30:396–403.

40. Grant JE, Chamberlain SR, Redden SR, Leppink EW, Odlaug BL, Kim SW. N-acetycysteine in the treatment of excoriation disorder: a randomized clinical trial. *JAMA Psychiatry.* 2016;73(5):490–496.

41. Schlosser S, Black DW, Blum N, Goldstein RB. The demography, phenomenology, and family history of 22 persons with compulsive hair pulling. *Ann Clin Psychiatry.* 1994;6(3):147–152.

42. Keuthen NJ, Altenburger EM, Pauls D. A family study of trichotillomania and chronic hair pulling. *Am J Med Genet B Neuropsychiatr Genet.* 2014;165B(2):167–174.

43. Odlaug BL, Grant JE. Pathologic skin picking. In: Grant JE, Stein DH, Woods DW, Keuthen NJ, eds., *Trichotillomania, Skin Picking, and Other Body-Focused Repetitive Behaviors.* Washington, DC: American Psychiatric Association Publishing; 2012:21–41.

44. Bienvenu OJ, Wang Y, Shugart YY, et al. Sapap3 and pathological grooming in humans: results from the OCD collaborative genetics study. *Am J Med Genet B: Neuropsychiatr Genet.* 2009;150B:710–720.

45. Grant JE, Odlaug BL, Kim SW. A clinical comparison of pathologic skin picking and obsessive-compulsive disorder. *Compr Psychiatry.* 2010;51(4):347–352.

46. Chamberlain SR, Menzies LA, Fineberg NA, et al. Grey matter abnormalities in trichotiilomani: morphometric magnetic resonance imagine study. *Br J Psychiatry.* 2008;193(3):216–221.

47. White MP, Shirer WR, Molfino MJ, Tenison C, Damoiseaux JS, Greicius MD. Disordered reward processing and functional connectivity in trichotillomania: a pilot study. *J Psychiatr Res.* 2013;47(9):1264–1272.

48. Chamberlain SR, Hampshire A, Menzies LA, et al. Reduced brain white matter integrity in trichotillomania: a diffusion tensor imaging study. *Arch Gen Psychiatry.* 2010;67(9):965–971.

49. Grant JE, Odlaug BL, Hampshire A, Schreiber LR, Chamberlain SR. White matter abnormalities in skin picking disorder: a diffusion tensor imaging study. *Neuropsychopharmacology.* 2013;38(5):763–769.

50. Chamberlain SR, Odlaug BL, Boulougouris V, Fineberg NA, Grant JE. Trichotillomania: neurobiology and treatment. *Neurosci Biobehav Rev.* 2009;33(6):831–842.

51. Odlaug BL, Hampshire A, Chamberlain SR, Grant JE. Abnormal brain activation in excoriation (skin-picking) disorder: evidence from an executive planning fMRI study. *Br J Psychiatry.* 2016;208(2):168–174.

52. Roberts S, O'Connor K, Belanger C. Emotion regulation and other psychological models for body-focused repetitive behaviors. *Clin Psychol Rev.* 2013;33(6):745–762.

53. Shusterman A, Feld L, Baer L, Keuthen N. Affective regulation in trichotillomania: evidence from a large-scale internet survey. *Behav Res Ther.* 2009;47(8):637–644.

54. O'Connor K, Brisebois H, Brault M, Robillard S, Loiselle J. Behavioral activity associated with onset in chronic tic and habit disorder. *Behav Res Ther.* 2003;41(2):241–249.

55. Greer JM, Capecchi MR. Hoxb8 is required for normal grooming behavior in mice. *Neuron.* 2002;33:23–34.

56. Welch JM, Lu J, Rodriguiz RM, et al. Cortico-striatal synaptic defects and OCD-like behaviours in Sapap3-mutant mice. *Nature.* 2007;448:894–990.

Chapter 29

Stereotypic Movement Disorder

Dan J. Stein

Introduction

Stereotypic movement disorder (SMD) is classified in the *Diagnostic and Statistical Manual of Mental Disorders*, fifth edition (DSM-5) as a neurodevelopmental disorder, and is characterized by repetitive, seemingly driven and apparently purposeless motor behavior [1]. At the same time, stereotypic behavior is widely seen in the animal kingdom, and is found in a broad range of human psychiatric conditions [2]. This chapter reviews clinical aspects of SMD, drawing on a translational approach to address transdiagnostic aspects of this condition. It makes the argument that a more complete understanding of SMD may be useful for conceptualizing and managing a broad range of compulsive behavior.

Recent Research Findings

Diagnosis

The stereotypies that characterize SMD are characterized by the DSM-5 as repetitive, seemingly driven and apparently purposeless [1]. Typical examples are hand shaking or waving, body rocking, head banging, self-biting and hitting one's own body. While similar rhythmical movements may be seen across individuals, each individual may have an individually patterned set of symptoms. Multiple movements may be combined (e.g., cocking the head, rocking the torso, waving a small string repetitively in front of the face).

Stereotypic movements may last a few seconds to several minutes or longer, and their frequency may vary from multiple occurrences in a single day to several weeks elapsing between episodes. Different patterns of self-injurious behavior may be seen in different genetic disorders associated with intellectual disability [3]. Stereotypic behaviors may be precipitated by both hyper- (e.g., excitement) or hypo-arousal (e.g., fatigue). While DSM-5 notes that the movements are apparently purposeless, the manual admits that such associations suggests that they do serve a function [1], such as regulating arousal or decreasing anxiety.

DSM-5 diagnostic criteria also emphasize that these symptoms begin early in life; indeed, this is the basis for the inclusion of SMD in the DSM-5 chapter on neurodevelopmental disorders. Simple stereotypic movements (e.g., rocking) are common in typically developing children in the first three years of life, may play a role in learning movements, and typically resolve. Complex stereotypic movements occur in around 3–4%, with about 80% having symptoms before two years of age [1]. Prevalence is considerably higher in individuals with intellectual disability (4–16%), and even higher in autistic disorder [4], and in a number of genetic syndromes associated with intellectual disability and self-injurious behavior [3,5].

DSM-5 also includes a standard clinical criterion and hierarchy criterion. The repetitive motor behavior must interfere with social, academic or other activities and may result in self-injury. The repetitive motor behavior must not be attributable to a substance of abuse, to a neurological condition, mental disorder or another neurodevelopmental disorder. Examples listed in DSM-5 are obsessive-compulsive disorder (OCD) and trichotillomania. SMD should also be differentiated from drug-induced disorders with abnormal movements, such as tardive dyskinesia and akathisia.

DSM-5 also notes two possible specifiers for SMD [1]. First, there is a specifier for self-injury; when the individual has self-injurious behavior, or behavior that would result in an injury if preventive measures were not used. Second, there is a specifier for SMD that is associated with a known medical or genetic condition, neurodevelopmental disorder or environmental factor. As examples, DSM-5 lists Lesch–Nyhan syndrome, intellectual disability and intrauterine alcohol exposure.

There is arguably a contradiction between the hierarchy criterion in DSM-5 and the association specifier. On the one hand, the diagnostic criteria do not allow SMD to be diagnosed in the presence of another condition (the hierarchy criterion). In contrast, the association specifier indicates that another condition may indeed be present. That said, the examples listed under the hierarchy criterion (say, trichotillomania) are quite different from those listed under the associated specifier criterion (say, Lesch–Nyhan syndrome).

Skin picking in Prader-Willi syndrome may be a useful exemplar to consider in this context, and is discussed in the DSM-5 diagnostic section on excoriation (skin picking) disorder [1]. While patients with skin-picking disorder have a somewhat variable age of onset, this condition most commonly begins during adolescence [6]. Prader-Willi syndrome is a neurodevelopmental condition and characteristic symptoms, including skin picking, begin very early in life [7].

While many patients with SMD have intellectual disability, there are reports of SMD in children and adults of normal intelligence. In pediatric neurology, there are well-characterized case series of intellectually normal patients with symptoms such as head nodding and hand waving [8]. Stereotypies in children with normal intelligence may have an early age of onset, chronicity and high prevalence of comorbid difficulties, including tics, obsessive-compulsive behaviors and attention deficit and hyperactivity disorder. There are also well-described series of adult patients with SMD, again with a high prevalence of comorbid mood and anxiety disorders [9].

These considerations raise the question of whether typical stereotypic symptoms (e.g., body rocking, head banging) may be a form of compulsivity that is particularly common in neurodevelopmental disorders, while in intellectually normal individuals such compulsivity presents more often in a different form (e.g., hair pulling, skin picking). Hypothetically, there may be similar psychobiological characteristics underlying such compulsivity, including the involvement of particular neurocircuits and neurochemistry and precipitation of behavior by similar sets of cues. This idea is explored in more detail later in this chapter.

Treatment

The literature on SMD notes the importance of careful assessment to individualize therapy, and the possible value of both pharmacological and psychotherapeutic interventions [10]. Where the stereotypy is associated with a known genetic or neurological condition, a specific pathophysiology may be known and targeted. Lesch–Nyhan syndrome, for example, represents a specific genetic defect of purine metabolism, which can be targeted by particular agents such as allopurinol [11]. At the same time, even in such a disorder, broader psychobiological dysfunctions are present, and may respond to less specific interventions [12,13].

Animal models of stereotypy emphasize the possible mediating role of dopaminergic and serotonergic neurocircuitry, suggesting the potential of dopamine blockers and selective serotonin reuptake inhibitors (SSRIs) in the treatment of human SMD. There is a relative paucity of randomized controlled trials, but Castellanos and colleagues reported a few cases in which the serotonergic antidepressant clomipramine seemed more effective than the noradrenergic antidepressant desipramine in adults of normal intellect with SMD [9]. Small case series suggest that SSRIs may also be useful in some cases [14].

There have also been a number of randomized controlled trials of various psychotropic medications for SMD in the context of intellectual disability and autistic disorder [15,16]. The SSRI fluoxetine, for example, was found more efficacious than placebo in reducing repetitive symptoms in patients with autistic disorder [17]. There is also some evidence that fluoxetine in low doses is more effective than placebo in the treatment of repetitive behaviors in childhood autism [18]. Nevertheless, not all data are consistent, and there are concerns about publication bias in this area [16]. Other medications studied in this context include dopamine blockers, D-cycloserine, valproate and oxytocin [19,20]. A number of agents, including levetiracetam, guanfacine and atomoxetine appear not to be useful for stereotypy in autistic disorder [20].

A behavioral literature has emphasized the relevance of understanding cues that precipitate stereotypy, and the value of habit reversal therapy [8]. Habit reversal therapy includes a focus on increasing awareness of precipitating cues, replacing stereotypic behavior with more adaptive behavior, and the potential value of rewarding such behavior. A meta-analysis based on 575 participants in 18 studies found habit reversal therapy to be an efficacious intervention for a wide variety of maladaptive repetitive behaviors [21]. A range of behavioral work has also focused on reducing stereotypy and self-injury in intellectual disability and autistic disorder [22,23,24,25,26].

Cross-Diagnostic Approaches and Diagnosis

An animal literature on stereotypy has been useful in emphasizing that stereotypy ranges from simple stereotypies (e.g., repetitive self-grooming) to more complex stereotypies or habits (e.g., repeating a series of behaviors) [27]. There has been growing work focused on understanding the relevant neurocircuitry and neurochemistry of simple stereotypy, as well as of more complex habits [10,28,29,30,31,32,33,34]. This work perhaps provides a basis for reconsidering our nosological approach to a range of conditions characterized by stereotypy.

Striatal circuitry seems to play a particularly important role in mediating stereotypic behavior, including grooming behaviors [35,36], although a range of other brain regions may also be important [29]. Corticostriatal circuitry includes a range of neurochemical systems, including dopaminergic and serotonergic circuitry. While D_1 and D_2 receptors may play somewhat different roles in modulating stereotypic behavior [37], there is evidence that dopamine agonism increases grooming while D_2 blockers decrease grooming [29].

Serotonin reuptake inhibitors (SRIs) also decrease stereotypy in a number of animal models [38,39,40]. Glutamatergic, GABA-ergic and opioid systems likely also contribute to mediating stereotypy and grooming [29]. Furthermore, there is increased understanding of a range of molecules, including neuroinflammatory and scaffolding proteins, which contribute to stereotypy and self-injurious behavior [40,41]. There is also a growing understanding of the neurobiological mechanisms underlying the relationship between exposure to stressors and increased stereotypy [42,43,44].

This literature provides the basis for a translational neuroscience approach to understanding stereotypic behavior in the clinic. In animals, simple stereotypy arises commonly in confined environments (e.g., pacing in large mammals confined to small cages). In humans, simple stereotypy is most likely to emerge in patients with intellectual disability, where it may manifest in the form of symptoms such as body rocking and head banging. Stereotypies may, however, also emerge in cases of sensory deprivation or social isolation [45]. Frustrative non-reward may be a particularly important cue for self-injurious behavior [24].

Trichotillomania and skin-picking disorder have features in common with simple stereotypies [46,47]. Cues often include hyper- and hypo-arousal; such behaviors may have useful self-soothing or emotional regulation properties. Certainly, in animals, grooming behaviors have a range of adaptive functions, that go beyond mere cleaning [48,49]. Pharmacotherapy of trichotillomania and skin-picking disorder may address the neurocircuitry and neurochemistry underlying these grooming behaviors, while psychotherapy uses the principles of habit reversal to modify the relevant behavior.

OCD is arguably characterized by more complex stereotypic behavior. Ethologically informed observations in patients with OCD have emphasized the extent to which classical compulsions are repetitive and invariant [49,50]. Recent work has focused on abnormal habit processes in patients with OCD; compulsivity may represent an imbalance between goal-directed and habit-learning systems, for example, with excessive stimulus-response habit learning or deficient goal-directed control over action and response inhibition [51,52,53].

Stereotypic behavior is not confined to the obsessive-compulsive and related disorders. From the perspective of the Research Domain Criteria (RDoC) framework, it is notable that stereotypic and self-injurious behavior is characteristic of a number of neurodevelopmental conditions, including autistic disorder [54,55]. Stereotypic motoric behavior may also emerge in a range of other conditions (e.g., pacing and related symptoms in psychotic disorders, stereotypic movements in dementia). Stereotypic cognitive behavior may be seen in an even broader range of conditions (e.g., stereotypic thoughts in eating disorders). It may be hypothesized that there are some overlaps in the mediating neurocircuitry and neurochemistry across these different disorders.

DSM-5 includes the new category of self-injurious non-suicidal behaviors. These are defined as repetitive intentional self-inflicted damage to the surface of the body of a sort likely to induce bleeding, bruising or pain (e.g., cutting, burning, stabbing, hitting, excessive rubbing), with the expectation that the injury will not lead to severe physical harm (i.e., there is no suicidal intent). From a translational neuroscience perspective, these behaviors may again have a good deal in common with simple stereotypy. It is notable that self-injurious non-suicidal behaviors are often triggered by negative emotional states, and that they may respond to specific pharmacotherapies (e.g., SSRIs), and to particular forms of psychotherapy [56,57].

Cross-Diagnostic Approaches and Treatment

Serotonergic medications seem more efficacious than noradrenergic medications in a broad range of conditions characterized by stereotypic behavior, including trichotillomania [58]. Although SSRIs have been disappointing in trichotillomania, there is some evidence that these agents are efficacious for skin-picking disorder [59]. As noted earlier, SRIs have been studied for SMD in intellectually normal individuals [9], as well as for stereotypies in the context of intellectual disability [15] and autistic disorder [16,20]; although there are some signals of efficacy, not all data are consistent, and there is evidence of publication bias.

Dopamine blockers decrease stereotypy in animal models as well as in the clinical context. Low-dose dopamine blockers have been found efficacious for the augmentation of SSRIs in OCD [60], and may also be useful in conditions such as trichotillomania and skin-picking disorder [61]. While there is some evidence for the value of dopamine blockers for the treatment of stereotypies and self-injurious behavior in the context of intellectual disability and autistic disorder, not all data are consistent [15,20], and risk–benefit ratio must be carefully considered [62].

Glutamatergic agents may be useful in trichotillomania and skin-picking disorder, and have been used as augmenting agents in OCD [63]. D-cycloserine was effective in improving stereotypic symptoms in older adolescents and young adults with autism spectrum disorders [64]. Further work is needed on the potential role of glutamatergic agents for the treatment of stereotypy and self-injurious behavior in the context of intellectual disability and autistic disorder.

Opioid agents may decrease stereotypy in animal models [28]. Such agents have also been suggested to be useful in OCD, trichotillomania and skin-picking disorder, although there have been few rigorous randomized controlled trials to date [46]. The role of the opioid system in non-suicidal self-injurious behavior has long been mooted [65]. Naltrexone has been studied for the treatment of self-injurious behavior in individuals with intellectual disability, with some evidence for efficacy [15]. Opioid agents certainly warrant further investigation in compulsivity, stereotypy and self-injurious behavior.

Behavioral principles appear useful in conceptualizing and treating SMD, as well as a range of obsessive-compulsive and related disorders. As above, habit reversal therapy is an efficacious intervention for a wide variety of maladaptive repetitive behaviors [21]. It has been suggested that most forms of stereotypy are maintained by automatic reinforcement; antecedent (e.g., environmental enrichment) and consequent (e.g., differential reinforcement of alternative behavior) interventions may lead to reductions in stereotypy and self-injury, including both lower-order and higher-order repetitive behaviors in intellectual disability and autistic disorder [22,23,24,25,26].

There is a small literature on the use of electroconvulsive therapy for stereotypies; for example, in individuals with autistic disorder and intractable self-injurious behavior [66]. This raises the question of whether other forms of brain stimulation, including deep brain stimulation, may also be effective for these symptoms [67], perhaps targeting the neural circuitry thought to underlie stereotypy and self-injury. Further studies in this area seem warranted.

Future Directions

This chapter has explored the entity of SMD, which is classified in the DSM-5 chapter on neurodevelopmental disorder. At the same time, it has noted an extensive animal and basic neuroscience literature, which includes the notion that stereotypies fall on a spectrum between simple and complex. This raises the question of whether an RDoC-like approach should include a spectrum of stereotypic and self-injurious behavior that cuts across various diagnostic categories. From this perspective, a range of neurodevelopmental, obsessive-compulsive and related disorders, as well as other psychiatric conditions, are characterized by simple and complex stereotypic behavior.

This perspective may be particularly useful to the extent that it helps understand overlapping neurocircuitry and neurochemical mechanisms across different diagnostic entities, and to the extent that this in turn provides useful targets for pharmacotherapy and psychotherapy. We have noted that certain medications may be selectively efficacious for simple and complex stereotypic symptoms across different diagnostic conditions. Similarly, behavioral principles including habit reversal and reinforcement of alternative behavior, appear efficacious for simple and complex stereotypic symptoms across diagnoses. The hope is that as the translational neuroscience of stereotypy and self-injury advances, so too will our clinical assessments and interventions.

Translational neuroscience of stereotypy may well benefit from current advances in animal models, in brain imaging and in neurogenetics. Further phenotypic and molecular exploration of a range of animal models of stereotypy and self-injury is needed to provide a more detailed understanding of the functional pathways and systems biology underlying these behaviors [22,68,69,70]. It may be useful to supplement behavioral analyses of repetitive behaviors with physiological measures [71].

Collaborative brain imaging investigations are providing new insights into the neurobiology of OCD [72], and may ultimately lead to a better understanding of the neurocircuitry of compulsivity and stereotypy in general. Similarly, collaborative investigations have advanced our understanding of the genetic architecture of OCD [73], and may eventually lead to advances in understanding the pathophysiology of compulsivity and stereotypy. Such work may ultimately provide a useful foundation for a personalized approach to intervention for SMD and self-injurious behavior.

References

1. American Psychiatric Association. *Diagnostic and Statistical Manual of Mental Disorders,* 5th ed. Washington, DC: APA; 2013.
2. Stein D, Christenson G. Stereotypic movement disorder: a neglected problem. *Psychiatr Ann.* 1998;28(6):304.
3. Huisman S, Mulder P, Kuijk J, et al. Self-injurious behavior. *Neurosci Biobehav Rev.* 2018;84:483–491.
4. Bodfish JW, Symons FJ, Parker DE, Lewis MH. Varieties of repetitive behavior in autism: comparisons to mental retardation. *J Autism Dev Disord.* 2000;30(3):237–243.
5. Oliver C, Licence L, Richards C. Self-injurious behaviour in people with intellectual disability and autism spectrum disorder. *Curr Opin Psychiatry.* 2017;30(2):97–101.
6. Grant JE, Odlaug BL, Chamberlain SR, Keuthen NJ, Lochner C, Stein DJ. Skin picking disorder. *Am J Psychiatry.* 2012;169(11):1143–1149.
7. Stein DJ, Keating J, Zar HJ, Hollander E. A survey of the phenomenology and pharmacotherapy of compulsive and impulsive-aggressive symptoms in Prader-Willi syndrome. *J Neuropsychiatry Clin Neurosci.* 1994;6(1):23–29.
8. Muthugovindan D, Singer H. Motor stereotypy disorders. *Curr Opin Neurol.* 2009;22(2):131–136.
9. Castellanos FX, Ritchie GF, Marsh WL, Rapoport JL. DSM-IV stereotypic movement disorder: persistence of stereotypies of infancy in intellectually normal adolescents and adults. *J Clin Psychiatry.* 1996;57(3):116–122.
10. Stein DJ, Chamberlain SR, Fineberg N. An A-B-C model of habit disorders: hair-pulling, skin-picking, and other stereotypic conditions. *CNS Spectr.* 2006;11(11):824–827.
11. Schretlen DJ, Ward J, Meyer SM, et al. Behavioral aspects of Lesch–Nyhan disease and its variants. *Dev Med Child Neurol.* 2005;47(10):673–677.
12. Olson L, Houlihan D. A review of behavioral treatments used for Lesch-Nyhan syndrome. *Behav Modif.* 2000;24(2):202–222.
13. Zilli EA, Hasselmo ME. A model of behavioral treatments for self-mutilation behavior in Lesch–Nyhan syndrome. *Neuroreport.* 2008;19(4):459–462.
14. Stein DJ, Bouwer C, Niehaus DJ. Stereotypic movement disorder. *J Clin Psychiatry.* 1997;58(4):177–178.
15. Gormez A, Rana F, Varghese S. Pharmacological interventions for self-injurious behaviour in adults with intellectual disabilities: abridged republication of a Cochrane systematic review. *J Psychopharmacol.* 2014;28(7):624–632.
16. Carrasco M, Volkmar FR, Bloch MH. Pharmacologic treatment of repetitive behaviors in autism spectrum disorders: evidence of publication bias. *Pediatrics.* 2012;129(5):e1301–e1310.
17. Hollander E, Soorya L, Chaplin W, et al. A double-blind placebo-controlled trial of fluoxetine for repetitive behaviors and global severity in adult autism spectrum disorders. *Am J Psychiatry.* 2012;169(3):292–299.
18. Hollander E, Phillips A, Chaplin W, et al. A placebo controlled crossover trial of liquid fluoxetine on repetitive behaviors in childhood and adolescent autism. *Neuropsychopharmacology.* 2005;30(3):582–589.
19. Soorya L, Kiarashi J, Hollander E. Psychopharmacologic interventions for repetitive behaviors in autism spectrum disorders. *Child Adolesc Psychiatr Clin N Am.* 2008;17(4):753–771.
20. Rajapakse T, Pringsheim T. Pharmacotherapeutics of Tourette syndrome and stereotypies in autism. *Semin Pediatr Neurol.* 2010;17(4):254–260.
21. Bate KS, Malouff JM, Thorsteinsson ET, Bhullar N. The efficacy of habit reversal therapy for tics, habit disorders, and stuttering: a meta-analytic review. *Clin Psychol Rev.* 2011;31(5):865–871.

22. Rapp JT, Vollmer TR. Stereotypy I: a review of behavioral assessment and treatment. *Res Dev Disabil.* 2005;26(6):527–547.

23. Boyd BA, McDonough SG, Bodfish JW. Evidence-based behavioral interventions for repetitive behaviors in autism. *J Autism Dev Disord.* 2012;42(6):1236–1248.

24. Furniss F, Biswas AB. Recent research on aetiology, development and phenomenology of self-injurious behaviour in people with intellectual disabilities: a systematic review and implications for treatment. *JIDR.* 2012;56(5):453–475.

25. Denis J, Van den Noortgate W, Maes B. Self-injurious behavior in people with profound intellectual disabilities: a meta-analysis of single-case studies. *Res Dev Disabil.* 2011;32(3):911–923.

26. Matson JL, Lovullo SV. A review of behavioral treatments for self-injurious behaviors of persons with autism spectrum disorders. *Behav Modif.* 2008;32(1):61–76.

27. Ridley RM. The psychology of perserverative and stereotyped behaviour. *Prog Neurobiol.* 1994;44(2):221–231.

28. Rapp JT, Vollmer TR. Stereotypy II: a review of neurobiological interpretations and suggestions for an integration with behavioral methods. *Res Dev Disabil.* 2005;26(6):548–564.

29. Kalueff AV, Stewart AM, Song C, Berridge KC, Graybiel AM, Fentress JC. Neurobiology of rodent self-grooming and its value for translational neuroscience. *Nat Rev Neurosci.* 2016;17(1):45–59.

30. Whitehouse CM, Lewis MH. Repetitive behavior in neurodevelopmental disorders: clinical and translational findings. *Behav Anal.* 2015;38(2):163–178.

31. Lewis MH, Tanimura Y, Lee LW, Bodfish JW. Animal models of restricted repetitive behavior in autism. *Behav Brain Res.* 2007;176(1):66–74.

32. Muehlmann AM, Lewis MH. Abnormal repetitive behaviours: shared phenomenology and pathophysiology. *JIDR.* 2012;56(5):427–440.

33. Smith KS, Graybiel AM. Habit formation. *Dialogues Clin Neurosci.* 2016;18(1):33–43.

34. Burguiere E, Monteiro P, Mallet L, Feng G, Graybiel AM. Striatal circuits, habits, and implications for obsessive-compulsive disorder. *Curr Opin Neurobiol.* 2015;30:59–65.

35. Ahmari SE, Spellman T, Douglass NL, et al. Repeated cortico-striatal stimulation generates persistent OCD-like behavior. *Science.* 2013;340(6137):1234–1239.

36. Burguiere E, Monteiro P, Feng G, Graybiel AM. Optogenetic stimulation of lateral orbitofronto-striatal pathway suppresses compulsive behaviors. *Science.* 2013;340(6137):1243–1246.

37. Eilam D, Talangbayan H, Canaran G, Szechtman H. Dopaminergic control of locomotion, mouthing, snout contact, and grooming: opposing roles of D1 and D2 receptors. *Psychopharmacology.* 1992;106(4):447–454.

38. Hugo C, Seier J, Mdhluli C, et al. Fluoxetine decreases stereotypic behavior in primates. *Prog Neuropsychopharmacol Biol Psychiatry.* 2003;27(4):639–643.

39. Korff S, Stein DJ, Harvey BH. Stereotypic behaviour in the deer mouse: pharmacological validation and relevance for obsessive compulsive disorder. *Prog Neuropsychopharmacol Biol Psychiatry.* 2008;32(2):348–355.

40. Welch JM, Lu J, Rodriguiz RM, et al. Cortico-striatal synaptic defects and OCD-like behaviours in Sapap3-mutant mice. *Nature.* 2007;448(7156):894–900.

41. Symons FJ. Self-injurious behavior in neurodevelopmental disorders: relevance of nociceptive and immune mechanisms. *Neurosci Biobehav Rev.* 2011;35(5):1266–1274.

42. Taylor SB, Anglin JM, Paode PR, Riggert AG, Olive MF, Conrad CD. Chronic stress may facilitate the recruitment of habit- and addiction-related neurocircuitries through neuronal restructuring of the striatum. *Neuroscience.* 2014;280:231–242.

43. Martin LJ, Spicer DM, Lewis MH, Gluck JP, Cork LC. Social deprivation of infant rhesus monkeys alters the chemoarchitecture of the brain: I. Subcortical regions. *J Neurosci.* 1991;11(11):3344–3358.

44. Knowlton BJ, Patterson TK. Habit formation and the striatum. *Curr Top Behav Neurosci.* 2018;37:275–295.

45. Barry S, Baird G, Lascelles K, Bunton P, Hedderly T. Neurodevelopmental movement disorders – an update on childhood motor stereotypies. *Dev Med Child Neurol.* 2011;53(11):979–985.

46. Stein DJ, Grant JE, Franklin ME, et al. Trichotillomania (hair pulling disorder), skin picking disorder, and stereotypic movement disorder: toward DSM-V. *Depress Anxiety.* 2010;27(6):611–626.

47. Stein DJ, Woods DW. Stereotyped movement disorder in ICD-11. *Rev Bras Psiquiatr.* 2014;36(Suppl 1):65–68.

48. Hoppe L, Ipser J, Lochner C, Thomas K, Stein D. Should there be a category: "grooming disorders"? In: Kalueff A, LaPorte J, CL B, eds. *Neurobiology of Grooming Behavior.* New York: Cambridge University Press; 2010:226–251.

49. Stein DJ, Hermesh H, Eilam D, et al. Human compulsivity: a perspective from evolutionary medicine. *Eur Neuropsychopharmacol.* 2016;26(5):869–876.

50. Eilam D, Zor R, Szechtman H, Hermesh H. Rituals, stereotypy and compulsive behavior in animals and humans. *Neurosci Biobehav Rev.* 2006;30(4):456–471.

51. Gillan CM, Papmeyer M, Morein-Zamir S, et al. Disruption in the balance between goal-directed behavior and habit learning in obsessive-compulsive disorder. *Am J Psychiatry.* 2011;168(7):718–726.

52. Voon V, Reiter A, Sebold M, Groman S. Model-based control in dimensional psychiatry. *Biol Psychiatry.* 2017;82(6):391–400.

53. Cuzen NL, Fineberg NA, Stein DJ. Unconscious habit systems in compulsive and impulsive disorders. *Behav Brain Sci.* 2014;37(2):141.

54. Anagnostou E, Chaplin W, Watner D, et al. Factor analysis of repetitive behaviors in Autism as measured by the Y-BOCS. *J Neuropsychiatry Clin Neurosci.* 2011;23(3):332–339.

55. Devine DP. Self-injurious behaviour in autistic children: a neuro-developmental theory of social and environmental isolation. *Psychopharmacology.* 2014;231(6):979–997.

56. McKay D, Andover M. Should nonsuicidal self-injury be a putative obsessive-compulsive-related condition? A critical appraisal. *Behav Modif.* 2012;36(1):3–17.

57. Schiavone FL, Links PS. Common elements for the psychotherapeutic management of patients with self injurious behavior. *Child Abuse Negl.* 2013;37(2–3):133–138.

58. Swedo SE, Leonard HL, Rapoport JL, Lenane MC, Goldberger EL, Cheslow DL. A double-blind comparison of clomipramine and desipramine in the treatment of trichotillomania (hair pulling). *N Engl J Med.* 1989;321(8):497–501.

59. Simeon D, Stein DJ, Gross S, Islam N, Schmeidler J, Hollander E. A double-blind trial of fluoxetine in pathologic skin picking. *J Clin Psychiatry.* 1997;58(8):341–347.

60. Ipser JC, Carey P, Dhansay Y, Fakier N, Seedat S, Stein DJ. Pharmacotherapy augmentation strategies in treatment-resistant anxiety disorders. *Cochrane Database Syst Rev.* 2006(4):CD005473.

61. Lochner C, Roos A, Stein DJ. Excoriation (skin-picking) disorder: a systematic review of treatment options. *Neuropsychiatr Dis Treat.* 2017;13:1867–1872.

62. McDonough M, Hillery J, Kennedy N. Olanzapine for chronic, stereotypic self-injurious behaviour: a pilot study in seven adults with intellectual disability. *JIDR.* 2000;44(Pt 6):677–684.

63. Kariuki-Nyuthe C, Gomez-Mancilla B, Stein DJ. Obsessive compulsive disorder and the glutamatergic system. *Curr Opin Psychiatry.* 2014;27(1):32–37.

64. Urbano M, Okwara L, Manser P, Hartmann K, Herndon A, Deutsch SI. A trial of D-cycloserine to treat stereotypies in older adolescents and young adults with autism spectrum disorder. *Clin Neuropharmacol.* 2014;37(3):69–72.

65. Kirtley OJ, O'Carroll RE, O'Connor RC. The role of endogenous opioids in non-suicidal self-injurious behavior: methodological challenges. *Neurosci Biobehav Rev.* 2015;48:186–189.

66. D'Agati D, Chang AD, Wachtel LE, Reti IM. Treatment of severe self-injurious behavior in autism spectrum disorder by neuromodulation. *J ECT.* 2017;33(1):7–11.

67. Park HR, Kim IH, Kang H, et al. Nucleus accumbens deep brain stimulation for a patient with self-injurious behavior and autism spectrum disorder: functional and structural changes of the brain: report of a case and review of literature. *Acta Neurochir (Wien).* 2017;159(1):137–143.

68. Moy SS, Riddick NV, Nikolova VD, et al. Repetitive behavior profile and supersensitivity to amphetamine in the C58/J mouse model of autism. *Behav Brain Res.* 2014;259:200–214.

69. Tanimura Y, Yang MC, Ottens AK, Lewis MH. Development and temporal organization of repetitive behavior in an animal model. *Dev Psychobiol.* 2010;52(8):813–824.

70. Kazdoba TM, Leach PT, Yang M, Silverman JL, Solomon M, Crawley JN. Translational mouse models of autism: advancing toward pharmacological therapeutics. *Curr Top Behav Neurosci.* 2016;28:1–52.

71. Rapp JT, Lanovaz MJ. Introduction to the special issue: assessment and treatment of stereotypy. *Behav Modif.* 2014;38(3):339–343.

72. de Wit SJ, Alonso P, Schweren L, et al. Multicenter voxel-based morphometry mega-analysis of structural brain scans in obsessive-compulsive disorder. *Am J Psychiatry.* 2014;171(3):340–349.

73. Stewart SE, Yu D, Scharf JM, et al. Genome-wide association study of obsessive-compulsive disorder. *Mol Psychiatry.* 2013;18(7):788–798.

Chapter 30

The Clinical Neuropsychiatry of "Organic" Obsessive-Compulsive Disorder

Leonardo F. Fontenelle

Introduction

Mind–brain dualism has affected the status of psychiatry both as a science and a medical specialty for centuries. Sadly, as the specific etiologies of different mental disorders are unveiled, psychiatry has progressively lost territory to other areas of medicine, particularly neurology. This phenomenon, which has happened in neurosyphilis, pellagra, *mixedema madness*, and many other neuropsychiatric disorders, is unfortunate, both for patients, who were then precluded from having their illnesses managed by doctors who specialized in behavioral problems, and for medicine as a whole, as psychiatrists have seen their medical skills shrinking throughout the last century. Thus, for the sake of our patients' health, psychiatrists need to develop the ability to diagnose and treat the conditions that have been variably known as "organic", "secondary", or "symptomatic" mental disorders, including obsessive-compulsive disorder (OCD) and obsessive-compulsive related disorders (OCRDs).

As a general guideline, a few features may help differentiating "primary" (idiopathic) from "organic" OCRDs [1], including the temporal relationship between the psychiatric syndrome and the underlying neurological or medical condition (although OCRDs may be the first "symptom" of a medical condition that appears only later), the atypicality of presentation (e.g., late or super-late onset OCRDs, suddenly developed OCRDs, *de novo* cognitive impairment, or the appearance of OCRDs with focal neurological signs), and the fact that obsessions or compulsions are not better explained by a "primary" OCRD, such as the lack of a family history or a premorbid cluster C personality disorder (although some might consider these latter conditions as risk factors for "secondary" OCRDs as well). One study suggested indifference to illness, a lack of motivation for treatment, absence of depression/anxiety, rigid and concrete thinking, and treatment refractoriness to be particularly evident in "organic" OCD [2].

Rather than discussing the evidence for brain involvement in, for example, "primary" OCRDs (e.g., volumetric abnormalities, neurocognitive deficits, and the presence of neurological soft signs, among others), the findings of these studies are used to provide a conceptual framework for this chapter. Structural, spectroscopic, and functional studies performed at rest, during symptom provocation, and after treatment all support the involvement of the so-called corticostriatothalamocortical circuit in the pathophysiology of primary OCD. Thus, this chapter discusses the occurrence of obsessions, compulsions, and related phenomena, particularly OCD, across a range of neurological conditions that affect key structures of the above-mentioned neurocircuit, namely, the striatum, orbitofrontal, anterior cingulate and prefrontal cortices, and the temporal lobe disorders.

Striatal Disorders

In general, basal ganglia disorders express themselves clinically as abnormal movements that can be further classified into akinetic rigid or hyperkinetic syndromes [3]. Although these syndromes have been associated with OCRDs to differing extents, a general discussion of the ways of conceptualizing them clinically may be helpful. It is important to mention that patients often show a combination of different akinetic rigid and hyperkinetic syndromes, which may alternate and predominate according to disease stage and medication status [3]. However, determining the predominant syndrome and its associated features is an important initial diagnostic step, as it restricts the range of the differential diagnoses.

Akinetic Rigid Syndromes

Although akinetic rigid syndromes include different combinations and degrees of slowness (bradykinesia) or poverty (hypokinesia)[1] of movements, its critical component has been hypothesized as being the progressive fatiguing and decrease of repetitive alternating movements (elicited by, for instance, up to 64 repetitions of finger or foot tapping) [3]. Thus, prompting these symptoms can be time consuming. Typically, brady- and hypokinesia interfere with "reactive" (automatic) and "expressive" movements, the latter of which are thought to reflect the patient's underlying affective life and to include the facial expression and gesticulation of the individual's arms, hands, and upper trunk [4,5]. A few authors have also considered akinesia and hypokinesia to be the inability to initiate and a delay in initiating motor responses, respectively [6].

Before discussing the OCRDs that can be associated with akinetic rigid symptoms, it is also important to mention that a few OCRDs can mimic akinetic rigid symptoms, including the so-called "obsessional slowness" (slowness due to overt, time-consuming, compulsive behaviors, or more strictly, to covert symptoms) [7] and some forms and symptoms of catatonia that can be found in patients with OCD [8]. *Formes frustes* of catatonia have been described in patients with OCD resulting from compulsive posturing (bizarre posturing in response to obsessive thoughts), comorbid neuropsychiatric disorders (e.g., mania), drug intoxication (e.g., antipsychotics), and Tourette's disorder; the latter being common in OCD patients and sharing typical symptoms with catatonia, such as echophenomena [8]. Mild bradykinetic symptoms were reported in up to 34% of patients with OCD and were also associated with repeating rituals and lower intelligence quotient [9].

Despite sharing the striatum as a major pathophysiological hub with OCD, it is still doubtful whether patients with Parkinson's disease show increased rates and severities of OCD or obsessive-compulsive symptoms (OCS) compared with matched controls [10,11,12,13]. Although there have been suggestions that OCS may be particularly severe in severe Parkinson's disease [14,15], the association between OCS and a particular aspect of motor involvement is unclear [14,16]. Genetic factors may contribute to this heterogeneity. For instance, patients with Parkinson's disease who have PARKIN-1 and -2 mutations endorsed OCS to a *lesser* extent than non-carriers with Parkinson's disease, whereas asymptomatic relatives with mutations endorsed OCS to a *greater* extent than asymptomatic relatives who did not carry mutations [17]. We have not found systematic investigations assessing OCD or clearly defined OCS (other than case reports) in other rigid akinetic syndromes [18,19,20,21].

The so-called "Parkinsonian personality" [22], a construct characterized by industriousness, inflexibility, punctuality, cautiousness, and lack of novelty seeking [22,23], has been suggested as heralding a diagnosis of Parkinson's disease. Clearly, the "Parkinsonian personality" has some conceptual overlaps with obsessive-compulsive personality disorder (OCPD). Thus, not surprisingly, an increased prevalence of OCPD in both medicated (long duration) [23] and treatment naïve (short-duration) [24] patients with Parkinson's disease has been described. More recently, however, similar rates of OCPD were found in Parkinson's disease and progressive supranuclear palsy, thus suggesting that OCPD may reflect a common impairment of specific parts of the frontostriatal circuits [25]. However, there is no well-controlled longitudinal study showing either "Parkinsonian personality" or OCPD to antedate Parkinson's disease, progressive supranuclear palsy, or any other akinetic rigid syndrome, so the concept of a premorbid Parkinsonian personality is speculative.

Further important, yet relatively poorly understood phenomena having some similarities with OCRDs are the impulse control disorders that develop as complications of dopaminergic treatment for akinetic rigid syndromes. In a two-year prospective study assessing impulse control disorders in patients with Parkinson's disease (n = 1000) [26], prevalence was relatively stable across time (approximately 28–33% depending on the diagnostic instrument employed). Patients with impulse control disorders who also had Parkinson's disease were younger and more often male; they also had an earlier age at onset, a longer duration of illness and more severe non-motor symptoms, among other features [26]. Although the factors that determine what types of impulse control disorder subtypes patients with Parkinson's disease

[1] I acknowledge some might consider this subdivision to be confusing, as, terminologically, akinesia could be considered as an extreme form of hypokinesia.

will develop as a consequence of treatment are still unclear, there is some evidence suggesting that PARKIN mutations may play a role. For instance, biallelic PARKIN mutations have been associated with drug-induced compulsive shopping, binge eating, and punding/hobbyism [27,28].[2]

The syndrome known as "psychic akinesia" or "loss of psychic self-activation" [29] can be clinically translated as an extreme form of behavioral inertia that is transiently reversible by external stimulation [30]. It results from damage to striatothalamoprefrontal circuits [30]. This condition has been included in the spectrum of "athymhormia"[3] and other disorders of motivation [32]. Other associated features include descriptions (but not complaints) of "mental emptiness", blunted affectivity, and "compulsive-like activities" such as mental compulsions (e.g., counting), and motor behaviors that ranged from simple (e.g., finger snapping, moving, or sucking) to complex (e.g., painting pictures) [29,30]. To Laplane and colleagues, authors of the first report, compulsive behaviors developed on the mental vacuum left by damage to the basal ganglia, a hypothesis deemed consistent with Pierre Janet's concept of OCD ("psychasthenia") [29]. Later, however, compulsive behaviors were thought not to be essential for the diagnosis [32].

Hyperkinetic Syndromes

Hyperkinetic (or dyskinetic) syndromes are more pleomorphic than the akinetic rigid syndromes [3]. Though hyperkinesias have been specifically defined as "involuntary" movement disorders characterized by "excessive amplitude of movement" [33], some clinicians have provided broader and somewhat simpler definitions of hyperkinetic syndromes, such as "too much movement" [3]. Hyperkinesias have been further subdivided into jerky (e.g., chorea, tics, and myoclonus) and non-jerky (e.g., dystonia and tremor) [3]. Early clinicians stretched the spectrum of hyperkinesias to include excessive expressive and reactive movements shown by patients with motility psychosis, catatonia, and other psychotic conditions [5]. Indeed, clinicians often perceive the differential diagnosis of hyperkinetic syndromes as more challenging than akinetic rigid syndromes [3].

It is important to characterize and differentiate jerky hyperkinetic syndromes from one another. A myoclonus is a sudden, rhythmic or nonrhythmic, predictable or not, "shock-like" involuntary movement, which usually affects the same part of the body and is caused by either muscle contractions (positive myoclonus) or relaxations (negative myoclonus: asterixis) [3]. Despite also being sudden, a chorea is unpredictable, nonrhythmic, and involuntary; it affects alternating parts of the body and appears as "randomly flowing jerks" [3]. A tic is a sudden, predictable (or "stereotyped"[4]) [34] nonrhythmic movement or vocalization that is also temporarily suppressible (semi-voluntary), and is associated with the relief of an uncomfortable, often premonitory, "sensory phenomena" [3]. It can be simple (e.g., blinking or grunting) or complex (e.g., echopraxia or echolalia). When a slow and prolonged movement follows a tic, the latter is called dystonic [3] (for a discussion on OCD and tics [35] see Chapter 27).

Among the non-jerky hyperkinetic syndromes, only dystonia seems relevant to our discussion, as tremors are not apparently specifically related to OCS or OCD. A dystonia is characterized by sustained or intermittent muscle contractions causing abnormal, often repetitive, movements, postures, or both [36]. It can affect the neck, limbs, trunk, eyelids, face, or vocal cords [37]. Cervical and limb dystonic syndromes are characterized by the presence of dystonic postures and movements (e.g., dystonic tremors); the performance of alleviating tricks (*gestes antagonistes*), such as touching the cheek to improve cervical dystonia; the so-called "mirror dystonia" (which is provoked by a task, such as piano movements, performed by the opposite non-affected body region), and the "overflow phenomena" (dystonia extending beyond the commonly involved body regions) [38]. However, these signs are not very useful in diagnosing cranial and laryngeal dystonias [38].

[2] Punding can be defined as complex and pointless repetitive behaviors which captivate the individual's attention and resemble his/her previous occupation, hobbies and pastimes [27].

[3] Athymhormia, meaning "absence of mood to move forward", was a term coined by Dide and Giraud to describe the amotivational syndrome found among patients with schizophrenia [31].

[4] In DSM-5, the expression "stereotyped" is reserved for "stereotypic movement disorder" [34].

Immune Mediated Movement Disorders

The group of immune mediated movement disorders includes encephalitis lethargica, lupus/antiphospholipid syndrome chorea, Sydenham chorea, pediatric autoimmune neuropsychiatric disorders associated with streptococcal infections (PANDAS), and a few paraneoplastic disorders [39,40]. Among these conditions, only Sydenham chorea [41,42] PANDAS [39,41], and opsoclonus–myoclonus [43] have been consistently associated with OCD. Sydenham chorea is a symptom of acute rheumatic fever, a condition related to exposure to a group A streptococcal infection [44]. It is the most common cause of chorea in children, particularly girls in developing countries [44]. Sydenham chorea generally remits after a few months, only to recur in almost 50% of the cases, often after an infectious trigger [44]. One study found OCD in 38.4% of cases of Sydenham chorea, and the most common OCS to be aggressive (63%) and checking (53%) symptoms [45]. In general, OCS peaks in two months after rheumatic fever, but can occur before, concomitantly, or after the onset of Sydenham chorea [46]. As a group, OCRDs are more frequent in rheumatic fever than in controls regardless of the presence of Sydenham chorea [47].

The PANDAS concept was etiologically related to Sydenham chorea, although only fine movements of the fingers when the child maintains stressed postures (choreiform movements), and not frank chorea, could be present [48]. Both OCD and tics were core to the first descriptions of PANDAS, which was also assessed as a potential subtype of OCD for DSM-5 [49]. In 2015, however, PANDAS was renamed to pediatric acute neuropsychiatric syndrome (PANS) to reflect a greater understanding of the phenomenon [44]. Accordingly, its criteria have been reshaped by: (i) an extra emphasis on the *foudroyant* (lightning-like) onset or recurrence of OCD and/or restricted food intake (rather than of OCD and/or tics);[5] (ii) the recognition that the syndrome is frequently associated with other neuropsychiatric symptoms, including emotional, behavioral, academic, neurologic, and somatic abnormalities (yet not attributable to Sydenham chorea or other recognized disorders); and (iii) the exclusion of the requirement of prepubertal onset and of an evidence of a previous group A streptococcal infection [48].

Paraneoplastic syndromes are rare autoimmune non-metastatic complications of cancer [52,53]. The group of paraneoplastic syndromes with abnormal movements as its most noticeable component includes opsoclonus–myoclonus syndrome (OMS), movement disorders associated with CRMP-5/CV2 antibodies, stiff person syndrome, and cerebellar degeneration, among others. However, only OMS [41] and chorea associated with CRMP-5/CV2 antibodies [54] have been associated with OCD. The distinguishing features of OMS (or dancing eyes syndrome) are bursts of conjugate, chaotic eye movements (opsoclonus), myoclonus and/or ataxia, and behavioral and/or sleep disturbance [55]. In children, paraneoplastic OMS has been related to the presence of neuroblastoma, and in adults, to an underlying small-cell lung cancer and cancer of the breast and ovary. In one survey of OMS cases across the United States, "obsessions and compulsions" were reported by the parents of up to 58% of patients with OMS, and were the greatest residual problem in 9% of the cases [43].

Huntington Disease

In a systematic review on the co-occurrence of hyperkinetic disorders and OCD/OCS [42], Huntington disease was associated with increased rates of OCD/OCS in clinically manifested and non-manifesting gene carriers. However, this review also found that OCS severity tended to remain at a subthreshold level at all stages of disease progression (e.g., less than one hour daily spent on OCS), with some fluctuations. In contrast, in one study [56], the group of participants closest to onset of illness (i.e., those with the most neuropathology) had the lowest ratings of OCS endorsement, although it is unclear whether this finding results from the natural progression of illness, to a decrease in insight, to the ability to self-report symptoms due to cognitive dysfunction, or to a combination of these factors. According to the same systematic review reported above [42], the whole range of typical OCS dimensions (e.g., checking) were present among patients with Huntington disease.

[5] While the exclusion of tics as part of PANS was based on the difficulties "distinguishing the 'acute, dramatic onset' of tics in the PANDAS subgroup from the typically 'acute' onset of tics in non-PANDAS tic disorders" [48], the inclusion of restricted food intake as a symptom of PANS reflected the reports of anorexia nervosa developing after group A streptococcal infections [50,51].

Neuroacanthocytosis

The term neuroacanthocytosis refers to a group of syndromes characterized by abnormal movements (including chorea, dystonia, Parkinsonism, or tics) and acanthocytes (red blood cells). They include chorea acanthocytosis, McLeod syndrome, pantothenate kinase-associated neurodegeneration (PKAN) and Huntington disease-like 2 [57]. Chorea acanthocytosis is an autosomal recessive disorder associated with abnormalities in the *VPS13A* gene located on chromosome 9q21.2, and with frequent lip, cheek, and tongue mutilation. McLeod syndrome is an X-linked disorder resulting from defects on the *XK* gene, which leads to a decrease in Kell antigens and elevated creatine kinase levels. PKAN is an autosomal recessive disorder resulting from abnormalities in the *PANK2* gene, located on chromosome 20p13. It leads to iron accumulation in the basal ganglia (visualized as the "eye of the tiger sign" on brain scans). Broadly speaking, these conditions are associated with neuropsychiatric symptoms, particularly OCD and psychosis, in 60–80% of cases [57].[6]

Benign Hereditary Chorea

Benign hereditary chorea (BHC) is a childhood-onset, non-progressive autosomal dominant chorea without cognitive impairment, which is due to mutations in *NKX2.1* (14q13.3), a gene involved in the embryogenesis of brain, lung and thyroid tissue [59]. Therefore, BHC has often been associated with pulmonary dysfunction and hypothyroidism, forming a triad also known as brain–lung–thyroid syndrome [59]. In the largest cohort of patients with BHC to date ($n = 10$), a few additional features have been described, including skeletal abnormalities and, in one patient, severe OCD as a psychiatric comorbidity [60]. The most distinguishing features in this patient were fear of harm and need to touch [60]. Although the co-occurrence of BHC and OCD in this cohort may represent a chance finding, the authors of this report pondered whether the similarity between BHC phenotype and other movement disorders associated with OCD supports a true relationship between these conditions.

Dystonic Disorders

The classification of dystonia includes a clinical axis, where syndromes are classified according to age at onset (e.g., late adulthood), body distribution (e.g., focal), temporal pattern (e.g., progressive), and associated features (e.g., presence of another movement disorder); and an etiological axis, which defines syndromes on the basis of neuropathology (e.g., neurodegeneration), heritability (or lack of thereof), and absence of an identifiable cause (sporadic or familial) [61,62]. Syndromes deemed relevant to our discussion include: (i) dystonia–Parkinsonism, which is also sometimes accompanied by pyramidal signs or other neurological deficits and is usually inherited (e.g., dopa-responsive dystonia and Wilson's disease); (ii) myoclonus dystonia, whose onset is on childhood years; and (iii) focal or segmental isolated dystonia with onset in adulthood, which is usually sporadic (e.g., cervical dystonia, blepharospasm, and writer's cramp) [41].

Dopa-responsive dystonia (Segawa syndrome or DYT5) is an early-onset form of dystonia with diurnal fluctuation and a dramatic response to levodopa [63]. It is frequently caused by an autosomal dominant mutation in the *GCH1* gene (14q22.2), which is involved in the conversion of tyrosine to levodopa [63]. A systematic review found OCD in 9% of 70 published cases, a rate that is much higher than those reported in the general population [64]. In contrast, Wilson's disease is caused by an autosomal recessive defect of the gene *ATP7B* (13q14.3) leading to accumulation of copper in liver, brain and other tissues [41]. Although there are a few case reports of OCD among patients with Wilson's disease [65,66,67,68,69,70], the lack of systematic research on the topic precludes us from reaching any conclusion about the approximate rates of OCD in this population.

Myoclonus dystonia is a condition comprising an alcohol responsive myoclonus plus a dystonia, usually affecting arms, trunk, and neck [71]. It is frequently ascribed to mutations of the *sarcoglycan epsilon* gene (*SGCE*) [72], which have also been associated with greater prevalence of alcohol dependence and OCD than in *SGCE* non-carriers [73] and disability-matched patients (essential tremor) [74]. Finally, the relationship between focal/segmental dystonia and OCD is still unsettled, as studies found either no difference [75,76,77] or greater [78,79] presence and severity of OCS among cervical dystonia,

[6] The only exception to this rule of thumb is Huntington disease-like 2, a condition resulting from a CTG/CAG expansion mutation of the *Junctophilin-3* gene on chromosome 16q24.3, which has been less frequently associated with OCD [58].

blepharospasm, and writer's cramp compared with appropriately matched controls (e.g., hemifacial spasm). In one of the positive studies, severity of depression was the main driver of high OCS, irrespective of neurological diagnosis [78].

Frontal, Anterior Cingulate and Temporal Lobe Disorders

Frontotemporal Lobar Degeneration (Pick's Disease)

In 2011, the International Behavioural Variant FrontoTemporal Dementia Criteria Consortium reviewed older guidelines that were considered to be too strict and insensitive for the early stages of frontotemporal dementia (FTD), the moment when disease-modifying agents were thought to be most effective. This consortium proposed newer and more flexible diagnostic criteria, which were organized on three different levels, including "possible" behavioral variant FTD (bvFTD; at least three behavioral/cognitive criteria), "probable" bvFTD (the former criteria plus significant functional decline and neuroimaging consistent with bvFTD), and "definite" bvFTD, defined by one of the two previous criteria plus histopathological evidence of frontotemporal lobar degeneration (FTLD) or mutations of pathogenic genes, such as genes encoding microtubule-associated protein tau, charged multivesicular body protein 2B, valosin-containing protein and progranulin [80].

The behavioral/cognitive criteria for bvFTD proposed by the consortium included: (i) executive dysfunction; (ii) hyperorality and dietary changes; (iii) early behavioral disinhibitions; (iv) early apathy or inertia; (v) early loss of sympathy or empathy; and, notably, (vi) early perseverative, stereotyped or compulsive/ritualistic behaviors [80]. The last group of symptoms are reminiscent of OCRDs and comprise simple repetitive movements (including, *inter alia*, tapping, picking at skin, or throat clearing) [80], stereotypy of speech (i.e., "single words, phrases or entire themes or stories that the patient habitually repeats") [80], or complex, compulsive, or ritualistic behaviors (such as checking, washing, ordering, counting, hoarding, and repetitive trips to the bathroom, among others) [80]. The *Diagnostic and Statistical Manual of Mental Disorders*, fifth edition (DSM-5) criteria for the behavior variant of major or mild frontotemporal neurocognitive disorder [34] were clearly influenced by these guidelines.

Almost in parallel with the publication of the International Behavioural Variant FrontoTemporal Dementia Criteria Consortium, another group of experts published a consensus on primary progressive aphasia (PPA), a different clinical expression of FTLD [81]. The consensus proposed clinical, imaging supported, or definite pathologic diagnosis for a PPA non-fluent/agrammatic variant (agrammatism in language production and effortful speech are the core features), a semantic variant (with anomia and single-word comprehension deficits as the core features), and a logopenic variant (characterized by word retrieval in spontaneous speech and confrontation naming and sentence repetition deficits) [81]. The DSM-5 criteria for the language variant of major or mild frontotemporal neurocognitive disorder ("Prominent decline in language ability, in the form of speech production, word finding, object naming, grammar, or word comprehension") largely overlapped with the concept of PPA [34].

Regardless of the actual phenotype (bvFTD or PPA), it seems that a dysfunction of the temporal lobes and/or striatum in the presence of preserved frontal lobe functions is important in generating complex compulsive behaviors in FTLD. In one study in patients with bvFTD [82], severity of associated OCS correlated with decreased gray matter in the bilateral globus pallidus, left putamen, and lateral temporal lobe, particularly the left middle and inferior temporal gyri. Similarly, temporal lobe atrophy and asymmetry of atrophy were independently associated with complex compulsive behaviors in a (probably mixed) sample of patients with FTD [83]. Indeed, although one study [84] found repetitive behaviors to be equally common in both bvFTD and semantic dementia, repetitive behaviors with a more compulsive quality were reported in semantic dementia (or semantic variant of PPA) and included clockwatching tendencies, rigid adherence to a fixed routine, carrying out tasks in precisely the same way, and preoccupation with a limited range of topics leading to repetitive conversational themes.

From the diagnostic point of view, the concept of "organic OCD" in the presence of FTLD is a controversial issue. For instance, many case reports [85,86,87,88,89], case series [90], and controlled studies [91,92] suggest that "organic" OCD can escort or herald the appearance of FTLD. However, the fact that complex, compulsive or ritualistic behaviors can be indistinguishable from idiopathic OCD but also core to the diagnosis of FTLD suggests that an additional diagnosis of "organic OCD" or OCRD due to another medical condition may be redundant and unnecessary. One additional word of caution is the possibility that what looks like "organic OCD" may be actually a "pseudo-organic OCD". For instance, based on observations of a single case [93] we have speculated that lifelong "idiopathic" subclinical OCD could be simply "unmasked" (or converted into full-blown OCD) by unspecific factors, such as the cognitive decline or the underlying neurodegenerative process, in patients who develop dementia.

Stroke

For reasons that are not completely clear, OCD has been described as the least common anxiety disorder (when it was classified as such) that can develop after stroke [94]. As expected, most published studies have described OCD after lesions in structures that pertained to the corticostriatothalamocortical circuit, including the basal ganglia [95–100], the thalamus [96,101], and the orbitofrontal cortex [101]. This is not to say that post-stroke OCD does not appear after lesions in other areas, but only that this is found less frequently. For instance, post-stroke OCD and other atypical OCRDs (including punding/hoarding [102]) have been described after lesions affecting the brainstem [103,104], the cerebellum [105] and the left middle cerebral artery territory [106].

Interestingly, vascular lesions of the fronto-subcortical systems have also reactivated OCS in association with the emergence of *de novo* motor/phonic tics and mental compulsions in elderly patients who have experienced spontaneous or therapeutically induced remission of idiopathic OCD for decades [107]. However, just as ablative procedures may be performed to manage otherwise treatment-refractory OCD [107,108,109], vascular lesions of the frontostriatal systems may also be "strategically" located to lead to remission of OCRD symptoms. For instance, there are cases of OCD or trichotillomania symptoms resolution after basal ganglia [110,111] and nondominant frontoparietal infarct [112]. Post-stroke OCD cases have been successfully treated with both serotonin reuptake inhibitors (SRIs) [102,113] and atypical antipsychotics [114].

Epilepsy

Although OCD and OCS occur in patients with epilepsy at rates that are significantly higher (11–34.5%) than those found in healthy controls (0–3%), the reasons that determine their appearance seem to be highly dependent on the specific studies and/or samples under study [115,116,117,118,119,120]. One study found depression, interictal epileptiform discharges on electroencephalogram recordings, and underlying etiology ("symptomatic" epilepsy") to be the major predictors of OCS in a highly heterogeneous outpatient sample of patients with epilepsy [120]. There has been a proclivity toward greater frequency/severity of OCD/OCS among patients with temporal lobe epilepsy as compared with healthy controls [118] and patients with idiopathic generalized epilepsy [116,119]. However, the relationships between OCD/OCS and lateralization of foci have been equivocal, and no study associated the former with specific neuropathological etiologies.

We have noted that most patients with epilepsy with OCD/OCS can be tentatively classified into interictal or peri-ictal OCD cases [121]. For example, interictal OCD can be ascribed to a chance association (where OCD and epilepsy follow independent courses), to shared electrical mechanisms (e.g., where OCD reflects continuous epileptiform activity or, alternatively, forced normalization[7]) [122], or to a common anatomical abnormality affecting the corticostriatothalamocortical circuit [121]. In contrast, peri-ictal "OCD-like" symptoms (including pre-ictal, ictal, and post-ictal cases) [123] comprise "forced thoughts" or motor automatisms that reflect continuing epileptiform activity and are not necessarily related to a diagnosis of OCD. It is important to consider that interictal symptoms may be exacerbated during the peri-ictal period [123].

Although the borders of interictal and peri-ictal periods are often indistinct [124], there may be therapeutic implications of such tentative classification. For instance, a simple chance association between epilepsy and OCD could indicate simultaneous treatment for both conditions (e.g., antiepileptic drugs and SRIs,

[7] Forced normalization refers to the emergence of psychiatric symptoms on electrical normalization of the electroencephalogram [122].

respectively). The presence of continuous epileptiform activity could predict response to antiepileptic drugs [125], whereas forced normalization could be treated by the reduction of antiepileptic drugs, the use of drugs that lower seizure threshold, or even by electroconvulsive therapy [126]. A common anatomical abnormality (e.g., a tumor) could be corrected, for instance, by neurosurgery [127]. As peri-ictal OCD-like states are dependent on continuing epileptiform activity, they are amenable to treatment with antiepileptic drugs [128].

The so-called "epileptic personality" is a controversial concept that has been debated for decades in the psychiatric literature. Also known as Gastaut Geschwind syndrome, epileptic personality includes hyperreligiosity, hypergraphia (compulsive writing), hyposexuality, viscosity, and irritability [129]. Bear and Fedio developed an instrument to assess the interictal personality features [130], which were found to differ between patients with temporal lobe epilepsy and healthy controls [130], but to be similar to patients with non-epileptic seizures [131]. Yaryura-Tobias and Neziroglu [132] perspicaciously noted several areas of overlap between the "epileptic personality" and OCPD, including scrupulosity (concerns with right or wrong, cautiousness, preciseness and hesitation), perfectionism, meticulosity, and perseveration. It is surprising that no research on this relationship exists.

Traumatic Brain Injury

A 2016 systematic review suggested that prevalence rates of OCD following traumatic brain injury (TBI) are quite variable, as it affects anywhere from 2% to 30% of all TBI survivors [133]. However, lower estimates are probably more realistic, as exceedingly high rates of OCD in this population may simply reflect misleading interpretations of studies that employed the Symptoms Check List 90 Revised (e.g., Hoofien et al. [134]), a scale that was not developed to diagnose OCD and has shown poor divergent validity [115]. Typically, post-TBI OCS emerges during the very early acute phase (one week to two months) until two years post-TBI [135]. One classical study with ten patients with post-TBI OCD found them to exhibit OCS that are similar to idiopathic OCD, but also to have an overrepresentation of obsessional slowness (three cases) and compulsive exercising (three cases) [136]. Although the whole post-TBI OCD group was more impaired on executive, attention, memory, language and intelligence tests than matched controls, patients with obsessional slowness were particularly compromised in these tests [136].

One of the challenges met by clinicians assessing patients with TBI is the difficult disentangling post-TBI OCS (such as checking, rigidity, and obsessional slowness) from "understandable" behaviors that emerge as attempts to cope with common cognitive difficulties that characterize post-TBI states (including memory, executive dysfunction, or poor information processing speed; i.e., a "pseudo post-TBI OCD") [135]. However, once post-TBI OCS are suspected, it may be difficult to ascribe, in a single case, whether the observed cognitive difficulties are related to TBI itself, to post-TBI OCD, or to other conditions that are frequently comorbid with TBI and/or OCD. Hypothetically, the importance of this differentiation rests on the fact that "pseudo post-TBI OCD" may predict responses to cognitive rehabilitation, whereas true post-TBI OCD may respond to traditional anti-OCD treatments, such as cognitive behavioral therapy and/or SRIs.

Generalized Brain Disorders

Tumors

Unfortunately, there is not much information on the frequency of OCRDs (particularly OCD) among patients diagnosed with different types of brain tumors [137]. However, we found a proclivity toward left-sided tumoral lesions (including the left frontoparietal region [138], the left frontal region near the midline [139], and the left posterior insula [140]) among the published cases of "organic OCD" due to more anatomically discrete tumors. Further midline regions such as the midbrain [141] and the pineal regions have also been implicated [142]. There are some instances, however, where OCD is associated with lesions generalized across many different encephalic structures [143–147]. From the histopathological point-of view, "organic" OCD has been caused by arachnoid cysts [138], low- [140,141] and high-grade [139,144] astrocytomas, germinomas [142,143,145], and nodules and tubers [146,147]. We speculate that slow-growing tumors, which are known to produce changes in the personality realms, may allow subclinical OCD to manifest itself clinically [137].

In contrast, a well-documented and often overlooked possibility is the occurrence of OCS after resection of brain neoplasms in areas deemed relevant for the pathophysiology of OCD, including the right frontal lobe [148], the left frontotemporal region [149], the right parietal vertex [150], the brain stem [151], and the cerebellar vermis [152]. In these cases, we believe that OCS may stem from a local "hyperfunction" that results from the removal of the tumoral noxious effects over one particular region of the brain. In a group of neurosurgical patients assessed preoperatively and three months to one year after the operation, worsening of obsessionality has been noted in women after removal of left-sided tumors [153]. The occurrence of OCD in oncological patients should also entertain the possibilities of distant effects of a tumor [154], the effect of drugs initiation (e.g., interferon) [155], or withdrawal (e.g., dexamethasone) [154], a paraneoplastic syndrome (e.g., limbic encephalitis) [156], and obviously the stressful situation of having a severe medical illness diagnosed [157].

Substance and Medication-Induced Obsessive-Compulsive Disorder

There are reports of OCD being attributed to the use of, or intoxication with, drugs of abuse, such as amphetamine [158], meta-amphetamine [158], cocaine [159], and ecstasy [160]; medications, such as atypical antipsychotics (e.g., clozapine, olanzapine, and risperidone) [161], antiparkinsonians (e.g., dopaminergic agonists) [162], anticonvulsants (e.g., topiramate) [163], tuberculostatics (e.g., isoniazid) [164], immune modulators (i.e., interferon) [165]; opioids (codeine) [166]; toxins (carbon monoxide) [167]; and biological poisons (e.g., wasp sting) [168]. A diagnosis of OCD due to meta-amphetamine was reported in 6.9% of all meta-amphetamine abusers but was not predicted by any socio-demographic nor illness-related factors [169]. SRIs have led to skin-picking behaviors in patients with OCD [171]. However, withdrawal states from benzodiazepines [170], alcohol [172], and clozapine [173] have also been reported to lead to OCD.

Although there are many epidemiological studies showing an association between OCD and drugs of abuse [174], most of the findings of these cross-sectional studies not do allow any conclusion regarding direction of causality. However, there is evidence that OCS can lead to cannabis problems via coping motives, even after controlling for anxiety, depression, and stress [175]. Other drugs, including alcohol, may be used for similar purposes. In contrast, at least one follow-up epidemiological study suggested that certain substances (e.g., marijuana and cocaine) can predispose to OCD in the long term [176], or at least lead to a greater persistence of OCD (alcohol abuse) [177]. Whether these OCD cases are caused rather than just predisposed by previous drug use is debatable though (see discussion below).

Current Diagnostic Criteria For "Organic Obsessive-Compulsive Disorder"

In DSM-5, the conditions described in this chapter are, for the most part, diagnosable as either OCRDs due to another medical conditions or substance/medication-induced OCRDs [34]. While clinicians can specify whether OCRDs due to another medical condition display OCD-like symptoms, appearance preoccupations, hoarding symptoms, hair-pulling symptoms, or skin-picking symptoms, they can only specify substance/medication-induced OCRDs as having an onset during intoxication, during withdrawal, or after medication use. What DSM-5 means by OCD-like symptoms is unclear and could result in an exaggerated expansion of the concept of OCRD due to another medical condition. Of note, while the DSM-IV referred to non-psychiatric medical conditions as "general medical conditions", DSM-5 refers to them as "*other* medical conditions" based on the fact that, according to DSM-5, psychiatric disorders should be considered as medical conditions as well [178].

In DSM-5, both OCRDs due to another medical condition and substance/medication-induced OCRDs share criterion A, which mentions a clinical picture dominated by obsessions, compulsions, skin picking, hair pulling, other body-focused repetitive behaviors, or other OCRDs symptom [34]. In contrast, a criterion B, which is more "etiologically" based, differs between the two disorders [34]. It mentions the evidence from the history, physical examination, or laboratory findings that: (i) the disturbance is the direct pathophysiological consequence of another medical condition, in the case of OCRDs due to another medical condition; or that (ii) symptoms in criterion A developed during or soon afterwards substance intoxication or withdrawal or after exposure to medication that is recognized as capable of producing symptoms in criterion

A (although the specific drugs that are able to do so are not mentioned) [34].

Criterion C also aimed to exclude other conditions as explanations for "organic OCRDs", such as: (i) "another mental disorder", for OCRDs due to another medical condition; and (ii) "an OCRD that is not substance/medication induced" for substance/medication-induced OCRDs, as evidenced by the fact that OCRD symptoms precede, persist after a substantial amount of time (e.g., one month) or follow an independent course from substance/medication use [34]. Finally, the last two criteria are the same for both disorders (i.e., while criterion D requires OCRDs not to occur exclusively during the course of a delirium, criterion E requires OCRDs to cause clinically significant distress or impairment in social, occupational or other important areas of functioning) [34]. One should keep in mind that these disorders may be broader than the concept of "Organic OCRDs" though. For instance, while skin picking due to eczema may be classified as an OCRD according to DSM-5, it probably does not fit very well with the concept of "organic OCD".

"Organic Obsessive-Compulsive Disorder": The Diagnostic Process

One question that is often asked is that, once one identifies an OCS and suspects an organic cause, how should the clinician proceed to diagnose "organic OCD". In fact, a workup to rule out an "organic" etiology in every new patient with psychosis has been proposed and, with a few adaptations, might be of some applicability in the context of obsessions and compulsions [1], including: (i) a thorough medical history (including, for instance, complaints of sore throat in childhood-onset OCD); (ii) a thorough neurological examination (to identify, for instance, subtle extrapyramidal signs); and (iii) laboratory examinations, such as blood count and erythrocyte sedimentation rate (which may disclose recent infections), glucose and electrolytes (as hypocalcemia has been associated with "organic" OCD) [179], liver and renal tests (which may be abnormal in Wilson's disease and kidney disease) [66,180], electroencephalography (to investigate the presence of epilepsy) [181], and urinary drug screen (e.g., to disclose recent use of cocaine) [176]. Further tests are probably best guided by suspicion of a specific underlying "organicity".

Cross-Diagnostic Approaches and Their Implications for Classification and Diagnosis

Any reorganization on the way OCD is classified or diagnosed in non-psychiatric medical disorders should be based on the existence of some sort of *continuity* or *discontinuity* between symptom resulting from "organic" OCD compared with "idiopathic" OCD. From the clinical standpoint [182], "organic" OCD should only be diagnosed as OCD if it resembles the "idiopathic" form of the disorder on its defining features. For instance, it is important to differentiate true OCS from phenomena that lack the more "OCD-ish" subjective components, such as "organic rigidity" and "sterile" repetitions (e.g., stereotypies) that are common in coarse brain disorders (for a few additional examples, see Chapter 1). Curiously, there are a few "idiopathic" psychiatric disorders that are both reminiscent of these symptoms and considered as related to OCD, such as OCPD (and its underlying rigidity), and low-order ("motorically focused") OCRDs.[8]

Another important aspect that is often ignored in the "organic" OCD literature is whether the latter is actually *caused* or just *triggered* by a specific neurological insult or medication in a susceptible individual [182]. Unfortunately, we believe the current state of knowledge does not allow us to answer this question. For instance, one could speculate that only predisposed individuals would present with an OCD after, for instance, a stroke affecting the head of the caudate. To answer this important question, researchers would have to, for instance, compare the frequencies of different risk factors for OCD (such as family history of OCRDs [183] or the presence of serotonin transporter polymorphism 5-HTTLPR or HTR2A polymorphism rs6311, or rs6313 [184]) between carefully matched groups, including patients with "organic" OCD arising in the context of a specific neurological condition (e.g., caudate stroke), patients without OCD, but with the same neurological condition, and patients with idiopathic OCD. If, for instance, those with "organic OCD" and "idiopathic" OCD share a similar family history, one could argue that we are actually dealing with the same condition.

[8] Skin-picking (excoriation) disorder and trichotillomania (hair-pulling disorder) are often described in this way.

The findings that the rates of drug-induced OCD in patients with schizophrenia were dependent on the variations and interactions between a series of polymorphisms of the *SCL1A1* [185,186], *GRIN2B* [185,187], and *DLGAP3* [187] genes, suggest that atypical antipsychotics could lead to OCD in patients with schizophrenia who were genetically susceptible. However, one important aspect that is worth mentioning is that different neurological conditions may differ in their relationship with OCD. For instance, while Huntington disease might be considered a cause of OCD (for resulting in obsessions and/or compulsions in patients who were not susceptible to idiopathic OCD), a stroke of the basal ganglia may be considered to be one of few possible triggers for OCD (i.e., risk factors that contribute to the development of OCD in a genetically predisposed individual). The first scenario would be more consistent with an OCD due to another medical condition and the second would be more coherent with an "idiopathic" OCD precipitated by stroke.

Clinical Implications of Cross-Diagnostic Approaches for Treatment and Prevention

When "organic OCD" is diagnosed, it is appropriate to target the underlying medical condition (group A streptococcal infection), the substance use disorder (with substance use-focused psychotherapy and/or medication), or to discontinue the causative medication [34]. However, this "knee-jerk" approach may not be fully effective when the underlying medical condition is neither curable nor treatable (e.g., a neurodegenerative disease), when the substance causing OCD is not continuously abused (e.g., there is no substance use disorder), or when the underlying medication cannot be stopped for medical reasons (e.g., interferon for cancer). Thus, in many cases, the approach to the underlying etiologic of "organic OCD" should be paralleled by the specific remediation of obsessions and/or compulsions. In fact, the most intuitive implication of a cross-diagnostic approach to "organic OCD" is that it should be treated similarly to idiopathic OCD, thus including the use of SRIs and/or exposure and response prevention as first-line alternatives. However, this tactic remains a challenge, as indicators of underlying organicity in patients with OCD have also been linked to resistance to conventional anti-OCD treatments [2]. It is also unclear whether organic patients need (or tolerate) a critical component of the pharmacotherapy for OCD symptoms (i.e., high-dose SRIs), as do most patients with idiopathic OCD. For instance, high-dose SRIs may lower the seizure threshold and complicate the treatment of patients with OCD who have concomitant epilepsy. Antipsychotics may prove useful for OCD in the context of hyperkinetic disorders other than Tourette's disorder. In terms of behavior therapy, however, exposure and response prevention therapy has been successfully used in antipsychotic-induced OCD and does not appear to have any major contraindications [188]. The efficacy and tolerability of innovative treatments for treatment-resistant idiopathic OCD, such as transcranial magnetic stimulation, deep brain stimulation, and even functional neurosurgery, remains unknown in patients with organic disorder, as clinical trials generally exclude "organic OCD" from their samples.

Future Directions

Future studies should assess the presence of OCD symptoms and their impact on the outcomes across a range of neurological disorders. However, given the plethora of conditions that can cause OCS, developments in the field are highly dependent on the elucidation of pathophysiological mechanisms and treatment advances of each particular illness underlying OCS. Clearly, there is a pressing need to conduct clinical trials in individuals exhibiting OCS as a result of neurological disorders. Ideally, future studies would need to focus on OCD caused by circumscribed, etiologically homogeneous neuropathologies, although unknown prevalence rates in individuals with these disorders may challenge recruitment of research subjects.

References

1. Keshavan MS, Jindal RD. Neurobiology and etiology of primary schizophrenia: current status. In: Sachdev PS, Keshavan MS, eds. *Secondary Schizophrenia*. Cambridge University Press; 2010:3–11.
2. Yaryura-Tobias JA, Anderson MC, Neziroglu FA. Organicity in obsessive-compulsive disorder. *Behav Modif.* 2000;24(4):553–565.
3. Abdo WF, van de Warrenburg BP, Burn DJ, Quinn NP, Bloem BR. The clinical approach to movement disorders. *Nat Rev Neurol.* 2010;6(1):29–37.
4. Fish F. *Clinical Psychopathology.* (M. Hamilton, ed.). Bristol: John Wright; 1985.

5. Leonhard K. *Classification of Endogenous Psychoses and Their Differential Etiology*, 2nd ed. Wien: Springer; 1999.
6. Heilman KM, Watson RT. Intentional motor disorders. In: Levin HS, Eisenberg HM, Benton AL, eds. *Frontal Lobe Function and Dysfunction*. Oxford University Press; 1991:199–213.
7. Ganos C, Kassavetis P, Cerdan M, et al. Revisiting the syndrome of "obsessional slowness". *Mov Disord Clin Pract*. 2015;2(2):163–169.
8. Fontenelle LF, Lauterbach EC, Telles LL, Versiani M, Porto FH, Mendlowicz MV. Catatonia in obsessive-compulsive disorder: etiopathogenesis, differential diagnosis, and clinical management. *Cogn Behav Neurol*. 2007;20(1):21–24.
9. Pasquini M, Fabbrini G, Moretti G, et al. Bradykinesia in patients with obsessive-compulsive disorder. *Eur Psychiatry*. 2010;25(7):378–381.
10. Muller N, Putz A, Kathmann N, Lehle R, Gunther W, Straube A. Characteristics of obsessive-compulsive symptoms in Tourette's syndrome, obsessive-compulsive disorder, and Parkinson's disease. *Psychiatry Res*. 1997;70(2):105–114.
11. Maia AF, Pinto AS, Barbosa ER, Menezes PR, Miguel EC. Obsessive-compulsive symptoms, obsessive compulsive disorder, and related disorders in Parkinson's disease. *J Neuropsychiatry Clin Neurosci*. 2003;15(3):371–374.
12. Harbishettar V, Kumar PP, Janardhan RYC, Thennarasu K. Is there a relationship between Parkinson's disease and obsessive-compulsive disorder? *Parkinsonism Rel Disord*. 2005;11(2):85–88.
13. Sharp ME, Caccappolo E, Mejia-Santana H, et al. The relationship between obsessive-compulsive symptoms and PARKIN genotype: the CORE-PD study. *Mov Disord*. 2015;30(2):278–283.
14. Tomer R, Levin BE, Weiner WJ. Obsessive-compulsive symptoms and motor asymmetries in Parkinson's disease. *Cogn Behav Neurol*. 1993;6(1):26–30.
15. Alegret M, Junque C, Valldeoriola F, Vendrell P, Marti MJ, Tolosa E. Obsessive-compulsive symptoms in Parkinson's disease. *J Neurol Neurosurg Psychiatry*. 2001;70(3):394–396.
16. Maia AF, Pinto AS, Barbosa ER, Menezes PR, Miguel EC. Obsessive-compulsive symptoms, obsessive-compulsive disorder, and related disorders in Parkinson's disease. *J Neuropsychiatry Clin Neurosci*. 2003;15(3):371–374.
17. Sharp ME, Caccappolo E, Mejia-Santana H, et al. The relationship between obsessive compulsive symptoms and PARKIN genotype: the CORE-PD study. *Mov Disord*. 2015;30(2):278–283.
18. Destee A, Gray F, Parent M, et al. Obsessive-compulsive behavior and progressive supranuclear palsy. *Rev Neurol (Paris)*. 1990;146(1):12–18.
19. Fukui T, Lee E, Hosoda H, Okita K. Obsessive-compulsive behavior as a symptom of dementia in progressive supranuclear palsy. *Dement Geriatr Cogn Disord*. 2010;30(2):179–188.
20. Karnik NS, D'Apuzzo M, Greicius M. Non-fluent progressive aphasia, depression, and OCD in a woman with progressive supranuclear palsy: neuroanatomical and neuropathological correlations. *Neurocase*. 2006;12(6):332–338.
21. Yamamoto T, Oishi K, Oya Y, Ogawa M, Kawai M. Compulsive repetition of movements in a case of progressive supranuclear palsy. *Rinsho Shinkeigaku*. 2002;42(10):925–929.
22. Ishihara L, Brayne C. What is the evidence for a premorbid parkinsonian personality: a systematic review. *Mov Disord*. 2006;21(8):1066–1072.
23. Nicoletti A, Luca A, Raciti L, et al. Obsessive compulsive personality disorder and Parkinson's disease. *PLoS One*. 2013;8(1):e54822.
24. Nicoletti A, Luca A, Luca M, et al. Obsessive-compulsive personality disorder in drug-naive Parkinson's disease patients. *J Neurol*. 2015;262(2):485–486.
25. Nicoletti A, Luca A, Luca M, et al. Obsessive compulsive personality disorder in progressive supranuclear palsy, multiple system atrophy and essential tremor. *Parkinsonism Relat Disord*. 2016;30:36–39.
26. Antonini A, Barone P, Bonuccelli U, Annoni K, Asgharnejad M, Stanzione P. ICARUS study: prevalence and clinical features of impulse control disorders in Parkinson's disease. *J Neurol Neurosurg Psychiatry*. 2017;88(4):317–324.
27. O'Sullivan SS, Evans AH, Lees AJ. Punding in Parkinson's disease. *Pract Neurol*. 2007;7(6):397–399.
28. Morgante F, Fasano A, Ginevrino M, et al. Impulsive-compulsive behaviors in parkin-associated Parkinson disease. *Neurology*. 2016;87(14):1436–1441.
29. Laplane D, Baulac M, Widlocher D, Dubois B. Pure psychic akinesia with bilateral lesions of basal ganglia. *J Neurol Neurosurg Psychiatry*. 1984;47(4):377–385.
30. Laplane D, Dubois B. Auto-activation deficit: a basal ganglia related syndrome. *Mov Disord*. 2001;16(5):810–814.
31. Dide M, Guiraud P. *Psychiatrie du médecin praticien*. Paris: Masson; 1922.
32. Habib M. Athymhormia and disorders of motivation in basal ganglia disease. *J Neuropsychiatry Clin Neurosci*. 2004;16(4):509–524.

33. Larner AJ. *A Dictionary of Neurological Signs*. New York, NY: Springer; 2016.

34. American Pyschiatric Association. *Diagnostic and Statistical Manual of Mental Disorders*, 5th ed. Washington, DC: APA; 2013.

35. Goodman WK, Storch EA, Geffken GR, Murphy TK. Obsessive-compulsive disorder in Tourette syndrome. *J Child Neurol*. 2006;21(8):704–714.

36. Albanese A, Bhatia K, Bressman SB, et al. Phenomenology and classification of dystonia: a consensus update. *Mov Disord*. 2013;28(7):863–873.

37. Campbell WW. *Pocket Guide and Toolkit to DeJong's Neurologic Examination*. Philadelphia, PA: Lippincott Williams and Wilkins; 2008.

38. Albanese A, Lalli S. Is this dystonia? *Move Disord*. 2009;24(12):1725–1731.

39. Dale RC. Immune-mediated extrapyramidal movement disorders, including Sydenham chorea. *Handb Clin Neurol*. 2013;112:1235–1241.

40. Panzer J, Dalmau J. Movement disorders in paraneoplastic and autoimmune disease. *Curr Opin Neurol*. 2011;24(4):346–353.

41. Ben-Pazi H, Jaworowski S, Shalev RS. Cognitive and psychiatric phenotypes of movement disorders in children: a systematic review. *Dev Med Child Neurol*. 2011;53(12):1077–1084.

42. Fibbe LA, Cath DC, van den Heuvel OA, Veltman DJ, Tijssen MA, van Balkom AJ. Relationship between movement disorders and obsessive-compulsive disorder: beyond the obsessive-compulsive-tic phenotype. A systematic review. *J Neurol Neurosurg Psychiatry*. 2012;83(6):646–654.

43. Tate ED, Allison TJ, Pranzate MR, Verhu SJ. Neuroepidemiologic trends in 105 US cases of pediatric opsoclonus-myoclonus syndrome. *J Pediatr Oncol Nurs*. 2005;22(1):8–19.

44. Williams KA, Swedo SE. Post-infectious autoimmune disorders: Sydenham's chorea, PANDAS and beyond. *Brain Res*. 2015;1617:144–154.

45. Asbahr FR, Garvey MA, Snider LA, Zanetta DM, Elkis H, Swedo SE. Obsessive-compulsive symptoms among patients with Sydenham chorea. *Biol Psychiatry*. 2005;57(9):1073–1076.

46. Asbahr FR, Negrao AB, Gentil V, et al. Obsessive-compulsive and related symptoms in children and adolescents with rheumatic fever with and without chorea: a prospective 6-month study. *Am J Psychiatry*. 1998;155(8):1122–1124.

47. Hounie AG, Pauls DL, Mercadante MT, et al. Obsessive-compulsive spectrum disorders in rheumatic fever with and without Sydenham's chorea. *J Clin Psychiatry*. 2004;65(7):994–999.

48. Swedo SE, Leckman JF, Rose NR. From research subgroup to clinical syndrome: modifying the PANDAS criteria to describe PANS (pediatric acute-onset neuropsychiatric syndrome). *Pediatr Therapeut 2*. 2013;2(113) doi: 10.4172/2161-0665.1000113.

49. Leckman JF, Denys D, Simpson HB, et al. Obsessive–compulsive disorder: a review of the diagnostic criteria and possible subtypes and dimensional specifiers for DSM-V. *Depress Anxiety*. 2010;27(6):507–527.

50. Sokol MS. Infection-triggered anorexia nervosa in children: clinical description of four cases. *J Child Adolesc Psychopharmacol*. 2000;10(2):133–145.

51. Sokol MS, Gray NS. Case study: an infection-triggered, autoimmune subtype of anorexia nervosa. *J Am Acad Child Adolesc Psychiatry*. 1997;36(8):1128–1133.

52. Grant R, Graus F. Paraneoplastic movement disorders. *Mov Disord*. 2009;24(12):1715–1724.

53. Dalmau J, Rosenfeld MR. Paraneoplastic syndromes of the CNS. *Lancet Neurol*.7(4):327–340.

54. Muehlschlegel S, Okun MS, Foote KD, Coco D, Yachnis AT, Fernandez HH. Paraneoplastic chorea with leukoencephalopathy presenting with obsessive–compulsive and behavioral disorder. *Mov Disord*. 2005;20(11):1523–1527.

55. Pike M. Opsoclonus–myoclonus syndrome. *Handb Clin Neurol*. 2013;112:1209–1211.

56. Beglinger LJ, Paulsen JS, Watson DB, et al. Obsessive and compulsive symptoms in prediagnosed Huntington's disease. *J Clin Psychiatry*. 2008;69(11):1758–1765.

57. Walterfang M, Evans A, Looi JC, et al. The neuropsychiatry of neuroacanthocytosis syndromes. *Neurosci Biobehav Rev*. 2011;35(5):1275–1283.

58. Fischer CA, Licht EA, Mendez MF. The neuropsychiatric manifestations of Huntington's disease-like 2. *J Neuropsychiatry Clin Neurosci*. 2012;24(4):489–492.

59. Peall KJ, Kurian MA. Benign hereditary chorea: an update. *Tremor Other Hyperkinet Mov (N Y)*. 2015;5:314.

60. Peall KJ, Lumsden D, Kneen R, et al. Benign hereditary chorea related to NKX2.1: expansion of the genotypic and phenotypic spectrum. *Dev Med Child Neurol*. 2014;56(7):642–648.

61. Albanese A, Bhatia K, Bressman SB, et al. Phenomenology and classification of dystonia: a consensus update. *Mov Disord*. 2013;28(7):863–873.

62. Jinnah HA, Albanese A. The new classification system for the dystonias: why was it needed and how was it developed? *Mov Disord Clin Pract*. 2014;1(4):280–284.

63. Tadic V, Kasten M, Bruggemann N, Stiller S, Hagenah J, Klein C. Dopa-responsive dystonia revisited: diagnostic delay, residual signs, and nonmotor signs. *Arch Neurol.* 2012;69(12):1558–1562.

64. Ruscio AM, Stein DJ, Chiu WT, Kessler RC. The epidemiology of obsessive-compulsive disorder in the National Comorbidity Survey Replication. *Mol Psychiatry.* 2010;15(1):53–63.

65. Arruda WO, Munhoz RP, de Bem RS, et al. Pathogenic compound heterozygous ATP7B mutations with hypoceruloplasminaemia without clinical features of Wilson's disease. *J Clin Neurosci.* 2014;21(2):335–336.

66. Duggal HS, Nizamie HS. Wilson's disease presenting with obsessive-compulsive disorder. *Indian J Psychiatry.* 2000;42(3):312–316.

67. Kumawat BL, Sharma CM, Tripathi G, Ralot T, Dixit S. Wilson's disease presenting as isolated obsessive-compulsive disorder. *Indian J Medical Sciences.* 2007;61(11):607–610.

68. Rosenblatt A, Leroi I. Neuropsychiatry of Huntington's disease and other basal ganglia disorders. *Psychosomatics.* 2000;41(1):24–30.

69. Sahu JK, Singhi P, Malhotra S. Late occurrence of isolated obsessive-compulsive behavior in a boy with Wilson's disease on treatment. *J Child Neurol.* 2013;28(2):277.

70. Woerwag-Mehta S, Hindley P, Hedderly T, Dhawan A. Complex psychiatric presentation in adolescent onset Wilson's disease. *BMJ Case Rep.* 2011;2011:pii: bcr0120102628.

71. Kinugawa K, Vidailhet M, Clot F, Apartis E, Grabli D, Roze E. Myoclonus-dystonia: an update. *Mov Disord.* 2009;24(4):479–489.

72. Zimprich A, Grabowski M, Asmus F, et al. Mutations in the gene encoding [epsiv]-sarcoglycan cause myoclonus-dystonia syndrome. *Nat Genet.* 2001;29(1):66–69.

73. Peall KJ, Dijk JM, Saunders-Pullman R, et al. Psychiatric disorders, myoclonus dystonia and SGCE: an international study. *Ann Clin Transl Neurol.* 2016;3(1):4–11.

74. Peall KJ, Smith DJ, Kurian MA, et al. SGCE mutations cause psychiatric disorders: clinical and genetic characterization. *Brain.* 2013;136(1):294–303.

75. Dias FM, Doyle F, Kummer A, Cardoso F, Fontenelle LF, Teixeira AL. Frequency of psychiatric disorders in blepharospasm does not differ from hemifacial spasm. *Acta Neuropsychiatr.* 2010;22(5):223–227.

76. Fontenelle LF, Pacheco PG, Nascimento PM, et al. Obsessive-compulsive symptoms among patients with blepharospasm and hemifacial spasm. *Gen Hosp Psychiatry.* 2011;33(5):476–481.

77. Fabbrini G, Berardelli I, Moretti G, et al. Psychiatric disorders in adult-onset focal dystonia: a case-control study. *Mov Disord.* 2010;25(4):459–465.

78. Lehn A, Mellick G, Boyle R. Psychiatric disorders in idiopathic-isolated focal dystonia. *J Neurol.* 2014;261(4):668–674.

79. Barahona-Correa B, Bugalho P, Guimaraes J, Xavier M. Obsessive-compulsive symptoms in primary focal dystonia: a controlled study. *Mov Disord.* 2011;26(12):2274–2278.

80. Rascovsky K, Hodges JR, Knopman D, et al. Sensitivity of revised diagnostic criteria for the behavioural variant of frontotemporal dementia. *Brain.* 2011;134(9):2456–2477.

81. Gorno-Tempini ML, Hillis AE, Weintraub S, et al. Classification of primary progressive aphasia and its variants. *Neurology.* 2011;76(11):1006–1014.

82. Perry DC, Whitwell JL, Boeve BF, et al. Voxel-based morphometry in patients with obsessive-compulsive behaviors in behavioral variant frontotemporal dementia. *Eur J Neurol.* 2012;19(6):911–917.

83. Rosso SM, Roks G, Stevens M, et al. Complex compulsive behaviour in the temporal variant of frontotemporal dementia. *J Neurol.* 2001;248(11):965–970.

84. Snowden JS, Bathgate D, Varma A, Blackshaw A, Gibbons ZC, Neary D. Distinct behavioural profiles in frontotemporal dementia and semantic dementia. *J Neurol Neurosurg Psychiatry.* 2001;70(3):323–332.

85. Tonkonogy JM, Smith TW, Barreira PJ. Obsessive-compulsive disorders in Pick's disease. *J Neuropsychiatry Clin Neurosci.* 1994;6(2):176–180.

86. Nakaaki S, Murata Y, Shinagawa Y, et al. A case of late-onset obsessive compulsive disorder developing frontotemporal lobar degeneration. *J Neuropsychiatry Clin Neurosci.* 2007;19(4):487–488.

87. Pompanin S, Perini G, Toffanin T, et al. Late-onset OCD as presenting manifestation of semantic dementia. *Gen Hosp Psychiatry.* 2012;34(1):102.e101–102.e104.

88. Sabbe T, Vandenbulcke M. Obsessive-compulsive behaviour in two patients with right temporal variant frontotemporal dementia. *Tijdschr Psychiatrie.* 2014;56(10):685–688.

89. Slachevsky A, Munoz-Neira C, Nunez-Huasaf J, Stern TA, Blesius CR, Atri A. Late-onset cinephilia and compulsive behaviors: harbingers of frontotemporal dementia. *Prim Care Companion CNS Disord.* 2011;13(3):pii: PCC.10f01115.

90. Mateen FJ, Josephs KA. The clinical spectrum of stereotypies in frontotemporal lobar degeneration. *Mov Disord.* 2009;24(8):1237–1240.

91. Mendez MF, Perryman KM, Miller BL, Swartz JR, Cummings JL. Compulsive behaviors as presenting symptoms of frontotemporal dementia. *J Geriatr Psychiatry Neurol.* 1997;10(4):154–157.
92. Mendez MF, Shapira JS, Miller BL. Stereotypical movements and frontotemporal dementia. *Mov Disord.* 2005;20(6):742–745.
93. Frydman I, Ferreira-Garcia R, Borges MC, Velakoulis D, Walterfang M, Fontenelle LF. Dementia developing in late-onset and treatment-refractory obsessive-compulsive disorder. *Cogn Behav Neurol.* 2010;23(3):205–208.
94. Cumming TB, Blomstrand C, Skoog I, Linden T. The high prevalence of anxiety disorders after stroke. *Am J Geriatr Psychiatry.* 2016;24(2):154–160.
95. Carmin CN, Wiegartz PS, Yunus U, Gillock KL. Treatment of late-onset OCD following basal ganglia infarct. *Depress Anxiety.* 2002;15(2):87–90.
96. Khairkar P, Diwan S. Late-onset obsessive-compulsive disorder with comorbid narcolepsy after perfect blend of thalamo-striatal stroke and post-streptococcal infection. *J Neuropsychiatry Clin Neurosci.* 2012;24(4):E29-31.
97. Lopez-Rodriguez F, Gunay I, Glaser N. Obsessive compulsive disorder in a woman with left basal ganglia infarct: a case report. *Behav Neurol.* 1997;10(2):101–103.
98. Rodrigo Escalona P, Adair JC, Roberts BB, Graeber DA. Obsessive-compulsive disorder following bilateral globus pallidus infarction. *Biol Psychiatry.* 1997;42(5):410–412.
99. Katz BS, Flemming KD. Obsessive compulsive disorder due to a cavernous malformation hemorrhage in the dominant caudate head. *J Clin Neurosci.* 2015;22(2):398–399.
100. Thobois S, Jouanneau E, Bouvard M, Sindou M. Obsessive-compulsive disorder after unilateral caudate nucleus bleeding. *Acta Neurochirurg.* 2004;146(9):1027–1031; discussion 1031.
101. Cooper JJ, Grant J. Refractory OCD due to thalamic infarct with response to dronabinol. *J Neuropsychiatry Clin Neurosci.* 2017;29(1):77–78.
102. Nguyen FN, Pauly RR, Okun MS, Fernandez HH. Punding as a complication of brain stem stroke? Report of a case. *Stroke.* 2007;38(4):1390–1392.
103. Kim KW, Lee DY. Obsessive-compulsive disorder associated with a left orbitofrontal infarct. *J Neuropsychiatry Clin Neurosci.* 2002;14(1):88–89.
104. Matsui T, Saxena S, Kawabe J, et al. Secondary obsessive-compulsive disorder related to diaschisis after pontine infarction, successfully treated with paroxetine. *Psychiatry Clin Neurosci.* 2007;61(2):186–189.
105. Tessier A, Cosin C, Mayo W, Pfeuty M, Misdrahi D, Sibon I. Impulsive aggressive obsessions following cerebellar strokes: a case study. *J Neurol.* 2015;262(7):1775–1776.
106. Mahendran R. Obsessive compulsive disorder following left middle cerebral artery infarct. *Singapore Med J.* 2000;41(10):498–499.
107. Salinas C, Davila G, Berthier ML, Green C, Lara JP. Late-life reactivation of obsessive-compulsive disorder associated with lesions in prefrontal-subcortical circuits. *J Neuropsychiatry Clin Neurosci.* 2009;21(3):332–334.
108. Lopes AC, Greenberg BD, Canteras MM, et al. Gamma ventral capsulotomy for obsessive-compulsive disorder: a randomized clinical trial. *JAMA Psychiatry.* 2014;71(9):1066–1076.
109. Lopes AC, Greenberg BD, Pereira CA, Noren G, Miguel EC. Notice of retraction and replacement. Lopes et al. gamma ventral capsulotomy for obsessive-compulsive disorder: a randomized clinical trial. *JAMA Psychiatry.* 2014;71(9):1066–1076. *JAMA Psychiatry.* 2015;72(12):1258.
110. Yaryura-Tobias JA, Neziroglu F. Basal ganglia hemorrhagic ablation associated with temporary suppression of obsessive-compulsive symptoms. *Rev Bras Psiquiatr.* 2003;25:40–42.
111. Ferrão YA, Scheidt B. Basal ganglia hemorrhagic ablation causing temporary suppression of trichotillomania symptoms. *Rev Bras Psiquiatr.* 2003;25(4):262–263.
112. Diamond A, Ondo WG. Resolution of severe obsessive--compulsive disorder after a small unilateral nondominant frontoparietal infarct. *Int J Neurosci.* 2011;121(7):405–407.
113. Muneoka K, Shirayama Y, Kon K, Kawabe M, Kimura S. Delayed-onset obsessive-compulsive symptoms after brain infarctions treated with paroxetine. *Clin Neuropharmacol.* 2011;34(6):260–261.
114. Sun CH, Lu CH, Huang TL. Clozapine for blepharospasm, obsessive-compulsive symptoms, and psychotic symptoms in a patient of old brain infarction. *Clin Neuropharmacol.* 2006;29(6):368–370.
115. de Oliveira GN, Kummer A, Salgado JV, et al. Psychiatric disorders in temporal lobe epilepsy: an overview from a tertiary service in Brazil. *Seizure.* 2010;19(8):479–484.
116. Ertekin BA, Kulaksizoglu IB, Ertekin E, et al. A comparative study of obsessive-compulsive disorder and other psychiatric comorbidities in patients with temporal lobe epilepsy and idiopathic generalized epilepsy. *Epilepsy Behav.* 2009;14(4):634–639.
117. Hamed SA, Elserogy YM, Abd-Elhafeez HA. Psychopathological and peripheral levels of

neurobiological correlates of obsessive-compulsive symptoms in patients with epilepsy: a hospital-based study. *Epilepsy Behav.* 2013;27(2):409–415.

118. Isaacs KL, Philbeck JW, Barr WB, Devinsky O, Alper K. Obsessive-compulsive symptoms in patients with temporal lobe epilepsy. *Epilepsy Behavior.* 2004;5(4):569–574.

119. Monaco F, Cavanna A, Magli E, et al. Obsessionality, obsessive-compulsive disorder, and temporal lobe epilepsy. *Epilepsy Behavior.* 2005;7(3):491–496.

120. Seo JH, Lee WK, Park SP. Obsessive-compulsive symptoms and their impacts on psychosocial functioning in people with epilepsy. *J Clin Neurol.* 2014;10(2):125–132.

121. Fontenelle L, Marques C, Piedade RA, Figueira I, Nardi AE, Versiani M. The relationship between obsessive-compulsive disorder and epilepsy. *J Bras Psiquiatr.* 1998;47(11):591–598.

122. Krishnamoorthy ES, Trimble MR. Forced normalization: clinical and therapeutic relevance. *Epilepsia.* 1999;40(Suppl 10):S57–S64.

123. Mula M, Monaco F. Ictal and peri-ictal psychopathology. *Behav Neurol.* 2011;24(1):21–25.

124. Fisher RS, Scharfman HE, deCurtis M. How can we identify ictal and interictal abnormal activity? *Adv Exp Med Biol.* 2014;813:3–23.

125. Kroll L, Drummond LM. Temporal lobe epilepsy and obsessive-compulsive symptoms. *J Nerv Ment Dis.* 1993;181(7):457–458.

126. Green AL, Harmon PH, Boyer FA, Detyniecki K, Motlagh MG, Gligorovic PV. Forced normalization's converse as nature's model for use of ECT in the management of psychosis: an observational case series. *Epilepsy Behav Case Rep.* 2016;6:36–38.

127. Levin B, Duchowny M. Childhood obsessive-compulsive disorder and cingulate epilepsy. *Biol Psychiatry.* 1991;30(10):1049–1055.

128. Koopowitz LF, Berk M. Response of obsessive compulsive disorder to carbamazepine in two patients with comorbid epilepsy. *Ann Clin Psychiatry.* 1997;9(3):171–173.

129. Trimble M, Freeman A. An investigation of religiosity and the Gastaut-Geschwind syndrome in patients with temporal lobe epilepsy. *Epilepsy Behav.* 2006;9(3):407–414.

130. Bear DM, Fedio P. Quantitative analysis of interictal behavior in temporal lobe epilepsy. *Arch Neurol.* 1977;34(8):454–467.

131. Tremont G, Smith MM, Bauer L, et al. Comparison of personality characteristics on the bear-fedio inventory between patients with epilepsy and those with non-epileptic seizures. *J Neuropsychiatry Clin Neurosci.* 2012;24(1):47–52.

132. Yaryura-Tobias JA, Neziroglu FA. *Obsessive-Compulsive Disorder Spectrum: Pathogenesis, Diagnosis, and Treatment.* Washington, DC: American Psychiatric Association Publishing; 1997.

133. Stefan A, Mathe JF. What are the disruptive symptoms of behavioral disorders after traumatic brain injury? A systematic review leading to recommendations for good practices. *Ann Phys Rehab Med.* 2016;59(1):5–17.

134. Hoofien D, Gilboa A, Vakil E, Donovick PJ. Traumatic brain injury (TBI) 10–20 years later: a comprehensive outcome study of psychiatric symptomatology, cognitive abilities and psychosocial functioning. *Brain Inj.* 2001;15(3):189–209.

135. Rydon-Grange M, Coetzer R. What do we know about obsessive-compulsive disorder following traumatic brain injury? *CNS Spect.* 2015;20(5):463–465.

136. Berthier ML, Kulisevsky JJ, Gironell A, Lopez OL. Obsessive compulsive disorder and traumatic brain injury: behavioral, cognitive, and neuroimaging findings. *Neuropsychiatry Neuropsychol Behav Neurol.* 2001;14(1):23–31.

137. Mellado-Calvo N, Fleminger S. Cerebral tumours. In: David A, David AS, Fleminger S, Kopelman M, Lovestone S, Mellers J, eds. *Lishman's Organic Psychiatry: A Textbook of Neuropsychiatry.* Oxford: Wiley; 2012:281–308.

138. Hegde A, Ghosh A, Grover S, Kumar A, Chabbra R. Arachnoid cyst masquerades as late onset obsessive-compulsive disorder. *Gen Hosp Psychiatry.* 2014;36(1):125.e127–125.e129.

139. John G, Eapen V, Shaw GK. Frontal glioma presenting as anxiety and obsessions: a case report. *Acta Neurol Scand.* 1997;96(3):194–195.

140. Shuren JE, Flynn T, Fennell E, Crosson B. Insula and obsessive-compulsive disorder. *Can J Psychiatry.* 1995;40(2):112.

141. Wu MS, Horng B, Storch EA. A case report on obsessive-compulsive disorder and low-grade astrocytomas. *Ann Clin Psychiatry.* 2013;25(4):309–310.

142. De Nadai AS, Storch EA, Alvaro JL. Development of obsessive-compulsive disorder following a pineal germinoma: a case report. *Am J Psychiatry.* 2011;168(5):550–551.

143. Mordecai D, Shaw RJ, Fisher PG, Mittelstadt PA, Guterman T, Donaldson SS. Case study: suprasellar germinoma presenting with psychotic and obsessive-compulsive symptoms. *J Am Acad Child Adolesc Psychiatry.* 2000;39(1):116–119.

144. Kumar V, Chakrabarti S, Modi M, Sahoo M. Late-onset obsessive compulsive disorder associated with possible gliomatosis cerebri. *World J Biol Psychiatry.* 2009;10(4 Pt 2):636–639.

145. Gamazo-Garran P, Soutullo CA, Ortuno F. Obsessive-compulsive disorder secondary to brain dysgerminoma in an adolescent boy: a positron emission tomography case report. *J Child Adolesc Psychopharmacol.* 2002;12(3):259–263.

146. Rao SA, Rao MG, Rao NP, Varambally S, Gangadhar BN. Successful treatment of tuberous sclerosis with psychosis and obsessive-compulsive disorder: a case report. *Psychiatry Clin Neurosci.* 2015;69(8):504–505.

147. Hassan IK, Looi JC, Velakoulis D, et al. Psychosis with obsessive-compulsive symptoms in tuberous sclerosis. *J Clin Neurosci.* 2014;21(5):867–869.

148. Liu J, Zhang X, Liu J. Obsessions appear after the removal a brain tumor in the right frontal lobe. *Gen Hosp Psychiatry.* 2014;36(4):450.e453–450.e454.

149. Rogers MP, Mendoza AY. Development of obsessive-compulsive disorder after brain tumor surgery and radiation. *Psychosomatics.* 1994;35(4):402–406.

150. Paradis CM, Friedman S, Hatch M, Lazar RM. Obsessive-compulsive disorder onset after removal of a brain tumor. *J Nerv Ment Dis.* 1992;180(8):535–536.

151. Moriarty J, Trimble M, Hayward R. Obsessive-compulsive disorder onset after removal of a brain tumor. *J Nerv Ment Dis.* 1993;181(5):331.

152. Sathe H, Karia S, De Sousa A, Shah N. Obsessive-compulsive symptoms in an adolescent appearing after cerebellar vermian mass resection. *J Clin Diagn Res.* 2016;10(5):Vd01–Vd02.

153. Mainio A, Hakko H, Niemelä A, Salo J, Koivukangas J, Räsänen P. Level of obsessionality among neurosurgical patients with a primary brain tumor. *J Neuropsychiatry Clin Neurosci.* 2005;17(3):399–404.

154. Morris DR, Meighen KG, McDougle CJ. Acute onset of obsessive-compulsive disorder in an adolescent with acute lymphoblastic leukemia. *Psychosomatics.* 2005;46(5):458–460.

155. Mavrogiorgou P, Juckel G. Interferon-induced obsessive-compulsive symptoms in malignant melanoma. *Pharmacopsychiatry.* 2012;45(1):28–30.

156. Scheid R, Voltz R, Guthke T, Bauer J, Sammler D, von Cramon DY. Neuropsychiatric findings in anti-Ma2-positive paraneoplastic limbic encephalitis. *Neurology.* 2003;61(8):1159–1161.

157. Rajarethinam RP, Abelson JL, Himle JA. Acute onset and remission of obsessions and compulsions following medical illnesses and stress. *Depress Anxiety.* 2000;12(4):238–240.

158. Iyo M, Sekine Y, Matsunaga T, Tsukamoto T, Takei N, Mori N. Methamphetamine-associated obsessional symptoms and effective risperidone treatment: a case report. *J Clin Psychiatry.* 1999;60(5):337–338.

159. Satel SL, McDougle CJ. Obsessions and compulsions associated with cocaine abuse. *Am J Psychiatry.* 1991;148(7):947.

160. Marchesi C, Tonna M, Maggini C. Obsessive-compulsive disorder followed by psychotic episode in long-term ecstasy misuse. *World J Biol Psychiatry.* 2009;10(4 Pt 2):599–602.

161. Fonseka TM, Richter MA, Müller DJ. Second generation antipsychotic-induced obsessive-compulsive symptoms in schizophrenia: a review of the experimental literature. *Curr Psychiatry Rep.* 2014;16(11):510.

162. Weintraub D, David AS, Evans AH, Grant JE, Stacy M. Clinical spectrum of impulse control disorders in Parkinson's disease. *Mov Disord.* 2015;30(2):121–127.

163. Thuile J, Even C, Guelfi JD. Topiramate may induce obsessive-compulsive disorder. *Psychiatry Clin Neurosci.* 2006;60(3):394.

164. Baytunca MB, Erermis S, Bildik T, Kayahan B. Isoniazid-induced psychosis with obsessive-compulsive symptoms (schizo-obsessive disorder) in a female child. *J Child Adolesc Psychopharmacol.* 2015;25(10):819–820.

165. DeRosse P, Szeszko PR, Malhotra AK. Interferon-induced obsessive-compulsive disorder. *Gen Hosp Psychiatry.* 2006;28(4):357–358.

166. Senjo M. Obsessive-compulsive disorder in people that abuse codeine. *Acta Psychiatr Scand.* 1989;79(6):619–620.

167. Laplane D, Baulac M, Pillon B, Panayotopoulou-Achimastos I. Loss of psychic self-activation. Compulsive activity of obsessional type. Bilateral lenticular lesion (author's transl). *Rev Neurol.* 1982;138(2):137–141.

168. Laplane D, Widlocher D, Pillon B, Baulac M, Binoux F. Obsessional-type compulsive behavior caused by bilateral circumscribed pallidostriatal necrosis. Encephalopathy caused by a wasp sting. *Rev Neurol.* 1981;137(4):269–276.

169. Shakeri J, Farnia V, Karimi AR, et al. The prevalence and clinical features of amphetamine-induced obsessive compulsive disorder. *Drug Alcohol Depend.* 2016;160:157–162.

170. Denys D, van Megen HJ, Westenberg HG. Emerging skin-picking behaviour after serotonin reuptake inhibitor-treatment in patients with obsessive-compulsive disorder: possible mechanisms and implications for clinical care. *J Psychopharmacol.* 2003;17(1):127–129.

171. Drummond LM, Matthews HP. Obsessive-compulsive disorder occurring as a complication in benzodiazepine withdrawal. *J Nerv Ment Dise.* 1988;176(11):688–691.

172. Cardoso F, Vargas AP. Persistent dyskinesia and obsessive-compulsive behavior following alcohol withdrawal. *Neurology.* 1996;47(3):844.

173. Poyurovsky M, Bergman Y, Shoshani D, Schneidman M, Weizman A. Emergence of obsessive--compulsive symptoms and tics during clozapine withdrawal. *Clin Neuropharmacol.* 1998;21(2):97–100.

174. Cuzen NL, Stein DJ, Lochner C, Fineberg NA. Comorbidity of obsessive-compulsive disorder and substance use disorder: a new heuristic. *Hum Psychopharmacol.* 2014;29(1):89–93.

175. Spradlin A, Mauzay D, Cuttler C. Symptoms of obsessive-compulsive disorder predict cannabis misuse. *Addict Behav.* 2017;72:159–164.

176. Crum RM, Anthony JC. Cocaine use and other suspected risk factors for obsessive-compulsive disorder: a prospective study with data from the Epidemiologic Catchment Area surveys. *Drug Alcohol Depend.* 1993;31(3):281–295.

177. Nelson E, Rice J. Stability of diagnosis of obsessive-compulsive disorder in the Epidemiologic Catchment Area study. *Am J Psychiatry.* 1997;154(6):826–831.

178. Phillips KA, Stein DJ. Other obsessive-compulsive and related disorders in DSM-5. In: Phillips KA, Stein DJ, eds. *Handbook on Obsessive-Compulsive and Related Disorders.* Washington, DC: American Psychiatric Association Publishing; 2015:181–198.

179. Kara T, Akaltun İ. A 12-year-old boy with Fahr disease accompanying a diagnosis of obsessive compulsive disorder. *Nord J Psychiatry.* 2017:1–2.

180. Yousefichaijan P, Sharafkhah M, Rafeie M, Salehi B. Obsessive Compulsive Inventory-Child Version (OCV-CI) to evaluate obsessive compulsive disorder in children with early stages of chronic kidney disease: a case control study. *Nephrourol Mon.* 2016;8(1):e34017.

181. Kaplan PW. Epilepsy and obsessive-compulsive disorder. *Dialogues Clin Neurosci.* 2010;12(2):241–248.

182. Berrios GE. Trastorno obsesivo-compulsivo y enfermedad neurológica: estado actual de la cuestión. In: Ruiloba JV, Berrios GE, eds. *Estados Obsesivos,* 3rd ed. Barcelona: Masson; 2006:487–519.

183. Fontenelle LF, Hasler G. The analytical epidemiology of obsessive-compulsive disorder: risk factors and correlates. *Prog Neuropsychopharmacology Biol Psychiatry.* 2008;32(1):1–15.

184. Sinopoli V, Burton CL, Kronenberg S, Arnold PD. A review of the role of serotonin system genes in obsessive-compulsive disorder. *Neurosci Biobehav Rev.* 2017;80:372–381.

185. Cai J, Zhang W, Yi Z, et al. Influence of polymorphisms in genes SLC1A1, GRIN2B, and GRIK2 on clozapine-induced obsessive-compulsive symptoms. *Psychopharmacology.* 2013;230(1):49–55.

186. Kwon JS, Joo YH, Nam HJ, et al. Association of the glutamate transporter gene SLC1A1 with atypical antipsychotics-induced obsessive-compulsive symptoms. *Arch Gen Psychiatry.* 2009;66(11):1233–1241.

187. Ryu S, Oh S, Cho EY, et al. Interaction between genetic variants of DLGAP3 and SLC1A1 affecting the risk of atypical antipsychotics-induced obsessive-compulsive symptoms. *Am J Medi Genet B, Neuropsychiatr Genet.* 2011;156b(8):949–959.

188. Tundo A, Salvati L, Cieri L, et al. Cognitive behavioral therapy for obsessive-compulsive disorder secondary to second-generation antipsychotics. *Psychother Psychosom.* 2015;84(3):188–189.

Chapter 31

Behavioral Addictions

Samuel R. Chamberlain and Jon E. Grant

Introduction

Certain centrally acting chemicals, such as cocaine or amphetamine, affect the brain's reward pathways, particularly the nucleus accumbens "reward center" and linked dopamine and opioid systems [1,2,3]. Repeated consumption of such substances, for vulnerable individuals, can lead to escalating cycles of intake and functional impairment, termed addiction. Addiction encompasses a number of core features, as highlighted in the *Diagnostic and Statistical Manual of Mental Disorders*, fifth edition (DSM-5), including impaired top-down control (unsuccessful attempts to reduce intake), narrowing of interests, risky use (continued use despite knowledge of damaging consequences) and physiologic aspects (tolerance and withdrawal) [4]. As psychoactive substances including alcohol and cocaine have high addictive potential by virtue of their effects on the brain's reward pathways, so too do certain types of behavior. This has led to the proposal that some mental disorders can be conceptualized as behavioral addictions [5,6]. Most people who engage in these behaviors will not become addicted, but some individuals will. Individuals with behavioral addictions exhibit impaired control, functional impairment and persisting engagement in the behavior despite negative consequences. In addition, evidence also suggests that people with behavioral addictions experience tolerance (e.g., the need to gamble with greater amounts of money over time, having riskier sex to produce the same degree of euphoria) and withdrawal (e.g., agitation, insomnia, irritability, when unable to do the behavior) [7].

Many of these potentially addictive behaviors have been recognized for centuries [8]. Gambling, and its potentially untoward consequences, is mentioned in ancient religious texts such as the Koran and the Talmud. Ancient dice were discovered in caves dating back to 3500BC, while gambling has been documented in ancient cultures including in Egypt, Rome and China. Excessive sexual behavior and compulsive stealing are likely as old as humankind. The term "kleptomania" was created around 1816, when an apparent epidemic of young, wealthy women stealing clothes in Paris was reported in newspapers. Compulsive sexual behavior was described in the late 1700s and led to the terms nymphomania (for females), and satyrism (for males) both of which referred to excessive sex drive and/or activity. Compulsive shopping as a concept dates back to nineteenth-century America or earlier, and was referred to at that time as oniomania.

The "behavioral addiction" model has contributed to major changes in psychiatric nosology in recent times. In DSM-5, gambling disorder was officially recognized in the category of "substance related and addictive disorders" based on considerable evidence (discussed later in this chapter) as to overlapping comorbidity, phenomenology, neurobiology and treatment response with substance addictions [9]. Other conditions are recognized in DSM-5 but are currently placed in other diagnostic categories. Kleptomania (compulsive stealing) is listed in "disruptive, impulse control, and conduct disorders". Although "sex addiction" (excessive sexual drive and/or excessive sex acts) and compulsive buying disorder are not formally recognized in the DSM-5, the International Classification of Diseases 11th Revision Working Group on Obsessive-Compulsive and Related Disorders recommended that compulsive sexual behavior be recognized as a mental health disorder.

For the purposes of this chapter, we consider the above-listed as candidate behavioral addictions, with the caveat that evidence as to their precise definition and validity is incomplete: in the case of many candidate behavioral addictions this is due to a relative lack of studies rather than negative findings from available data. What is clear is that, far from being rare, many of these candidate behavioral addictions are common. By definition, these disorders are associated with marked functional impairment.

Recent Research Findings

Diagnostic Status and Operational Criteria

DSM-5 criteria for gambling disorder are derived from substance use disorder criteria. For the diagnosis, an individual needs to endorse four or more of the following criteria (12-month period): gambling increasing amounts over time, restless/irritability when trying to cut back, difficulty cutting back, preoccupation (e.g., obsessing about one's next gambling venture), gambling when feeling emotionally distressed, chasing losses, lying about gambling to others, risking job/relationship/educational opportunities due to gambling and relying on others to fund gambling [4]. Gambling due to other mental health disorders, such as a manic episode, would preclude the diagnosis. Defining a mental disorder with such a range of criteria is advantageous in the sense that many types of pathology will be captured rather than overlooked; but it does raise the question of where to place the diagnostic threshold. This approach also assigns equal importance to each criterion, whereas it is unlikely that each criterion would be – in reality – equally associated with functional impairment, or a given biological aspect of the disorder such as reward system dysfunction (assuming this could be objectively measured).

Kleptomania is diagnosed on the basis of recurrent irresistible urges to steal, tension before stealing and relief/gratification when stealing (or after stealing) [4]. Stealing that is undertaken because items are needed (such as stealing clothes for one's children) or because of their intrinsic monetary value (e.g., stealing items to sell to fund drugs) are exempted from the diagnosis. Kleptomania should also not be diagnosed when stealing is better explained by another mental health condition (such as mania, or antisocial personality disorder) or where it is undertaken for the purposes of revenge or relief from anger.

For the conditions not currently recognized in DSM-5, there are operational diagnostic criteria that can be used. Compulsive buying disorder is characterized by a maladaptive preoccupation with buying items (e.g., irresistible impulses to buy, frequent preoccupation with buying), and consequent functional impairment and/or distress [10]. Buying must occur outside the setting of hypomanic/manic episodes to warrant the diagnosis. Compulsive sexual behavior (also known as sex addiction) is characterized by repetitive and intense preoccupations with sexual thoughts and/or behaviors, and consequent functional impairment or distress to the affected individual [11]. Again, sexual thoughts and behaviors that are due to another condition (e.g., mania, organic disease) would not support the diagnosis.

In general, diagnosing one or more behavioral addictions in someone can be problematic as affected individuals may minimize their problems; for example, a person may feel ashamed or be worried about the potential consequences of divulging information (such as upsetting a loved one, or getting into legal trouble). Emphasizing the confidential nature of the clinician–patient relationship can be helpful (of course, also explaining the limits of confidentiality), as can obtaining collateral information from others with consent when possible. It is important to assess the current patterns of the problem behavior (antecedents, nature of behaviors and consequences), the individual's readiness for change, and any relevant medical, psychiatric, substance use and medication history.

Epidemiology and Clinical Aspects of Behavioral Addictions

The lifetime prevalence estimates for different behavioral addictions are summarized in Table 31.1. Of these disorders, most epidemiological research has been conducted for gambling disorder – mainly thanks to large-scale studies in the US and Europe.

Gambling Disorder

Surveys have demonstrated that the prevalence of gambling disorder in the general US population ranges from 0.4% to 2.1%, with similar rates reported globally [12,13]. To put that in perspective with other psychiatric disorders, about 0.8% have bipolar disorder, and 2% have a substance use disorder. These estimates refer to gambling disorder; rates are higher when also considering sub-syndromal gambling problems. Studies have identified an intermediate form of gambling pathology which, despite not fulfilling the current diagnostic threshold in DSM-5 for gambling disorder, is nonetheless associated with impaired quality of life and some degree of cognitive

Table 31.1 Lifetime prevalence of behavioral addictions, based largely on community survey data [8].

Disorder	Lifetime Prevalence Estimate (%)
Gambling Disorder	0.4–2.1
Kleptomania (Compulsive stealing)	0.4–0.9
Compulsive Buying	3.6–5.8
Compulsive Sexual Behavior	2.0–3.7

impairment [14]. Gambling disorder is more common among younger and middle-age persons than among older adults, but it can occur at any age. The types of gambling activities people engage in is contingent on age, local culture and availability. In a systematic review and meta-analysis, gambling disorder was highly comorbid with mood disorders, substance use disorders (especially alcohol and nicotine) and anxiety disorders [15].

Gambling disorder is more common in men than in women, but women appear to be more likely to seek treatment. Men tend to start gambling earlier in life, are more likely to report marital consequences from gambling, and are more likely to have antisocial personality traits or substance use difficulties. For women, even though gambling starts (on average) later in life, the behavior seems to progress more rapidly to a pathological level than in men, which is referred to as the "telescoping phenomenon" [16], although this may be restricted to treatment rather than community settings [17]. Men prefer "strategic" forms of gambling (e.g., sports betting, poker, blackjack) whereas women prefer "non-strategic" forms of gambling (slot machines, bingo, lottery).

Kleptomania

Little is known about the epidemiology of kleptomania, as people are reluctant to discuss their kleptomania by virtue of the illegal nature of stealing, and few researchers have focused on this topic. The National Epidemiologic Survey on Alcohol and Related Conditions assessed rates of stealing (not a formal diagnosis of kleptomania) among 43,000 adults and found that the lifetime prevalence of shoplifting in the US population was 11.3%. Most shoplifters steal sporadically, for their own consumption (unlike people with kleptomania), and have never been caught or subjected to legal consequences. Less than 5% of people who shoplift would meet diagnostic criteria for kleptomania (stealing for financial reasons or because items are needed would not warrant a diagnosis) [18]. The actual prevalence of kleptomania is unknown, but has been estimated at 0.6% in the United States [19].

Kleptomania typically begins during adolescence (though there are case reports of it starting aged 4 years, or as late as 77 years), but if individuals seek treatment at all, this comes much later (average age at clinical evaluation 35 years) [18]. Kleptomania appears to be more common in women than in men [19], and shows high comorbidity with depression and (to a smaller extent) with anxiety and eating disorders [20]. Kleptomania often follows a chronic course, and the typical affected individual steals twice per week, but experiences urges to steal most days. Unfortunately, being apprehended for stealing only temporarily reduces these urges. Individuals with kleptomania could nearly always afford to buy the things they steal, and do not even necessarily keep the stolen items (often they might secretly return them to the store, or give them away); hence, the urge appears intrinsic to the stealing itself, rather than the desire to keep items [21]. Examples of commonly stolen objects in kleptomania include sweets, newspapers, food, books and clothes.

Compulsive Buying

There is a large pool of data regarding the epidemiology of compulsive buying. In a meta-analysis of the literature (40 studies), the point prevalence of compulsive buying disorder in adults was 4.9%, being highest in university students (8.3%) [22]. The prevalence was found to be similar across different countries but was more common in women than in men, and declined with advancing age. The prevalence of compulsive buying is, overall, increasing over time, based on European data [23,24].

The onset of compulsive buying begins in the early 20s, but people do not present for treatment typically (if at all) until much later, after the buying has led to debts, legal problems or severe family upset [25]. Individuals with compulsive buying disorder commonly buy goods but never use them – the main focus is on the process of acquisition. Some buy anonymously, whereas others engage with more exclusive stores and seem to be as driven by the interactions with sales staff as they are with the items they purchase. Approximately 90% of people with compulsive buying disorder report a history of one or more other mental health disorders, and the most common comorbidities are depressive and anxiety disorders, as well as compulsive hoarding [23,24]. Substance use disorders and eating disorders (especially binge eating) also appear to be relatively highly comorbid in compulsive buying disorder.

Compulsive Sexual Behaviors

Evaluating the epidemiology of compulsive sexual behavior is problematic, because it is often hidden, and definitions abound [26]. No large epidemiological studies have been performed, but the estimated prevalence rate of compulsive sexual behavior is 3–6% [27]. For example, in a college survey in the United States, 3.7% of students reported symptoms consistent with compulsive sexual behavior [28]. Another, in a US university setting, found that 2.0% (3.0% for men, 1.2% for women) met the diagnostic criteria [29].

Based on clinical samples, compulsive sexual behavior tends to begin during adolescence, and affects both men and women. In the majority of cases, gratification or pleasure is experienced from sexual behavior, but this is commonly replaced by a sense of shame/regret [30]. The typical individual has multiple types of compulsive sexual behavior which may include excessive masturbation, compulsive use of pornography and promiscuity [31]. Most people with compulsive sexual behavior have other mental disorders, with depression and substance use disorders being especially common [26,31].

Evidence-Based Treatments

When compared with other major mental disorders, the evidence base for treating behavioral addictions is partial, characterized by only a handful of rigorously conducted high quality trials. However, certain medications found useful for treating substance use disorders also show promise for one or more of the behavioral addictions. Here, we focus on placebo-controlled, double-blind trials.

Different types of medications have been investigated in the management of gambling disorder. These have included serotonin reuptake inhibitors (SRIs), opioid antagonists, glutamatergic agents and the anti-dopaminergic medication olanzapine. For SRIs, findings have been mixed. One trial used sertraline, and found an approximately 70% treatment response in both the active and placebo treatment arms (no benefit of active treatment over placebo) [32]. Two studies examined fluvoxamine and two studies examined paroxetine; in the case of each medication, one trial identified significant benefit versus placebo, and one trial was negative overall [33,34,35,36]. Positive results have been reported for opioid antagonists. Naltrexone showed significant benefit over placebo in two trials [37,38]. Nalmefene showed significant benefit over placebo in two trials, albeit one of these trials did not yield a significant benefit when a more conservative intent-to-treat approach was used [39,40].

Another promising area is glutamatergic medications. N-acetyl cysteine (NAC), a glutamate modulating agent, was highly superior to placebo (83.3% still met responder criteria at the end of the double-blind phase, compared with only 28.6% of those assigned to placebo) in one trial [41]. Another study, this time in nicotine-dependent pathological gamblers, found that initial treatment with NAC and psychotherapy was associated with lower gambling symptoms some months later (after treatment had ended), compared with initial treatment with placebo and psychotherapy [42]. Topiramate did not differentiate from placebo in one study, but this may reflect the relatively mixed chemical actions of this agent which also has problematic adverse effects (i.e., its actions are not solely glutamatergic) [43]. Two trials found that olanzapine was no more effective than placebo for gambling disorder [44,45].

There have been only a few randomized, placebo-controlled studies of medication for the treatment of the other behavioral addictions considered herein. For kleptomania, one trial reported that naltrexone was superior to placebo given over eight weeks [46]. In a study that used open-label escitalopram (an SRI), when participants were then randomized to double-blind escitalopram or placebo, relapse rates did not differ between the treatment arms [47]. For compulsive buying disorder, all double-blind placebo-controlled trials used SRIs. Two trials in compulsive buying reported that fluvoxamine was not superior to placebo [48,49]. In a study that used open-label active treatment followed by double-blind discontinuation, relapse rates did not differ significantly between escitalopram and placebo [50]. For compulsive sexual behavior, the only published double-blind, placebo-controlled trial found that citalopram (over 12 weeks) reduced desire for sex, frequency of masturbation and frequency of pornography use, compared with placebo [51]. No overall benefits on risky behaviors were observed, but this could reflect the difficulties measuring this construct.

In our experience, close monitoring is needed in the treatment of compulsive sexual behavior because the reduction in sex drive using SRIs could in turn lead some people to undertake riskier sexual acts to overcome the blunted sexual desire.

Cross-Diagnostic Approaches

Brain Imaging: Dopaminergic Dysregulation Measured Using Radioligands

It is established from animal and human data that the addictive potential of certain psychoactive substances (e.g., cocaine) arises from their effects on dopaminergic and opioid neurochemical pathways, implicating brain regions including the ventral striatum (nucleus accumbens) [52,53,54,55]. For some substances, this model is reinforced by findings from human radioligand studies which allow neurochemical systems to be probed in vivo [56]. Positron emission tomography and single-photon emission computed tomography have been used in conjunction with various ligands in substance disorder research, including D_2/D_3 receptor ligands (e.g., fallypride, raclopride). Using these methodologies, studies have found that substance-dependent individuals have a blunted dopaminergic response to amphetamine or methylphenidate challenge (which would ordinarily increase extracellular dopamine levels by blocking reuptake and triggering release) [57]. Sufficient research has been conducted in the context of stimulant dependence to conduct a meta-analysis. Ashok and colleagues examined total 31 studies, and confirmed a significant blunting of striatal dopamine release in patients compared with controls with a medium–large effect size [56]. There was also a significant decrease in dopamine D_2/D_3 receptor availability with medium–large effect size.

The behavioral addiction field is lagging behind the substance addiction field in terms of the number of radioligand neuroimaging studies that have been conducted. Clinically, pro-dopaminergic medication has been linked with apparent new onset (or worsening of) behavioral addictions (e.g., shopping, sex, gambling) in some individuals treated for Parkinson's disease [58,59,60], thereby providing evidence for a role for dopamine in behavioral addictions. Nearly all the available radioligand studies in behavioral addictions have focused on gambling disorder. One study measured the effects of amphetamine administration on dopamine release (indexed using a D_3 preferring radioligand) in patients with gambling disorder (n = 12) compared with healthy controls (n = 11) [61]. Gambling disorder was associated with higher, rather than lower, dopamine response in the striatum compared with controls, suggesting a hyperdopaminergic state in patients, in marked contrast to the earlier findings reported in substance use disorders [61]. In a sample of 16 patients with gambling disorder and 15 healthy controls, gamblers who lost money on the Iowa gambling task had significantly increased dopamine release in the left ventral striatum compared with controls [62]. The same research group also found, in another study (18 patients with gambling disorder and 16 controls), that gamblers reported higher excitement levels than controls, and that excitement correlated with dopamine release only in the patients [63]. Elsewhere, using radioligand positron emission tomography (12 patients with gambling disorder and 12 controls), imaging showed that striatal dopamine was released during gambling, irrespective of gambling outcome, and similarly between cases and controls [64]. However, greater gambling severity was associated with more dopamine release, even though the group comparison was non-significant.

Another trial examined dopamine function using raclopride in patients with Parkinson's disease who were given a dopamine agonist. Patients with Parkinson's disease who also had gambling disorder (n = 7) showed greater dopamine increase during gambling than those without gambling disorder (n = 7) [65]. Lastly, again using raclopride but this time without a drug challenge, men with gambling disorder (n = 9) did not differ from controls (n = 9) in terms of striatal dopamine D_2/D_3 receptor availability. Urgency was negatively correlated with striatal dopamine receptor binding potentials in the patients [66]. Viewed collectively, these findings suggest that patients with gambling disorder, especially at the more severe end, may have an overactive striatal dopaminergic system, which is in contrast with findings in substance dependence, which tends to be characterized by a blunted dopaminergic system.

To the authors' knowledge, there are no radioligand studies that have assessed the dopamine system in groups of patients with compulsive sexual behavior, kleptomania or compulsive buying disorder. However, one study examined the dopamine system using raclopride in a collection of patients with Parkinson's disease who had multiple impulse control disorders

(n = 10), one impulse control disorder (n = 7) or no impulse control disorders (n = 9) [67]. Those with impulse control disorders showed significantly greater ventral striatal dopamine release in response to reward cues. Disorders in the impulsive disorder groups included compulsive sexual behavior, gambling disorder, binge-eating and compulsive buying.

Brain Imaging: Structural and Functional Changes

There is a growing body of literature examining structural and functional brain abnormalities in gambling disorder [68,69,70,71,72,73,74]. The majority of studies have focused on functional rather than structural neuroimaging abnormalities. Most functional imaging studies using attentional and inhibitory control tasks (such as Stroop, or go/no-go paradigms) have indicated hypoactivation of key frontal regions in groups of patients with gambling disorder compared with controls [75,76,77,78]. In a 2017 meta-analysis of functional imaging studies using monetary reward tasks (25 studies), gambling disorder was associated with hypoactivation of the striatum versus controls (which may relate to a baseline hyperdopaminergic state), as contrasted with substance use disorder, which was associated with hyperactivation [79]. In one of the largest studies to date, which also controlled for substance use disorders, Zois and colleagues reported decreases in frontal gray-matter volumes (medial and orbitofrontal) in patients with gambling disorder (n = 107) compared with controls (n = 98) [80]. Similarly, we found reduced predominantly right frontal cortical thickness in people with gambling disorder (n = 16) compared with controls (n = 17), in a sample that carefully excluded substance use disorders [81]. The average diminution in cortical thickness in the affected region was approximately 20%. In a study in treatment-resistant gambling disorder (16 patients and 15 controls), patients had reduced fractional anisotropy (suggestive of disorganized white matter) in the corpus callosum and superior longitudinal fasciculus [82].

The neural correlates of kleptomania, compulsive buying and compulsive sexual behavior disorder are virtually unstudied. In one neuroimaging study, kleptomania (n = 10) was associated with significantly reduced fractal anisotropy (suggestive of disorganized and/or damaged white-matter tracts) in frontal brain regions compared with controls (n = 10) [83]. To our knowledge, there are no imaging studies of compulsive buying disorder. In a pilot study, people with compulsive sexual behavior (n = 8) showed lower white-matter diffusivity in superior frontal brain regions compared with controls (n = 8), coupled with impulsive behavioral performance on a go/no-go paradigm [84]. Voon and colleagues reported enhanced neural responses to erotic videos in the dorsal anterior cingulate cortex, nucleus accumbens and amygdala, in compulsive sexual behavior (n = 19) compared to controls (n = 19) [85]. Compulsive sexual behavior (n = 23) was associated with greater left amygdala gray-matter volumes and reduced resting state connectivity between amygdala and prefrontal cortex, compared with controls (n = 69) [86].

Cognition

Objective measurable traits that deconstruct top-level phenotypes into meaningful markers more closely related to the underlying etiology, if identified, would be invaluable for understanding the behavioral addictions. Symptoms of behavioral addictions (e.g., escalating use over time, fixation on disorder-relevant stimuli, risky or inappropriate decisions, narrowing of the behavioral repertoire) are themselves suggestive of underlying cognitive abnormalities. Furthermore, cognitive dysfunction has been heavily implicated in the pathophysiology of substance use disorders include failures of top-down control, lack of planning, risky decision making and cognitive inflexibility [87]. Some of these impairments for substance use disorders appear to constitute vulnerability markers, rather than arising due to toxic effects of chronic drug consumption [88]. If behavioral addictions share overlapping neurobiology with substance addictions, one would anticipate impairments of similar cognitive domains [68,89].

Consistent with overlapping profiles between behavioral and substance addictions, multiple studies have found that people with gambling disorder experience cognitive deficits relating to inhibition, working memory, planning, cognitive flexibility and time management/estimation [74,90,91]. Although studies of gambling disorder demonstrate that the behavior is associated with diminished performance, a temporal relationship has not been established between cognitive deficits and clinically significant symptoms. It is highly likely that some cognitive deficits predispose, but that other deficits occur, as a consequence of recurrent engagement in gambling itself. Individuals with intermediate forms of gambling behaviors (falling short of a full diagnosis of gambling disorder) showed impaired decision making on a cognitive test (the Cambridge Gambling Test) dependent on the orbitofrontal and insular cortices [14]. In contrast, other domains (set-shifting and response inhibition) were only impaired in people with the full disorder [92].

One study has explored cognition in people with kleptomania, but did not include a control group, so performance was interpreted relative to normative data [93]. The authors found that the mean cognitive scores for the kleptomania group were within 0.5 standard deviations from the normative standard for age. However, worse symptom severity was associated with worse Wisconsin Card Sorting Test global performance. In a study evaluating cognitive abilities in a group of people who had shoplifted over the preceding year, deficits were found on the hardest level of a working memory task, compared with the normative group [94]. Shoplifters also gambled more points on the Cambridge Gambling Task, but appeared relatively intact on the other neurocognitive domains that were examined. One study indicated that individuals with compulsive buying had impairments in response inhibition (stop-signal task), risk adjustment during decision making and spatial working memory [95]. In a relatively small study of people with compulsive sexual disorder, no significant cognitive differences were found on set shifting, stop-signal, gambling or working memory tasks [96].

Distillation and Implications of Cross-Diagnostic Approaches

The nascent field of behavioral addictions research and treatment has seen some progress but mainly in relation to gambling disorder. Little is known about the neurobiological underpinnings of the other conditions. Gambling disorder, for the most part, is associated with over-responsive sub-cortical dopamine release in response to reward (i.e., gambling). What is not known is whether this is cause or effect: do gamblers gamble because the reward they experience in the brain is disproportionately high, or do repeated gambling episodes over time have an effect on baseline dopamine functioning? Several substance use disorders have been associated with a hypodopaminergic state, with blunted response to drug-relevant rewarding information, and the data thus far indicate that gambling disorder and substance use disorders share overlapping neural regions but with an opposite direction of abnormality with respect to dopamine release in response to challenge. Of course, none of the imaging studies with radioligands examines the dopamine system directly; they rely on assuming an underlying dopaminergic change based on observed displacement of the radioligand (such as displacement of a radioligand from D_2/D_3 receptors after methamphetamine has been administered). We hypothesize that other behavioral addictions are likely to be associated with excessive dopaminergic responses to disorder-specific environmental information, but radioligand studies are lacking. These types of studies are expensive and rely on many statistical assumptions, which make it difficult to replicate methodologies between studies (a hallmark of good science), even though meta-analysis is possible.

Turning to other types of neuroimaging, decreased volumes/thickness of frontal gray matter have been observed in gambling disorder, even up to 20% reductions in cortical thickness (on average) compared with controls [81]. Consistent with this, hypoactivation during functional imaging paradigms in frontal regions have been robustly identified using meta-analysis [79], indicating a high degree of replicability. Executive dysfunction has also been widely reported across different studies of gambling disorder, including working memory, inhibitory control and flexible responding [74,90,91]. Decision-making deficits appear to be particularly strong as candidate vulnerability markers (candidate endophenotypes) [14,97]. To our minds, these tiers of evidence indicate that gambling disorder is biologically tractable and constitutes a useful model for behavioral addictions to better understand implicated neural pathways and cognitive dysfunction more widely. Gambling addiction also represents a useful model for exploring the "cause versus effect" issue in addiction more broadly, since chronic gambling is presumably unlikely to exert toxic effects on the brain, as compared with chronic substance misuse. The emerging picture of markedly different direction of effect in terms of brain activation and dopamine functioning from substance use disorders indicates that gambling disorder is not equivalent to substance addiction biologically. Could most of the findings in substance use disorder have been driven by deleterious effects of repeated substance use on brain function, rather than constituting vulnerability markers? Further research is needed to address these issues.

Future Directions

As seen from this chapter, any neurobiological or cognitive abnormalities in the other behavioral addictions considered here have not been much examined. When abnormalities have been identified in groups of such patients compared with reference groups, researchers have generally not yet sought to replicate these results. Until results are shown to hold true across different studies of the same disorder, we caution against any firm conclusions. That replication studies are few in number is unsurprising: research funding to examine these conditions is sparse as they are not viewed as high priority by funding bodies; recruitment can also be difficult due to their nature; for example, patients often feel ashamed about their behavioral addiction, and/or are reluctant to disclose such problems (e.g., due to legal issues in the case of kleptomania or some types of compulsive sex behaviors).

Pharmacological treatment options for these behavioral addictions include consideration of opioid antagonists (e.g., naltrexone) or glutamate modulating agents (e.g., NAC). Direct evidence to support the use of these compounds is strongest for gambling disorder. Given the high comorbidity between these behavioral addictions and other mental disorders (especially depressive, anxiety, obsessive-compulsive and substance use disorders) the clinician should be careful to screen and treat these, as well as focusing on the behavioral addiction itself. While outside the scope of this chapter, there also exist various psychological treatment options for these conditions (for reviews see Dowling [98], Rash and Petry [99] and Rogers [100]).

Acknowledgments

This chapter is partly based on Grant JE and Chamberlain SR. Pharmacotherapy for behavioral addictions. *Curr Behav Neurosci Rep.* 2016;3(1):67–72. Dr. Chamberlain's involvement in this work was funded by a Wellcome Trust Clinical Fellowship (110049/Z/15/Z). Dr. Chamberlain consults for Cambridge Cognition and Shire.

Dr. Grant has research grants from the National Institute on Drug Abuse, National Institute on Alcohol Abuse and Alcoholism, the National Center for Responsible Gaming, the American Foundation for Suicide Prevention, the Trichotillomania Learning Center, Brainsway, Takeda and Psyadon Pharmaceuticals. He receives yearly compensation from Springer Publishing for acting as Editor-in-Chief of the *Journal of Gambling Studies* and has received royalties from Oxford University Press, American Psychiatric Publishing, Inc., Norton Press and McGraw Hill.

References

1. Goodman A. Neurobiology of addiction. An integrative review. *Biochem Pharmacol.* 2008;75(1):266–322.
2. Vetulani J. Drug addiction. Part II. Neurobiology of addiction. *Pol J Pharmacol.* 2001;53(4):303–317.
3. Volkow ND, Fowler JS, Wang GJ. The addicted human brain viewed in the light of imaging studies: brain circuits and treatment strategies. *Neuropharmacology.* 2004;47(Suppl 1):3–13.
4. American Psychiatric Association. *Diagnostic and Statistical Manual of Mental Disorders,* 5th ed. Washington, DC: APA; 2013.
5. Goodman A. Diagnosis and treatment of sexual addiction. *J Sex Marital Ther.* 1993;19(3):225–251.
6. Grant JE, Brewer JA, Potenza MN. The neurobiology of substance and behavioral addictions. *CNS Spectr.* 2006;11(12):924–930.
7. el-Guebaly N, Mudry T, Zohar J, Tavares H, Potenza MN. Compulsive features in behavioural addictions: the case of pathological gambling. *Addiction.* 2012;107(10):1726–1734.
8. Grant JE, Chamberlain, SR, Odlaug BL. *Clinical Guide to Obsessive Compulsive and Related Disorders.* New York, NY: Oxford University Press; 2014.
9. Chamberlain SR, Lochner C, Stein DJ, et al. Behavioural addiction-a rising tide? *Eur Neuropsychopharmacol.* 2016;26(5):841–855.
10. McElroy SL, Keck PE Jr, Pope HG Jr, et al. Compulsive buying: a report of 20 cases. *J Clin Psychiatry.* 1994;55(6):242–248.
11. Fong TW, Reid RC, Parhami I. Behavioral addictions: where to draw the lines? *Psychiatric Clin N Am.* 2012;35(2):279–296.
12. Hodgins DC, Stea JN, Grant JE. Gambling disorders. *Lancet.* 2011;378(9806):1874–1884.
13. Shaffer HJ, Hall MN, Vander Bilt J. Estimating the prevalence of disordered gambling behavior in the United States and Canada: a research synthesis. *Am J Public Health.* 1999;89(9):1369–1376.
14. Grant JE, Chamberlain SR, Schreiber LR, et al. Selective decision-making deficits in at-risk gamblers. *Psychiatry Res.* 2011;189(1):115–120.
15. Dowling NA, Cowlishaw S, Jackson AC, et al. Prevalence of psychiatric co-morbidity in

treatment-seeking problem gamblers: a systematic review and meta-analysis. *Aust N Z J Psychiatry.* 2015;49(6):519–539.

16. Tavares H, Zilberman ML, Beites FJ, et al. Gender differences in gambling progression. *J Gambl Stud.* 2001;17(2):151–159.
17. Slutske WS, Piasecki TM, Deutsch AR, et al. Telescoping and gender differences in the time course of disordered gambling: evidence from a general population sample. *Addiction.* 2015;110(1):144–151.
18. Aboujaoude E, Gamel N, Koran LM. Overview of kleptomania and phenomenological description of 40 patients. *Prim Care Companion J Clin Psychiatry.* 2004;6(6):244–247.
19. Goldman MJ. Kleptomania: making sense of the nonsensical. *Am J Psychiatry.* 1991;148(8): 986–996.
20. McElroy SL, Pope HG Jr, Hudson JI, et al. Kleptomania: a report of 20 cases. *Am J Psychiatry.* 1991;148(5):652–657.
21. Grant JE, Odlaug BL, Chamberlain, S. *Why Can't I Stop? Reclaiming Your Life from a Behavioral Addiction.* Baltimore, MD: Johns Hopkins University Press; 2016.
22. Maraz A, Griffiths MD, Demetrovics Z. The prevalence of compulsive buying: a meta-analysis. *Addiction.* 2016;111(3):408–419.
23. Muller A, Claes L, Georgiadou E, et al. Is compulsive buying related to materialism, depression or temperament? Findings from a sample of treatment-seeking patients with CB. *Psychiatry Res.* 2014;216(1):103–107.
24. Muller A, Mitchell JE, de Zwaan M. Compulsive buying. *Am J Addict.* 2015;24(2):132–137.
25. Christenson GA, Faber RJ, de Zwaan M, et al. Compulsive buying: descriptive characteristics and psychiatric comorbidity. *J Clin Psychiatry.* 1994;55(1):5–11.
26. Derbyshire KL, Grant JE. Compulsive sexual behavior: a review of the literature. *J Behav Addict.* 2015;4(2):37–43.
27. Coleman E. Is your patient suffering from compulsive sexual behavior? *Psychiatric Annals.* 1992;22(6):320–325.
28. Odlaug BL, Grant JE. Impulse-control disorders in a college sample: results from the self-administered Minnesota Impulse Disorders Interview (MIDI). *Prim Care Companion J Clin Psychiatry.* 2010;12(2):ii.
29. Odlaug BL, Lust K, Schreiber LR, et al. Compulsive sexual behavior in young adults. *Ann Clin Psychiatry.* 2013;25(3):193–200.
30. Coleman E, Raymond N, McBean A. Assessment and treatment of compulsive sexual behavior. *Minn Med.* 2003;86(7):42–47.
31. Black DW, Kehrberg LL, Flumerfelt DL, et al. Characteristics of 36 subjects reporting compulsive sexual behavior. *Am J Psychiatry.* 1997;154(2):243–249.
32. Saiz-Ruiz J, Blanco C, Ibáñez A, et al. Sertraline treatment of pathological gambling: a pilot study. *J Clin Psychiatry.* 2005;66(1):28–33.
33. Hollander E, DeCaria CM, Finkell JN, et al. A randomized double-blind fluvoxamine/placebo crossover trial in pathologic gambling. *Biol Psychiatry.* 2000;47(9):813–817.
34. Blanco C, Petkova E, Ibáñez A, et al. A pilot placebo-controlled study of fluvoxamine for pathological gambling. *Ann Clin Psychiatry.* 2002;14(1):9–15.
35. Grant JE, Kim SW, Potenza MN, et al. Paroxetine treatment of pathological gambling: a multi-centre randomized controlled trial. *Int Clin Psychopharmacol.* 2003;18(4):243–249.
36. Kim SW, Grant JE, Adson DE, et al. A double-blind placebo-controlled study of the efficacy and safety of paroxetine in the treatment of pathological gambling. *J Clin Psychiatry.* 2002;63(6):501–507.
37. Grant JE, Kim SW, Hartman BK. A double-blind, placebo-controlled study of the opiate antagonist naltrexone in the treatment of pathological gambling urges. *J Clin Psychiatry.* 2008;69(5):783–789.
38. Kim SW, Grant JE, Adson DE. Double-blind naltrexone and placebo comparison study in the treatment of pathological gambling. *Biol Psychiatry.* 2001;49(11):914–921.
39. Grant JE, Odlaug BL, Potenza MN, et al. Nalmefene in the treatment of pathological gambling: multicentre, double-blind, placebo-controlled study. *Br J Psychiatry.* 2010;197(4):330–331.
40. Grant JE, Potenza MN, Hollander E, et al. Multicenter investigation of the opioid antagonist nalmefene in the treatment of pathological gambling. *Am J Psychiatry.* 2006;163(2):303–312.
41. Grant JE, Kim SW, Odlaug BL. N-acetyl cysteine, a glutamate-modulating agent, in the treatment of pathological gambling: a pilot study. *Biol Psychiatry.* 2007;62(6):652–657.
42. Grant JE, Odlaug BL, Chamberlain SR, et al. A randomized, placebo-controlled trial of N-acetylcysteine plus imaginal desensitization for nicotine-dependent pathological gamblers. *J Clin Psychiatry.* 2014;75(1):39–45.
43. Berlin HA, Braun A, Simeon D, et al. A double-blind, placebo-controlled trial of topiramate for pathological gambling. *World J Biol Psychiatry.* 2013;14(2):121–128.

44. Fong T, Kalechstein A, Bernhard B, et al. A double-blind, placebo-controlled trial of olanzapine for the treatment of video poker pathological gamblers. *Pharmacol Biochem Behav.* 2008;89(3):298–303.

45. McElroy SL, Nelson EB, Welge JA, et al. Olanzapine in the treatment of pathological gambling: a negative randomized placebo-controlled trial. *J Clin Psychiatry.* 2008;69(3):433–440.

46. Grant JE, Kim SW, Odlaug BL. A double-blind, placebo-controlled study of the opiate antagonist, naltrexone, in the treatment of kleptomania. *Biol Psychiatry.* 2009;65(7):600–606.

47. Koran LM, Aboujaoude EN, Gamel NN. Escitalopram treatment of kleptomania: an open-label trial followed by double-blind discontinuation. *J Clin Psychiatry.* 2007;68(3):422–427.

48. Black DW, Gabel J, Hansen J, et al. A double-blind comparison of fluvoxamine versus placebo in the treatment of compulsive buying disorder. *Ann Clin Psychiatry.* 2000;12(4):205–211.

49. Ninan PT, McElroy SL, Kane CP, et al. Placebo-controlled study of fluvoxamine in the treatment of patients with compulsive buying. *J Clin Psychopharmacol.* 2000;20(3):362–366.

50. Koran LM, Aboujaoude EN, Solvason B, et al. Escitalopram for compulsive buying disorder: a double-blind discontinuation study. *J Clin Psychopharmacol.* 2007;27(2):225–227.

51. Wainberg ML, Muench F, Morgenstern J, et al. A double-blind study of citalopram versus placebo in the treatment of compulsive sexual behaviors in gay and bisexual men. *J Clin Psychiatry.* 2006;67(12):1968–1973.

52. Everitt BJ, Robbins TW. Neural systems of reinforcement for drug addiction: from actions to habits to compulsion. *Nat Neurosci.* 2005;8(11):1481–1489.

53. Everitt BJ, Robbins TW. From the ventral to the dorsal striatum: devolving views of their roles in drug addiction. *Neurosci Biobehav Rev.* 2013;37(9 Pt A):1946–1954.

54. Kalivas PW, Volkow ND. The neural basis of addiction: a pathology of motivation and choice. *Am J Psychiatry.* 2005;162(8):1403–1413.

55. Volkow ND, Fowler JS, Wang GJ, et al. Imaging dopamine's role in drug abuse and addiction. *Neuropharmacology.* 2009;56(Suppl 1):3–8.

56. Ashok AH, Mizuno Y, Volkow ND, et al. Association of stimulant use with dopaminergic alterations in users of cocaine, amphetamine, or methamphetamine: a systematic review and meta-analysis. *JAMA Psychiatry.* 2017;74(5):511–519.

57. Del Campo N, Chamberlain SR, Sahakian BJ, et al. The roles of dopamine and noradrenaline in the pathophysiology and treatment of attention-deficit/hyperactivity disorder. *Biol Psychiatry.* 2011;69(12):e145–e157.

58. Ambermoon P, Carter A, Hall WD, et al. Impulse control disorders in patients with Parkinson's disease receiving dopamine replacement therapy: evidence and implications for the addictions field. *Addiction.* 2011;106(2):283–293.

59. Bugalho P, Oliveira-Maia AJ. Impulse control disorders in Parkinson's disease: crossroads between neurology, psychiatry and neuroscience. *Behav Neurol.* 2013;27(4):547–557.

60. Poletti M, Logi C, Lucetti C, et al. A single-center, cross-sectional prevalence study of impulse control disorders in Parkinson disease: association with dopaminergic drugs. *J Clin Psychopharmacol.* 2013;33(5):691–694.

61. Boileau I, Payer D, Chugani B, et al. In vivo evidence for greater amphetamine-induced dopamine release in pathological gambling: a positron emission tomography study with [(11)C]-(+)-PHNO. *Mol Psychiatry.* 2014;19(12):1305–1313.

62. Linnet J, Peterson E, Doudet DJ, et al. Dopamine release in ventral striatum of pathological gamblers losing money. *Acta Psychiatr Scand.* 2010;122(4):326–333.

63. Linnet J, Møller A, Peterson E, et al. Dopamine release in ventral striatum during Iowa Gambling Task performance is associated with increased excitement levels in pathological gambling. *Addiction.* 2011;106(2):383–390.

64. Joutsa J, Johansson J, Niemelä S, et al. Mesolimbic dopamine release is linked to symptom severity in pathological gambling. *Neuroimage.* 2012;60(4):1992–1999.

65. Steeves TD, Miyasaki J, Zurowski M, et al. Increased striatal dopamine release in Parkinsonian patients with pathological gambling: a [11C] raclopride PET study. *Brain.* 2009;132(Pt 5): 1376–1385.

66. Clark L, Stokes PR, Wu K, et al. Striatal dopamine D(2)/D(3) receptor binding in pathological gambling is correlated with mood-related impulsivity. *Neuroimage.* 2012;63(1):40–46.

67. Wu K, Politis M, O'Sullivan SS, et al. Single versus multiple impulse control disorders in Parkinson's disease: an (1)(1)C-raclopride positron emission tomography study of reward cue-evoked striatal dopamine release. *J Neurol.* 2015;262(6):1504–1514.

68. Grant JE, Chamberlain SR. Expanding the definition of addiction: DSM-5 vs. ICD-11. *CNS Spectr.* 2016;21(4):300–303.

69. Potenza MN. The neural bases of cognitive processes in gambling disorder. *Trends Cogn Sci.* 2014;18(8):429–438.

70. Meng YJ, Deng W, Wang HY, et al. Reward pathway dysfunction in gambling disorder: a meta-analysis of functional magnetic resonance imaging studies. *Behav Brain Res.* 2014;275C:243–251.

71. Clark L, Limbrick-Oldfield EH. Disordered gambling: a behavioral addiction. *Curr Opin Neurobiol.* 2013;23(4):655–659.

72. Conversano C, Marazziti D, Carmassi C, et al. Pathological gambling: a systematic review of biochemical, neuroimaging, and neuropsychological findings. *Harv Rev Psychiatry.* 2012;20(3):130–148.

73. van Holst RJ, van den Brink W, Veltman DJ, et al. Brain imaging studies in pathological gambling. *Curr Psychiatry Rep.* 2010;12(5):418–425.

74. Goudriaan AE, Yücel M, van Holst RJ. Getting a grip on problem gambling: what can neuroscience tell us? *Front Behav Neurosci.* 2014;8:141.

75. Potenza MN, Leung HC, Blumberg HP, et al. An FMRI Stroop task study of ventromedial prefrontal cortical function in pathological gamblers. *Am J Psychiatry.* 2003;160(11):1990–1994.

76. de Ruiter MB, Oosterlaan J, Veltman DJ, et al. Similar hyporesponsiveness of the dorsomedial prefrontal cortex in problem gamblers and heavy smokers during an inhibitory control task. *Drug Alcohol Depend.* 2012;121(1–2):81–89.

77. Goudriaan AE, de Ruiter MB, van den Brink W, et al. Brain activation patterns associated with cue reactivity and craving in abstinent problem gamblers, heavy smokers and healthy controls: an fMRI study. *Addict Biol.* 2010;15(4):491–503.

78. de Ruiter MB, Veltman DJ, Goudriaan AE, et al. Response perseveration and ventral prefrontal sensitivity to reward and punishment in male problem gamblers and smokers. *Neuropsychopharmacology.* 2009;34(4):1027–1038.

79. Luijten M, Schellekens AF, Kühn S, et al. Disruption of reward processing in addiction: an image-based meta-analysis of functional magnetic resonance imaging studies. *JAMA Psychiatry.* 2017; 74(4):387–398.

80. Zois E, Kiefer F, Lemenager T, et al. Frontal cortex gray matter volume alterations in pathological gambling occur independently from substance use disorder. *Addict Biol.* 2017;22(3):864–872.

81. Grant JE, Odlaug BL, Chamberlain SR, et al. Reduced cortical thickness in gambling disorder: a morphometric MRI study. *Eur Arch Psychiatry Clin Neurosci.* 2015;265(8):655–661.

82. Grant JE, Odlaug BL, Hampshire A, et al. White matter abnormalities in skin picking disorder: a diffusion tensor imaging study. *Neuropsychopharmacology.* 2013;38(5):763–769.

83. Grant JE, Correia S, Brennan-Krohn T, et al. White matter integrity in kleptomania: a pilot study. *Psychiatry Res.* 2006;147(2–3):233–237.

84. Miner MH, Raymond N, Mueller BA, et al. Preliminary investigation of the impulsive and neuroanatomical characteristics of compulsive sexual behavior. *Psychiatry Res.* 2009;174(2):146–151.

85. Voon V, Mole TB, Banca P, et al. Neural correlates of sexual cue reactivity in individuals with and without compulsive sexual behaviours. *PLoS One.* 2014;9(7):e102419.

86. Schmidt C, Morris LS, Kvamme TL, et al. Compulsive sexual behavior: prefrontal and limbic volume and interactions. *Hum Brain Mapp.* 2017;38(3):1182–1190.

87. Yucel M, Lubman DI, Solowij N, et al. Understanding drug addiction: a neuropsychological perspective. *Aust N Z J Psychiatry.* 2007;41(12):957–968.

88. Ersche KD, Turton AJ, Chamberlain SR, et al. Cognitive dysfunction and anxious-impulsive personality traits are candidate endophenotypes for drug dependence. *Am J Psychiatry.* 2012;169(9):926–36.

89. Grant JE, Chamberlain SR. Impulsive action and impulsive choice across substance and behavioral addictions: cause or consequence? *Addict Behav.* 2014;39(11):1632–1639.

90. Clark L. Decision-making during gambling: an integration of cognitive and psychobiological approaches. *Philos Trans R Soc Lond B Biol Sci.* 2010;365(1538):319–330.

91. Verdejo-Garcia A, Chong TT, Stout JC, et al. Stages of dysfunctional decision-making in addiction. *Pharmacol Biochem Behav.* 2018;164:99–105.

92. Odlaug BL, Chamberlain SR, Kim SW, et al. A neurocognitive comparison of cognitive flexibility and response inhibition in gamblers with varying degrees of clinical severity. *Psychol Med.* 2011;41(10):2111–2119.

93. Grant JE, Odlaug BL, Wozniak JR, et al. Neuropsychological functioning in kleptomania. *Behav Res Ther.* 2007;45(7):1663–1670.

94. Grant JE, Chamberlain SR, Schreiber LR, et al. Neurocognitive deficits associated with shoplifting in young adults. *Compr Psychiatry.* 2012;53(8):1049–1055.

95. Derbyshire KL, Chamberlain SR, Odlaug BL, et al. Neurocognitive functioning in compulsive buying disorder. *Ann Clin Psychiatry.* 2014;26(1):57–63.

96. Derbyshire KL, Grant JE. Neurocognitive findings in compulsive sexual behavior: a preliminary study. *J Behav Addict*. 2015;4(2):35–36.
97. Goodie AS, Fortune EE. Measuring cognitive distortions in pathological gambling: review and meta-analyses. *Psychol Addict Behav*. 2013;27(3):730–743.
98. Dowling NA, Merkouris SS, Lorains FK. Interventions for comorbid problem gambling and psychiatric disorders: advancing a developing field of research. *Addict Behav*. 2016;58:21–30.
99. Rash CJ, Petry NM. Psychological treatments for gambling disorder. *Psychol Res Behav Manag*. 2014;7:285–295.
100. Rogers RD. Review: psychological treatments improve pathological gambling in the short and long term. *Evid Based Ment Health*. 2006;9(2):44.

Chapter 32

Other Obsessive-Compulsive Related Disorders

Ygor Arzeno Ferrão

Introduction

We expect the transdiagnostic approach to mental distress to result in a paradigm shift in psychiatry for not being strictly linked to categorical diagnosis, as currently listed on the official *Diagnostic and Statistical Manual of Mental Disorders*, fifth edition (DSM-5) [1] or International Classification of Diseases (ICD) nosological systems [2]. We also consider it will allow a practice that is closer to reality, as patients who seek treatment frequently do not present all symptoms of a specific disease or disorder. This chapter covers some conditions that have not been accommodated comfortably by the current DSM/ICD systems. However, the prevalence of some of these disorders may not be negligible. They may be also relevant for the clinical practice not only because of the resulting incapacitation but also because of their ability to complicate the correct diagnostic process of other well-established disorders.

In this chapter, we discuss the following conditions from a transdiagnostic perspective: (i) body dysmorphic disorder (BDD) with actual flaws (BDD-AF), a form of BDD that may be of particular interest of non-psychiatrists; (ii) BDD-like disorder without repetitive behavior (BDD-WRB); (iii) obsessional jealousy, also described as a presentation of pathological jealousy; (iv) shubo-kyofu, one subtype of the Japanese taijin-kyofusho (TKS) and (v) koro, a culture-bound syndrome endemic in East Asia. Both BDD-AF and -WRB may be conceptualized as variants of the classical BDD (see Chapter 23). Obsessional jealousy is not captured by the concept of delusional disorder and is probably related to obsessive-compulsive disorder (OCD). Shubo-kyofu may not be adequately subsumed by an existing category in Western systems, and may involve a blend of social anxiety, obsessional and delusional aspects shaped by cultural factors.

Recent Research Findings

Epidemiology, Clinical Picture, Diagnosis and Treatment

Body Dysmorphic Disorder With Actual Flaws

As described in Chapter 23, BDD is classified according to DSM-5 [1] as an obsessive-compulsive related disorder (OCRD) and it is best described as a distressing or impairing preoccupation with nonexistent or slight defect in one's physical appearance. However, through BDD-AF, one is able to realize that the absence of a real defect may not be the sole determinant of the pathological character of the so-called body image disorders. Instead, the patient's psychological reaction to the flaw may be more critical. Although the clinical picture of BDD-AF remains elusive, we can make a number of predictions. For instance, differently from BDD, BDD-AF will be less likely to be characterized as delusional, as the patient's belief in the defect in their appearance will probably be shared by others.

It remains unclear though, whether BDD-AF thoughts, preoccupations or images about the flaws will be characterized as intrusive as an obsession, or dominating as an overvalued idea. Conceptually, like most mental disorders, BDD-AF does probably result in significant emotional distress or impairment in social, occupational or other important areas of functioning [1]. One can speculate that patients with BDD-AF, as those with BDD, will also exhibit camouflaging, excessive use of cosmetics and "do-it-yourself" surgeries. However, as they do have unequivocal physical flaws, patients with BDD-AF may eventually display less-compulsive or confirmatory behaviors, including recurrent mirror checking and reassurance seeking.

Dermatologists, plastic surgeons and orthodontists are non-psychiatric specialists who may frequently come across BDD-AF, especially in patients with acne, psoriasis, dermatitis or vitiligo, or with conditions needing facial/rhinoplastic surgery or orthodontic treatments [3,4]. In fact, attempts to refer these patients to psychiatrists or mental health professionals may be met with surprise and may prove to be difficult for different reasons. For instance, patients with BDD-AF may actually perceive the referral as unjustifiable, given the undisputable evidence of a flaw in their appearance, as a proof of lack of empathy from their doctors, who may not put themselves in their patients' shoes (e.g., "anyone would be distressed with these appearance flaws") or as a loss of focus on the main problem to be treated or fixed.

The individual seeking treatment for severe acne may be considered the prototypical patient with BDD-AF in dermatology [5,6]. However, it is unfortunate that most BDD prevalence studies to date have excluded patients with moderate or severe acne *a priori* [7,8,9]. It is reasonable to assume, however, that most patients with severe acne do show levels of preoccupation and distress that would otherwise fulfill the criteria for BDD, but their evident facial lesions rule out the classical criteria for this diagnosis [10]. Bowe et al. investigated patients from an outpatient dermatology clinic for the treatment of acne vulgaris with the BDD Questionnaire Dermatology Version [11], and an objective assessment of acne severity. From the total of 128 patients (72% female), 43% fulfilled BDD criteria; of the 11 patients with the most severe acne, 9 (81.8%) met BDD criteria [10].

Other epidemiological studies found prevalence rates of BDD ranging from 8.8% to 11.1% in acne dermatology clinics [3], although BDD-AF cases were not specifically described. It is also possible that other relevant psychosomatic skin diseases, such as eczema, dermatitis artefacta, contamination dermatitis, and even lichen simplex chronicus, possess prominent obsessive-compulsive characteristics that overlap the BDD-AF diagnosis [12]. BDD-AF prevalence in cosmetic clinics has not yet been described, but it is expected to occur much more frequently than classical BDD.

Although the prevalence of BDD in patients seeking facial plastic surgery is not well documented, Joseph and colleagues assessed a total of 597 patients from facial plastic and oculoplastic surgery services for BDD and found that 58 (9.7%) screened positive for BDD according to the BDD Questionnaire, although real flaws rates have not been described [13]. In contrast, Dey et al., who also did not describe the real flaw rates in their study, found a lower prevalence (1.8%) of BDD among the 234 patients who underwent a reconstructive surgery [14]. According to a systematic review from Veale et al. [3], five of seven studies that investigated BDD in rhinoplasty surgery used instruments to verify real flaws, but the instruments were generally used to exclude patients with real flaws for not having BDD according to DSM criteria.

Although it seems reasonable to assume that BDD-AF would disappear together with the treatment of the primary appearance flaw, there is no good quality evidence to confirm or refute this possibility. Future studies are needed to investigate whether BDD-AF does respond positively to cognitive behavior therapy (CBT) [15,16] and selective serotonin reuptake inhibitors (SSRIs), similarly to classical BDD [16,17]. The inference based approach, through which the patient learns to rely on sensory information instead of obsessive thoughts, has been used in BDD. However, its usefulness in BDD-AF remains elusive, as sensory information may actually confirm the patient's concerns. Recent non-invasive techniques, such as repetitive or deep transcranial magnetic stimulation (TMS), and transcranial direct current stimulation, need further investigation, since no specific case of BDD-AF treated with them have been described yet. Based on existing imaging studies [18,19], we speculate that stimulating the reachable areas of the orbitofrontal and temporal cortex with high-frequency repetitive TMS or reaching deeper structures with deep TMS may be potentially beneficial. Both procedures may increase or modulate dopamine function [20] in the neural networks, possibly related to some BDD neurocognitive dysfunction, as face recognition and emotion identification [21].

Body Dysmorphic Disorder-Like Disorder Without Repetitive Behaviors

Differently from BDD-AF, the patient with BDD-WRB should fulfill all the criteria for BDD according to DSM-5 [1], with the exception of the "B" criterion (repetitive behaviors, such as mirror checking or camouflaging). As in OCD, however, the clinician should bear in mind that patients believed to have BDD-WRB may actually have classical BDD with hidden (covert) rituals, such as mentally checking and/or comparing their own appearance with others; imagining that they are camouflaging the flaw or defect; trying to remember their own appearance when it was perfect or mentally fixing their flaw. In cases where motor acts and/or mental rituals are missing, BDD-WRB may resemble depression, delusional BDD or even BDD plus the inattentive type of attention deficit and hyperactivity disorder.

If BDD and BDD-WRB do belong to the same spectrum, BDD-WRB may be actually a milder form of BDD characterized by greater ability to resist performing the repetitive rituals/behaviors. In such cases, lack of rituals can be ascribed, for instance, to preserved metacognitive abilities [22] or preserved visual perception [23]. Alternatively, BDD-WRB may be conceptualized as a more severe, delusional form of BDD where the degree of certainty about the physical flaw is so high that the patient does not need to check his or her own appearance and confirm the presence of the flaw [12]. Regardless of the exact interpretation, future studies should investigate the response of BDD-WRB to SSRIs, CBT (e.g., psychoeducation, social skills training, cognitive restructuring, as well as behavioral experiments, especially graded exposure and response prevention), or metacognitive therapies [22].

Obsessional Jealousy

Jealousy can be defined as a reaction aimed at eliminating the threat of losing a loved partner to a real or imagined rival [24]. It is a complex phenomenon that includes affective, cognitive and behavioral components [25,26], and is consistently seen across different cultures. Jealousy can be considered pathological if intense and persistent, and is further classified along a spectrum of insight into obsessional (more ego-dystonic), overvalued or delusional (more ego-syntonic) [27,28]. It is unclear, though, whether these forms may fluctuate between one and another. So far, there are no empirical data on the prevalence of pathological jealousy and its forms. In this chapter, we focus on obsessional forms of pathological jealousy (obsessional jealousy).

Obsessional jealousy involves persistent, intrusive and unwanted images or doubts about being betrayed by a loved one. From the cognitive point of view, intolerance of uncertainty is thought to play a significant role in obsessional jealousy. Although the individual suffering from obsessional jealousy generally shows preserved insight in relation to the content of their beliefs, they tend to show increased distress to situations where the fidelity of the partner is not in question. Such symptoms are followed by attempts to: (i) elicit "proofs" of the infidelity, such as checking the partner's belongings, clothes, telephones messages and social media messages or (ii) to seek reassurance from the partner that they are really loved and that no betrayals have ever occurred and will not ever occur [29].

Avoidance of jealousy-provoking situations (e.g., restrictions of the freedom of the partner who is not allowed to leave the house or to contact persons of the opposite sex) resembles avoidance seen in OCD [29]. Thus, obsessional jealousy can also be clearly conceptualized as a monothematic form of OCD [29]. Although aggressive outbursts are frequently described in individuals with pathological jealousy, it is unclear whether the former is more or less frequent in delusional compared with obsessional jealousy. However, differently from typical OCD, where aggressive behavior generally occurs in response to relatives' or partners' noncompliance with OCD-motivated instructions, aggression in pathological jealousy is probably more likely to result in tragic outcomes (e.g., homicide and/or suicide) [30].

There has been interest in a syndrome known as relational OCD that, similarly to obsessional jealousy, has been characterized by obsessive-compulsive symptoms involving the perceived flaws of one's relationship or partner [31]. However, unlike obsessive jealousy, relationship-centered obsessions do not assume the existence of a potential competitor and are less likely to involve monitoring and checking of partner's behaviors for cues indicating infidelity [31]. While delusional jealousy can be an independent type of delusional disorder, it can also be seen in schizophrenia spectrum and other psychotic disorders. In contrast, pathological jealousy involving overvalued ideas can be part of a paranoid personality disorder [30].

It is unfortunate that very little research has been performed on the neurobiological underpinnings of pathological jealousy. Further, we are not aware of studies comparing obsessional and delusional forms of jealousy. In a functional magnetic resonance imaging study in healthy volunteers, infidelity situations led to more intense activation in men in areas related to sexual and aggressive behavior, such as the amygdala and hypothalamus, and, in women, in areas related to the perception of social rules transgression, such as the posterior superior temporal sulcus [32]. One study compared obsessional jealousy patients with healthy controls and found the former group to exhibit reduced density of a platelet serotonin transporter [33].

The treatment of pathological jealousy has been based on the administration of SSRIs [34,35,36] or antipsychotics [37], depending on whether patients exhibit obsessional or delusional symptoms, respectively. Unfortunately though, the evidence supporting the prescription of these drugs is not of high quality, being based mostly on case reports. It is also unclear whether antipsychotics are effective in patients with obsessional jealousy partly responsive to SSRIs, as in OCD, or ineffective as in BDD. Although exposure and response prevention is a well-established first-line therapy for the treatment of OCD [38], its efficacy in obsessional jealousy has been shown only in case reports [39,40]. In contrast, while evidence supporting schema-focused in pathological jealousy was stronger, differential responses in obsessional jealousy were not reported [41].

Shubo-Kyofu

Culture-bound syndromes illustrate how cultural influences on psychopathology patterns render them difficult to be placed in Western nosological classifications [42]. One of these syndromes, TKS (fear of interpersonal relations) is unique, or almost unique, to East Asian societies. In the local Japanese diagnostic classification system, TKS includes several different subtypes, such as sekimen-kyofu (phobia of blushing), jiko-shisen-kyofu (phobia of one's own glance), jiko-shu-kyofu (phobia of one's own foul body odor) and shubo-kyofu (phobia of a deformed face/body), among others [43]. Accordingly, there have been attempts at operationalizing the TKS diagnosis based on DSM-IV criteria for social anxiety disorder, but it is unclear whether these diagnoses are redundant.

The community-wide prevalence of shubo-kyofu is still unknown. In Japan, however, clinical studies have yielded prevalence rates of TKS ranging from 7.8% in treatment seeking "neurotic" patients, to 45.5% in traditional clinics specialized in the so-called Morita therapy [44]. It has been suggested that the number of rules governing social behaviors in Eastern cultures may facilitate transgression and/or detection of TKS and possibly shubo-kyofu, thus increasing their prevalence [44,45,46]. Most patients with TKS who seek treatment are males in their teens or 20s [44]. We are not aware of long-term studies or community based studies of TKS (or shubo-kyofu) but there has been a consensus among specialists that the prognosis for TKS is generally good [44].

There have also been attempts to classify TKS along a spectrum of severity, in which shubo-kyofu and jiko-shu-kyofu are among the most severe forms. One such attempt has listed: (i) a transient and mild form typically manifested during adolescence; (ii) a form that is almost indistinguishable from social anxiety disorder; (iii) a "borderline" form of social anxiety disorder with ideas of reference ("severe social phobia") and (iv) a delusional form, with fixed ideas [47]. While the first two types are not offensive and usually involve fears of blushing and trembling, the "borderline" and delusional forms fall within the most severe and offensive category and include fears of having physical defects or emanating an unpleasant body odor. Notably, these severe, end-state, TKS syndromes have already been discussed within the realm of OCRDs as BDD-like syndrome and olfactory reference syndrome.

It is beyond the scope of this chapter to discuss olfactory reference syndrome, which has been addressed in Chapter 23. However, shubo-kyofu has often been considered a BDD-like syndrome as it is characterized by: (i) the belief that one displays physical defects and/or socially inappropriate behaviors and (ii) fear of offending others because of these physical defects and/or socially inappropriate behaviors (allocentric focus) [48]. However, BDD differs from shubo-kyofu as it involves fears of being rejected by, rather than offending, others. Also, unlike BDD, shubo-kyofu does not lead to desires for surgical correction [49]. However, these social fears frequently coexist across cultures. Choy et al. found shubo-kyofu symptoms in up to 75% of US and Korean patients with social anxiety disorder, who also proved to be more socially anxious, depressive and disabled [48].

The evidence reviewed above suggests that treatments proved effective for BDD, OCRDs or social anxiety disorder may also be useful in the management of TKS and shubo-kyofu syndromes. Not surprisingly, a few open studies have indicated the potential utility of SSRIs [50,51] and selective serotonin and noradrenaline reuptake inhibitors [52] on the treatment of TKS. It is unclear whether antipsychotics augment TKS syndromes that are partly responsive to SSRIs or serotonin–norepinephrine reuptake inhibitors, or actually treat delusional forms of the disorder. Similarly, it is also unclear whether different subtypes of TKS, including shubo-kyofu, show different responses to different treatments. Morita therapy, a mindfulness-based form of therapy, has been traditionally prescribed to patients with TKS [53].

Koro

Koro is a syndrome characterized by an episode of sudden and intense fear that the genitalia (generally the penis, but sometimes the nipples or vulva) is retracting and will result in death [54,55]. Koro attacks occurs mostly during the night when patients are indoors [56]. Almost half of sufferers complain of a feeling of body heat prior to a koro attack [57]. It was initially reported in Asian countries (mainly in South-East Asia and China). The syndrome usually has acute, self-limited course [57,58]. However, it can also follow a chronic or recurrent course, lasting from days to weeks, months or even years [59].

The fear of genital retraction that characterizes koro bears a striking resemblance to obsessions involving somatic and/or sexual themes [60], particularly when followed by: (i) checking compulsions (such as verifying the penis length with a rule), or the repetitive manipulation of the genitalia with hands or instruments to impede the feared outcome; (ii) avoidance of marriage, dating or casual sexual intercourse, of touching or looking at one's own genitalia or even of visiting the bathroom [61–63] or (iii) using jelling, vacuum pumps or stretching devices. Thus, koro may well be characterized as an Eastern form of OCD.

Sometimes koro may occur as an epidemic involving several hundreds to thousands of people within a short period of time, taking the form of "mass panic" [64,65,66], or "mass hysteria" [67]. Evaluating 214 epidemics of koro in China, Tseng et al. [65] found that the victims were characterized by low intelligence quotient and strong acceptance of koro-related beliefs, suggesting that preexisting beliefs in the culturally related concepts make people more vulnerable to koro, which can also be triggered by social crisis or tension [66]. It is more prevalent in men [56,57] and may lead to impotence. However, it can also lead to frigidity in women [57,67,68].

Although most cases do not exhibit significant premorbid or sexual psychopathology [69], one in every four patients has a history of an extramarital affair, sexually transmitted disease or scrotal filariasis [70]. In some cases, recent cannabis or alcohol use [57,71–73], or alcohol withdrawal [57,73], has precipitated the syndrome. Koro has been reported in patients with mood disorders [74,75]; generalized anxiety and panic disorders [76]; schizophrenia [59,77,78]; HIV [79]; genital pain [80] and prostatic enlargement [81]. Curiously, no comorbidity with OCD or BDD was reported.

If one conceptualizes koro as a culture-bound form of OCD, a high-dose SSRI may potentially be useful [74,82,83,84]. Further, as koro may share symptoms with the so-called "penile dysmorphic disorder" (a special form of BDD), techniques used in the management of BDD (e.g., exposure and response prevention) may also be attempted; always bearing in mind that sexual/somatic symptoms may be sensitive themes to address. The use of antipsychotics has been reported in the context of schizophrenia or when koro presented as a delusional form [85,86]. It is unclear whether antipsychotics may prove useful in patients who are partly responsive to SSRIs [57].

Cross-Diagnostic Approaches and Their Implications for Classification and Diagnosis

The current interest in the dimensional diagnostic approach has its foundation in the reductionism of categorical models and the problems that clinicians face daily in their practice. First, despite attempts to identify homogeneous psychiatric phenotypes, patients frequently present heterogeneous clinical pictures. Second, despite insistence on categorical models since the first classificatory systems, diagnostic criteria continue to change. Third, different types of cognitions, emotions, behaviors and interpersonal styles are repeatedly seen across different diagnostic categories. Fourth, clinicians have already noted that the more rigid the evaluation criteria, the more it is evident that patients meet criteria for multiple mental disorders, making comorbidity almost a rule in psychiatric diagnosis.

A transdiagnostic approach may be more intuitively applicable to cases that blend features of other, well-established or valid disorders or do not fulfill all the criteria for a specific disorder, such as the previously known "not otherwise specified group". According to the prevailing purely categorical approach, if a given patient presents a clinical picture characterized by a mix of two different syndromes (say, OCD and social anxiety disorder), the clinician will either: (i) diagnose a third disorder (e.g., BDD) that encapsulates the former conditions or (ii) diagnose not two, but three conditions, thus multiplying diagnostic entities. Table 32.1 summarizes the

Table 32.1 Summary of transdiagnostic characteristics and their implications for classification of obsessive-compulsive and related disorders, delusional/psychotic disorders, mood and anxiety disorders.

Transdiagnostic Aspects	Body Dysmorphic Disorder With Actual Flaws	BDD-Like Disorder Without Repetitive Behavior	Obsessional Jealousy	Shubo-Kyofu	Koro
Obsessive-compulsive disorder	+++	+++	+++	+	+
Body dysmorphic disorder	++++	++++ / +++++	0	++++	+
Impulse-control disorders	0	0	+	0	0
Delusional disorder	+++	+	+[d]	+++	++
Schizophrenia	0	0	0	0	0
Major depression	+[a]	+[a]	+[e]	++[a]	++[a]
Dysthymia	++[a]	++[a]	0	++[a]	++[a]
Bipolar disorder	0	0	0	0	0
Social anxiety disorder	+[b]	+[b]	0	+++	+[g]
Panic disorder with or without agoraphobia	0	0	0	0	+++[h]
Simple phobia	0	0	0	+	+
Psychological factors affecting general medical conditions	++++	0	0	0	0
Functional somatic symptoms	+[c]	++[c]	0	0	++[c]
Personality disorders	0	0	++[f]	0	0

\+ Strength (1–5) of the descriptive psychopathological relation between the disorders.
0 There is no descriptive psychopathological interface between the disorders.
[a] Major depression and dysthymia are probably secondary to the primary condition.
[b] The avoidant behavior commonly seen in social anxiety disorder may be present in these conditions, but the avoidance is strictly linked to the perceived appearance/defect/flaw (core symptom of body dysmorphic disorder).
[c] Functional somatic symptoms (fibromyalgia, low back pain, headache, irritable bowel and insomnia, for example) may co-occur with body dysmorphic disorder, mainly as a depressive and/or anxious secondary manifestation of the condition chronicity.
[d] The ego-syntonic (but non-delusional) obsessional jealousy may be due to overvalued ideas secondary to poor insight.
[e] Secondary depressive symptoms may be due to the consequences of the condition or due to the low self-esteem.
[f] Especially the DSM-5 cluster B personality disorders (borderline, narcissistic, histrionic and antisocial personalities) and dependent personality disorder.
[g] The social isolation commonly seen in social anxiety disorder may be present in these conditions, but it is strictly linked to the perceived genitalia problem (core symptom of the koro).
[h] Attention may be given to the dissociative symptoms of both syndromes.

cross-diagnostic characteristics and the implications for classification of the disorders described in this chapter, especially regarding their interfaces with OCD and OCRD, delusional/psychotic disorders, mood and anxiety disorders.

In sum: (i) BDD-AF lies half way between classical BDD and DSM-5 psychological factors affecting general medical conditions (e.g., acne); (ii) BDD-WRB may be simply BDD with mental compulsions or prominent avoidance; (iii) obsessional jealousy is probably simply monothematic OCD, also having a "poor insight" presentation; (iv) shubo-kyofu seems to blend social anxiety disorder, OCD and delusional disorder features into a BDD variant and (v) koro may be one of the few conditions resting on a spectrum between OCRDs and "hysteria" (dissociative disorders). Although the lack of randomized controlled trials precludes definitive conclusions regarding the effectiveness of anti-OCD treatments in these conditions, lack of better alternatives and clinical similarities suggests that they are worth being investigated.

Table 32.2 Possible therapeutic strategies for transdiagnostic disorders.

Treatment Options	BDD-AF	BDD-WRB	Obsessional Jealousy	Shubo-Kyofu	Koro
Pharmacologic:					
Antidepressants	+++	+++	+++	+++	+++
SSRIs or SRIs	+	+	+	++	+++
SNRIs	++	+	+	+	++
Tricyclics					
Antipsychotics	+[a]	0	+[a]	++[g]	++[g]
Benzodiazepines	0	0	0	0	++
Mood stabilizers	0	0	++[d]	0	0
Psychotherapy:					
Cognitive behavior	+++	++++	+++[e]	+	++
Psychodynamic	0	0	+	0	0
Other	+[b]	++[c]	++[f]	++[h]	++[i]
Psychosocial approach:					
Family/couple therapy	0	0	++	0	0
Psychoeducation	++	++	++	+	+
Non-invasive brain stimulation:					
Transcranial magnetic stimulation	+	+	+	?	?
Transcranial direct current stimulation	?	?	?	?	?
Other	0	0	0	0	0
Invasive brain stimulation:					
Deep brain stimulation	0	0	0	0	0
Neurosurgery	0	0	0	0	0
Physical activity	+	+	?	+	++
Meditation/relaxation techniques:					
Mindfulness	+	++	?	?	?
Yoga	+	++	?	?	?
Tai-chi	?	?	?	?	?

BDD-AF, body dysmorphic disorder with actual flaws; BDD-WRB, body dysmorphic disorder-like disorder without repetitive behavior; SNRI, serotonin norepinephrine reuptake inhibitor; SRI, serotonin reuptake inhibitor; SSRI, selective serotonin reuptake inhibitor.
+ Strength (1–5) of the therapeutic possibility.
0 There is no evidence it may have effect.
? A possible effect is expected, but it has not been tested.
[a] Atypical antipsychotics may augment the effect of SSRIs or SRIs.
[b] Inference-based approach.
[c] Metacognitive psychotherapy.
[d] Lithium and anticonvulsants may help to control outbursts, when present.
[e] Exposure and response prevention and/or schema-focused treatment.
[f] For the delusional form of presentation.
[g] Morita psychotherapy.
[h] Supportive psychotherapy.

Clinical Implications of Cross-Diagnostic Approaches for Treatment and Prevention

Treatment is always guided by diagnosis, either categorical or dimensional. According to the traditional categorical approach, one single therapeutic strategy is prescribed to a passive and disempowered patient based on the best available evidence for a given disorder defined according to surface symptoms (evidence-based medicine). In contrast, in transdiagnostic (or dimensional) approaches, the patient's main syndromes are not the single therapeutic targets. The patient's whole existence, including their biography, personality traits and cognitive resources, should always be taken into consideration. Categorical and dimensional approaches are not mutually exclusive though, and should probably be integrated for a better practice.

For the disorders reviewed in the present chapter, it seems obvious that the current level of scientific evidence is not enough to lead to the recommendation of any specific psychotherapy or drug, for several reasons. First, patients with these disorders have been systematically excluded from high-quality research protocols (double-blind randomized clinical trials) as they do not fit into current categorical diagnosis. Second, treatment suggestions are based on single case reports or case series with small samples. Third, as these disorders are complex, it is unlikely that one single treatment will provide the only answer.

Finally, as the disorders discussed in the present chapter are situated at the crossroads of two or more psychopathological dimensions, it is reasonable to assume that they will demand more than one single therapeutic strategy, including different pharmacotherapies, psychotherapies, brain stimulation techniques, exercise or meditation. To illustrate our point, we have listed in Table 32.2 several potential therapeutic strategies for each of them, taking into account the scarce evidence and their psychopathological interfaces with well-known or consolidated categorical disorders. This information may provide the first step toward a rationale for future studies focusing on the treatment (or even prevention) of these disorders.

Future Directions

It will be important to gather information on the prevalence, risk factors, psychopathology and neurobiology of the OCRDs described in the present chapter. It will also be critical to determine whether and how these specificities will impact treatment responses. The identification of vulnerable populations can maximize recruitment for clinical trials. Taken together, these strategies will also allow us to determine if these disorders have more commonalities or differences in relation to other OCRDs. Multisite research across different areas of the world should also be prioritized to understand the impact of culture on these phenotypes and the variants (specifiers) of each disorder, if any.

Keeping in mind that the disorders listed in this chapter do vary in terms of epidemiological importance (probably higher in pathological jealousy and lower in koro), we specifically suggest: (i) the elaboration of multisite epidemiological surveys; (ii) the performance of Delphi surveys to learn from experts not only what should be defining characteristics of OCRDs but also whether and how comfortably the disorders discussed in the present chapter fit in this spectrum; (iii) developing and validating screening and/or diagnostic tools for these OCRDs; (iv) training and informing general practitioners, psychiatrists, psychologists and other actors about the existence and importance of these disorders and finally, (v) performing double-blind randomized trials with samples large enough to provide robust effect sizes.

References

1. American Psychiatric Association. *Diagnostic and Statistical Manual of Mental Disorders*, 5th ed. Washington, DC: APA; 2013.
2. World Health Organization. *ICD-10 Classifications of Mental and Behavioural Disorder: Clinical Descriptions and Diagnostic Guidelines*. Geneva: WHO; 1992.
3. Veale D, Gledhill LJ, Christodoulou P, et al. Body dysmorphic disorder in different settings: a systematic review and estimated weighted prevalence. *Body Image*. 2016;18:168–186.
4. Yassaei S, Moghadam MG, Aghili H, et al. Body dysmorphic disorder in Iranian orthodontic patients. *Acta Med Iran*. 2014;52(6):454–457.
5. Cotterill JA. Body dysmorphic disorder. *Dermatol Clin*. 1996;14:457–463.
6. Crerand CE, Phillips KA, Menard W, et al. Nonpsychiatric medical treatment of body dysmorphic disorder. *Psychosomatics* 2005;46:549–555.
7. Phillips KA, Dufresne Jr, RG, Wilkel CS, et al. Rate of body dysmorphic disorder in dermatology patients. *J Am Acad Dermatol*. 2000;42:436–441.

8. Uzun O, Basoglu C, Akar A, et al. Body dysmorphic disorder in patients with acne. *Compr Psychiatry.* 2003;44:415–419.

9. Conrado LA, Hounie AG, Diniz JB, et al. Body dysmorphic disorder among dermatologic patients: prevalence and clinical features. *J Am Acad Dermatol.* 2010;63(2):235–243.

10. Bowe WP, Leyden JJ, Crerand CE, et al. Body dysmorphic disorder symptoms among patients with acne vulgaris. *J Am Acad Dermatol.* 2007;57(2):222–230.

11. Dufresne RG, Phillips KA, Vittorio CC, et al. A screening questionnaire for body dysmorphic disorder in a cosmetic dermatologic surgery practice. *Dermatol Surg.* 2001;27:457–462.

12. Zhu TH, Nakamura M, Farahnik B, et al. Obsessive-compulsive skin disorders: a novel classification based on degree of insight. *J Dermatolog Treat.* 2017;28(4):342–346.

13. Joseph AW, Ishii L, Joseph SS, et al. Prevalence of body dysmorphic disorder and surgeon diagnostic accuracy in facial plastic and oculoplastic surgery clinics. *JAMA Facial Plast Surg.* 2017;19(4):269–274.

14. Dey JK, Ishii M, Phillis M, et al. Body dysmorphic disorder in a facial plastic and reconstructive surgery clinic: measuring prevalence, assessing comorbidities, and validating a feasible screening instrument. *JAMA Facial Plast Surg.* 2015;17(2):137–143.

15. Harrison A, Fernández de la Cruz L, Enander J, et al. Cognitive-behavioral therapy for body dysmorphic disorder: a systematic review and meta-analysis of randomized controlled trials. *Clin Psychol Rev.* 2016;48:43–51.

16. Phillipou A, Rossell SL, Wilding HE, et al. Randomised controlled trials of psychological and pharmacological treatments for body dysmorphic disorder: a systematic review. *Psychiatry Res.* 2016;245:179–185.

17. Arnold LM, Auchenbach MB, McElroy SL. Psychogenic excoriation. Clinical features, proposed diagnostic criteria, epidemiology and approaches to treatment. *CNS Drugs.* 2001;15(5):351–359.

18. Madsen SK, Zai A, Pirnia T, et al. Cortical thickness and brain volume analysis in body dysmorphic disorder. *Psychiatry Res.* 2015;232(1):115–122.

19. Buchanan B, Rosselll S, Maller JJ, Toh WL, Brennan S, Castle D. Regional brain volumes in body dysmorphic disorder compared to controls. *Aust N Z J Psychiatry.* 2014;46(7):654–662.

20. Tanaka T, Takano Y, Tanaka S, et al. Transcranial direct-current stimulation increases extracellular dopamine levels in the rat striatum. *Front Syst Neurosci.* 2013;7:6.

21. Beilharz F, Castle DJ, Grace S, Rossell SL. A systematic review of visual processing and associated treatments in body dysmorphic disorder. *Acta Psychiatr Scand.* 2017;136(1):16–36.

22. Zeinodini Z, Sedighi S, Rahimi MB, et al. Dysfunctional metacognitive beliefs in body dysmorphic disorder. *Glob J Health Sci.* 2016;8(3):10–16.

23. Toh WL, Rossell1 SL, Castle DJ. Body dysmorphic disorder: a review of current nosological issues and associated cognitive deficits. *Curr Psychiatry Rev.* 2009;5:261–270.

24. Torres AR, de Abreu Ramos-Cerqueira AT, da Silva Dias R. Jealousy as a symptom of obsessive-compulsive disorder. *Rev Brasil Psiquiatr.* 1999;21(3):165–173.

25. Marazziti D, Poletti M, Dell'Osso L, et al. Prefrontal cortex, dopamine, and jealousy endophenotype. *CNS Spectr.* 2013;18(1):6–14.

26. Marazziti D, Di Nasso E, Masala I. Normal and obsessional jealousy: a study of a population of young adults. *Eur Psychiatry.* 2003;18(3):106–111.

27. Tarrier N, Beckett R, Harwood S, et al. Morbid jealousy: a review and cognitive-behavioural formulation. *Br J Psychiatry.* 1990;157:319–326.

28. McKenna PJ. Disorders with overvalued ideas. *Br J Psychiatry.* 1984;145:579–585.

29. Ecker W. Non-delusional pathological jealousy as an obsessive-compulsive spectrum disorder: cognitive-behavioural conceptualization and some treatment suggestions. *J Obsess Compuls Relat Disord.* 2012;1:203–210.

30. De Koning E, Piette MHA. A retrospective study of murder-suicide at the Forensic Institute of Ghent University, Belgium: 1935–2010. *Med Sci Law.* 2014;54(2):88–98.

31. Doron G, Derby DS, Szepsenwol O. Relationship obsessive compulsive disorder (ROCD): a conceptual framework. *J Obsess Compul Relat Disord.* 2014;3(2):169–180.

32. Takahashi H, Matsuura M, Yahata N, et al. Men and women show distinct brain activations during imagery of sexual and emotional infidelity. *Neuroimage.* 2006;32(3):1299–1307.

33. Marazziti D, Rucci P, Di Nasso E, et al. Jealousy and subthreshold psychopathology: a serotonergic link. *Neuropsychobiology.* 2003;47(1):12–16.

34. Stein DJ, Hollander E, Josephson SC. Serotonin reuptake blockers for the treatment of obsessional jealousy. *J Clin Psychiatry.* 1994;55(1):30–33.

35. Batinic B, Duisin D, Barisic J. Obsessive versus delusional jealousy. *Psychiatr Danub.* 2013;25(3):334–339.

36. Wright S. Familial obsessive-compulsive disorder presenting as pathological jealousy successfully treated with fluoxetine. *Arch Gen Psychiatry.* 1994;51:430–431.
37. Bisol L, Lara DR. Low-dose risperidone for pathological jealousy: report of 3 cases. *J Clin Psychopharmacol.* 2008;28(5):595–596.
38. American Psychiatric Association. *Practice Guideline for the Treatment of Patients with Obsessive-Compulsive Disorder.* Washington, DC: APA; 2007.
39. Cobb JP, Marks IM. Morbid jealousy featuring as obsessive-compulsive neurosis: treatment by behavioural psychotherapy. *Br J Psychiatry.* 1979;34:301–305.
40. Parker G, Barrett E. Morbid jealousy as a variant of obsessive-compulsive disorder. *Aust N Z J Psychiatry.* 1997;31:133–138.
41. Dolan M, Bishay N. The effectiveness of cognitive therapy in the treatment of non-psychotic morbid jealousy. *Br J Psychiatry.* 1996;168(5):588–593.
42. Prince R, Tcheng-Laroche F. Culture-bound syndromes and international disease classifications. *Cult Med Psychiatry.* 1987;11(1):3–52.
43. Iwata Y, Suzuki K, Takei N, et al. Jiko-shisen-kyofu (fear of one's own glance), but not taijin-kyofusho (fear of interpersonal relations), is an East Asian culture-related specific syndrome. *Aust N Z J Psychiatry.* 2011;45(2):148–152.
44. Takahashi T. Social phobia syndrome in Japan. *Compr Psychiatry.* 1989;30:45–52.
45. Lim L. Taijin-kyofu-sho: a subtype of social anxiety. *Open J Psychiatry.* 2013;3:393–398.
46. Singelis TM, Sharkey WF. Culture, self-construal, and embarrassability. *J Cross-Cultural Psychol.* 1995;26:622–626.
47. Sharpless B, Balko AL, Grom JL. Taijin Kyofusho. In: Sharpless B, ed. *Unusual and Rare Psychological Disorders: A Handbook for Clinical Practice and Research.* New York, NY: Oxford University Press; 2017:177–195.
48. Choy Y, Schneier FR, Heimberg RG, et al. Features of the offensive subtype of Taijin-kyofu-sho in US and Korean patients with DSM-IV social anxiety disorder. *Depress Anxiety* 2008;25(3):230–240.
49. Tarumi S, Ichimiya A, Yamada S, et al. Taijin Kyofusho in university students: patterns of fear and predispositions to the offensive variant. *Transcult Psychiatry.* 2004;41:533–546.
50. Nagata T. An open trial of paroxetine for the "offensive subtype" of taijin kyofusho and social anxiety disorder. *Depress Anxiety.* 2006;23:168–174.
51. Matsunaga H, Kiriike N, Matsui T, et al. Taijin kyofusho: a form of social anxiety disorder that responds to serotonin reuptake inhibitors? *Int J Neuropsychopharmacol.* 2001;4:231–237.
52. Nagata T. Open trial of milnacipran for taijin kyofusho in Japanese patients with social anxiety disorder. *Int J Psychiatry Clin Pract.* 2003;7:107–112.
53. Maeda F, Nathan JH. Understanding taijin kyofusho through its treatment, morita therapy. *J Psychosom Res.* 1999;46:525–530.
54. Crozier I. Making up koro: multiplicity, psychiatry, culture, and penis-shrinking anxieties. *J Hist Med Allied Sci.* 2012;67(1):36–70.
55. Atalay H. Two cases of koro syndrome or anxiety disorder associated with genital retraction fear. *Turk Psikiyatri Derg.* 2007;18(3):282–285.
56. Dutta D, Phookan HR, Das PD. The koro epidemic in lower Assam. *Indian J Psychiatry.* 1982;24(4):370–374.
57. Ghosh S, Nath S, Brahma A, et al. Fifth koro epidemic in India: a review report. *WCPRR.* 2013;8(1):8–20.
58. Chakraborty S, Sanyal D. An outbreak of koro among 19 workers in a jute mill in South Bengal. *Ind Psychiatry J.* 2011;20(1):58–60.
59. Ntouros E, Ntoumanis A, Bozikas V, et al. Koro-like symptoms in two Greek men. *BMJ Case Rep.* 2010;2010:bcr08.2008.0679.
60. Davis DM, Steever AM, Terwilliger JM, Williams MT. The relationship between culture-bound syndrome koro and obsessive-compulsive disorder. In: Hayes GR, Bryant MH, eds. *Psychology of Culture.* New York, NY: Nova Science; 2012:213–221.
61. Mattelaer JJ, Jilek W. Koro: the psychological disappearance of the penis. *J Sex Med.* 2007;4(5):1509–1515.
62. Kar N. Chronic koro-like symptoms – two case reports. *BMC Psychiatry.* 2005;12(5):34.
63. Silva L, Raposo-Lima C, Soares C, Cerqueira JJ, Morgado P. Koro syndrome in an obsessive-compulsive disorder patient. *Eur Psychiatry.* 2016;33(Suppl):S618.
64. Atalay H. Two cases of koro syndrome or anxiety disorder associated with genital retraction fear. *Turk Psikiyatri Derg.* 2007;18(3):282–285.
65. Tseng WS, Mo KM, Li LS, et al. Koro epidemics in Guangdong, China. A questionnaire survey. *J Nerv Ment Dis.* 1992;180(2):117–123.
66. Bartholomew RE. The social psychology of "epidemic" koro. *Int J Soc Psychiatry.* 1994;40(1):46–60.
67. Jilek W, Jilek-Aall L. Mass-hysteria with koro-symptoms in Thailand. *Schweiz Arch Neurol Neurochir Psychiatr.* 1977;120(2):257–259.

68. Sachdev PS. Koro epidemic in north-east India. *Aust N Z J Psychiatry.* 1985;19(4):433–438.

69. Chowdhury AN. Biomedical potential for symptom choice in koro. *Int J Soc Psychiatry.* 1989;35(4):329–332.

70. Chowdhury AN, Bera NK. Koro following cannabis smoking: two case reports. *Addiction.* 1994;89(8):1017–1020.

71. Earleywine M. Cannabis-induced koro in Americans. *J Clin Psychiatry.* 2002;63(12):1182–1183.

72. Kalaitzi CK, Kalantzis A. Cannabis-induced koro-like syndrome. A case report and mini review. *Urol Int.* 2006;76(3):278–280.

73. Al-Sinawi H, Al-Adawi S, Al-Guenedi A. Ramadan fasting triggering koro-like symptoms during acute alcohol withdrawal: a case report from Oman. *Transcult Psychiatry.* 2008;45(4):695–704.

74. Freudenmann RW, Schonfeldt-Lecuona C. Koro-like symptoms in a recurrent depressive disorder. *Der Nervenarzt.* 2005;76:885–887.

75. Damodaran SS, Nizamie HS. Incomplete koro. A forerunner for mood disorder: two case reports. *Indian J Psychiatry.* 1993;35:60–62.

76. Al-Hmoud N. Koro-like syndrome in a Jordanian male. *Eastern Med Health J.* 1999;5:611–613.

77. Maslowski J. Koro-like syndrome in Maltese subject on the basis of chronic schizophrenia. *Bull Inst Marit Trop Medi Gdynia.* 1988;39:108–110.

78. Afonso P, Saraiva S, Gameiro Z. Schizophrenia presenting with koro-like symptoms. *J Neuropsychiatry Clin Neurosci.* 2013;25(1):E32.

79. Heyman I, Fahy TA. Koro-like symptoms in a man infected with the human immunodeficiency virus. *Br J Psychiatry.* 1992;160:119–121.

80. Caballero JM, Avila A, Cardona X, et al. Genital pain without urogenital pathology: the koro-like syndrome. *J Urol.* 2000;163:243.

81. Naim M, Aligarh JA. Penile retraction in non psychiatric patients [e-letter]. *BMJ Case Rep.* 2010: April 22. Available from: http://casereports.bmj.com/content/2010/bcr.08.2008.0679.abstract/reply#casereports_el_57 (accessed July 27, 2018).

82. Nakaya M. Fluvoxamine treatment of a Japanese patient with koro. *J Clin Psychiatry.* 2002;63(12):1182–1183.

83. Turnier L, Chouinard G. The anti-koro effect of a tricyclic antidepressant. *Can J Psychiatry.* 1990;35(4):331–333.

84. Hallak JE, Crippa JA, Zuardi AW. Treatment of koro with citalopram. *J Clin Psychiatry.* 2000;61:951.

85. Ramamourty P, Menon V, Aparna M. Koro presenting as acute and transient psychosis: implications for classification. *Asian J Psychiatr.* 2014;10: 116–117.

86. Rosca-Rebaudengo P, Durst R, Minuchin-Itzigsohn S. Transculturation, psychosis and koro symptoms. *Isr J Psychiatry Relat Sci.* 1996;33(1):54–62.

Index

Note: References to tables indicated with *italics*.

5-HT_3 antagonists, *190*, 192
5-hydroxytryptamine (5-HT) system, 187

ABGA (anti-basal ganglia antibodies), 54–55, 57
Acceptance and Commitment Therapy (ACT), 352, 353
acceptance-enhanced behavior therapy, 371
acute threat, *see* fear
addiction, 401, *see also* behavioral addictions
ADHD. *see* attention deficit hyperactivity disorder (ADHD)
adolescents. *see* children and adolescents
agency, 2, 8
agoraphobia, 115–17, 164–65
akinetic-rigid syndromes, 384–85
alcohol dependence, *see* substance use disorders (SUD)
alexithymia, 3
allergies, 165
allopurinol, 377
alpha-2 agonists, 186, 360
amitriptyline, 185
amygdala
  and BDD, 309
  and fear response and regulation, 96–97
  and hoarding behaviors, 335–36
  and negative reinforcement, 62–63, 67
  and OCD, 76, 77–78, 79, 96
  and PG, 63
  and reward processing, 96
  and SUD, 62–63
animal hoarding, 332
animal models
  and DBS, 66
  and excessive grooming, 32, 372–73
  and habit, 64
  and herbal remedies, 298
  and hoarding behaviors, 335
  and pharmacotherapy, 66, 187, 294, 301
  and PSP, 371
  and schedule-induced polydipsia, 63
  and stereotypy, 377, 378
  and stress, 41
anterior limb of the internal capsule (ALIC), 256–57, *258*, *259*
antibiotics, 56, 249–50, 377, 379
antibodies, 54–55
  anti-basal ganglia antibodies (ABGA), 54–55, 57
  anti-streptolysin O (ASO), 54
antidepressants, *see* selective serotonin reuptake inhibitors (SSRI); serotonin norepinephrine reuptake inhibitors (SNRI); serotonin reuptake inhibitors (SRI); tricyclic antidepressants (TCA); *specific drugs*
antiepileptics. *see also* lamotrigine; topiramate; valproate
  for ASD, 377
  for OCD, 191, 389–90
  for PG, 66
  for SMD, 377
  for SUD, 66
  for tic disorders, 360–61
antipsychotics, 231–32, *see also* aripiprazole; haloperidol; olanzapine; pimozide; quetiapine; risperidone
  for BDD, 193
  for koro, 417
  for OCD, 186, 187, 188–89, 231–32, 248
  for tic disorders, 186, 232, 360
  for TTM, 194, 232, 371
  side-effects, 232
anti-reward systems, *see* negative reinforcement
anxiety and anxiety disorders. *see also* agoraphobia; generalized anxiety disorder (GAD); post-traumatic stress disorder (PTSD); social anxiety disorder (SAD)
  excessive, and obsessional stimuli, 207
  and experiential avoidance, 339
  and fear response and regulation, 96–97
  and obsessions, 130
  as OCD comorbidity, 19, 116–17, 118, 165
  as OCD risk factor, 120
  as sub-clinical OCD comorbidity, 165
  relief, and compulsive rituals, 207
  risk factors, 121–23
  treatment-seeking behaviors, 115–16
Anxiety Disorder Interview Schedules (ADIS), 172
anxiety sensitivity, 176, 178, 339
Anxiety Sensitivity Index-3 (ASI-3), 176
appraisal model of OCD, 163, 220–21
aripiprazole
  in animal models, 65
  for BDD, 193
  for eating disorders, 65
  for OCD, 188, 189, 232
  for tic disorders, 360
ASD, *see* autistic spectrum disorder (ASD)
Ashwagandha, 298
ASO (anti-streptolysin), 54
assessment. *see also* classification and diagnosis; history taking; *specific assessment instruments*
  of cognitive control, 4
  of insight, 174
  of OCD, 172–74
  and RDoC, 2
association specifier, 376–77
athymhormia, 385
atomoxetine, 338
attention deficit hyperactivity disorder (ADHD)
  and HD, 339
  as OCD comorbidity, 19–20, 22–23, 146
  as sub-clinical OCD comorbidity, 165
  neuropathology, 77, *88*
  pharmacotherapy, 186, 360

attentional bias to threat, 6
autistic spectrum disorder (ASD), 77, 175, 333, 376, 377
autoimmune disease. *see* immune system: dysfunction, and autoimmune disease
avoidance, 6, 178

basal ganglia, 63, *see also* caudate nucleus; nucleus accumbens (NA); putamen; subthalamic nucleus; ventral striatum
BDD (BDDQ) questionnaire - dermatology version (DV), 414
bed nucleus stria terminalis (BST), 62–63, 67
behavior therapy, *see* cognitive behavioral therapy (CBT); exposure and response prevention (ERP)
behavioral addictions, 401–08, *see also* compulsive buying disorder; compulsive sexual behavior; gambling, pathological; kleptomania
  classification and diagnosis, 401
  cognitive dysfunction, 406–7
behavioral inflexibility, 63, *see also* flexibility and inflexibility
Behavioral Inhibition/Activation System (BIS/BAS) questionnaire, 65
benzodiazepines, 185
bifactor model of OCD, 176
binge eating disorder (BED), *see* eating disorders
biomarkers, for OCRDs, 139–40, 196, 255–56
bipolar disorders, 116, 118, 165
birth complications, and risk of OCD, 39, 40
body dysmorphic disorder (BDD). *see also* koro
  with actual flaws (BDD-AF), 413–14, 418, *418*, *419*
  without repetitive behaviors (BDD-WRB), 414–15, 418, *418*, *419*
  and acne, 414
  classification and diagnosis, 307, 310
  comorbidities, 308
  cosmetic surgery, 310, 414
  course and outcome, 147, 307–08, 310
  and effort valuation, 3
  and hyperreflexivity, 3
  and insight, 307, 308
  neuropathology, 77, *86*, 98, 309
  pharmacotherapy
    antidepressants, 192–93, 229, 310
    antipsychotics, 193
    drug augmentation, 193, 232
    incremental response, 193
    myo-inositol (MI), 297
  placebo response, blunted, 192–93
  prevalence, 307, 414
  psychotherapy
    CBT, 210, 235–36, 309–11
    IBA, 226
    mirror retraining, 309–10, 311
    visual training, 311–12
  and quality of life, 308
  and recurrent images, 4
  remission rate, 147
  and suicide, 308
  and visual processing abnormalities, 309, 310–11
body-focused repetitive behaviors, *see* skin picking, pathological (PSP); trichotillomania (TTM)
  as focused or automatic, 178
Borna disease virus, 53
bradykinesia, *see* akinetic-rigid syndromes
brain damage and injury, and pathogenesis of OCRDs
  stroke, 333, 390–91
  traumatic, 42, 119, 333, 390
  tumors, 390–91
brain imaging, *see* neuroimaging
brain models of OCD, 3–4, 74, *see also* cognitive models of OCRD
  and decision-making, 41, 76–77, 271
brain tumors, 390–91
Brown Assessment of Beliefs Scale (BABS), 174, 178, 308
buspirone, 185

cancer, 391
  brain, 390–91
candidate gene studies and gene polymorphisms, 30–31, *see also* epigenetics; genetics; Genome Wide Association Studies (GWAS)
  in dystonic syndromes, 387
  and glutamatergic system, 233
  in impulse control disorders, 384–85
  in OCD, 30–31, 32, 52, 53, 233
  in OCPD, 347–48
  in OCS, 384
  in onychophagia (animal models), 32
  in PD, 384–85
  in PSP, 373
  in rheumatic fever, 53
  splicing, 34–35
  and therapeutic response, 33–34
  in TTM (animal models), 32
cannabinoid agonists, 371
CANS (childhood acute neuropsychiatric symptoms), 53
capsulotomy, 257–58, 281–86
catatonia, 384
categorical approach, to diagnosis and treatment of OCRDs, vs. dimensional approach, 7, 420
caudal temporal regions, 75, 76
caudate nucleus, 75, 92, 96, 139–40, 255
cerebellum, 75
childhood experiences, and risk of OCRD, 44, 119, 121–22, 335
children and adolescents
  and history taking, 172, 173
  and OCD, *see* Obsessive-Compulsive Disorder (OCD): in children and adolescents
  and PSP, 369
  and stereotypic movement disorder, 376, 377
  and sub-clinical OCD, 165–66, 168
  and tic disorders, 357–58, 359–60
  and TTM, 155, 194, *295*, 368
chorea, 385
  Benign Hereditary Chorea (BHC), 387
  Sydenham chorea, 51, 53, 56–57, 386
cingulate cortex, 335
  anterior, 4, 92, 96, 97, 255
  and HD, 98, 335–36
  volume change, 75, 78–79
cingulotomy, 281, 287–88
citalopram
  with CBT, 313
  with clomipramine, 230
  for compulsive sexual behavior, 404–05
  for OCD, 185
  for OCPD, 349
  for ORD, 313
  for PSP, 371
  for TTM, 194
classification and diagnosis. *see also* assessment; International Classification of Functioning, Disability, and Health (ICF); *under specific disorders; specific DSMs; specific ICDs; specific instruments*
  assessment and diagnostic instruments, 120–21
  biomarkers, 139–40, 196, 255–56

cross-diagnostic approaches, 174–77
defined, 128
dimensional approach, to diagnosis and treatment of OCRDs, 195, 196–97, 351
vs. categorical approach, 7, 420
early systems, 133
and ego-dystonicity, 130
functional analysis, 214
role of treatment approaches, 195–96
specifiers, *see* association specifier; course of illness specifier; excessive acquisition specifier; insight specifier; obsessive-compulsive symptoms specifier; self-injury specifier; tic-related specifier
as symptoms, syndromes, and nosological entities, 129
as typification, 128
Clinical Global Impression-Improvement (CGI-I), 229
clomipramine
for BDD, 192–93, 310
with CBT, 242–46, *243*, 247, 313
for OCD, 185, 186, 242–46, 349
for OCPD, 349
for ORD, 313
for SMD, 377
with SSRIs, 230–31
for TTM, 194, 370
incremental response, 186
clorgyline, 185
Clutter Image Rating (CIR), 336
clutter, vs. hoarding, 333
cobalamin, 292–93
cognitive behavioral therapy (CBT). *see also* exposure and response prevention (ERP); psychotherapy
and brain structure and activity, 78–79, 99–100, 101–2
for BDD, 210, 235–36, 309–10, 311
for clinical perfectionism (CBT-P), 352
for HD, 155, 337
for hypochondriasis, 323–24
for OCD, *91*, 146–54, 209, 234–35, 242–44, 300
for OCPD, 349–50, 352
for ORD, 313
and pediatric patients, 78
with pharmacotherapy
antibiotics, 249–50
ketamine, 234–35
SRIs, 247–44, 248, 338
SSRIs, 230, 245, 246, 247, 313, 324
TCAs, *243*
with physical activity, 300
for phobias, 219
for PSP, 371
response prediction, 102, 235–36
cognitive confidence, 222–23, *see also* senses, distrust of in OCD
cognitive control, assessment of, 4
cognitive distortions, 176
cognitive dysfunction, in behavioral addictions, 406–7
cognitive inflexibility, 63, 64, 92–96, 97, 348, 372, *see also* flexibility and inflexibility
cognitive models of OCRD, *see* appraisal model of OCD; bifactor model of OCD; cognitive confidence; Inference-Based Approach (IBA) model; metacognitive model of OCD; network model
completeness, vs. harm avoidance, 176, 195
compulsions and compulsivity. *see also* obsessive-compulsive symptoms (OCS)
compulsive rituals, 5, 163, 207
and control loss, 15, 236
definitions and classification, 7–8, 14–16, 17, 131–33
desires to resist, 132
diagnostic instruments, 65
as dysfunctional behavior, 15–16, 17
as focused or automatic, 178
and free will, 15, 16
vs. impulsivity, 14–15, 175–76, 325, 350–51
treatment implications, 177–78, 195, 236, 271
mental compulsions, 176, 195
and negative reinforcement, 62–63, 67, 211
neurobiological basis, 97
observational perspective, 14–16
phenomenological perspective, 14–16, 17
and practical identity, 16–17
vs. repetitive behaviors, 175–76,
tics, 175–76, 361
as stereotyped behaviors, 131
and stress, 41
as subjective phenomena, 132–33
Compulsive Acquisition Scale, 336–37
compulsive buying disorder, 338, 402–4, 407
compulsive sexual behavior, 404–5, 406
computed tomography (CT), 74
conditioned associations, and OCD, 219–20
conditioning theory, 219
conflict detection, and sustained threat, 6
contingency-related flexibility, 63
control, loss of, and compulsivity, 15, 236
coprolalia, 358, *see also* tics
copropraxia, 358, *see also* tics
corpus callosum, 78
corpus striatum, 77, 98
correct-related negatives (CRN), 4
cortical thickness changes, 75, 77, 78, 79, 406
corticosteroids, 56–57
cortico-striato-thalamic circuits. *see also* basal ganglia; prefrontal cortex
CSTC model of OCD, 85–92, 99, 255
gray matter, 75
resting-state fMRI studies, 96, 255–56
and stereotypy, 378
and stress, 44
and therapeutic response, 45
white matter, 75–76
cortico-subcortical circuits, 3–4
cosmetic surgery, 310, 414
course of illness specifier, 156–57
culture-bound syndromes (CBS), 416–17, *418*
cytokines, 54, 55, 300–01

daily life, impairment, 115, *see also* quality of life
D-amphetamine, *190*
decision-making
and HD, 97–98, 101–02
and OCD, 97–98
and PG, 406–07
goal-directed vs. habit-based, 41, 76–77, 271
deep brain stimulation (DBS), 256–61, *see also* repetitive transcranial magnetic stimulation (rTMS)
complications, 286, 287
method, 256, 261, 286
and non-OCD compulsive behaviors, 259
for OCD, 66–67, 256–61
and orbitofrontothalamic fiber morphology, 79, 288
for Parkinson's disease, 259–60
post-surgery optimization, 261
RCT design, 261
and stereotypy, 379
for SUD, 66

deep brain stimulation (DBS) (*cont.*)
  for TD, 259, 287, 361
  target sites, 66–67, 256–59
    optimization, 260–61, 361
delusions, 3, 8, 313, 322
depressive disorders
  and gray matter volume changes, 76, 77
  and hyperreflexivity, 3
  vs. hypochondriasis, 322
  and immune dysfunction, 55
  as OCD comorbidity, 19, 21–22, 116, 164–65
    pharmacotherapy, 186
    sub-clinical OCD, 164–65
    temporal pattern, 118
  as OCD risk factor, 119–20
  risk factors, 121–23
desipramine, 186, 192–93, 194, 377
dexamphetamine, 192
diagnosis. *see* classification and diagnosis
Diagnostic and Statistical Manuals (DSM). *see also* classification and diagnosis
  DSM-I, 130, 131, 133
  DSM-II, 130, 133
  DSM-III and DSM-IIIR, 130, 131, 132, 133–34
  DSM-IV
    and compulsions, 131, 132
    and obsessions, 130
    and OCD, 120
    and poor insight specifier, 136–37
    and role of anxiety in obsessions, 130
  vs. RDoC, 2, 140
  DSM-5
    and addiction, 401
    and ADHD, 23
    and compulsions, 131, 132
    and Frontotemporal Neurocognitive Disorder, 388
    and hypochondriasis, 320–21
    and kleptomania, 401, 402
    and obsessions, 129–30
    and OCD, 3, 19, 23, 121, 135
    and OCPD, 345–46
    and OCRD cluster, 184, 196, 391–92
    and OCRD due to other medical causes, 42, 135, 391–92
    and PG, 401, 402
    and PSP, 367
    and role of anxiety in obsessions, 130
    and self-injurious non-suicidal behaviors, 378
    and SMD, 376–77
    and Substance/Medication-Induced OCRDs, 391–92
    and tic disorder and Tourette's Disorder, 358–59
    and TTM, 367
    specifiers in, 137, 376–77
  instruments, *see specific instruments*
diathesis-stress model, 52–54
diffusion magnetic resonance imaging, 79
dimensional approach, to diagnosis and treatment of OCRDs, 195, 196–97, 351
  vs. categorical approach, 7, 420
Dimensional Yale-Brown Obsessive Compulsive Scale (DY-BOCS), 173–74, 196
disgust, 85–92, 176–77, 178
Disgust Propensity and Sensitivity Scale-Revised (DPSS-R), 177
dissociative absorption, and OCD, 221–22, 223
distress tolerance, and CBT, 235–36
distrust of the senses, 222, 223–24
dopaminergic system
  abnormalities, 65, 231
  and antipsychotics, 231
  and glutamatergic signaling, 66
  and hoarding behaviors, 335
  and myo-inositol (MI), 294–97
  and OCD, 30
  and PG, 405, 407
  and stereotypy, 378
  and SUD, 405
dopaminergic treatments, 65, 250–51
  blockers, 30, 65, 377, 379
dorsal striatum, 7, 41, 64
doubt, 4, 8, 225
dronabinol, 371
drug therapy, *see* pharmacotherapy
DSM, *see* Diagnostic and Statistical Manuals (DSM)
dysfunctional beliefs, and gray matter volume changes, 76
dyskinetic syndromes, *see* hyperkinetic syndromes
dysmorphophobia
  olfactory, 312–14
  visual, *see* body dysmorphic disorder (BDD)
dysphoria, chronic, and SUD, 62–63
dystonic disorders, 385, 387–88

early treatment, advantages, 121, 147, 166, 188
eating disorders
  and behavioral inflexibility, 63
  classification and diagnosis, 310
  and cognitive inflexibility, 64
  and habit, 64
  neuropathology, 61–62, 77, 97
  as OCD comorbidity, 116–17
  pharmacotherapy, 65, 66
  psychosurgery
    ablative, 287
    DBS, 66, 67, 287
  psychotherapy, 225–26
  and punishment sensitivity, 62
  and reward processing, 61–62, 97
echolalia, 358, *see also* tics
echopraxia, 358, *see also* tics
educational level, and risk of OCD, 40
effort valuation, 3–4
ego-dystonicity
  and classification systems, 130
  vs. ego-syntonicity, 174–75, 350
  and hyperreflexivity, 3
ego-syntonicity, vs. ego-dystonicity, 174–75, 350
embarrassment. *see* shame and embarrassment
emotion regulation, 101–02, 339
endocannabinoids, 250–51
Environmental Cleanliness and Clutter Scale (ECCS), 336–37
environmental risk factors, *see* brain damage and injury, and pathogenesis of OCRDs; childhood experiences, and risk of OCRD; educational level, and risk of OCD; ethnicity, and risk of OCRDs; family studies; intelligence, and OCD risk; menarche, and pathogenesis of OCD; parental style, and risk of OCRD; pregnancy and postpartum period, and risk of OCRD; sexual abuse, and risk of OCD; social isolation, and risk of OCRD; sociodemographic factors, and risk of OCD; stress, and risk of OCD; traumatic life events, and risk of OCRD; twin studies
epigenetics, 34
epilepsy, 389–90
error avoidance, and OCD, 4
error-related negatives (ERN), 4, 96
escitalopram, 194, 404
ethnicity, and risk of OCRDs, 118, 347
excessive acquisition specifier, 332
excoriation disorder, *see* skin picking, pathological (PSP)
executive function, 96, 97, 348, *see also* flexibility and inflexibility
experiential avoidance, 339, 352, 353

exposure and response prevention (ERP), 208–12
  and conditioning theory, 219
  and low distress tolerance, 235–36
  contraindications, 211, 212, 217, 219, 220
  inhibitory learning, 208

Family Accommodation Scale for Obsessive-Compulsive Disorder (FAS), 177
family accommodation to symptomology, 40, 147–54, 177, 178
Family Impact Scale for Hoarding (FISH), 336–37
family studies. *see also* twin studies
  fMRI studies, *88*, 92–96
  heritability estimates, 25, 32
  of OCD and comorbidities, 19–20, 23, 25, 32
    sub-clinical OCD, 166
  of PSP, 372
  of tic disorders, 357
  of TTM, 372
fear, 6, 96–97
  extinction
    and ERP, 208–9, 212–13, 249, 250
    and pharmacotherapy, 249, 250–51
  response, and ERP, 208–9
five-factor model, 348, *see also* dimensional approach, to diagnosis and treatment of OCRDs
flexibility and inflexibility, 63–64, 76–77, *see also* behavioral inflexibility; cognitive inflexibility; contingency-related flexibility; executive function
Florida Obsessive-Compulsive Inventory (FOCI), 139
fluoxetine
  for ASD, 377
  augmentation, 230–31, 232
  for BDD, 232, 310
  effect on brain, 99
  for excessive grooming (animal models), 32
  for hypochondriasis, 324
  for OCD, *91*, 185
  for PSP, 194, 371
  for TTM, 194
fluvoxamine
  augmentation, 231, 232
  with behavior therapy, 245, 247
  for compulsive buying disorder, 404
  effect on brain, 78–79
  for hypochondriasis, 324
  for OCD, 185
  for OCPD, 348–49
  for PG, 404
  for PSP, 194, 232
folate deficiency, 42
free will, and compulsivity, 15, 16
frontal cortex, 255
fronto-cingulate system, and error processing, 96
frontoparietal network, and executive function, 96
frontotemporal lobe degeneration (FTLD), 388
functional magnetic resonance imaging (fMRI), 85–103, *88*
  and ADHD, *88*
  and BDD, *86*, 98
  and error processing, 96
  executive function studies, 96, 97
  family studies, *88*, 92–96
  and fear response, 96–97
  and HD, *88*, 97–98, 101–2
  and hypochondriasis, *88*
  and infidelity situations, 415
  and kleptomania, 406
  and OCD, *92*, 97–98, 99–101, 255–56
    cognitive activation studies, *88*, 92
    treatment effect studies, *91*, 257
  and panic disorder, *88*
  and PG, 406
  and PSP, *88*, 98–99, 372
  resting state studies, *93*, 96
  reward processing studies, 96, 97, 372
  and social anxiety disorder, *88*
  and SUD, *92*
  symptom provocation studies, 85–92, *86*, 97, 98–99
  therapeutic response studies, *91*, 99–102
  and TTM, *88*, 98–99, 372

GABA (Gamma-Aminobutyric Acid), 31, 66, 298
GABA receptor antagonists, 250–51
GABHS (group A beta-hemolytic Streptococcus), *see* streptococcal infections
GAD, *see* generalized anxiety disorder (GAD)
gambling, pathological (PG)
  behavioral addictions model, 401, 407
  classification and diagnosis, 401, 402
  and cognitive dysfunction, 63, 64, 406–7
  comorbidities, 403
  course and outcome, 403
  and dopaminergic system, 405, 407
  and glutamatergic signaling, 66
  epidemiology, 402–3
  neuropathology, 63, 406
  pharmacotherapy, 66, 191, 404
    glutamatergic agents, *295*
  prevalence, 402
  and punishment sensitivity, 62
  and reward processing, 97
  vs. substance use disorders, 405, 406, 407
gamma knife radiosurgery, 257–58, 281–86, 288
  complications, 281, 286
  early techniques, 281
gamma ventral capsulotomy (GVC), 286
gender differences
  and BDD, 307
  and kleptomania, 403
  and OCD, 20, 118–19, 145–46
  and OCPD, 346, 347
  and OCS, 21
  and ORD, 312
  and PG, 403
  and tic disorders, 357, 358
  and TTM, 368
gene polymorphisms, *see* candidate gene studies and gene polymorphisms
generalized anxiety disorder (GAD)
  and doubt, 8
  and error signals, 4
  and fear response and regulation, 96–97
  vs. hypochondriasis, 322
  as OCD comorbidity, 116–17, 165
  as sub-clinical OCD comorbidity, 165
  and treatment-seeking behaviors, 115–16
genetic association studies, *see* candidate gene studies and gene polymorphisms; Genome Wide Association Studies (GWAS)
genetics, *see* candidate gene studies and gene polymorphisms; epigenetics; Genome Wide Association Studies (GWAS); linkage studies; *under specific disorders*
genome scans, 29
Genome Wide Association Studies (GWAS), 34, *see also* genetic association studies
Gilles de la Tourette, Georges, 357–58
globus pallidus, 75, 388

glucocorticoids, 250–51
glutamatergic agents. *see also* ketamine; lamotrigine; memantine; N-acetylcysteine (NAC); riluzole; topiramate
  and CBT, 249–50
  in drug augmentation, 232–35
  for PSP, 66, 194, 233, 234, 294, *295*, 371
glutamatergic signaling, 66, 189, 233, 234
  and glycine, 297
  and NAC, 233, 294
  and zinc, 293
glutathione (GSH), 292–93, 294
glycine, 297, *see also* sarcosine
goal-directed behavior, 41, 76–77, 271
gray matter, 75, 76–79
  and age, 76
  and ASD, 77
  and CBT, 78
  and comorbid depression, 76
  and compulsive sexual behavior, 406
  and gamma ventral capsulotomy, 79
  and medication status, 76
  and OCS, 388
  and PG, 406
  and SSRIs, 78
  and TTM, 372
  as predictor of treatment response, 78–79
grooming, excessive, in animal models, 32, 372–73
gustatory cortex, 92

habit, 6–7, 64
habit reversal therapy (HRT), 211, 361–62, 370
  for PSP, 177–78, 211
  for skin picking disorder, 371
  for SMD, 377
  for tic disorders, 177–78
  for TTM, 177–78, 211, 370
hair ingestion (trichophagia), 369
hair-pulling disorder, *see* trichotillomania (TTM)
hallucinogens, 187, 192
haloperidol, 189, 232
harm avoidance, 176, 188, 195
HD Dimensional Scale (HD-D), 336
health anxiety disorder, *see* hypochondriasis
herbal medicines, 299
hippocampus, 6, 76, 335–36
history taking, 128–29, 140, 172, 173, 402, *see also* assessment
hoarding disorder (HD) and behavior, 331–40
  after brain damage or injury, 333, 389
  animal hoarding, 332
  and anxiety-related tendencies, 339
  classification and diagnosis, 331–34
    assessment and diagnostic instruments, 336–37
    diagnostic criteria (DSM-5), 211, 331–32
    differential diagnosis, 332–34
    home visit, 336
    specifiers, 332
  vs. collecting, 334
  comorbidities, 333, 334, 338–39
  and compulsive buying, 338
  course and outcome, 147–55, 188, 335, 337
  decision-making, 97–98
  epidemiology, 334–35
  fMRI studies, *88*, 97–98, 101–2
  genetic and environmental contributions, 29, 335
  heritability, 335
  hoarding vs. clutter, 333
  and immune dysfunction, 55
  neurocognitive correlates, 335–36
  vs. neurocognitive disorders, 334
  neuropathology, 97–98, 335–36
  pharmacotherapy
    atomoxetine, 338
    drug augmentation, 194, 229, 232, 340
    methylphenidate, 338
    SNRIs, 194, 338
    SRIs, 338
    SSRIs, 193–94, 229, 338
    stimulants, 194
  prevalence, 334
  psychosurgery, 287–88
  psychotherapy, 155, 212, 226, 337–38, 340
    ERP (unsuitability of), 212
  quality of life, 332
  in schizophrenia, 333
  squalor, 332, 333, 336–37
  and tics, 25
  treatment-seeking behaviors, 337–38
Hoarding Rating Scale (HRS), 336
Home Environment Index, 336–37
Huntington disease, 386
hyperactivity, and tic disorders, 359–60
Hypericum perforatum (St John's wort), 299
hyperkinetic syndromes, 385, *see also* tic disorders
hyperreflexivity, 3
hypochondriasis, 320–28
  classification and diagnosis, 320–21, 326
    differential diagnosis, 321–23, 325–26
  compulsivity and impulsivity in, 325
  fMRI studies, *88*
  and hyperreflexivity, 3
  and OCD, 324–26, 327
  prevalence, 323
  secondary hypochondriasis, 324
  treatment, 323
    CBT with pharmacotherapy, 230, 324
    pharmacotherapy, 324, 327
    psychotherapy, 323–24, 326–27
  treatment-seeking behaviors, 320
hypokinesia, *see* akinetic-rigid syndromes
hypothalamus, and hoarding behaviors, 335

ICD-10, 130, 131, 132, 135–36
ICD-11
  and compulsions, 131
  and compulsive sexual behavior, 401
  and HD, 331, 338
  and hypochondriasis, 321
  and obsessions, 129–30
  and OCD, 136
  and role of anxiety in obsessions, 130
  and tic disorders and TD, 359
identity, practical, 16–17
illness anxiety disorder (IAD), 320–21, *see also* hypochondriasis
images, recurrent, 4
imipramine, 185, 324
immersion, and OCD, 221–22, 223
immune system, 51–52, *see also* infections
  as mediator of OCS, 54–55
  dysfunction, and autoimmune disease, 54–55, *see also* PANDAS
    immune molecules and cells, 54–56
    and pathogenesis of OCD, 43, 52, 57, 386
    and pathogenesis of OCRDs, 386
    and pathogenesis of TD, 357
    rheumatic fever, 51, 53
    Sydenham chorea, 51, 53
  maternal, and pediatric OCD risk, 43
  microglia, 52, 55

impulse control disorders, *see* gambling, pathological; kleptomania; trichotillomania (TTM)
impulsivity
  vs. compulsivity. *see* compulsions and compulsivity: vs. impulsivity
  as risk factor for addiction, 8
  vs. urges, 129–30
incidental learning, 219–20
incompleteness, 176
infections. *see also* immune system
  Borna disease virus, 53
  streptococcal infections. *see* streptococcal infections
  toxoplasmosis, 53–54
Inference-Based Approach (IBA) model, 217–18, 222–23, *see also* senses, distrust of in OCD
Inference-Based Approach (IBA) therapy, 225–26
inferential confusion, 221–22, 223–24
inferior frontal gyrus, 75, 79, 309
inferior thalamic pendunche (ITP), *258*, 260
inflexibility, *see* flexibility and inflexibility
infralimbic cortex, 7
inhibitory control, lack of, 15, 236
inhibitory learning, 208
inositol, 294–97
insight. *see also* alexithymia; ego-syntonicity
  assessment, 174
  and BDD, 307, 308
  and effort valuation, 3
  and OCD, 3, 134, 136–37, 174
    as outcome predictor, 147–54
  and OCRDs, 137, 139
  and ORD, 313
  treatment implications, 177, 179, 308
insight specifier, 138, 332
insula, 92–96
intelligence, and OCD risk, 119
International Classification of Functioning, Disability, and Health (ICF), 167
intravenous immunoglobulin (IVIG), 56
intrusive thoughts, unwanted, 163, 185, *see also* appraisal model of OCD; metacognitive model of OCD

jealousy, obsessional, 415–16, 418, *418*, *419*

ketamine, 66, 189–91, *190*, 234–35, 250
kleptomania
  in children and adolescents, 403
  classification and diagnosis, 401, 402
  and cognition, 407
  course and outcome, 403
  neuropathology, 406
  pharmacotherapy, 191
  prevalence, 402–3
  vs. shoplifting, 403
  treatment-seeking behaviors, 403
koro, 417, 418, *418*, *419*

lamotrigine, *190*, 191, 195, 234, 371
lateral habenula, 62–63, 67
lenticular nucleus, 75, 76, 78
Lesch-Nyhan syndrome, 377
linkage studies, 29
lisdexamfetamine, 65
lithium, 185
Longitudinal Interval Follow-up Evaluation (LIFE), 144
loss (punishment) sensitivity, 62, 65
lymphocytes, 51–52, 54

magnetic resonance imaging (MRI), *see* diffusion magnetic resonance imaging; functional magnetic resonance imaging (fMRI); structural magnetic resonance imaging
major depressive disorder (MDD), *see* depressive disorders
medial forebrain bundle (MFB), *258*, 260
memantine, 66, 189, *190*, 234
memory, visual, 5
menarche, and pathogenesis of OCD, 39
menopause, and OCD prevalence, 40
mental compulsions, 134, 135
metacognitive model of OCD, 163, *see also* intrusive thoughts, unwanted
methylphenidate, 186, 192, 194, 338
microglia, 52, 55
migraines, 165
milk thistle, 298–99
mindfulness, 224, 292, 416–17
Mini International Neuropsychiatric Interview (MINI), 129
mirror retraining, 309–10, 311
mirtazapine, *190*, 192
miscarriage, and pathogenesis of OCD, 40
molecular studies, 29–31, *see also* candidate gene studies and gene polymorphisms
morphine, *190*
motivational interviewing, 177, 212, 337, 340
motives, conflicting, 16–17
movement disorders, 383–87, *see also* akinetic-rigid syndromes; dystonic disorders; hyperkinetic syndromes; neuroacanthocytosis; opsoclonus myoclonus syndrome (OMS); paraneoplastic syndromes (PNS); tic disorders
muscle dysmorphia, 307
myo-inositol (MI), 294–97

N-acetylcysteine (NAC), *190*, 233, 294–95
  for OCD, 191, 233, 294, *295*
  for PG, 404
  for PSP, 194, 294, *295*, 371
  side-effects, 294, 371
  for SUD, 294, *295*
  for TTM, 194, *295*, 371
nalmefene, 65, 404
naloxone, 191
naltrexone, 191–92
  for compulsive sexual behavior, 191
  for kleptomania, 191, 404
  for OCD, 340
  for PG, 191, 404
  for PSP, 195
  for self-injurious behavior, 379
  for SUD, 191
  for TTM, 194
National Institute of Mental Health Global Obsessive-Compulsive Scale (NIMH-GOCS), 173
negative reinforcement, 62–63, 67, 211
network model, 327–28
neuroacanthocytosis, 387
neuroanatomy and neuropathology. *see also* neuroimaging; specific brain regions; under specific disorders
  and cognitive control, 4
  and decision-making, 41
  and effort-resistance in OCD, 3–4
  and habit, 7
  and negative reinforcement, 62–63
  and punishment sensitivity, 62
  and reward processing, 5–6, 61–62
  and stress, 41, 44
  and sustained threat, 6
neurobiological models of OCD, 3–4, 74, *see also* cognitive models of OCRD

neuroimaging, 74–80, *see also* computed tomography (CT); diffusion magnetic resonance imaging; functional magnetic resonance imaging (fMRI); neuroanatomy and neuropathology; positron emission tomography (PET); single photon emission computed tomography (SPECT); structural magnetic resonance imaging
  algorithms, 74–75
  children and adolescents, 75, 76–77
  gray matter, *see* gray matter
  and identification of at-risk individuals, 79
  white matter. *see* white matter
neuromodulation
  DBS, *see* deep brain stimulation (DBS)
  rTMS, *see* repetitive transcranial magnetic stimulation (rTMS)
  transcranial direct current stimulation (tDCS), 268–70
neuropeptides, 250–51
neurosurgery, *see* psychosurgery
non-steroidal anti-inflammatories, 56–57
non-verbal memory, 5
nortriptyline, 185
nucleus accumbens (NA), 258–59, *258*, *259*, 335, 372
nutrient deficiencies in OCD, 42–43, 119, 292–93
nutrients and nutraceuticals, 292–97
  glycine, 297
  myo-inositol (MI), 294–97
  N-acetylcysteine (NAC), *see* N-acetylcysteine (NAC)
  sarcosine, 297
  vitamin B12 (cobalamin), 292–93
  zinc, 293

obsessional jealousy, 415–16, 418, *418*, *419*
obsessions and obsessionality. *see also* obsessive-compulsive symptoms (OCS)
  role of anxiety, 130
  classification, 129–31
  and cognitive symptoms, 8
  vs. delusions, 8
  obsessionality, 7–8
  vs. worries and ruminations, 174
Obsessive Beliefs Questionnaire (OBQ), 176
Obsessive Compulsive Inventory (OCI), 173
Obsessive-Compulsive Core Dimensions Questionnaire, 176
Obsessive-Compulsive Disorder (OCD), 217–19, *see also* obsessive-compulsive symptoms (OCS)
  age of onset, 114–15, 145–46, 155–56, 166
    as outcome predictor, 147–54
  and agency, 8
  as an anxiety disorder (appraisal model), 163, 220–21
  assessment, 172–74
  catatonia in, 384
  in children and adolescents, 145–46, 166
    course and outcome, 146, 147
    prevalence, 147
    treatment effectiveness, 188, 246, 248
  classification and diagnosis
    after traumatic brain injury, 42
    childhood acute-onset, *see* CANS; PANDAS; PANS
    Diagnostic and Statistical Manuals (DSM), 3, 19, 133–35, *see also* Diagnostic and Statistical Manuals (DSM)
    differential diagnosis, 8, 390, 391–92
    of "organic" OCD, 392
    Research Domain Criteria (RDoC), 8–11
    subdiagnostic OCD, 167
    transdiagnostic characteristics, *418*
    unsuitability of genetics for, 33
    with comorbid disorders, 133–35
  comorbidities, 116–18
    ADHD, 19–20, 22–23, 146
    allergies, 165
    anxiety and depressive disorders, 19, 21–22, 116–17, 118, 119–20, 165
    anxiety disorders, 186
    BDD, 308
    Benign Hereditary Chorea (BHC), 387
    bipolar disorders, 118
    cancer, 390–91
    dystonic syndromes, 387
    eating disorders, 116–17
    epilepsy, 389–90
    genetic and environmental contributions, 19
    HD, 19–20, 24–25, 334
    Huntington disease, 386
    hypochondriasis, 322
    migraines, 165
    as OCD risk factor, 119–20
    OCPD, 350
    ORD, 313
    as outcome predictors, 147–54, 188
    PTSD, 41, 116–17, 118
    SUD, 116–17, 118, 120, 165, 391
    TD, 19, 23, 55–56, 78, 358
    temporal pattern, 116–18
    tic disorders, 23–24, 78, 146, 186, 232
    treatment implications, 184–85
  course and outcome, 144–46, 187–88
    in children and adolescents, 146, 147
  in elderly, 147
  environmental risk factors. *see* environmental risk factors
  and error signals, 4
  gender differences, 20, 118–19, 145–46
  genetic and environmental contributions, 30–31, 32, 34, 52–53, 118–20, 233
    family studies, 19–20, 23
    stress, 40–42, 146
    twin studies, 19–21, 23, 24–25
  heritability, 25, 32
  and insight, *see* insight: and OCD
  and koro, *418*
  neuropathology, *86*, 97–98, 255–57, *see also* neuroanatomy and neuropathology
    cognitive control, 4
    complex motor acts, 7
    reward processing, 6, 63
  nutrient deficiencies in, 42–43, 119, 292–93
  and obsessional jealousy, *418*
  occupational functioning impairment, 115
  "organic" OCD, 388–89, 392
    treatment, 393
    vs. "primary" (idiopathic) OCD, 392–93
  outcome predictors, 147–54, 188
    in children and adolescents, 147, 188
  pathogenesis, *see* pathogenesis of OCRDs
  placebo response, blunted, 187
  prevalence, 20, 113–14
    gender differences, 118–19
    in children and adolescents, 147
    vs. sub-clinical OCD, 164, 165
  Relationship Obsessive-Compulsive Disorder (ROCD), 415

remission rate, 146, 147, 187–88
and shubo-kyofu, *418*
sub-clinical. *see also* obsessive-compulsive symptoms (OCS)
in children and adolescents, 165–66, 168
classification and diagnosis, 135
comorbidities, 164–65
course and outcome, 166, 168–69
family studies, 166
functioning impairment, 115
neuropsychology, 163–64
prevalence, 164–66
quality of life, 164
remission rate, 146
treatment, 167–68
treatment-seeking behaviors, 164
treatment
5-HT3 antagonists, 192
antibiotics, 56
antidepressants, other, 192
antidepressants, SNRIs, 194
antidepressants, SRIs, 2, 186, 246–44
antidepressants, SSRIs, 65–66, 185, 186–87, 229–30, 245, 247, 338, 349
antidepressants, TCAs, 185, 186, 242–46, 247, 349
antiepileptics, 191, 389–90
antipsychotics, 186, 187, 188–89, 231–32, 248
CBT, *91*, 146–54, 209, 242–44, 300
CBT with pharmacotherapy, 230, 234–35, 242–49
CBT with physical activity, 300
corticosteroids, 56–57
DBS, 66–67, 256–61
dopamine blockers, 379
dose-response relationship, 186–87
fear extinction modulators, 250–51
glutamatergic agents, 189–91, 233, 234–35, 250
glycine, 297
hallucinogens, 187, 192
herbal medicines, 298–99
incremental response, 186, 187
IVIG, 56
myo-inositol, 297
NAC, 294, *295*
opioid agonists, 192
opioid antagonists, 191–92
for "organic" OCD, 393
pharmacotherapy, 185–93, 229–35
physical activity and yoga, 299–300
plasma exchange, 56
probiotics, 301
psychosurgery, 281–86, 287
rTMS, *91*, 97, 262–68
sarcosine, 297
stimulants, 186, 192
tDCS, 268–70
vitamin B12, 293
zinc, 293
treatment-seeking behaviors, 115–16, 146, 185
vs. OCPD, 350–51
Obsessive-Compulsive Personality Disorder (OCPD), 345–53
classification and diagnosis, 345–46, 351
comorbidities, 350, 352
and compulsivity, 350–51
course and outcome, 347
and delayed reward, 351
and ego-syntonicity, 175, 350
'epileptic personality' in, 390
executive function, 348
and experiential avoidance, 352, 353
gender differences, 346, 347
genetic contributions, 347–48
impaired interpersonal functioning, 347
in children and adolescents, 347
neuropathology, 384
vs. OCD, 350–51
and Parkinson's disease, 384
and perfectionism, 175, 345–46, 351–52
and perseveration, 351
pharmacotherapy, 348–49
prevalence, 346–47
psychotherapy, 349–50, 352, 353
and serotonin, 347–48
treatment-seeking behaviors, 347
obsessive-compulsive related disorders (OCRD), *see specific disorders*
obsessive-compulsive symptoms (OCS), 66, *see also* compulsions and compulsivity; Obsessive-Compulsive Disorder (OCD)
classification
compulsions, 131–33
obsessions, 129–31
evolutionary basis, 163
gender differences, 21
genetic and environmental contributions, 21, 384
for HD, 194
neuropathology, 388
severity, and stress, 41
obsessive-compulsive symptoms specifier, 167
occipital cortex, lateral, 75
occupational functioning impairment, 115
olanzapine, 194, 231, 232, 371, 404
olfactory reference disorder (ORD), 312–14
onychophagia, animal models, 32
open interviews, 128–29, 140, *see also* history taking
opioid agonists, 192, *see also* morphine
opioid antagonists, 191–92, 371, 379, 404
naloxone, 191
naltrexone, *see* naltrexone
opsoclonus myoclonus syndrome (OMS), 386
orbitofrontal cortex (OFC), 41
and CBT, 78, 255
and cognitive inflexibility, 63, 92–96
dysconnectivity with ventral striatum, 255–56
and executive function, 96
hyperactivity, 75, 98, 255
and neuromodulation, 79, 262, *264*, 268, *269*
and pharmacotherapy, 255
and response inhibition, 92, 98
and treatment response prediction, 102, 255
volume changes, 76, 77, 78
"organic" vs. "primary" OCRDs, 383, 388–89, 392–93
oxytocin, as medication, 377

Padua Inventory, 65
palilalia, 358, *see also* tics
palipraxia, 358, *see also* tics
PANDAS (pediatric autoimmune neuropsychiatric disorders associated with streptococcal infections), 43, 53, 386
panic disorder. *see also* anxiety and anxiety disorders
and fear response and regulation, 96–97
fMRI studies, *88*
vs. hypochondriasis, 322
as OCD comorbidity, 116–17, 118
as OCD risk factor, 120
risk factors, 121–22
and treatment-seeking behaviors, 115–16
PANS (pediatric acute-onset neuropsychiatric syndrome), 53, 386, *see also* CANS; PANDAS
paraneoplastic syndromes (PNS), 386

parental and family accommodation to symptomology, 40, 147–54, 177, 178
parental style, and risk of OCRD, 40, 119, 122
parietal lobe, *88*, 99
Parkinson's disease (PD), 259–60, 384–85
paroxetine
  with CBT, 313
  for HD, 193–94
  for hypochondriasis, 324
  for OCD, 185
  for OCD with hoarding symptoms, 338
  for ORD, 313
  for PG, 404
pathogenesis of OCRDs
  brain tumors, 390–91
  environmental factors. *see* environmental risk factors
  genetic factors, *see* genetics
  immune system, 43, 52, 57, 386
  incidental learning, 219–20
  stroke, 389
  substances and medications, 391
pathological skin picking (PSP), *see* skin picking, pathological (PSP)
perception, 4–5
perceptual abnormalities, 309, 310–11
perfectionism, 176, 345–46, 351–52, 372
  and CBT, 352
perseverative behavior, 6, 351
pharmacogenetics, 33–34
pharmacotherapy, *see* under specific conditions; specific drug classes; specific drugs
phenelzine, 185
phobias, specific
  agoraphobia, 115–17, 164–65
  and fear response, 96–97
  as OCD comorbidity, 116–17
  as OCD risk factor, 120
  psychosurgery, 249–50
  psychotherapy, 213
  risk factors, 121–22
  treatment-seeking behaviors, 115–16
physical activity, 292, 299–300
Pick's disease, 388
pimozide, 193, 232
placebo response, blunted, 187, 192–93
planning, impaired, 96, 332, 339, 348, 406
plasma exchange, 56
positive reinforcement, 210, *see also* reward
positron emission tomography (PET), 55, 97, 99, 405
  and therapeutic response prediction, 102
post-traumatic stress disorder (PTSD). *see also* anxiety and anxiety disorders
  and fear response and regulation, 96–97
  as OCD comorbidity, 41, 116–17, 118
  neuropathology, 8, 96–97
  risk factors, 121–22
  and treatment-seeking behaviors, 115–16
potential threat (anxiety), 6
practical identity, 16–17
pramipexole, 65
prefrontal cortex
  and cognitive inflexibility, 92–96
  and compulsivity, 63
  and executive function, 96
  and fear response and regulation, 96–97
  and HD, 98
  medial prefrontal cortex (mPFC), 41, 262, *264*
  and response inhibition, 92
  and rTMS, 66, 262, *264*
  and tDCS, 268, *269*
  volume changes, 75, 77
    as predictor of treatment response, 79
pregnancy and postpartum period, and risk of OCRD, 39–40, 119, 123
  miscarriage, 40
  symptom severity, 39, 40, 123
premonitory sensation, 78
prenatal stress, and risk of OCRDs, 39
pre-supplementary motor area, 262–66, 268–69
probiotics, 301
psychasthenia, 4, 19, 385
psychedelic agents, 187, 192
psychic akinesia (athymhormia), 385
psychodynamic psychotherapy, 208, 349, 350
psychoeducation
  about anxiety sensitivity, 178
  for BDD, 309
  for hypochondriasis, 324
  for OCD, 246, 248
  for OCPD, 349–50, 352
  for TD, 360
psychosurgery, 279–88, *see also* under specific disorders
  capsulotomy, 257–58, 281–86
  cingulotomy, 281, 287–88
  early techniques, 280–81
  neuromodulation
    DBS, *see* deep brain stimulation (DBS)
    rTMS, *see* repetitive transcranial magnetic stimulation (rTMS)
    tDCS (transcranial direct current stimulation), 268–70
  radiosurgery
    gamma knife, *see* gamma knife radiosurgery
    radiofrequency, 281
  stereotactic, 280, 288
  suitability and contraindications, 279, 288
  target sites, 66–67, 75, 287
  ultrasound, 280, 288
psychotherapy. *see also* under specific disorders
  acceptance-enhanced behavior therapy, 371
  ACT, *see* Acceptance and Commitment Therapy (ACT)
  CBT, *see* cognitive behavioral therapy (CBT)
  HRT, *see* habit reversal therapy (HRT)
  IBA, *see* Inference-Based Approach (IBA) therapy
  mindfulness, 224, 292, 416–17
  mirror retraining, 309–10, 311
  psychodynamic, 208, 349, 350
  psychoeducation, *see* psychoeducation
  visual training programs, 311–12
PTSD, *see* post-traumatic stress disorder (PTSD)
punding, 384–85, 389
punishment sensitivity, 62, 65
putamen, 75, 76–77, 78, 388
  and behavior therapy, 255
  and reward processing, 6
  and SSRIs, 78, 255

quality of life. *see also* daily life, impairment
  and BDD, 308
  and HD, 332
  and OCD, 115
  and OCPD, 347
  and ORD, 313
  and PG, 402–3
  and sub-clinical OCD, 164
  and TTM, 368–69
quetiapine, 188–89, 231, 232

radiofrequency capsulotomy, 281, *see also* gamma knife radiosurgery
RDoC, *see* Research Domain Criteria (RDoC)

reasoning, in OCD, 221–23
recurrent images, 4
reflective consciousness, 3
Relationship Obsessive-Compulsive Disorder (ROCD), 415
repetitive behaviors, 178, 377
  body-focused, *see* skin picking, pathological (PSP); trichotillomania (TTM)
repetitive transcranial magnetic stimulation (rTMS), 261–68
  accelerated courses, 263
  EEG-linked, 263
  method, 261–62
  for OCD, *91*, 97, 262–68
  optimization, 263
  positioning, 263–68
  side-effects, 262
  for SUD, 66, 97
  theta burst, 263
Research Domain Criteria (RDoC), 2, 242
  and agency, 2
  and effort valuation, 3
  and habit, 6
  and neuromodulation, 271
  and obsessionality/compulsivity, 8–11
  and perception, 4
  and reward, 5
  and self-knowledge, 3
  and stereotypic and self-injurious behavior, 378
  and threat, 6
  vs. DSM/ICD, 2, 140
resistance, 3–4
response inhibition, 92, 98, 407
response-conflict tasks, 4
reversal learning studies, 92–96
reward, 5–6, 61–62, *see also* positive reinforcement
  and blunted placebo response, 187
  delayed, 351
  expectation, 5–6, 8, 61, 372
  fMRI studies, 96, 97, 372
  responsiveness, 5, 8
  self-report questionnaires, 65
  valuation, 5
  and ventral striatum activity, 61–62, 97, 187, 258
rheumatic fever, 51, 52–53, *see also* streptococcal infections; Sydenham chorea
riluzole, *190*, 191, 234
risperidone, 189, 232, 248, 360
Ritalin, 186, 192, 194, 338
rituals, compulsive, 5, 163, 207
rumination and worries, vs. obsession, 174
sarcosine, 297, *see also* glycine
Saving Cognitions Inventory, 336–37
Saving Inventory-Revised (SI-R), 336
Schedule for Affective Disorders and Schizophrenia for School-age Children (K-SADS), 172
schizophrenia
  and agency, 2–3, 8
  course specifier, 156
  and hoarding behavior, 333
  and hyperreflexivity, 3
selective serotonin reuptake inhibitors (SSRI). *see also* citalopram; escitalopram; fluoxetine; fluvoxamine; paroxetine; serotonin reuptake inhibitors (SRI); sertraline
  for ASD, 377
  for BDD, 192–93, 229, 310
  and behavior therapy, 245
  with CBT, 245, 246, 313, 324
    sequential treatment, 247
  for compulsive buying disorder, 404
  for compulsive sexual behavior, 404–05
  dose-response relationship, 186–87, 327
  for eating disorders, 66
  effect on brain, 78, 99
  for HD, 193–94, 229, 338
  increased dose, 188, 327, 417
  incremental response, 193
  for koro, 417
  for OCD, 65–66, 185, 186–87, 229–30, 245, 247, 338, 349
  for OCPD, 348–49
  for ORD, 313
  for PG, 404
  for PSP, 194, 229, 371
  response prediction, 102, 188, 255
  for TKS, 416
  for TTM, 194, 229
self-injury specifier, 376
self-knowledge, 3
Self-Rating Obsessive-Compulsive Personality Inventory (SROCPI), 349
senses, distrust of in OCD, 222, 223–24
Sensitivity to Punishment and Sensitivity to Reward Questionnaire (SPRSQ), 65
sensorimotor cortex, 76, 78
sensory phenomena, 4–5, 76, *see also* tics
separation anxiety disorder (SAD), 4, 22, 53
serotonin. *see also* selective serotonin reuptake inhibitors (SSRI); serotonin norepinephrine reuptake inhibitors (SNRI); serotonin reuptake inhibitors (SRI)
  and OCD, 30, 33, 292
  transmission abnormalities, 65–66, 347–48
  and Withania, 298
serotonin norepinephrine reuptake inhibitors (SNRI). *see also* venlafaxine
  for HD, 194, 338
  for TKS, 416
serotonin reuptake inhibitors (SRI). *see also* selective serotonin reuptake inhibitors (SSRI); serotonin norepinephrine reuptake inhibitors (SNRI)
  augmentation, 248
  and CBT, 247–44, 248, 338
  for HD, 338
  for kleptomania, 404
  mechanism of effect, 187
  for OCD, 2, 186, 246–44
  for PSP, 371
  and rate of remission, *146–54*
  response prediction, 186, 188
  response variability, 33, 34
  for SMD, 377
  for stereotypy, 378
  for TTM, 379
sertraline
  with CBT, 246, 313
  with clomipramine, 230
  increased dose, 188
  for OCD with comorbid depression, 186
  for OCPD, 349
  for ORD, 313
  for PG, 404
  and pharmacokinetic genes, 34
  for TTM, 194
sex addiction, *see* compulsive sexual behavior
sexual abuse, and risk of OCD, 41, 165
shame and embarrassment
  and compulsivity, 14, 15
  and symptom presentation, 314
  and treatment-seeking behaviors, 369, 402
  and TTM, 368–69
shubo-kyofo, 416–17, 418, *418*, *419*
Silybum marianum (milk thistle), 298–99
simulation heuristics, 221

single photon emission computed tomography (SPECT), 231, 405
skin picking, pathological (PSP), 210–11, 369
  age of onset, 155, 369
  in children and adolescents, 369
  classification and diagnosis, 367, 369–70
  comorbidities, 369–70
  course and outcome, 155, 369
  and dopaminergic system, 231
  as emotional regulation, 372
  genetic and environmental contributions, 44, 372, 373
  neuropathology, 372
  pharmacotherapy
    antiepileptics, 195, 371
    dopamine blockers, 379
    drug augmentation, 195, 232
    glutamatergic agents, 66, 194, 233, 234, 294, *295*, 371
    myo-inositol (MI), 297
    opioid antagonists, 195, 371
    SRIs, 371
    SSRIs, 194, 229, 371
  prevalence, 368
  psychosurgery, 288
  psychotherapy, 371
    ERP therapy (unsuit.), 211
    habit reversal therapy (HRT), 211
  treatment-seeking behaviors, 369
  triggers, 369, 372
SNRIs, *see* serotonin norepinephrine reuptake inhibitors (SNRI)
social anxiety disorder (SAD). *see also* anxiety and anxiety disorders; taijin-kyofu-sho (TKS)
  and error signals, 4
  and fear response and regulation, 96–97
  neuropathology, *88*
  as OCD comorbidity, 116–17, 165
  as sub-clinical OCD comorbidity, 164–65
  and treatment-seeking behaviors, 115–16
social functioning impairment, 115
social isolation, and risk of OCRD, 122–23, 378
sociodemographic factors, and risk of OCD, 40, 118–19
somatic symptom disorder (SSD), 165, 320–21, *see also* hypochondriasis
specifiers, *see* association specifier; course of illness specifier; excessive acquisition specifier; insight specifier; obsessive-compulsive symptoms specifier; self-injury specifier; tic-related specifier
splicing, 34–35
squalor, 332, 333, 336–37
SRIs, *see* serotonin reuptake inhibitors (SRI)
SSRIs, *see* selective serotonin reuptake inhibitors (SSRI)
St John's wort, 174
stereotactic psychosurgery, 268, 280
stereotypic movement disorder (SMD), 376–80
  age of onset, 376
  and body-focused repetitive behaviors, 378
  in children and adolescents, 376, 377
  classification and diagnosis, 376–77, 378
  comorbidities, 376, 377
  genetic and environmental contributions, 378
  molecular studies, 378
  neuropathology, 378
  pharmacotherapy, 377, 379
  psychosurgery, 379
  psychotherapy, 377, 379
  triggers, 376
stimulants, 186, 192
streptococcal infections, 43, 357
  PANDAS, 43, 53, 386
  Sydenham chorea, 51, 53, 56–57, 386
stress
  and gray matter volume changes, 76, 146
  immune response, 54, 57
  and OCRD symptom exacerbation, 41, 361, 378
  and risk of OCD, 40–42, 146
striato-thalamo-prefrontal circuits, 385
stroke, 389
structural magnetic resonance imaging, 74–75, 78, 79
Structured Interview for Hoarding Disorder (SIHD), 336
subdiagnostic OCD, *see* Obsessive-Compulsive Disorder (OCD): sub-clinical
subjective compulsions, 132–33
substance use disorders (SUD)
  and glutamatergic signaling, 66
  and habit, 64
  and inflexibility, 63, 64
  and negative reinforcement, 62–63
  neuropathology, 62–63, 77, 405
  as OCD comorbidity, 116–17, 120, 391
    sub-clinical, 165
    temporal pattern, 118
  as OCD risk factor, 120
  pharmacotherapy, 66
  psychosurgery
    DBS, 259
    neuromodulation, 66
    rTMS, 66, 97
  and reward processing, 61, 97
  risk factors, 121–22
subthalamic nucleus, 66–67, *258*, 259–60, *259*, *see also* cortico-striato-thalamic circuits
suicide, 308, 313
sulpiride, 65, 360
supplementary motor area (SMA), 262–66
sustained threat, 6, 8
Sydenham chorea, 51, 53, 56–57, 386, *see also* streptococcal infections
symmetry, 188, 333–34, 361
symptom provocation studies, 85–92, *86*, 97, 98–99

taijin-kyofu-sho (TKS) (fear of interpersonal relations), 416–17, *418*
task-switching studies, 96
temporal discounting, 351
temporal regions, 76, 79, 388
tetrabenazine, 360
thalamus, 75, 78, 92, 255, 335
therapeutic response, *see* treatment response
theta burst transcranial magnetic stimulation, 263
threat, 6, 8
  acute (fear), *see* fear
tic disorders, 357–63, *see also* tics; Tourette's Disorder (TD)
  and brain damage or injury, 389
  in children and adolescents, 357–58, 359–60
  classification and diagnosis, 358–60, 361
  course and outcome, 357–58
  and dopaminergic system, 357
  genetic and environmental contributions, 53, 55–56, 357
  heritability, 184, 357
  and hyperactivity, 359–60
  and incompleteness, 176
  intravenous immunoglobulin (IVIG), 56

neuropathology, 78, 357
as OCD comorbidity, 23–24, 78, 146, 186, 232
pharmacotherapy
alpha-2 agonists, 360
antibiotics, 56
antiepileptics, 233–34, 360–61
antipsychotics, 186, 232, 360
drug augmentation, 189, 362
glutamatergic agents, 360–61
sulpiride, 360
tetrabenazine, 360
plasma exchange, 56
prevalence, 357
psychotherapy, 360, 361–62
tic-related specifier, 137, 138
tics. *see also* tic disorders
defined, 385
expression, and environmental factors, 358
motor tics, 357–58
variability, 358
vocal tics, 358
topiramate, 66, 191, 233–34, 404
Tourette's disorder (TD). *see also* tic disorders
in children and adolescents, 357
classification and diagnosis, 357, 358–59, 361
comorbidities, 358
OCD, 19, 23, 55–56, 78, 358
and dopaminergic system, 231
genetic and environmental contributions, 357
and immune dysfunction, 55–56
neuropathology, 78
pharmacotherapy
alpha-2 agonists, 360
antiepileptics, 233–34
antipsychotics, 186, 232
drug augmentation, 56
glutamatergic agents, 234
indications, 360
prevalence, 357
psychosurgery, DBS, 259, 287, 361
psychotherapy, 360, 361–62
toxoplasmosis, 53–54
transcranial direct current stimulation (tDCS), 268–70
transcranial magnetic stimulation (TMS). *see* repetitive transcranial magnetic stimulation (rTMS)
traumatic brain injury (TBI). *see* brain damage and injury, and pathogenesis of OCRDs
traumatic life events, and risk of OCRD, 44, 121–22, 335
treatment response. *see also* treatment strategies
defined, *145*, 229
fMRI studies, *91*, 99–102
and gene polymorphisms, 33–34
of OCD vs. OCRDs, 235–36
and parental and family accommodation to symptomology, 40, 178
and poor insight, 177, 179, 308
prediction, 188
neuroimaging studies, 78–79, *92*, 102
and stress, 45
treatment strategies. *see also* treatment response; *under specific disorders*
categorical vs. dimensional approaches, 7, 420
herbal medicines, 298–99
intravenous immunoglobulin (IVIG), 56
nutrients and nutraceuticals. *see* nutrients and nutraceuticals
pharmacotherapy, *see* under specific disorders; specific drug classes; specific drugs
physical activity, 292, 299–300
plasma exchange, 56
probiotics, 301
psychoeducation, *see* psychoeducation
psychosurgery, *see* psychosurgery
psychotherapy, *see* psychotherapy
treatment-seeking behaviors, 185
in anxiety disorders, 115–16
in compulsive buying disorder, 403
in HD, 337–38
in hypochondriasis, 320
in kleptomania, 403
in OCD, 115–16, 146, 185
sub-clinical OCD, 164
in OCPD, 347
in ORD, 313, 314
in PSP, 371
in TTM, 369, 370
trichotillomania (TTM) (hair-pulling disorder)
age of onset, 155, 368
animal models, 32
in children and adolescents, 155, 194, *295*, 368
classification and diagnosis, 367
comorbidities, 369
course and outcome, 155, 370
and cytokines, 55
and dopaminergic system, 231
as emotional regulation, 372
epidemiology, 367–68
focused vs. automatic pulling, 210, 368
genetic and environmental contributions, 44, 372
and glutamatergic signaling, 66
habit reversal training, 211
hair ingestion (trichophagia), 369
medical complications, 369
neuropathology, 77, *88*, 98–99, 372
pharmacotherapy
antipsychotics, 194, 232, 371
cannabinoid agonists, 371
dopamine blockers, 379
drug augmentation, 194
for children and adolescents, 194
glutamatergic agents, 194, 233, 234, *295*, 371
milk thistle, 298
myo-inositol (MI), 297
opioid antagonists, 194
and positive reinforcement, 210
prevalence, 367–68
psychotherapy, 370
ERP therapy (unsuit.), 211
and quality of life, 368–69
treatment-seeking behaviors, 369, 370
triggers, 210, 368, 372
tricophagia, 369
tricyclic antidepressants (TCA). *see also* clomipramine; desipramine; imipramine; nortriptyline
for BDD, 192–93
and CBT, 242–46, *243*, 247, 313
for OCD, 185, 186, 349
for OCPD, 349
for ORD, 313
for SMD, 377
for TTM, 194
twin studies. *see also* family studies
of HD, 335
of OCD, OCS, and comorbidities, 19–21, *22*, 23–25
heritability estimates, 25
of OCPD, 347
of PSP, 372
typification, 128, *see also* classification and diagnosis

UCLA Hoarding Severity Scale (UHSS), 336
ultrasound surgery, 280, 288
urges, vs. impulses, 129–30

valproate, 377
venlafaxine, 194, 232, 338
ventral capsule, 257–58, *258*, *259*
ventral striatum, 66–67
  and DBS, 257–58, *258*, *259*
  dysconnectivity with orbitofrontal cortex, 255–56
  and habit, 64
  and punishment sensitivity, 62
  and reward processing, 61–62, 97, 187, 258
  and sub-clinical OCD, 79
  volume change, 76–77
ventral tegmental area, 335
visual (non-verbal) memory, 5
visual cortices, 309
visual dysmorphophobia. *see* body dysmorphic disorder (BDD)
visual processing abnormalities, and BDD, 309, 310–11
visual training programs, 311–12, *see also* mirror retraining
vitamin B12 (cobalamin), 292–93

washing symptoms, and immune dysfunction, 55
white matter, 75–76, 78
  and BDD, 309
  and compulsive sexual behavior, 406
  and kleptomania, 406
  and OCD, 75–76
  and PG, 406
  and PSP, 372
  and SSRIs, 78
  and TTM, 372
Withania somnifera, 298
working memory, impaired, 96, 348, 407
worries and rumination, vs. obsessions, 174

Yale-Brown Obsessive-Compulsive Scale (Y-BOCS), 139, 144, 172–73, 196, 229
yoga, 300

zinc, 293